New Frontiers in Breast Cancer

New Frontiers in Breast Cancer

Editor: Belinda Dormer

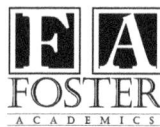

FA
FOSTER
ACADEMICS

www.fosteracademics.com

www.fosteracademics.com

FOSTER
ACADEMICS

Cataloging-in-Publication Data

New frontiers in breast cancer / edited by Belinda Dormer.
    p. cm.
Includes bibliographical references and index.
ISBN 978-1-63242-880-6
1. Breast--Cancer. 2. Mammary glands--Cancer. I. Dormer, Belinda.
RC280.B8 N49 2020
616.994 49--dc23

Foster Academics,
118-35 Queens Blvd., Suite 400,
Forest Hills, NY 11375, USA

ISBN 978-1-63242-880-6 (Hardback)

Contents

Preface

The main aim of this book is to educate learners and enhance their research focus by presenting diverse topics covering this vast field. This is an advanced book which compiles significant studies by distinguished experts in the area of analysis. This book addresses successive solutions to the challenges arising in the area of application, along with it; the book provides scope for future developments.

Breast cancer is the cancer which develops in the breast tissue. Being obese, lack of physical exercise, alcohol consumption, early puberty, not having children or having children late, and hormone replacement therapy can increase the risks of developing breast cancer. There is an element of genetic susceptibility to the disease, due to inheritance of BRCA1 and BRCA2 genes. Breast cancer can be ductal carcinomas or lobular carcinomas. Some of the indications of breast cancer are an inverted nipple, a breast becoming larger or lower, skin puckering or dimpling, discharge from nipple, swelling beneath the armpit, etc. Breast cancer is diagnosed to a reasonable accuracy with the aid of a mammography, fine needle aspiration and physical examination. A multidisciplinary approach to the management of breast cancer is generally adopted. It comprises of surgery, chemotherapy, monoclonal antibodies, hormone blocking therapy, radiotherapy, etc. This book provides comprehensive insights into the evaluation and management of breast cancer. It presents researches and studies performed by experts across the globe. It is meant for students who are looking for an elaborate reference text on oncology.

It was a great honour to edit this book, though there were challenges, as it involved a lot of communication and networking between me and the editorial team. However, the end result was this all-inclusive book covering diverse themes in the field.

Finally, it is important to acknowledge the efforts of the contributors for their excellent chapters, through which a wide variety of issues have been addressed. I would also like to thank my colleagues for their valuable feedback during the making of this book.

Editor

Proteolytic single hinge cleavage of pertuzumab impairs its Fc effector function and antitumor activity in vitro and in vivo

Hao-Ching Hsiao[†], Xuejun Fan[†], Robert E. Jordan, Ningyan Zhang[*] and Zhiqiang An[*] [iD]

Abstract

Background: Proteolytic impairment of the Fc effector functions of therapeutic monoclonal antibodies (mAbs) can compromise their antitumor efficacy in the tumor microenvironment and may represent an unappreciated mechanism of host immune evasion. Pertuzumab is a human epidermal growth factor receptor 2 (HER2)-targeting antibody and has been widely used in the clinic in combination with trastuzumab for treatment of HER2-overexpressing breast cancer. Pertuzumab susceptibility to proteolytic hinge cleavage and its impact on the drug's efficacy has not been previously studied.

Methods: Pertuzumab was incubated with high and low HER2-expressing cancer cells and proteolytic cleavage in the lower hinge region was detected by western blotting. The single hinge cleaved pertuzumab (scIgG-P) was purified and evaluated for its ability to mediate antibody-dependent cellular cytotoxicity (ADCC) in vitro and anti-tumor efficacy in vivo. To assess the cleavage of trastuzumab (IgG-T) and pertuzumab (IgG-P) when simultaneously bound to the same cancer cell surface, F(ab')$_2$ fragments of IgG-T or IgG-P were combined with the intact IgG-P and IgG-T, respectively, to detect scIgG generation by western blotting.

Results: Pertuzumab hinge cleavage occurred when the mAb was incubated with high HER2-expressing cancer cells. The hinge cleavage of pertuzumab caused a substantial loss of ADCC in vitro and reduced antitumor efficacy in vivo. The reduced ADCC function of scIgG-P was restored by an anti-hinge mAb specific for a cleavage site neoepitope. In addition, we constructed a protease-resistant version of the anti-hinge mAb that restored ADCC and the cell-killing functions of pertuzumab when cancer cells exressed a potent IgG hinge-cleaving protease. We also observed increased hinge cleavage of pertuzumab when combined with trastuzumab.

Conclusion: The reduced Fc effector function of single hinge-cleaved pertuzumab can be restored by an anti-hinge mAb. The restoration effect indicated that immune function could be readily augmented when the damaged primary antibodies were bound to cancer cell surfaces. The anti-hinge mAb also restored Fc effector function to the mixture of proteolytically disabled trastuzumab and pertuzumab, suggesting a general therapeutic strategy to restore the immune effector function to protease-inactivated anticancer antibodies in the tumor microenvironment. The findings point to a novel tactic for developing breast cancer immunotherapy.

Keywords: Pertuzumab, HER2, Antibody hinge cleavage, Fc effector function, Breast cancer, Tumor invasion of humoral immunity

* Correspondence: Ningyan.zhang@uth.tmc.edu; zhiqiang.an@uth.tmc.edu
†Equal contributors
Texas Therapeutics Institute, Brown Foundation Institute of Molecular Medicine, the University of Texas Health Science Center at Houston, 1825 Pressler St., Suite 532, Houston, TX 77030, USA

Background

Previous studies have indicated that pathogen-associated and tumor-associated proteases are capable of cleaving human IgG1 within or adjacent to the hinge region [1–6]. For example, a group of tumor-associated proteases such as matrix metalloproteinase MMP3, MMP7, MMP9, and MMP12 generate limited cleavage of human IgG1 in vitro, and in some cases demonstrably in vivo. Such cleavage can confer substantial functional impairment to therapeutic antibodies [2, 4, 6]. In addition to F(ab')$_2$ fragments with their Fc domains removed, IgG1 antibodies with a single proteolytic cleavage in the lower hinge region (scIgG1), but with the Fc domain remaining attached, also exhibit impaired antibody-dependent cell-mediated cytotoxicity (ADCC) and complement-dependent cytotoxicity (CDC) [6–8]. We have demonstrated this susceptibility for trastuzumab in clinical tumor samples as shown with detection of single hinge-cleaved trastuzumab (scIgG-T) in tumor tissues from patients with breast cancer treated with trastuzumab as neoadjuvant [9].

In related investigations, it was shown that anti-hinge antibodies (AHAs) that specifically bind to the neoepitope formed by enzymatic scission successfully restored Fc-dependent function to cleaved therapeutic antibodies [7, 8, 10]. Polyclonal AHAs purified from human intravenous immunoglobulin (IVIG) was shown to restore function to a set of antigen-specific therapeutic monoclonal antibodies disabled by proteolytic hinge cleavage [8]. In a separate study, we were able to demonstrate strong ADCC restoration of scIgG-T by a monoclonal AHA [7]. In a model system using the potent IdeS protease (expressed by *S. pyogenes*), AHAs were also found to be subject to proteolytic attack in the hinge region with a resulting loss of restorative capability [7]. To address this issue, we applied a protein engineering approach to derive a protease-resistant monoclonal antibody (mAb). This version of an otherwise proteolysis-susceptible mAb retained the required Fc function in protease-rich environments [7, 11].

Pertuzumab (IgG-P) is a humanized mAb targeting human epidermal growth factor receptor 2 (HER2) [12] at an epitope different from that of trastuzumab (IgG-T) [13, 14]. Specifically, IgG-P interacts with domain II of HER2 whereas IgG-T targets domain IV of the HER2 receptor [13, 14]. It has been reported that ADCC is an important IgG-P mechanism of action [15–20]. There have been no reports of any previous study of IgG-P susceptibility to proteolytic hinge cleavage.

In this study, we demonstrated the occurrence of hinge cleavage of IgG-P in cell cultures and that the scission of a single peptide bond in this region diminished the antitumor activity and ADCC functions of IgG-P. We also found enhanced hinge cleavage for HER2-bound IgG-P when combined with trastuzumab. The latter observation pointed to a conceptual model to incorporate observations

of basic biology, and suggests an application of that basic biological information to clinical situations in which polyclonal auto-antibodies are present against in situ tumor associated antigens (TAA). To this point, we investigated whether an AHA was effective at targeting both hinge cleaved IgG-T and IgG-P in combination to restore ADCC and antitumor activity. Taken together, our results suggest that using AHA to restore anticancer immunity is a promising strategy for developing a new class of breast cancer immunotherapy.

Methods
Cell culture and reagents

All cancer cell lines were obtained from the American Type Culture Collection (ATCC, Manassas, VA, USA) and maintained as previously described [7, 9]. Trastuzumab was obtained from a specialty pharmacy as previously described [7]. Pertuzumab with a single proteolytic cleavage in the lower hinge region (ScIgG-P) was prepared in house using a specific hinge cleavage proteinase (IdeS) (Sigma-Aldrich, St Louis, MO, USA). Intact IgG-P and protease-resistant IgG-P (PRIgG-P) were constructed based on variable sequences of pertuzumab, expressed in HEK293F cells, and purified using Protein A affinity chromatography as previously described [7]. Isotype control antibodies used in the study were prepared using the same expression system and protocols as the HER2 targeting IgG-P antibodies.

Preparation of scIgG-P and F(ab')$_2$ fragments

Both scIgG-T and scIgG-P were prepared using IdeS partial cleavage by monitoring the disappearance of intact IgG using non-reducing SDS-PAGE detection. After the partial cleavage of IgG hinge, the mixtures of scIgGs and F(ab')$_2$ fragments were separated using Protein A agarose (ThermoFisher, Waltham, MA, USA) to elute the bound scIgGs and free Fc fragment from unbound F(ab')$_2$. Then CaptureSelect™ Kappa XL Affinity Matrix (ThermoFisher) was used to further purify F(ab')$_2$ fragments from the flow through of the protein A purification step, while in a separate step the free Fc fragment from Protein A elution was removed to enrich scIgGs from the CaptureSelect™ Kappa XL affinity Matrix. The purity of both scIgG and the F(ab')$_2$ was > 95% as shown on fast protein liquid chromatography (FPLC) size exclusion chromatography.

IgG-P single-hinge cleavage when bound to a cancer cell line

SKBR3, BT474, MCF7-HER2, and MCF7 breast cancer cells and SKOV3 ovarian cancer cells were seeded on 6-well plates at 80% confluence and incubated for 24 h. The cancer cells were treated with 10 μg/ml of IgG-T, IgG-P, IgG-T F(ab')$_2$, or IgG-P F(ab')$_2$ for designated periods. Cells were harvested and lysed using radioimmunoprecipitation assay (RIPA) buffer (ThermoFisher) containing a 10% protease inhibitor cocktail (ThermoFisher). Monoclonal antibodies and F(ab')$_2$ fragments were enriched using Protein A (ThermoFisher) and their concentrations were determined as previously described [7]. Briefly, Protein A magnetic beads were incubated with cell lysates at 4 °C for 1 h, and the captured antibodies were collected in SDS containing sample buffer (Bio-Rad). Samples were subjected to SDS-PAGE and WB detection using a goat anti-human Fc-HRP conjugate (1:4000) (Jackson Immune Research Laboratory, West Grove, PA, USA) as previously described [7, 9].

Detection of HER2 expression in breast cancer cell lines by flow cytometry

The cancer cells were detached using non-enzymatic solution (Fisher Scientific) from a cell culture flask and blocked in PBS buffer with 1% BSA for 45 min at room temperature. IgG-P was used to stain HER2 and R-PE (phycoerythrin) conjugated F(ab')$_2$ goat anti-human IgG Fcγ (1:200) (Jackson Immune Research Laboratory) was used as detection antibody. For the determination of the anti-hinge antibody binding to scIgG-P and scIgG-T on cancer cell surfaces, AHA (mAb 2095–2) was biotinylated and the binding of the AHA was detected using R-PE conjugated streptavidin (1:200) (Jackson Immune Research laboratories). All stained cells were analyzed by a Guava easyCyte HT flow cytometer according to the manufacturer's instructions (Millipore, Hayward, CA, USA).

Detection of CD4, CD8 and CD56 expression level in human peripheral blood mononuclear cells (PBMCs) cells by flow cytometry

CD4, CD8, and CD56 positive cells in PBMCs isolated from healthy human donors were detected by flow cytometry on a fluorescence-activated cell sorter FACScan (Becton Dickinson, Walpole, MA, USA). Alexa Fluor 700 anti-CD4 (eBioscience, San Diego, CA, USA), anti-CD8-Per-CP-Cy5.5, and anti-CD56-Per-CP-Cy5.5 (BD Pharmingen, San Diego, CA, USA) antibodies were used to detect expression levels of CD4, CD8, and CD56, respectively. Approximately $1 \times 10^{\wedge 6}$ pelleted PBMC cells were blocked in PBS buffer with 1% BSA for 20 min at room temperature. The cells were then stained with antibodies at 4 °C for 30 min, washed twice in PBS buffer with 1% BSA and resuspended in 0.5 ml staining buffer for FACScan analysis.

Mouse xenograft tumor model

All animal procedures and care were conducted in accordance with the animal care and use guidelines and the protocol was approved by the Animal Welfare Committee (AWC) of the University of Texas Medical School at Houston. Breast cancer cells (BT474) with high HER2 expression were prepared and implanted into athymic nude mice ($Foxn1^{nu}/Fox1^{+}$ genotype, Envigo, East Millstone,

NJ, USA) subcutaneously (sc.) at the hind-leg fat pad to establish tumors as we described previously [7]. BT474 breast cancer cells (5×10^6 cells/mouse) were implanted into 6 to 8 week old mice and antibody treatment was initiated after one additional week. The mAb treatments were performed once a week by intraperitoneal (ip) injection for 5 weeks at a dosage of 10 mg/kg body weight. Tumor growth and mouse health were monitored twice per week. Tumor growth was quantified by measuring the size of tumors using a Vernier scale caliper.

Purification of human anti-hinge cleavage site antibodies from Octagam (IVIG)

A biotinylated human IgG1 hinge peptide analogue with the sequence biotin-THTCPPCPAPELLG (peptide 1981B) or a biotinylated IgG-P F(ab')$_2$ fragment (generated with the IdeS protease) were used as the absorbents to isolate human anti-hinge cleavage site autoantibodies from IVIG (pooled, purified IgGs from human plasma). The IVIG was diluted in PBS to a protein concentration of 1 mg/ml and was incubated with streptavidin agarose beads with bound peptide 1981B or biotinylated IgG-P F(ab')$_2$ for 1 h at 4 °C followed by three washes with PBS. Bound antibodies were eluted with 50 mM glycine (pH 2.6) then neutralized by adding 1/10th volume of 1 M Tris (pH 8.0). The antibody eluent was exchanged into PBS by adding 10× volume of PBS and concentrated using Amicon centrifugal filter units (MWCF, 30 kDa) (Millipore). Specificity enrichment of AHAP- F(ab')$_2$ was also performed by running the eluent through an additional affinity step with intact IgG-P linked on agarose. The flow through from the second enrichment step was buffer exchanged and concentrated using Amicon centrifugal filter units (MW, 30 kDa) (Millipore).

Antibody-dependent cellular cytotoxicity (ADCC) assay

Polyclonal human AHAs and the monoclonal AHA (2095–2) were examined for their ability to restore ADCC activity using a non-invasive gold microelectrode-based cell cytotoxicity assay by the xCELLigence instrument (ACEA Biosciences, San Diego, CA, USA) as described previously [7]. SKOV3 and SKBR3 cancer cells were used as target cells (T) and human PBMCs, freshly isolated from two healthy donors, were used as effector cells (E) with the E:T ratio at 25:1. The degree of ADCC restoration by AHA coupled with scIgG-P was by comparison to the cells treated with IgG-P (30 nM), or scIgG-P (30 nM), respectively, with or without AHA (60 nM). The ADCC rescuing efficacy of polyclonal human AHAs or monoclonal AHA (2095–2 mAb) was measured by adding scIgG-P alone or in combination with scIgG-T together with a twofold to tenfold excess of AHAs. The percentage of cell lysis was defined as: (cell index of control group − cell index of treatment group)/cell index of control group) × 100. All experiments were replicated three times ($n = 3$).

ELISA for assessing antibody binding to antigen HER2

A microtiter plate (ThermoFisher) was pre-coated with recombinantly expressed human HER2 extracellular domain protein (SinoBiological, Beijing, China) at 2 µg/ml overnight at 4 °C in PBS. Microtiter wells were washed with PBS and blocked with 200 µl/well of 3% BSA in PBS for 1 h at room temperature. Serial dilutions of IgG-P, PRIgG-P, or F(ab')$_2$ fragments were compared with the intact IgG-T/IgG-P antibodies for binding after incubating for 1 h at room temperature. After washing with PBS (three times), goat anti-human Fc-specific HRP conjugate (ThermoFisher) (1:4000) was used for detection with 3,3'-5,5' tetramethylbenzidin (TMB) (ThermoFisher) for 10 min incubation. The reaction was stopped by adding 50ul/well of 1 N H$_2$SO$_4$ and the individual wells were read for absorbance at 450 nm using a plate reader (SpectraMax M4, Molecular Devices, Sunnyvale, CA, USA).

Statistical analysis

The pair-wise Student t test was used for statistical analysis using GraphPad software. Statistical significance was defined as a p value ≤ 0.05.

Results

Detection of IgG-P hinge cleavage when incubated with high HER2-expressing cancer cells

As part of the ongoing investigation into whether antibody hinge cleavage represents a meaningful occurrence for IgG1 anticancer mAbs, we tested the hinge cleavage of pertuzumab (IgG-P) during incubation with high HER2-expressing cancer cells. As illustrated in Fig. 1a, the antibody with a single hinge cleavage (scIgG1) can be resolved into four components after separation by SDS-PAGE: light chain, full length heavy chain, hinge-cleaved heavy chain (scHC, upper fragment from the nicked hinge containing the Fab domain), and Fc monomer (Fc(m)). There was detectable Fc(m) in cell lysates after a 24-h incubation of IgG-P with high HER2-expressing cancer cells (BT474, SKOV3, SKBR3, and MCF7-HER2). IgG-P and scIgG-P were extracted from the cell lysates using Protein A beads and hinge cleavage, as indicated by presence of Fc(m), was tested by western blotting (WB) analysis using an anti-human Fc-specific detection antibody (Fig. 1b-e, top panels). SKBR3 cancer cells showed much stronger Fc(m) generation than the other high HER2-expressing cancer cell lines (Fig. 1d, top panel). In contrast, low HER2-expressing MCF7 cancer cells and IgG-P incubated with conditioned medium from cell culture did not have detectable levels of Fc (m) (Fig. 1f, top panel and g). High HER2 expression in BT474, SKOV3, SKBR3, and MCF7-HER2 cells (Fig. 1b-e, bottom panels) were detected by FACS. In contrast, no HER2 expression was detected in MCF7 cancer cells (Fig. 1f, bottom panel). The latter result indicates that antibody hinge cleavage preferentially

occurs on the cell surfaces when IgG-P engages its HER2 antigen target rather than in solution.

Single hinge cleavage impeded the anti-tumor function of IgG-P

It has been reported that ADCC is an important mechanism in the anticancer efficacy of pertuzumab [21]. To test whether proteolytic hinge cleavage of pertuzumab results in a loss of Fc-mediated cell killing function, we compared measurements of ADCC activity mediated by scIgG-P and intact IgG-P. We used a high HER2 expressing SKOV3 ovarian cancer cell line as the target and freshly isolated PBMCs as immune effector cells. The group treated with scIgG-P had significantly less lysis of cancer cells than the group treated with intact IgG-P (Fig. 2a). To compare scIgG-P antitumor function with the intact IgG-P in vivo, we adopted a murine xenograft tumor model in which mice were inoculated with an established high HER2-expressing cell line. Seven days after subcutaneous implantation of the cancer cells, tumor-bearing mice were randomly divided into groups ($n = 5$) for treatment with scIgG-P or IgG-P at a dose of 10 mg/kg, once weekly for five weeks. In addition to the isotype control IgG, IgG-P-N297A (IgG-P with a single amino acid mutation at position 297 to limit glycosylation of IgG-P) was used as a control group for a loss of Fc function. In comparison with the isotype control, all three pertuzumab antibody versions - scIgG-P, the N297A mutant, and intact IgG-P - inhibited tumor growth, but both scIgG-P and N297A mutant were significantly less effective than the intact IgG-P (Fig. 2b). With regard to the aglycosylated N297A mutant of IgG1, it has been established that this variant confers reduced Fc-mediated immune cell engagement and decreased ADCC due to impairment of Fc receptor binding [20]. Thus, the comparable reduction of tumor volume by scIgG-P and the aglycosylated IgG-P-N297A mutant pointed to a related mechanism of immune impairment (Fig. 2b). Tumor volumes at the end point of the xenograft study for individual mice in the four treatment groups are shown in Fig. 2c. The data further demonstrated that both the scIgG-P and the N297A mutant exhibited significantly less tumor inhibition efficacy than the intact IgG-P.

Anti-hinge cleavage site autoantibodies (AHA) rescued the ADCC activity of scIgG-P

In a previous study, human AHAs were purified using F(ab')$_2$ affinity chromatography [8]. Those purified autoantibodies from IVIG restored biological functions to F(ab')$_2$ generated from a variety of monoclonal antibodies. In this study, we enriched AHA from IVIG using a peptide analogue of the point of IdeS cleavage of the human IgG1 hinge (peptide 1981 sequence ending in PAPELLG-$_{COOH}$). AHA$_{1981}$ demonstrated a degree of restoration of the ADCC activity of scIgG-P diminished by the IdeS protease

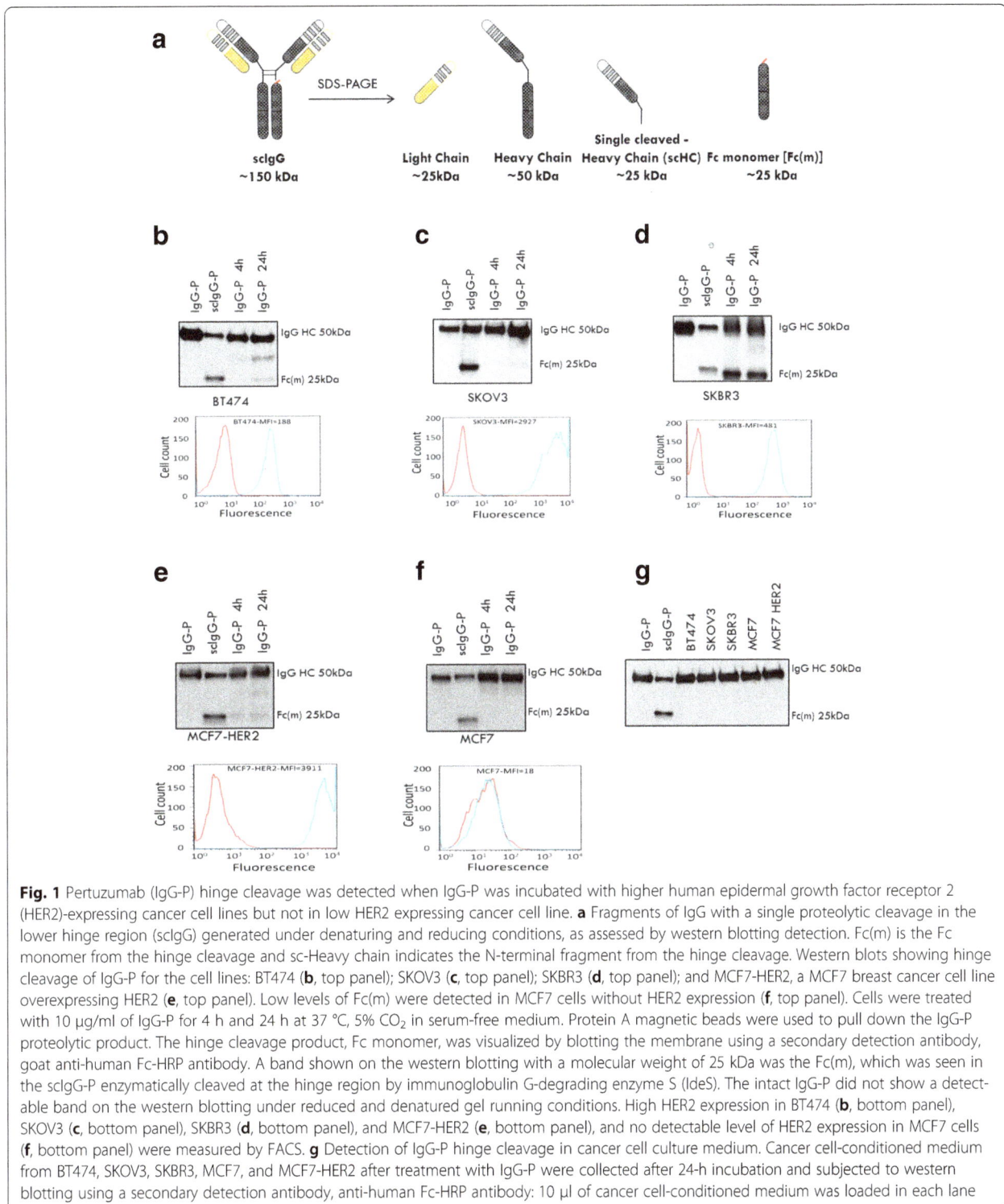

Fig. 1 Pertuzumab (IgG-P) hinge cleavage was detected when IgG-P was incubated with higher human epidermal growth factor receptor 2 (HER2)-expressing cancer cell lines but not in low HER2 expressing cancer cell line. **a** Fragments of IgG with a single proteolytic cleavage in the lower hinge region (scIgG) generated under denaturing and reducing conditions, as assessed by western blotting detection. Fc(m) is the Fc monomer from the hinge cleavage and sc-Heavy chain indicates the N-terminal fragment from the hinge cleavage. Western blots showing hinge cleavage of IgG-P for the cell lines: BT474 (**b**, top panel); SKOV3 (**c**, top panel); SKBR3 (**d**, top panel); and MCF7-HER2, a MCF7 breast cancer cell line overexpressing HER2 (**e**, top panel). Low levels of Fc(m) were detected in MCF7 cells without HER2 expression (**f**, top panel). Cells were treated with 10 µg/ml of IgG-P for 4 h and 24 h at 37 °C, 5% CO_2 in serum-free medium. Protein A magnetic beads were used to pull down the IgG-P proteolytic product. The hinge cleavage product, Fc monomer, was visualized by blotting the membrane using a secondary detection antibody, goat anti-human Fc-HRP antibody. A band shown on the western blotting with a molecular weight of 25 kDa was the Fc(m), which was seen in the scIgG-P enzymatically cleaved at the hinge region by immunoglobulin G-degrading enzyme S (IdeS). The intact IgG-P did not show a detectable band on the western blotting under reduced and denatured gel running conditions. High HER2 expression in BT474 (**b**, bottom panel), SKOV3 (**c**, bottom panel), SKBR3 (**d**, bottom panel), and MCF7-HER2 (**e**, bottom panel), and no detectable level of HER2 expression in MCF7 cells (**f**, bottom panel) were measured by FACS. **g** Detection of IgG-P hinge cleavage in cancer cell culture medium. Cancer cell-conditioned medium from BT474, SKOV3, SKBR3, MCF7, and MCF7-HER2 after treatment with IgG-P were collected after 24-h incubation and subjected to western blotting using a secondary detection antibody, anti-human Fc-HRP antibody: 10 µl of cancer cell-conditioned medium was loaded in each lane

(Fig. 3a). For comparison purposes, we also purified AHA from IVIG using IgG-P F(ab')$_2$ (generated with IdeS) as the absorbent and tested its ability to restore ADCC to F(ab')$_2$. As shown in Fig. 3b, AHA $_{P-F(ab')2}$ showed a comparable level of ADCC restoration to AHA$_{1981}$. In previous studies, a monoclonal antibody AHA (2095–2) was shown to restore ADCC activity to scIgG-T [7, 10]. In this study, we investigated the analogous potential of using AH-mAb (2095–2) to rescue the function of scIgG-P. Indeed, the AH-mAb 2095–2 was strongly bound to scIgG-P on high HER2-expressing cancer cells (Fig. 3c), and as expected, restored the ADCC activity of scIgG-P to a level comparable

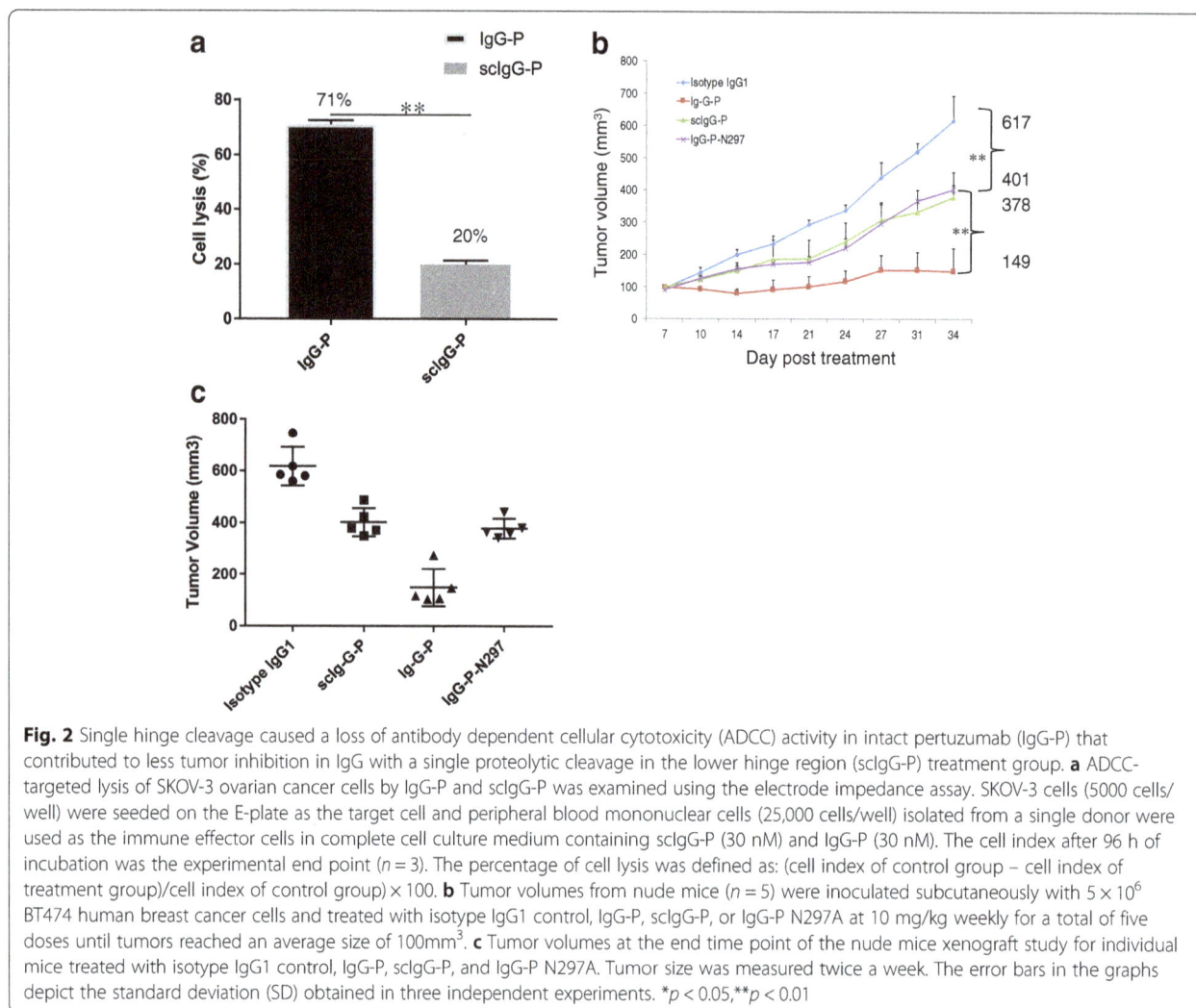

Fig. 2 Single hinge cleavage caused a loss of antibody dependent cellular cytotoxicity (ADCC) activity in intact pertuzumab (IgG-P) that contributed to less tumor inhibition in IgG with a single proteolytic cleavage in the lower hinge region (scIgG-P) treatment group. **a** ADCC-targeted lysis of SKOV-3 ovarian cancer cells by IgG-P and scIgG-P was examined using the electrode impedance assay. SKOV-3 cells (5000 cells/well) were seeded on the E-plate as the target cell and peripheral blood mononuclear cells (25,000 cells/well) isolated from a single donor were used as the immune effector cells in complete cell culture medium containing scIgG-P (30 nM) and IgG-P (30 nM). The cell index after 96 h of incubation was the experimental end point ($n = 3$). The percentage of cell lysis was defined as: (cell index of control group – cell index of treatment group)/cell index of control group) × 100. **b** Tumor volumes from nude mice ($n = 5$) were inoculated subcutaneously with 5×10^6 BT474 human breast cancer cells and treated with isotype IgG1 control, IgG-P, scIgG-P, or IgG-P N297A at 10 mg/kg weekly for a total of five doses until tumors reached an average size of 100mm³. **c** Tumor volumes at the end time point of the nude mice xenograft study for individual mice treated with isotype IgG1 control, IgG-P, scIgG-P, and IgG-P N297A. Tumor size was measured twice a week. The error bars in the graphs depict the standard deviation (SD) obtained in three independent experiments. *$p < 0.05$,**$p < 0.01$

with that of the intact IgG-P with SKOV3 ovarian cancer cells (Fig. 3d) or SKBR3 breast cancer cells (Fig. 3e) as the target cells.

A variant of IgG-P, engineered to resist protease hinge cleavage, confirmed the impact of local protease action on IgG function

An engineered Fc variant of trastuzumab (PRIgG-T) was previously shown to withstand protease attack and to retain ADCC function in a protease-rich environment compared to IgG-T [7]. In this study, we constructed a protease-resistant variant of pertuzumab (PRIgG-P) using the same experimental approach. PRIgG-P demonstrated strong resistance to IdeS proteolysis compared to IgG-P when incubated with the protease-expressing BT474-IdeS and SKOV3-IdeS cells (Fig. 4a). As expected, PRIgG-P had similar binding to the antigen HER2 extracellular domain (ECD) as IgG-P (Fig. 4b, c). We investigated PRIgG-P antibody-mediated ADCC activity in cells with elevated proteolytic activity. The SKOV3-IdeS cell line was used as

the target cell and PBMCs were used as the immune effector cell source. PRIgG-P clearly induced a higher percentage of cell lysis (> 60%) than IgG-P (< 20%) (Fig. 4d). Next, we examined the ADCC restorative function of a protease-resistant anti-hinge mAb, PR2095–2, in the IdeS-expressing cellular environment. Again, the SKOV3-IdeS cell line was used as the target cell and PBMCs were used as the source of immune effector cells. SKOV3-IdeS cells incubated with PR2095–2 and IgG-P had a higher percentage of cell lysis (~ 65%) than the group treated with 2095–2 and IgG-P (< 15%) at the end point of the experiment (96 h) (Fig. 4e). These results indicated a clear benefit of the engineered protease-resistant hinge for mAb-mediated ADCC in the IdeS protease-rich environment.

Elevated IgG-P hinge cleavage occurred when IgG-T and IgG-P were combined

IgG-T and IgG-P are often used in combination in patients with breast cancer with high HER2 expression. To investigate how the hinge impairment of IgG-T and IgG-P affects

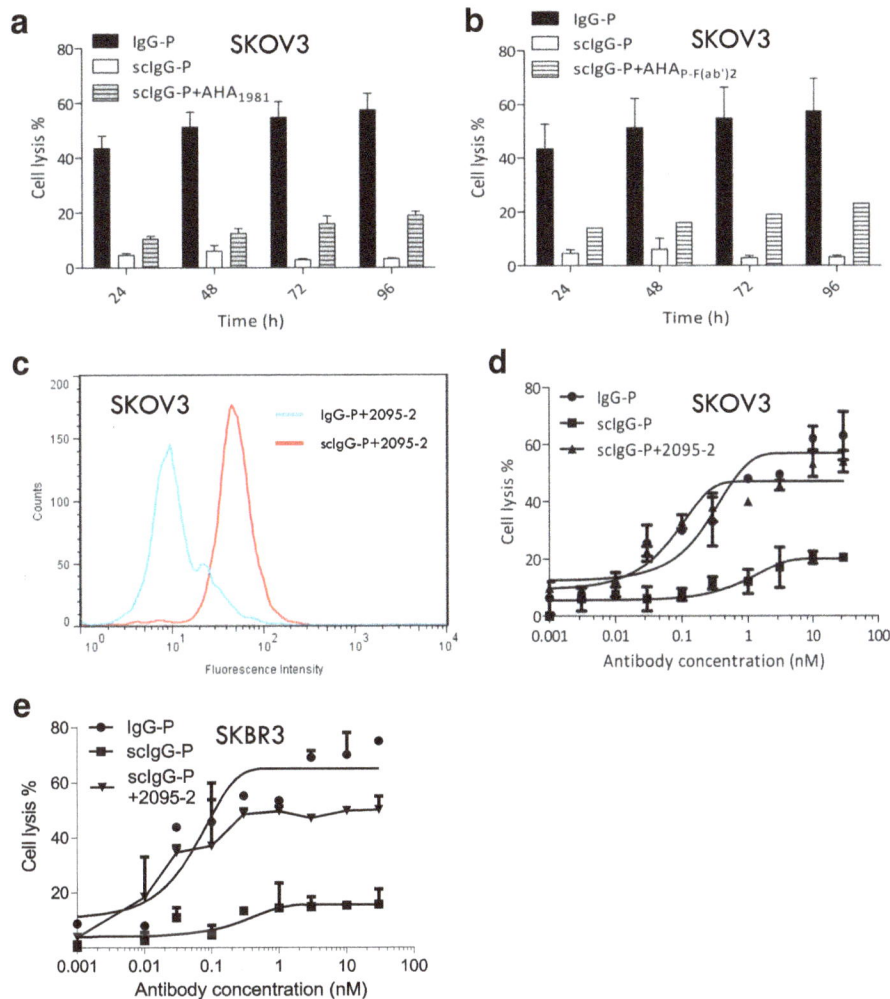

Fig. 3 Anti-hinge antibodies rescued antibody dependent cellular cytotoxicity (ADCC) activity for single hinge cleaved pertuzumab (scIgG-P). **a-b** Purified human anti-protease-induced, anti-hinge autoantibodies (AHA) using peptide analogues representing hinge-immunoglobulin G-degrading enzyme S (IdeS) cleavage sites, 1981 or F(ab')$_2$ generated by digesting immunoglobulin G (IgG-P) with IdeS as the absorbent, restored ADCC activity for scIgG-P. SKOV-3 cell (5000 cells/well) was seeded on the E-plate as the target cell and peripheral blood mononuclear cells PBMCs (25,000 cells/well) isolated from a single donor were used as the immune effector cell in complete cell culture medium containing scIgG-P (30 nM). The percentage of cell lysis was defined as: (cell index of control group – cell index of treatment group)/cell index of control group × 100. **c** Flow cytometry showing binding results for AH-mAb with IgG-P or scIgG-P on surfaces of high human epidermal growth factor receptor 2-expressing cancer cells. Biotinylated 2095–2 and streptavidin-PE conjugate were used for cell staining. **d-e** 2095–2 ADCC rescuing effect for scIgG-P at varying concentrations. A fixed concentration of 30 nM for IgG-P with threefold dilutions from 30 nM for 2095–2 were used in the ADCC assay. SKOV-3 cells (5000 cells/well) and SKBR3 cell (7000 cells/well) were used as the target cells and PBMCs isolated from a single donor were used as the immune effector cells at an effector (E)-target (T) ratio of 25:1

the combination treatment, we assessed the cleavage of antibodies when simultaneously bound to the same cancer cell surface. For detection of scIgG generation, F(ab')$_2$ fragments of IgG-T or IgG-P were combined with the intact IgG-P and IgG-T, respectively. After incubation with either the BT474 or the SKOV3 cancer cell line, any detected Fc(m) must have derived from the intact IgG. This additive test system was made possible by the similarity in the binding affinity for HER2 ECD between the F(ab')$_2$ fragments and the corresponding full-length version of either IgG-P or IgG-T (Fig. 5a). Although it was

not predicted in advance, the addition of the F(ab')$_2$ of IgG-T accelerated the generation of Fc(m) from IgG-P. This finding is unique in providing evidence for altered proteolytic kinetics of an antibody in a simultaneous binding circumstance. Intriguingly, there was not a corresponding increase in Fc(m) generation from IgG-T when combined with the F(ab')$_2$ of IgG-P (Fig. 5b). Structural rearrangements have been observed for IgG-T and IgG-P simultaneously interacting with HER2 ECD in an *in silico* analysis [22], which may explain the elevated IgG-P hinge cleavage in the presence of IgG-T.

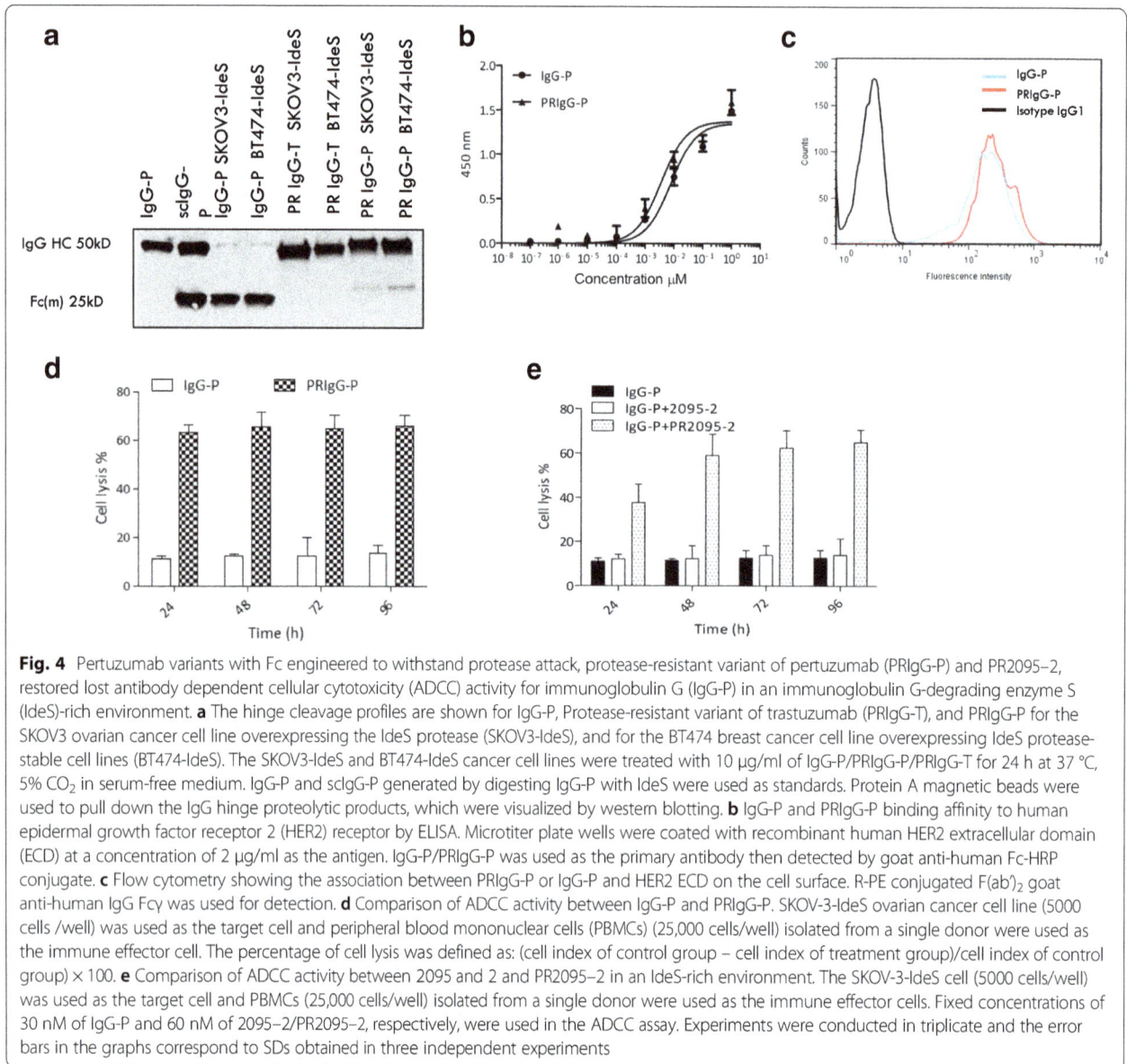

Fig. 4 Pertuzumab variants with Fc engineered to withstand protease attack, protease-resistant variant of pertuzumab (PRIgG-P) and PR2095–2, restored lost antibody dependent cellular cytotoxicity (ADCC) activity for immunoglobulin G (IgG-P) in an immunoglobulin G-degrading enzyme S (IdeS)-rich environment. **a** The hinge cleavage profiles are shown for IgG-P, Protease-resistant variant of trastuzumab (PRIgG-T), and PRIgG-P for the SKOV3 ovarian cancer cell line overexpressing the IdeS protease (SKOV3-IdeS), and for the BT474 breast cancer cell line overexpressing IdeS protease-stable cell lines (BT474-IdeS). The SKOV3-IdeS and BT474-IdeS cancer cell lines were treated with 10 µg/ml of IgG-P/PRIgG-P/PRIgG-T for 24 h at 37 °C, 5% CO_2 in serum-free medium. IgG-P and scIgG-P generated by digesting IgG-P with IdeS were used as standards. Protein A magnetic beads were used to pull down the IgG hinge proteolytic products, which were visualized by western blotting. **b** IgG-P and PRIgG-P binding affinity to human epidermal growth factor receptor 2 (HER2) receptor by ELISA. Microtiter plate wells were coated with recombinant human HER2 extracellular domain (ECD) at a concentration of 2 µg/ml as the antigen. IgG-P/PRIgG-P was used as the primary antibody then detected by goat anti-human Fc-HRP conjugate. **c** Flow cytometry showing the association between PRIgG-P or IgG-P and HER2 ECD on the cell surface. R-PE conjugated F(ab')2 goat anti-human IgG Fcγ was used for detection. **d** Comparison of ADCC activity between IgG-P and PRIgG-P. SKOV-3-IdeS ovarian cancer cell line (5000 cells /well) was used as the target cell and peripheral blood mononuclear cells (PBMCs) (25,000 cells/well) isolated from a single donor were used as the immune effector cell. The percentage of cell lysis was defined as: (cell index of control group – cell index of treatment group)/cell index of control group) × 100. **e** Comparison of ADCC activity between 2095 and 2 and PR2095–2 in an IdeS-rich environment. The SKOV-3-IdeS cell (5000 cells/well) was used as the target cell and PBMCs (25,000 cells/well) isolated from a single donor were used as the immune effector cells. Fixed concentrations of 30 nM of IgG-P and 60 nM of 2095–2/PR2095–2, respectively, were used in the ADCC assay. Experiments were conducted in triplicate and the error bars in the graphs correspond to SDs obtained in three independent experiments

Anti-hinge cleavage site antibodies rescued ADCC activity with a mixture of scIgG-T and scIgG-P

To determine whether the AHA can restore ADCC of scIgG-T and scIgG-P when used together on a HER2-expressing cell, we added purified human polyclonal anti-hinge autoantibodies (AHA$_{P- F(ab')2}$ or AHA$_{1981}$) to a combination of scIgG-T and scIgG-P. As expected, the combination of scIgG-T, scIgG-P, and purified polyclonal human AHA produced a higher percentage of cell lysis than the target cell line (SKOV3) treated with the combination of scIgG-T and scIgG-P alone (Fig. 6a). Next, we examined the ADCC rescuing effect of AH-mAb (2095–2) for the scIgG-T and scIgG-P combination treatment. The target cell line (SKOV3) treated with scIgG-P and scIgG-T combined with 2095–2 showed a similar level of cell lysis as the group treated with intact IgG-P and IgG-T at all time points (Fig. 6b). This indicated that 2095–2 was able to access the single hinge cleavage site of the therapeutic antibodies in combination on the same cell surface and receptor. These results were extended to an examination of the restoration phenomenon in a protease-enriched setting. For this, the IdeS-expressing SKOV-IdeS cell line was used for the anti-HER2 combination and the parental and the protease-resistant versions of 2095–2 anti-hinge mAb were tested for ADCC restoration. In this case, PR2095–2, but not 2095–2, successfully rescued ADCC activity with the combination treatment (Fig. 6c). Thus, cell lytic functions of combined hinge-cleaved anti-HER2 mAbs were recovered by polyclonal and monoclonal anti-hinge antibodies in multiple settings.

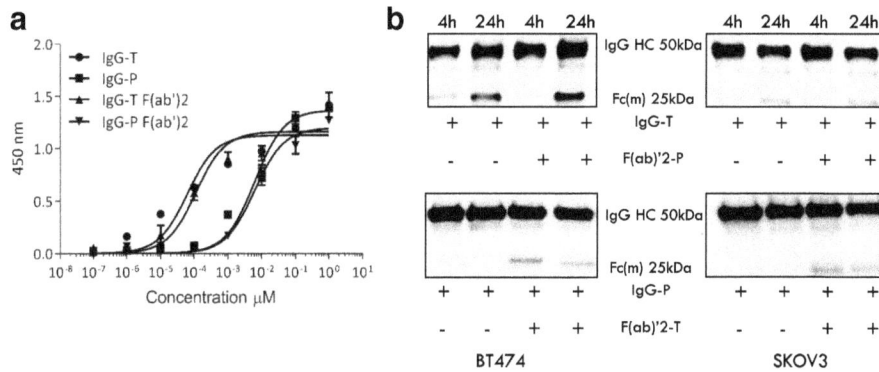

Fig. 5 Intact trastuzumab (IgG-T) and intact pertuzumab (IgG-P) combination treatment increased IgG-P cleavage. **a** The binding affinity to human epidermal growth factor receptor 2 (HER2) extracellular domain (ECD) for IgG-P, IgG-T and F(ab')$_2$ fragments of IgG-T and IgG-P. Microtiter plate wells were coated with HER2 ECD at a concentration of 2 µg/ml as the antigen. Threefold dilutions of IgG-P, IgG-T and the F(ab')$_2$ fragments of IgG-T and IgG-P were each applied to microtiter wells coated with recombinant human HER2 ECD. Goat anti-human kappa light chain-HRP conjugate was used as the detection antibody. **b** IgG-T and IgG-P proteolytic cleavage profile with/without addition of IgG-P-F(ab')$_2$ fragment and IgG-T-F(ab')$_2$ fragment, respectively. BT474 breast cancer cell line or SKOV3 ovarian cancer cell line were treated with IgG-T (10 µg/ml) with/without F(ab')$_2$ fragment of IgG-P (10 µg/ml) or vice versa for 4 h and 24 h at 37 °C, 5% CO_2 in serum-free medium. Protein A magnetic beads were used to pull down the IgG-P proteolytic product. The hinge cleavage product, Fc monomer, was visualized by blotting the membrane using a secondary detection antibody, goat anti-human Fc-HRP antibody

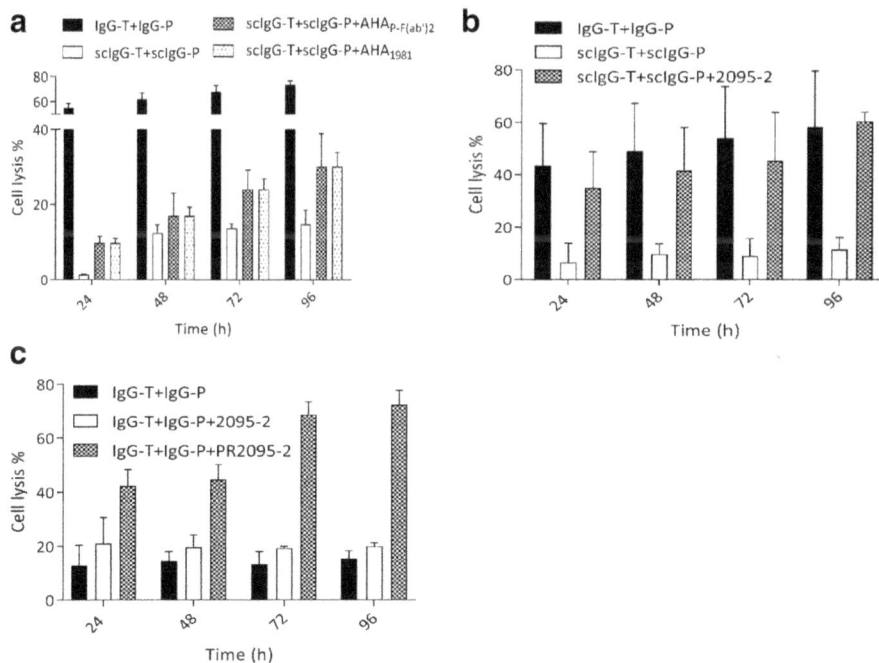

Fig. 6 Anti-hinge cleavage site antibodies rescued antibody dependent cellular cytotoxicity (ADCC) activity for a mixture of single hinge cleaved trastuzumab (scIgG-T) and single hinge cleaved pertuzumab (scIgG-P). SKOV-3 cells (5000 cells/well) were seeded on the E-plate as the target cell and peripheral blood mononuclear cells (25,000 cells/well) isolated from a single donor were used as the immune effector cells in complete cell culture medium containing a mixture of intact pertuzumab (IgG-P) (30 nM) and intact trastuzumab (IgG-T) (30 nM), or scIgG-P (30 nM) and scIgG-T (30 nM) with and without anti-hinge antibody (AHA) (120 nM). The percentage of cell lysis was defined as: (cell index of control group − cell index of treatment group)/cell index of control group) × 100. **a** ADCC activity for a combination of IgG-T and IgG-P (black bar), a combination of scIgG-P and scIgG-T (white bar), and a combination of scIgG-T and scIgG-P using human anti-protease-induced AHA using peptide analogues representing hinge-immunoglobulin G-degrading enzyme S (IdeS) cleavage sites, 1981B (dark gray bar) or F(ab')$_2$ generated by digesting IgG-P with IdeS as the absorbent (light gray bar). **b** ADCC activity for a combination of IgG-T and IgG-P (black bar), a combination of scIgG-P and scIgG-T (white bar), and a combination of scIgG-T and scIgG-P using the anti-hinge mAb 2095–2 (dark gray bar). **c** ADCC cell lysis of the IdeS-expressing SKOV3-IdeS cell line by a combination of IgG-T and IgG-P (black bar), a combination of IgG-T and IgG-P + anti-hinge mAb 2095–2 (white bar), and a combination of IgG-T, IgG-P, and protease-resistant PR2095–2 (dark gray bar)

Discussion

The susceptibility of IgGs to functional inactivation by proteolytic enzymes has been studied in various ways including purified systems using cancer-associated enzymes, endogenous proteases expressed by tumor cells, and model cell lines with enhanced protease secretion. The present investigation touched on these aspects as they might relate to the considerable complexity of the in vivo tumor environment and therapeutic approaches used to treat it.

Pertuzumab (IgG-P) is often administered to patients with HER2-positive breast cancer together with trastuzumab (IgG-T) as combination therapy [12, 18, 20, 21]. Both IgG-P and IgG-T target HER2 but interact with different domains of HER2 [13, 14]. The present findings demonstrated that there was enhancement of IgG-P cleavage on the cell surface by endogenous proteolytic action when the mAb was used in combination with trastuzumab. In addition, the inherent sensitivity of IgG-P to the hinge cleavage was different from that for IgG-T. Substantial levels of hinge proteolysis of IgG-P were detected when IgG-P was incubated with SKBR3 cells, while IgG-T had lower sensitivity on this high HER2-expressing cancer cell line [9]. *In silico* data suggest a structural rearrangement of IgG-T and IgG-P when both mAbs are bound to the HER2 receptor simultaneously [22]. The present finding of interdependent protease susceptibility further extends the topological dynamics of the receptor. For example, the formation of the HER2-pertuzumab complex may cause rearrangement of the receptor-antibody complex to expose previously inaccessible proteolytic sites buried inside the antibody protein structure [5]. Structure-based methodologies likely will be needed to detail the interactions among the targeted antigen, therapeutic antibodies, and proteases.

Studies have implicated the involvement of Fc-mediated ADCC activity in IgG-P-mediated inhibition of tumor growth [15, 16, 20]. We earlier showed that the cleavage of a single peptide bond in the hinge caused a partial loss of the ADCC function of IgG-T in vitro and in vivo [7, 9]. In this study, we showed a similar reliance on Fc structural integrity for IgG-P-mediated ADCC effector function and tumor inhibition in vitro and in vivo. The single hinge cleaved IgG-P and an engineered immune cell engagement deficient mutant of pertuzumab (IgG-P N297A) showed decreased tumor inhibition. Our results suggest that IgG-P with a cleaved hinge partially impedes tumor inhibition due to the loss of Fc effector function. The partial inhibition of tumor growth by scIgG can be attributed to a lack of interference with the Fc-independent pathway of pertuzumab cell killing via HER2 antigen engagement.

We and others have reported that MMPs are associated with antibody hinge cleavage in tumor tissues [4, 9]. Numerous proteases coexist in a tumor microenvironment. This poses a hurdle for attributing IgG functional loss to particular enzymes or mixtures of enzymes [23].

Consequently, an alternative and well-defined model system was considered to be essential for the present study. The specificity and potency of IdeS for cleaving the IgG hinge enabled this attempt [6, 24–26]. This was confirmed by the demonstration that IgG-P was enzymatically cleaved at the hinge when incubated with IdeS expressing cancer cell lines and in the solution-phase. The precise peptide bond specificity of IdeS in targeting the hinge region of human IgGs led to the development or isolation of antibodies that specifically detect the presence of the hinge cleavage site. By extension of these findings, it is possible to consider therapeutic options for restoring IgG function by the association of a functional anti-hinge IgG to the site of IgG proteolysis in cell-bound IgGs. The concept is not limited to IdeS and can apply to physiologically relevant, cancer-related proteases in the tumor environment.

Anti-hinge autoantibodies can be found in healthy individuals and patients with inflammatory diseases [5, 27]. Indeed, purified autoantibodies prepared from serum IgGs using immobilized F(ab')$_2$ generated from IdeS-cleaved IgG-P as the absorbent or using immobilized peptide possessing the "...PAPELLG" sequence with the free C-terminal glycine showed modest restoration of ADCC activity to scIgG-P in vitro. These findings support the concept that endogenous anti-hinge autoantibodies, especially at enhanced levels, might be efficacious in certain disease circumstances. Further, the development of anti-hinge monoclonal antibodies to rescue compromised Fc-mediated functions in hinge-cleaved mAbs is a readily achievable approach for this purpose [6–8]. The monoclonal AHA 2095–2 used in this study targets the neoepitope of IdeS cleaved IgG [10] and can restore the ADCC activity of scIgG-T in vitro and also the inhibition of tumor growth by administering scIgGT in vivo [7, 10]. This study demonstrated that AHA 2095–2 restored ADCC activity of scIgG-P as well. Moreover, mAb 2095–2 restored function to both scIgG-T and scIgG-P when the two distinct, dysfunctional anti-HER2 mAbs were used in combination. Thus, these interconnected findings suggest substantial flexibility for AHA as a therapeutic approach for cancer treatment. In addition, a promising alternative strategy using an engineered protease-resistant hinge in trastuzumab was capable of overcoming the protease susceptibility of the original IgG. In protease-expressing cellular settings, PRIgG-T conferred resistance to proteolytic hinge cleavage both in vitro and in vivo [7]. In the present study, the concept was applied successfully to pertuzumab and to the anti-hinge mAb 2095–2 and suggests broad generality for this approach within the tumor environment.

Conclusions

This study showed a readily detectable level of IgG-P hinge cleavage when incubated with high HER2-expressing breast cancer cell lines (but not with low HER2-expressing cells) and suggests that IgG proteolysis is facilitated when bound to the cell surface. ScIgG-P showed substantial loss of ADCC activity compared to un-cleaved IgG-P in vitro and was less potent against tumor growth in vivo. The loss of ADCC activity of scIgG-P can be restored by anti-hinge antibodies. An Fc engineering approach to derive a protease-resistant platform was shown to be applicable in two ways: (1) for directly maintaining IgG-P ADCC function in a protease-rich environment by engineering resistance into the heavy chain of IgG-P and (2) by the indirect method of engineering protease resistance into the AHA 2095–2. Both of these approaches afforded substantial protection in model systems to IgG-T and IgG-P singly or in combination. Taken together, the anti-hinge antibody and protease-resistant hinge suggest a powerful and versatile solution for overcoming the ability of tumor cells to evade the killing functions of targeted cancer immunotherapies.

Abbreviations
ADCC: Antibody-dependent cellular cytotoxicity; AHA: Ant-hinge antibody; ATCC: American Type Culture Collection; AWC: Animal Welfare Committee; BSA: Bovine serum albumin; CDC: Complement-dependent cytotoxicity; ECD: Extracellular domain; ELISA: Enzyme-linked immunosorbent assay; Fab: Fragment antigen binding; FBS: Fetal bovine serum; Fc: Fragment crystallizable; $Fc_{(m)}$: Fc monomer; HER2: Human epidermal growth factor receptor 2; HRP: Horseradish peroxidase; IdeS: Immunoglobulin G-degrading enzyme S; IgG: Immunoglobulin G; IgG-P: Intact pertuzumab; IgG-T: Intact trastuzumab; IVIG: Intravenous immunoglobulin; mAb: Monoclonal antibody; MMP: Matrix metalloproteinase; PBMC: Human peripheral blood mononuclear cells; PBS: Phosphate-buffered saline; PRIgG-P: Protease-resistant variant of pertuzumab; PRIgG-T: Protease-resistant variant of trastuzumab; RPMI 1640: Cell culture medium developed at Roswell Park Memorial Institute; scIgG-P: Single hinge cleaved pertuzumab; scIgG-T: Single hinge cleaved trastuzumab; SDS-PAGE: Sodium dodecyl sulfate polyacrylamide gel electrophoresis; TAA: Tumor-associated antigen; WB: Western blotting

Acknowledgements
We thank Drs. Wei Xiong and Xun Gui for their technical help in antibody production, and Dr. Georgina T. Salazar, Dr. Ahmad S. Salameh for their suggestions and discussion during the preparation of the manuscript.

Funding
Financial support: Cancer Prevention and Research Institute of Texas (RP150230) and the Welch Foundation (AU-0042-20030616).

Authors' contributions
H-CH participated in the study design and writing the draft manuscript, and conducted the in vitro studies. XF participated in the study design and writing the "Methods" sections, and conducted the mouse tumor xenograft studies. REJ contributed to study design, results interpretation, and editing the manuscript. NZ designed experiments, supervised in vitro and in vivo assay development, and edited the manuscript. ZA conceived the study, interpreted data, and edited the manuscript. All authors read and approved the final manuscript.

Competing interests
The authors declare that they have no competing interests.

References
1. Agniswamy J, Lei B, Musser JM, Sun PD. Insight of host immune evasion mediated by two variants of group a Streptococcus mac protein. J Biol Chem. 2004;279(50):52789–96.
2. Biancheri P, Brezski RJ, Di Sabatino A, Greenplate AR, Soring KL, Corazza GR, Kok KB, Rovedatti L, Vossenkamper A, Ahmad N, et al. Proteolytic cleavage and loss of function of biologic agents that neutralize tumor necrosis factor in the mucosa of Patients with inflammatory bowel disease. Gastroenterology. 2015;149(6):1564–74.
3. Gearing AJ, Thorpe SJ, Miller K, Mangan M, Varley PG, Dudgeon T, Ward G, Turner C, Thorpe R. Selective cleavage of human IgG by the matrix metalloproteinases, matrilysin and stromelysin. Immunol Lett. 2002;81(1):41–8.
4. Zhang N, Deng H, Fan X, Gonzalez A, Zhang S, Brezski RJ, Choi BK, Rycyzyn M, Strohl W, Jordan R, et al. Dysfunctional antibodies in the tumor microenvironment associate with impaired anticancer immunity. Clin Cancer Res. 2015;21(23):5380–90.
5. Falkenburg WJ, van Schaardenburg D, Ooijevaar-de Heer P, Tsang ASMW, Bultink IE, Voskuyl AE, Bentlage AE, Vidarsson G, Wolbink G, Rispens T. Anti-hinge antibodies recognize IgG subclass- and protease-restricted neoepitopes. J Immunol. 2017;198(1):82–93.
6. Ryan MH, Petrone D, Nemeth JF, Barnathan E, Bjorck L, Jordan RE. Proteolysis of purified IgGs by human and bacterial enzymes in vitro and the detection of specific proteolytic fragments of endogenous IgG in rheumatoid synovial fluid. Mol Immunol. 2008;45(7):1837–46.
7. Fan X, Brezski RJ, Deng H, Dhupkar PM, Shi Y, Gonzalez A, Zhang S, Rycyzyn M, Strohl WR, Jordan RE, et al. A novel therapeutic strategy to rescue the immune effector function of proteolytically inactivated cancer therapeutic antibodies. Mol Cancer Ther. 2015;14(3):681–91.
8. Brezski RJ, Luongo JL, Petrone D, Ryan MH, Zhong D, Tam SH, Schmidt AP, Kruszynski M, Whitaker BP, Knight DM, et al. Human anti-IgG1 hinge autoantibodies reconstitute the effector functions of proteolytically inactivated IgGs. J Immunol. 2008;181(5):3183–92.
9. Fan X, Brezski RJ, Fa M, Deng H, Oberholtzer A, Gonzalez A, Dubinsky WP, Strohl WR, Jordan RE, Zhang N, et al. A single proteolytic cleavage within the lower hinge of trastuzumab reduces immune effector function and in vivo efficacy. Breast Cancer Res. 2012;14(4):R116.
10. Brezski RJ, Kinder M, Grugan KD, Soring KL, Carton J, Greenplate AR, Petley T, Capaldi D, Brosnan K, Emmell E, et al. A monoclonal antibody against hinge-cleaved IgG restores effector function to proteolytically-inactivated IgGs in vitro and in vivo. MAbs. 2014;6(5):1265–73.
11. Kinder M, Greenplate AR, Grugan KD, Soring KL, Heeringa KA, McCarthy SG, Bannish G, Perpetua M, Lynch F, Jordan RE, et al. Engineered protease-resistant antibodies with selectable cell-killing functions. J Biol Chem. 2013; 288(43):30843–54.
12. Baselga J, Cortés J, Kim SB, Im SA, Hegg R, Im YH. Pertuzumab plus trastuzumab plus docetaxel for metastatic breast cancer. N Engl J Med. 2012;366:109–19.
13. Cho HS, Mason K, Ramyar KX, Stanley AM, Gabelli SB, Denney DW Jr, Leahy DJ. Structure of the extracellular region of HER2 alone and in complex with the Herceptin Fab. Nature. 2003;421(6924):756–60.
14. Franklin MC, Carey KD, Vajdos FF, Leahy DJ, de Vos AM, Sliwkowski MX. Insights into ErbB signaling from the structure of the ErbB2-pertuzumab complex. Cancer Cell. 2004;5(4):317–28.
15. El-Sahwi K, Bellone S, Cocco E, Cargnelutti M, Casagrande F, Bellone M, Abu-Khalaf M, Buza N, Tavassoli FA, Hui P, et al. In vitro activity of pertuzumab in combination with trastuzumab in uterine serous papillary adenocarcinoma. Br J Cancer. 2010;102(1):134–43.
16. Nahta R, Hung MC, Esteva FJ. The HER-2-targeting antibodies trastuzumab and pertuzumab synergistically inhibit the survival of breast cancer cells. Cancer Res. 2004;64(7):2343–6.
17. Scheuer W, Friess T, Burtscher H, Bossenmaier B, Endl J, Hasmann M. Strongly enhanced antitumor activity of trastuzumab and pertuzumab combination treatment on HER2-positive human xenograft tumor models. Cancer Res. 2009;69(24):9330–6.
18. Yamashita-Kashima Y, Iijima S, Yorozu K, Furugaki K, Kurasawa M, Ohta M, Fujimoto-Ouchi K. Pertuzumab in combination with trastuzumab shows significantly enhanced antitumor activity in HER2-positive human gastric cancer xenograft models. Clin Cancer Res. 2011;17(15):5060–70.
19. Takai N, Jain A, Kawamata N, Popoviciu LM, Said JW, Whittaker S, Miyakawa I, Agus DB, Koeffler HP. 2C4, a monoclonal antibody against HER2, disrupts the HER kinase signaling pathway and inhibits ovarian carcinoma cell growth. Cancer. 2005;104(12):2701–8.

20. Phillips GD, Fields CT, Li G, Dowbenko D, Schaefer G, Miller K, Andre F, Burris HA 3rd, Albain KS, Harbeck N, et al. Dual targeting of HER2-positive cancer with trastuzumab emtansine and pertuzumab: critical role for neuregulin blockade in antitumor response to combination therapy. Clin Cancer Res. 2014;20(2):456–68.

21. Richard S, Selle F, Lotz JP, Khalil A, Gligorov J, Soares DG. Pertuzumab and trastuzumab: the rationale way to synergy. An Acad Bras Cienc. 2016; 88(Suppl 1):565–77.

22. Fuentes G, Scaltriti M, Baselga J, Verma CS. Synergy between trastuzumab and pertuzumab for human epidermal growth factor 2 (Her2) from colocalization: an in silico based mechanism. Breast Cancer Res. 2011;13(3):R54.

23. Kessenbrock K, Plaks V, Werb Z. Matrix metalloproteinases: regulators of the tumor microenvironment. Cell. 2010;141(1):52-67.

24. Jarnum S, Bockermann R, Runstrom A, Winstedt L, Kjellman C. The bacterial enzyme IdeS cleaves the IgG-type of B cell receptor (BCR), abolishes BCR-mediated cell signaling, and inhibits memory B Cell activation. J Immunol. 2015;195(12):5592–601.

25. Vincents B, von Pawel-Rammingen U, Bjorck L, Abrahamson M. Enzymatic characterization of the streptococcal endopeptidase, IdeS, reveals that it is a cysteine protease with strict specificity for IgG cleavage due to exosite binding. Biochemistry. 2004;43(49):15540–9.

26. Wenig K, Chatwell L, von Pawel-Rammingen U, Bjorck L, Huber R, Sondermann P. Structure of the streptococcal endopeptidase IdeS, a cysteine proteinase with strict specificity for IgG. Proc Natl Acad Sci U S A. 2004;101(50):17371–6.

27. Ruppel J, Brady A, Elliott R, Leddy C, Palencia M, Coleman D, Couch JA, Wakshull E. Preexisting antibodies to an F(ab')2 antibody therapeutic and novel method for immunogenicity assessment. J Immunol Res. 2016;2016: 2921758.

2

Key regulators of lipid metabolism drive endocrine resistance in invasive lobular breast cancer

Tian Du[1,2], Matthew J. Sikora[1,3], Kevin M. Levine[1,4], Nilgun Tasdemir[1,5], Rebecca B. Riggins[6], Stacy G. Wendell[5], Bennett Van Houten[1,5] and Steffi Oesterreich[1,5*] [iD]

Abstract

Background: Invasive lobular breast carcinoma (ILC) is a histological subtype of breast cancer that is characterized by loss of E-cadherin and high expression of estrogen receptor alpha (ERα). In many cases, ILC is effectively treated with adjuvant aromatase inhibitors (AIs); however, acquired AI resistance remains a significant problem.

Methods: To identify underlying mechanisms of acquired anti-estrogen resistance in ILC, we recently developed six long-term estrogen-deprived (LTED) variant cell lines from the human ILC cell lines SUM44PE (SUM44; two lines) and MDA-MB-134VI (MM134; four lines). To better understand mechanisms of AI resistance in these models, we performed transcriptional profiling analysis by RNA-sequencing followed by candidate gene expression and functional studies.

Results: MM134 LTED cells expressed ER at a decreased level and lost growth response to estradiol, while SUM44 LTED cells retained partial ER activity. Our transcriptional profiling analysis identified shared activation of lipid metabolism across all six independent models. However, the underlying basis of this signature was distinct between models. Oxysterols were able to promote the proliferation of SUM44 LTED cells but not MM134 LTED cells. In contrast, MM134 LTED cells displayed a high expression of the sterol regulatory element-binding protein 1 (SREBP1), a regulator of fatty acid and cholesterol synthesis, and were hypersensitive to genetic or pharmacological inhibition of SREBPs. Several SREBP1 downstream targets involved in fatty acid synthesis, including *FASN*, were induced, and MM134 LTED cells were more sensitive to etomoxir, an inhibitor of the rate-limiting enzyme in beta-oxidation, than their respective parental control cells. Finally, *in silico* expression analysis in clinical specimens from a neo-adjuvant endocrine trial showed a significant association between the increase of *SREBP1* expression and lack of clinical response, providing further support for a role of SREBP1 in the acquisition of endocrine resistance in breast cancer.

Conclusions: Our characterization of a unique series of AI-resistant ILC models identifies the activation of key regulators of fatty acid and cholesterol metabolism, implicating lipid-metabolic processes driving estrogen-independent growth of ILC cells. Targeting these changes may prove a strategy for prevention and treatment of endocrine resistance for patients with ILC.

Keywords: Invasive lobular breast, Endocrine resistance, LTED, SREBP1, Fatty acid, Cholesterol

* Correspondence: oesterreichs@upmc.edu
[1]Women's Cancer Research Center, UPMC Hillman Cancer Institute, Magee Womens Research Institute, 204 Craft Avenue, Pittsburgh, PA 15213, USA
[5]Department of Pharmacology and Chemical Biology, University of Pittsburgh, Pittsburgh, PA 15213, USA
Full list of author information is available at the end of the article

Background

Accounting for 10–15% of all breast cancers, invasive lobular breast carcinoma (ILC) is the second most common histological subtype of breast cancer after invasive ductal cancer (IDC) [1, 2]. Tumor cells in classic ILC are small and round and invade the stroma in a discohesive single-file pattern, which can be attributed largely to the loss of E-cadherin (CDH1) [1]. Comparative analysis of luminal A ILC and IDC identified genomic and transcriptional differences between the two histological subtypes, including frequency of FOXA1 and GATA3 mutations, and activation of immune and metabolism pathways [3, 4]. ILC generally exhibits low rates of Ki67 and HER2 positivity, and more than 90% of ILC tumors are estrogen receptor–positive (ER$^+$) [1–3]. Paradoxically, despite these favorable prognostic and predictive features, there is accumulating evidence that some patients with ILC have worse long-term survival compared with stage/grade-matched IDC [5–9].

Anti-estrogen therapy, targeting ER signaling, is an important part of the treatment for patients with ER$^+$ breast cancer; however, its efficacy is often limited by intrinsic and acquired endocrine resistance. Mediators of endocrine resistance include loss of expression or genomic aberration (for example, mutations) of ER, altered expression of ER co-regulators and cell cycle signaling molecules, increased signaling of growth factor receptor pathways, and enhanced autophagy [10–12]. There have been only a limited number of studies testing the mechanism of anti-estrogen resistance in ILC, identifying potential roles for signaling through estrogen-related receptor gamma (ERRγ) [13], ERβ [14], FGFR1 [15, 16], and MAPK1 [17]. However, mechanisms of endocrine resistance in this understudied subtype of breast cancer remain largely unknown.

We have recently described a set of genes that are uniquely estrogen-regulated in ILC cells [15] and specifically identified WNT4 as an important mediator of estrogen-induced growth in ILC cells [18]. To test whether WNT4 played a similar role in anti-estrogen resistance in ILC, we generated long-term estrogen-deprived (LTED) MDA-MB-134VI (MM134) and SUM44PE (SUM44) ILC cell lines to mimic resistance to aromatase inhibitors (AIs) in the clinic and subsequently showed WNT4 overexpression in a subset of these models [18]. The objective of this study was to perform a comprehensive and unbiased characterization of these ILC LTED cell line models with the goal of identifying potential mechanisms of resistance. Here, we show that ILC LTED cells activate drivers of fatty acid/cholesterol metabolism, which could have therapeutic consequences and thus should pave the way for additional studies on unique cellular metabolism in lobular breast cancer.

Methods
Cell culture and reagents

SUM44PE (Asterand Bioscience, Detroit, MI, USA) cells were maintained as described previously [15]. MDA-MB-134VI (MM134) (American Type Culture Collection [ATCC], Manassas, VA, USA) cells were cultured in 1:1 Dulbecco's modified Eagle's medium (DMEM) (11,965; Life Technologies, Carlsbad, CA, USA): L-15 (11,415; Life Technologies) + 10% fetal bovine serum (FBS) (26,140; Life Technologies). LTED cell lines were generated as recently described [18]. Briefly, SUM44PE cells were cultured in 1:1 DMEM: L-15 + 10% FBS for 3 months to generate SUM44F cells, which have a stronger proliferative response to 17β-estradiol (E2) [18]. SUM44F and MM134 cells were hormone-deprived and then maintained in improved minimal essential medium (IMEM) (A10488; Life Technologies; Richter's modification, no Phenol Red, no Gentamycin) + 10% charcoal-stripped FBS (CSS) (12,676, lot 1,747,185; Life Technologies) for 6–12 months to acquire endocrine resistance (Additional file 1: Figure S1). Four MM134 LTED variants (LTED-A, -B, -D, and -E) and two SUM44 LTED variants (LTED-A and -B) were generated independently. SUM44F was used as the parental cell line for SUM44 LTED cells in this study. CSS lot 1,747,185 was used for the majority of the experiments herein, but owing to unavailability of the same lot after its depletion, some studies were performed using FBS that was charcoal-stripped in our laboratory using a previously described methodology (26,140, lot 1,715,928; Life Technologies) [19]. The majority of experiments were repeated in both CSS lots to ensure consistent phenotypes. All cell lines were incubated at 37 °C in 5% carbon dioxide. Cell lines were authenticated at the University of Arizona Genetics Core and confirmed to be mycoplasma-negative with a MycoAlert Mycoplasma Detection Kit (LT07; Lonza, Basel, Switzerland). Authenticated cells were in continuous culture for less than 8 months (except during the establishment of LTED models).

For hormone deprivation, cells were washed twice daily for 3 days. For each wash, cells were rinsed twice with serum-free IMEM and then cultured in IMEM + 10% CSS. A minimum 1-h interval was kept between two washes.

E2 (E8875; Sigma-Aldrich, St. Louis, MO, USA), 25-hydroxycholesterol (25-HC) (SC-214091; Santa Cruz, Dallas, TX, USA), and 27-hydroxycholesterol (27-HC) (SC-358756; Santa Cruz) were dissolved in ethanol. PF429242 (SML0667; Sigma-Aldrich) was dissolved in double-distilled water (ddH$_2$O). ICI 182,780 (ICI/fulvestrant) (1047; Tocris Bioscience, Avonmouth, Bristol, UK), etomoxir (E1905; Sigma-Aldrich), orlistat (O4139; Sigma-Aldrich), Fatostatin (F8932; Sigma-Aldrich), and TOFA (T6575; Sigma-Aldrich) were dissolved in dimethylsulfoxide (DMSO) (4-X; ATCC).

Growth assays, dose response, and two-dimensional colony formation

For growth assays, 16,000 cells were seeded per well in 96-well plates. Parental cells were hormone-deprived before seeding. Day 0 was set as 24 h after seeding. Cells were harvested each day from day 0 to day 5. For dose response, cells were treated with vehicle (control) or a different concentration of drugs 24 h after seeding. Cell proliferation was quantified by using the Fluoreporter double-stranded DNA quantification kit (F2692; Life Technologies) in accordance with the instructions of the manufacturer. Fluorescence was assessed by using a VICTOR X4 plate reader (PerkinElmer, Waltham, MA, USA). The half maximal inhibitory concentration (IC_{50}) was quantified with GraphPad Prism version 5.04 (GraphPad Software, La Jolla, CA, USA) using non-linear regression (log(inhibitor) versus response; three parameters).

For the two-dimensional (2D) colony formation, 5,000 cells per well were evenly seeded in six-well plates, media was changed once per week, and cells were harvested on day 15. Cells were washed twice with cold phosphate-buffered saline (PBS) and then fixed for 10 min with ice-cold 100% methanol. Fixed cells were stained with 0.5% crystal violet (C3886; Sigma-Aldrich. Dissolved in 25% methanol) for 10 min and further washed with H_2O. Pictures of each well were taken with a SZX16 Stereo Microscope (Olympus, Tokyo, Japan). Colonies with radium of more than 25 μM were counted with cellSens Dimension version 1.9 (Olympus).

RNA interference

Small interfering RNA (siRNA) was reverse-transfected into cells 24 h after cell seeding using Lipofectamine RNAiMAX transfection reagents (13,778,150; Life Technologies) in accordance with the instructions of the manufacturer. Specifically, for each well in a 96-well plate, cells were treated with 1 pmol *SREBP1* siRNA and 1 pmol *SREBP2* siRNA or with 2 pmol non-target siRNA. SiRNA sequences are provided in Additional file 2: Table S1.

Q-RT-PCR

RNA was extracted with a Qiagen RNeasy kit (74,106; Qiagen, Hilden, Germany). iScript reverse transcription supermix (1,708,841; Bio-Rad Laboratories, Hercules, CA, USA) was used to generate cDNA. Quantitative polymerase chain reaction (PCR) was then carried out with a CFX384 Real-Time PCR Detection System (Bio-Rad Laboratories) using SsoAdvanced SYBR Green Master Mix (Bio-Rad Laboratories). *RPLP0* was used as the internal control to normalize gene expression. Primer sequences are provided in Additional file 2: Table S1.

Immunoblotting

For whole cell lysis, cells were lysed with RIPA buffer supplied with Halt Protease and Phosphatase inhibitor (78,842; Thermo Fisher Scientific, Waltham, MA, USA). Nuclear proteins were extracted with NE-PER™ Nuclear and Cytoplasmic Extraction Reagents (78,833; Thermo Fisher Scientific) in accordance with the instructions of the manufacturer. Proteins were separated by SDS-PAGE and transferred to polyvinylidene difluoride (PVDF) membranes. Protein bands were detected by fluorescence with Odyssey CLX imaging system (LI-COR Biosciences, Lincoln, NE, USA). The following primary antibodies were used: anti-ERα (8644; Cell Signaling Technology, Danvers, MA, USA; dilution 1:1000), anti-SREBP1 (SC-13551; Santa Cruz; dilution 1:200), anti-β-actin (A5441; Sigma-Aldrich; dilution 1:2500), and anti-FASN (3180S; Cell Signaling Technology; dilution 1:1000). Anti-PCNA (NA03; EMD Millipore, Billerica, MA, USA; dilution 1:1000) was kindly provided by Yi Huang (UPMC Hillman Cancer Center) and used as the internal control for nuclear protein.

RNA-sequencing and differential expression analysis

Parental and LTED MM134 and SUM44 cells were seeded in triplicates in six-well plates. Parental cells were hormone-deprived for 3 days before cell collection. RNA was isolated by using an Illustra RNAspin Mini Kit (25–0500-72; GE Healthcare, Little Chalfont, UK). RNA-sequencing (RNA-Seq) was carried out by Illumina HiSeq 2000. Raw sequence data were mapped to hg38 genome (ensemble release version 82) and gene counts were quantified with Salmon (version 0.6.0) [20] using default settings. RNA-Seq mapping rates are provided in Additional file 3: Table S2. Differentially expressed (DE) analysis was performed with R package DESeq2 [21] in MM134 cells and SUM44 cells independently. DE genes in individual LTED variants were called using the following criteria: absolute log2(-fold change) > log2(1.5) and Benjamini-Hochberg–adjusted P value of less than 0.001. The complete list of DE genes is available in Additional file 4: Table S3. RNA-Seq raw sequence data are available via GSE116744 from gene expression omnibus (GEO) (http://ncbi.nlm.nih.gov/geo/).

The gene expression (microarray) data of SUM44 tamoxifen-resistant (SUM44 TamR) and parental cells (SUM44PE) were downloaded from GEO [GSE12708]. Probes with the highest interquartile range were selected for genes that matched to multiple probes. DE analysis was performed with R package Limma [22], and a Benjamini-Hochberg–adjusted P value of less than 0.05 was used to call DE genes in SUM44 TamR cells.

Heatmap clustering

The Salmon output of gene-level transcript per million (TPM) counts was used, first transforming by log2 (TPM + 1). The top 1000 most variable genes in MM134 or SUM44 cells (by interquartile range) were used for the heatmap. Relative expression values were calculated as fold change to the average expression level in parental cells. Hierarchical clustering of genes was conducted by using the heatmap.3 function (https://raw.githubusercontent.com/obigriffith/biostar-tutorials/master/Heatmaps/heatmap.3.R) under R version 3.2.2. The relationship between genes in terms of expression patterns across different samples was quantified with a Euclidean distance measure and visualized with complete-linkage clustering.

Pathway analysis

Pathway analysis was conducted with Ingenuity Pathway Analysis (IPA) using genes that were differentially expressed in at least three MM134 LTED variants or both SUM44 LTED variants. Complete pathway analysis results are shown in Additional file 5: Table S4. *GseaPreranked* function in Gene Set Enrichment Analysis (GSEA) (version 2.2.2, Broad Institute, Cambridge, MA, USA) was performed using the Reactome cholesterol synthesis signature (Additional file 5: Table S4), downloaded from the Molecular Signature Database (MsigDB, version 6.0, Broad Institute). DE genes ranked by their log2(fold change) were used as input. Default settings in *GseaPreranked* were used except the following parameters: "Enrichment statistic" was "Classic" and "Min size: exclude smaller sets" was set to be 0.

LC-MS/MS analysis

Cells were washed twice with cold PBS, scratched off the plate, and resuspended in cold PBS, and cell suspensions for each sample were spiked with cholesterol-d$_7$ (1.27 nmoles) and 16:0-cholesterol ester-d$_7$ (1.58 nmoles) internal standards and extracted using two volumes of isopropanol/chloroform/formic acid (50/50/0.1). Samples were centrifuged at 3000 revolutions per minute at room temperature for 10 min. The bottom layer (organic) was transferred to a clean vial and dried under N$_2$. Samples were reconstituted in 150 μL of chloroform/methanol (1:2) for high-performance liquid chromatography-electrospray ionization tandem mass spectrometry analysis (LC-MS/MS).

Samples were analyzed on a Sciex 5000 triple quadrupole coupled to a Shimadzu/CTC Leap HPLC system (Sciex, Framingham, MA, USA). Cholesterol and metabolites (for example, 27-HC) were separated by a Luna C18(2) reversed-phase column (5 μ, 2 X 100 mm; Phenomenex, Torrence, CA, USA) at a flow rate of 0.63 mL/min using a linear gradient. Solvent A consisted of water/acetonitrile/formic acid (50/50/0.1), and solvent B consisted of acetonitrile/iso-propanol/formic acid (40/60/0.1). The gradient started at 50% B and increased over 6 min to 100% B, which was maintained for 5 min and followed by a 4-min equilibration at initial conditions. Cholesterol esters were separated using the same column and flow rate, but the solvent system consisted of water/acetonitrile/formic acid (10/90/0.1) for solvent A and acetonitrile/isopropanol//formic acid (20/80/0.1) for solvent B. The gradient started at 55% B and increased over 9 min to 100% B, which was maintained for 4 min and followed by a 4-min equilibration at initial conditions. Samples were analyzed in positive ion mode using the following MS source and compound parameters: collision gas 5, curtain gas 40, ion source gas 1 55, ion source gas 2, 50, ion spray voltage 5500, temperature 600 °C, de-clustering potential 90, entrance potential 5, collision exit potential 10, and a collision energy of 25. The following transitions were used for cholesterol, 27-hydroxylcholesterol, and cholesterol esters: 369.3➔161.3 cholesterol and cholesterol esters, 376.4➔161.3 cholesterol-d$_7$ and 16:0-cholesterol ester-d$_7$, and 385.3➔215.1 27-hydroxylcholesterol. Cholesterol was quantified by using a standard curve developed with standards and the cholesterol-d$_7$ internal standard. Cholesterol esters were reported by integrating the total peak areas for cholesterol ester species detected and quantified using the 16:0-cholesterol ester and 16:0-cholesterol ester-d$_7$ standard curve. Cholesterol, 27-hydroxylcholesterol, and cholesterol esters are reported as nanomoles per 1000,000 cells for cell lysate.

Analysis of clinical samples

Gene expression microarray data of ER$^+$ breast cancers treated with letrozole were obtained from the GEO database [GEO: GSE20181] [23]. Gene expression changes after 3-month treatment with letrozole were determined for genes of interest in responders and non-responders, as defined by tumor volume reduction by 50%. Pearson's chi-squared test was used to check the dependence of the gene expression change and the response to letrozole.

Results

Growth and hormone response of MM134 and SUM44 LTED cells

The MM134 and SUM44 LTED cells were generated by growing parental cells in hormone-deprived serum (IMEM + 10% charcoal-stripped FBS, CSS) over 6–12 months until the emergence of several estrogen-independent clones, which were subsequently maintained in this medium [18] (Additional file 1: Figure S1). Growth analyses showed that all of the LTED clones had significantly increased growth rates as compared with their parental lines grown in CSS (Parental [CSS]) (Fig. 1a), confirming their estrogen-independent growth. While the LTED cells proliferated more slowly than their respective parental lines grown in FBS (Parental [FBS]) over 5 days (Fig. 1a),

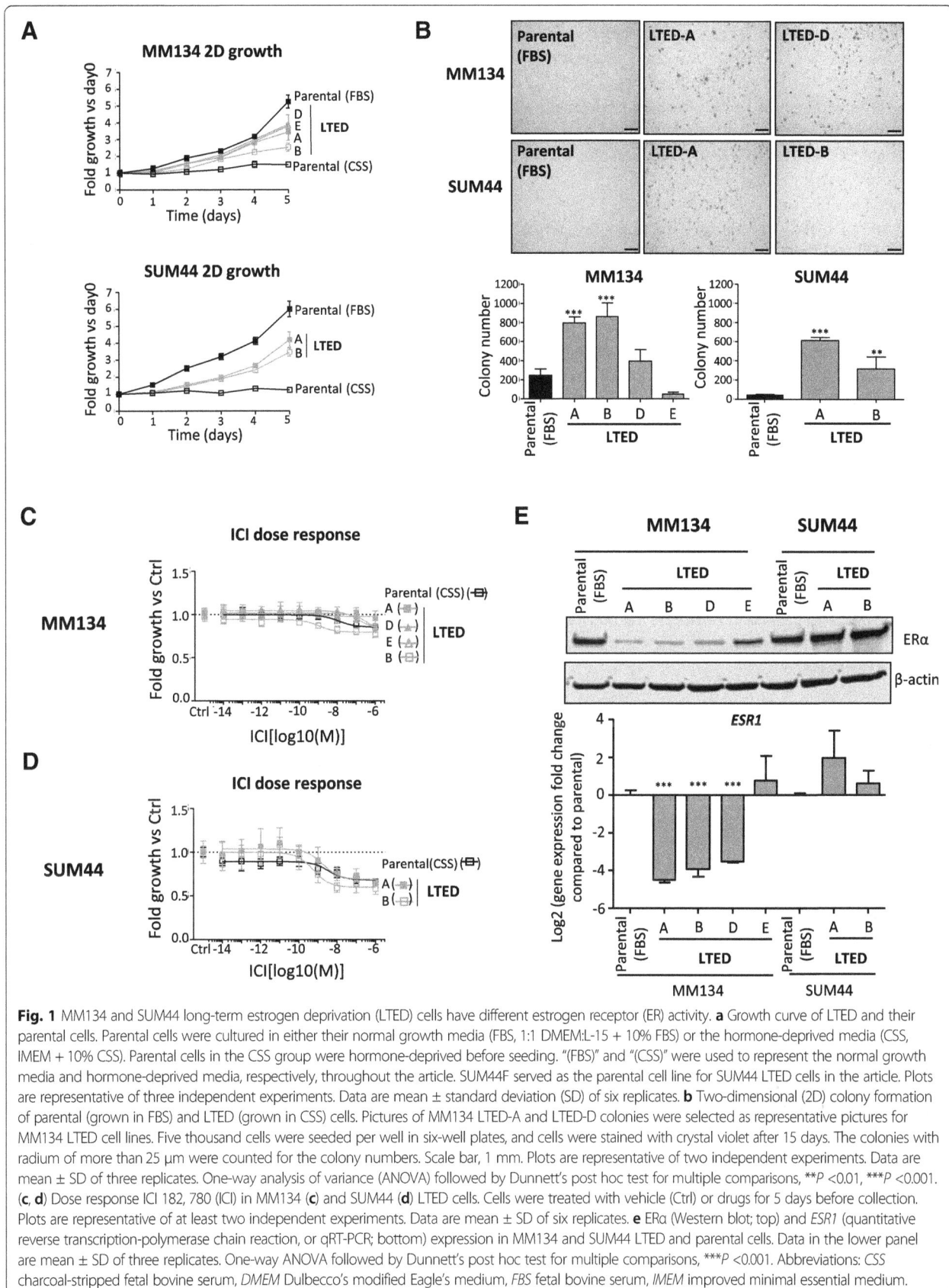

Fig. 1 MM134 and SUM44 long-term estrogen deprivation (LTED) cells have different estrogen receptor (ER) activity. **a** Growth curve of LTED and their parental cells. Parental cells were cultured in either their normal growth media (FBS, 1:1 DMEM:L-15 + 10% FBS) or the hormone-deprived media (CSS, IMEM + 10% CSS). Parental cells in the CSS group were hormone-deprived before seeding. "(FBS)" and "(CSS)" were used to represent the normal growth media and hormone-deprived media, respectively, throughout the article. SUM44F served as the parental cell line for SUM44 LTED cells in the article. Plots are representative of three independent experiments. Data are mean ± standard deviation (SD) of six replicates. **b** Two-dimensional (2D) colony formation of parental (grown in FBS) and LTED (grown in CSS) cells. Pictures of MM134 LTED-A and LTED-D colonies were selected as representative pictures for MM134 LTED cell lines. Five thousand cells were seeded per well in six-well plates, and cells were stained with crystal violet after 15 days. The colonies with radium of more than 25 μm were counted for the colony numbers. Scale bar, 1 mm. Plots are representative of two independent experiments. Data are mean ± SD of three replicates. One-way analysis of variance (ANOVA) followed by Dunnett's post hoc test for multiple comparisons, **P <0.01, ***P <0.001. (**c, d**) Dose response ICI 182, 780 (ICI) in MM134 (**c**) and SUM44 (**d**) LTED cells. Cells were treated with vehicle (Ctrl) or drugs for 5 days before collection. Plots are representative of at least two independent experiments. Data are mean ± SD of six replicates. **e** ERα (Western blot; top) and *ESR1* (quantitative reverse transcription-polymerase chain reaction, or qRT-PCR; bottom) expression in MM134 and SUM44 LTED and parental cells. Data in the lower panel are mean ± SD of three replicates. One-way ANOVA followed by Dunnett's post hoc test for multiple comparisons, ***P <0.001. Abbreviations: *CSS* charcoal-stripped fetal bovine serum, *DMEM* Dulbecco's modified Eagle's medium, *FBS* fetal bovine serum, *IMEM* improved minimal essential medium.

3/4 MM134 and 2/2 SUM44 LTED clones showed significantly increased growth or colony number (or both) in colony formation assays over 15 days, suggesting that LTED cells have higher clonogenic ability (Fig. 1b). Neither parental cells nor LTED variants, however, were able to form colonies in soft agar when grown in CSS (Additional file 1: Figure S2A). These results are likely due to different signaling pathways governing 2D and 3D growth in CSS versus FBS.

To comprehensively characterize the endocrine response of the LTED cell lines, we performed dose response assays with E2 and ICI 182,780 (ICI). These growth assays showed that MM134 and SUM44 LTED cells do not respond to E2 (Additional file 1: Figure S2B). In SUM44 LTED cells, we observed some weak growth inhibition with estradiol; however, this was a weak effect that varied with different lots of CSS (Additional file 1: Figure S2B, bottom panel). ICI had no effect on MM134 LTED (Fig. 1c) but did result in growth inhibition of SUM44 LTED cells (Fig. 1d). These results were supported by analysis of ER protein levels in MM134 and SUM44 LTED cells, showing decreased and increased ER expression compared with their parental cells, respectively (Fig. 1e). Collectively, these data suggest that the two ILC LTED cell line models differ in their hormone response; MM134 LTED cells had very low ER protein levels and lacked a hormone response, whereas SUM44 LTED cells maintained high ER expression and had some response to ICI.

Activation of lipid synthesis-related pathways in ILC LTED cells

To better understand the gene expression and pathway changes in LTED cells, we performed transcriptional profiling by RNA-Seq on LTED clones and their respective parental cells. Heatmap (Fig. 2a) and principal component analysis (Fig. 2b) showed that the different LTED variants were similar to each other and distinct from their parental cells by gene expression. Three thousand three hundred fifty-nine DE genes (upregulated $n = 1653$ and downregulated $n = 1706$) were shared in at least three MM134 LTED cell lines (Additional file 1: Figure S3A; Additional file 4: Table S3), and 2106 genes were shared in all four lines (P <2.2e-16). Three thousand two hundred sixteen DE genes (upregulated $n = 1448$, downregulated $n = 1768$) were shared by the two SUM44 LTED variants (P <2.2e-16) (Additional file 1: Figure S3B; Additional file 4: Table S3). Whereas MM134 LTED and SUM44 LTED cells shared a significant number of DE genes ($n = 437$, P <2.2e-16), the majority of DE genes were unique for MM134 LTED or SUM44 LTED cells (Additional file 1: Figure S3C), indicating that the two cell line models have acquired some shared but also many different mechanisms of endocrine resistance.

To identify pathways activated in the two resistant models, we applied IPA using the DE genes from MM134 and SUM44 LTED cells (Fig. 2c, Additional file 5: Table S4). The most strongly enriched pathways in MM134 versus SUM44 were distinct, again suggesting at least some differences in mechanisms of endocrine resistance. In MM134 LTED cells, the most enriched pathways were related to activation of immune functions and metabolism. Intriguingly, the enriched metabolic pathways were all related to lipid synthesis and lipid metabolism, such as "Ketogenesis" and "Superpathway of Cholesterol Biosynthesis" (indicated in bold in Fig. 2c). Similar pathways were not the primary pathways enriched in SUM44 LTED cells, which in contrast showed activation of DNA repair mechanisms and pathways related to cell cycle checkpoints. This finding was supported by the results from the GSEA, showing significant enrichment of an E2F signature in SUM44 LTED cells (Fig. 3a) but not in MM134 LTED cells (data not shown). These data suggest that one mechanism of endocrine resistance in SUM44 LTED cells is E2F-mediated activation of cell proliferation, previously described for other endocrine-resistant models [24].

We noted that although cholesterol-related signatures were not among the top 10 activated pathways in SUM44 LTED cells, the "Superpathway of Cholesterol Biosynthesis" pathway was still significantly enriched in this model ($P = 0.023$, corrected $P = 0.18$). A possible activation of cholesterol synthesis in MM134 and SUM44 LTED cells was further suggested by results from GSEA, which identified a modest enrichment of a cholesterol synthesis signature (Fig. 3b).

"Ketogenesis" involves β-oxidation of fatty acids [25], whereas the "Superpathway of cholesterol biosynthesis", "LXR/RXR Activation", and "Hepatic Cholestasis" are closely associated with both cholesterol and fatty acid transport and metabolism [26, 27]. We did not detect differences in total intracellular free cholesterol and cholesterol esters between parental MM134 or SUM44 and LTED cells (Additional file 1: Figure S4). As cholesterol metabolites (for example, 27-HC) were increased in endocrine-resistant IDC cells [28, 29], we investigated their potential role in our ILC LTED models. Although we were unable to quantify 27-HC because the levels were below the limit of detection in our assays, growth assays showed that the cholesterol metabolites 25-HC and 27-HC could promote the proliferation of SUM44 LTED cells, as well as MM134 and SUM44 parental cells grown in CSS, suggesting a potential similar role of cholesterol metabolites in endocrine-resistant ER+ ILC models (Fig. 3c).

Upregulation of sterol regulatory element-binding factor SREBP1 and other fatty acid synthesis enzymes in LTED ILC cells

Lipid homeostasis is closely regulated by sterol regulatory element-binding factors (SREBPs/SREBFs) [30, 31]. The

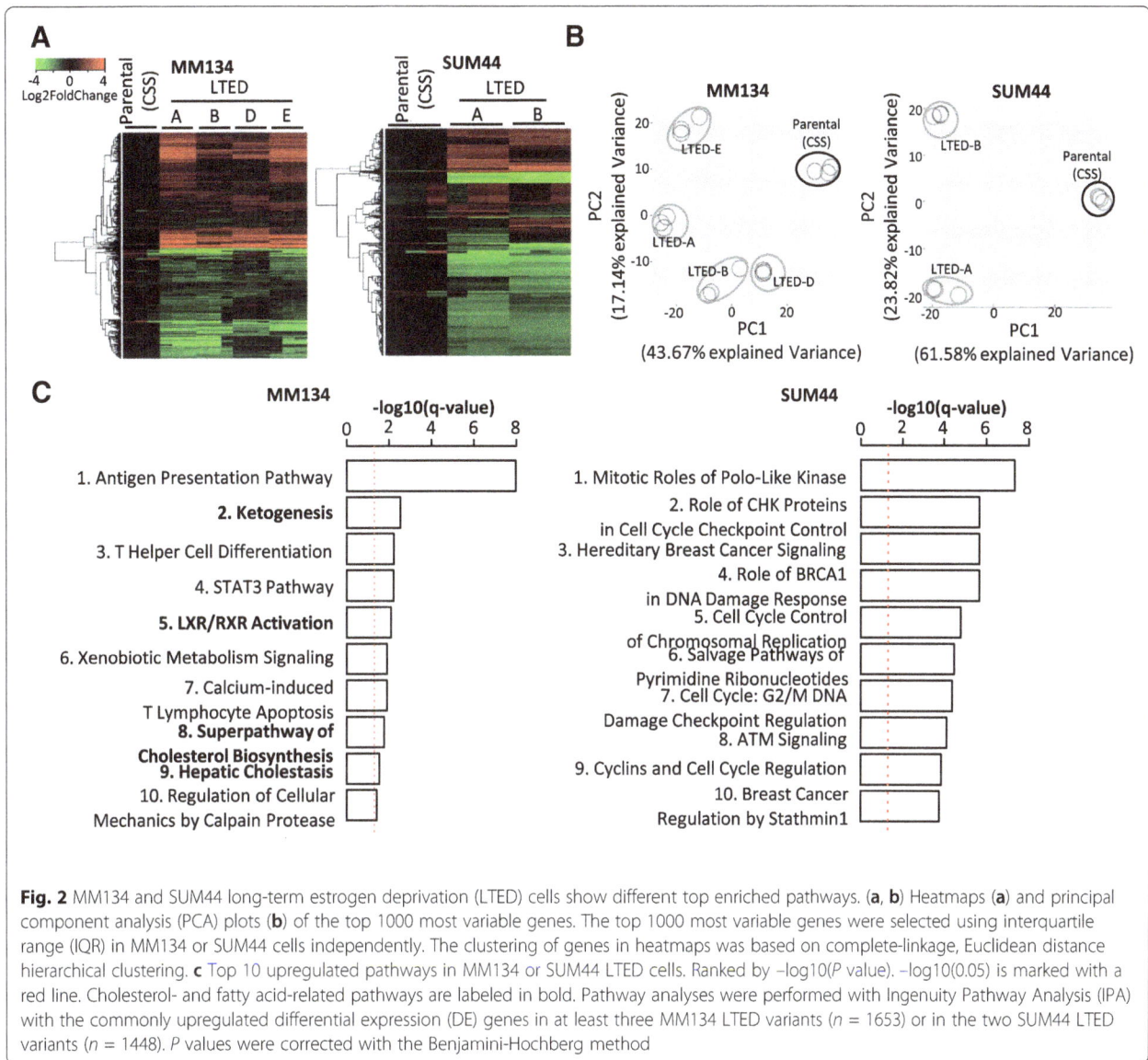

Fig. 2 MM134 and SUM44 long-term estrogen deprivation (LTED) cells show different top enriched pathways. (**a, b**) Heatmaps (**a**) and principal component analysis (PCA) plots (**b**) of the top 1000 most variable genes. The top 1000 most variable genes were selected using interquartile range (IQR) in MM134 or SUM44 cells independently. The clustering of genes in heatmaps was based on complete-linkage, Euclidean distance hierarchical clustering. **c** Top 10 upregulated pathways in MM134 or SUM44 LTED cells. Ranked by –log10(P value). –log10(0.05) is marked with a red line. Cholesterol- and fatty acid-related pathways are labeled in bold. Pathway analyses were performed with Ingenuity Pathway Analysis (IPA) with the commonly upregulated differential expression (DE) genes in at least three MM134 LTED variants (n = 1653) or in the two SUM44 LTED variants (n = 1448). P values were corrected with the Benjamini-Hochberg method

SREBP family that has been proposed to have roles in tumor differentiation, metastasis, and dormancy [32–34] contains two genes, *SREBP1* and *SREBP2*, which encode three protein isoforms: SREBP1a, SREBP1c, and SREBP2. Functionally, SREBP1c and SREBP2 regulate fatty acid synthesis and cholesterol synthesis, respectively, while SREBP1a regulates both of these pathways [35, 36]. We identified *SREBP1* as one of the only five genes (*SREBP1, FASN, FGFR4, AKR7A3*, and *FKBP11*) that were commonly upregulated in MM134 LTED, SUM44 LTED, and SUM44 TamR cells (previously described by Riggins et al. [13]). Further supporting a role for the SREBP family in endocrine resistance in ILC, IPA upstream regulator analysis showed that SREBP1, SREBP2, and SCAP (SREBP cleavage-activating protein) were activated in the ILC LTED models (Fig. 3d). Expression analysis of the three SREBP isoforms (SREBP1a, SREBP1c, and SREBP2)

showed upregulation of *SREBP1a* in all MM134 and SUM44 LTED lines (Fig. 4a, and Additional file 1: Figure S5). At the protein level, the precursor SREBP1 (pre-SREBP1) was increased in MM134 LTED but not in SUM44 LTED cells (Fig. 4b, left panel). Pre-SREBP1 is processed into mature SREBP1 (mSREBP1), which activates the transcription of target genes by binding to the sterol response element in nucleus (Additional file 1: Figure S6). Our cell fractionation and immunoblot analyses showed upregulation of mSREBP1 in the nucleus in MM134 LTED cells compared with parental cells (Fig. 4b, right panel), supporting increased transcriptional activity in endocrine-resistant MM134 cells.

Given the known role of SREBP1 in fatty acid synthesis [30, 31], we asked whether FASN, a key enzyme regulating fatty acid synthesis and direct target gene of SREBP1, was also induced in LTED cells. RNA and protein analysis showed significant upregulation of *FASN*

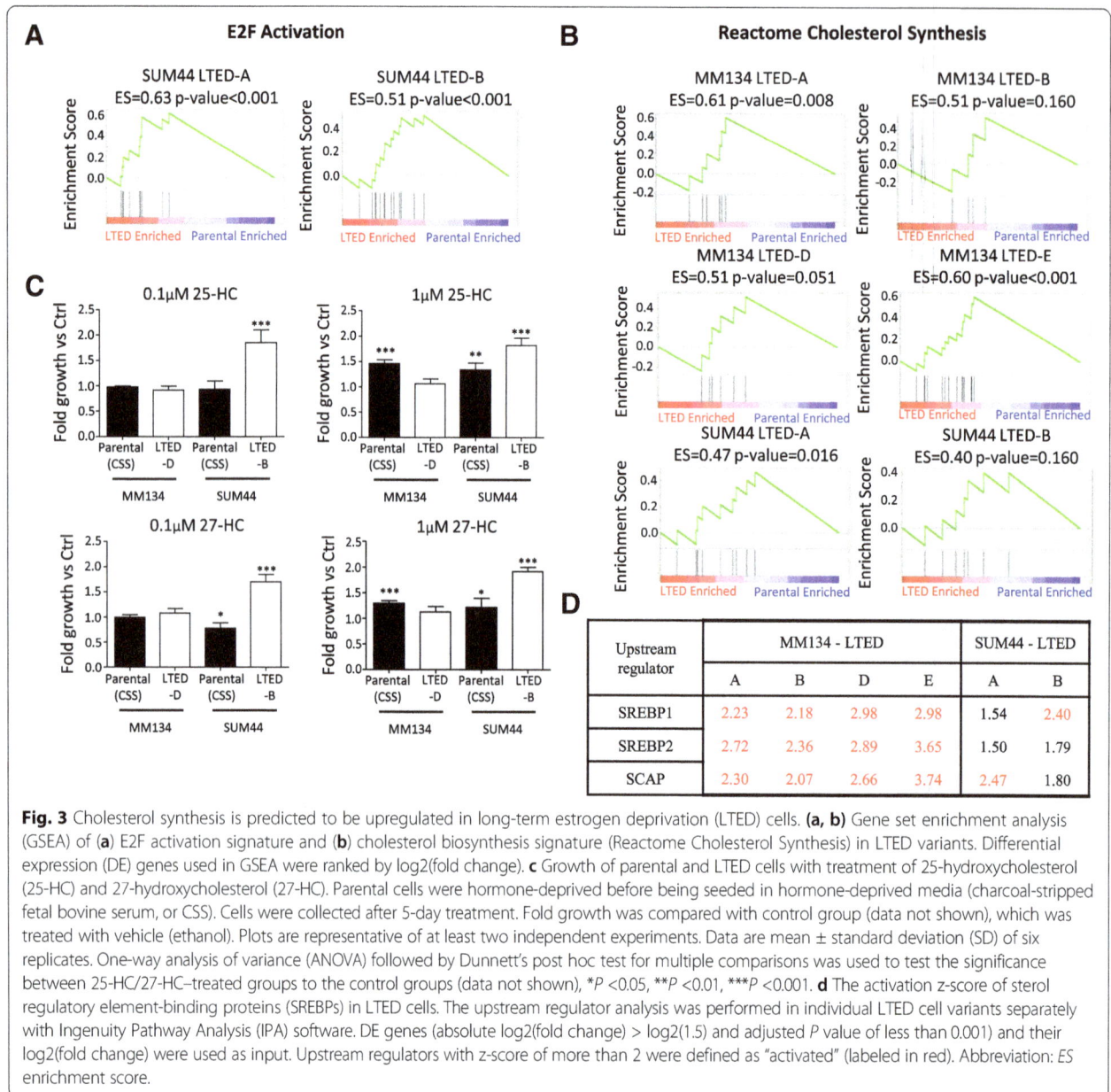

A E2F Activation

SUM44 LTED-A
ES=0.63 p-value<0.001

SUM44 LTED-B
ES=0.51 p-value<0.001

B Reactome Cholesterol Synthesis

MM134 LTED-A
ES=0.61 p-value=0.008

MM134 LTED-B
ES=0.51 p-value=0.160

MM134 LTED-D
ES=0.51 p-value=0.051

MM134 LTED-E
ES=0.60 p-value<0.001

SUM44 LTED-A
ES=0.47 p-value=0.016

SUM44 LTED-B
ES=0.40 p-value=0.160

C

0.1μM 25-HC

1μM 25-HC

0.1μM 27-HC

1μM 27-HC

D

Upstream regulator	MM134 - LTED				SUM44 - LTED	
	A	B	D	E	A	B
SREBP1	2.23	2.18	2.98	2.98	1.54	2.40
SREBP2	2.72	2.36	2.89	3.65	1.50	1.79
SCAP	2.30	2.07	2.66	3.74	2.47	1.80

Fig. 3 Cholesterol synthesis is predicted to be upregulated in long-term estrogen deprivation (LTED) cells. (**a, b**) Gene set enrichment analysis (GSEA) of (**a**) E2F activation signature and (**b**) cholesterol biosynthesis signature (Reactome Cholesterol Synthesis) in LTED variants. Differential expression (DE) genes used in GSEA were ranked by log2(fold change). **c** Growth of parental and LTED cells with treatment of 25-hydroxycholesterol (25-HC) and 27-hydroxycholesterol (27-HC). Parental cells were hormone-deprived before being seeded in hormone-deprived media (charcoal-stripped fetal bovine serum, or CSS). Cells were collected after 5-day treatment. Fold growth was compared with control group (data not shown), which was treated with vehicle (ethanol). Plots are representative of at least two independent experiments. Data are mean ± standard deviation (SD) of six replicates. One-way analysis of variance (ANOVA) followed by Dunnett's post hoc test for multiple comparisons was used to test the significance between 25-HC/27-HC–treated groups to the control groups (data not shown), *P <0.05, **P <0.01, ***P <0.001. **d** The activation z-score of sterol regulatory element-binding proteins (SREBPs) in LTED cells. The upstream regulator analysis was performed in individual LTED cell variants separately with Ingenuity Pathway Analysis (IPA) software. DE genes (absolute log2(fold change) > log2(1.5) and adjusted P value of less than 0.001) and their log2(fold change) were used as input. Upstream regulators with z-score of more than 2 were defined as "activated" (labeled in red). Abbreviation: *ES* enrichment score.

in all four MM134 LTED lines (Fig. 4c), and there was a trend toward higher expression in the SUM44 LTED cells (Additional file 1: Figure S7A). Significant *FASN* upregulation was also previously reported in SUM44 TamR cells [13]. Expression of other key enzymes in the fatty acid synthesis pathway (*ACACA*, *ACLY*, and *SCD*) was also upregulated but with variation among the different LTED cell lines (Additional file 1: Figure S7B).

FASN plays an important role in the *de novo* synthesis of long-chain fatty acids, which promotes the progression of tumors by fueling both membrane synthesis and energy production through β-oxidation [37, 38]. Since the pathway analysis also suggested activation of "Ketogenesis", which

involves the β-oxidation of fatty acids [25], we set out to determine whether the LTED cells were more dependent on fatty acid synthesis compared with their parental cells. Therefore, we treated the cells with various inhibitors of fatty acid synthesis and fatty acid oxidation. There was no significant difference between parental and LTED cells upon treatment with orlistat and TOFA, inhibitors of FASN and ACACA, respectively (Additional file 1: Figure S8A, B). However, MM134 LTED cells were significantly more sensitive to etomoxir, an inhibitor of carnitine palmitoyltransferase 1 (CPT-1), the rate-limiting enzyme in β-oxidation, than their parental cells (Fig. 4d, Additional file 1: Figure S8B). Collectively, these data suggest that the ILC LTED

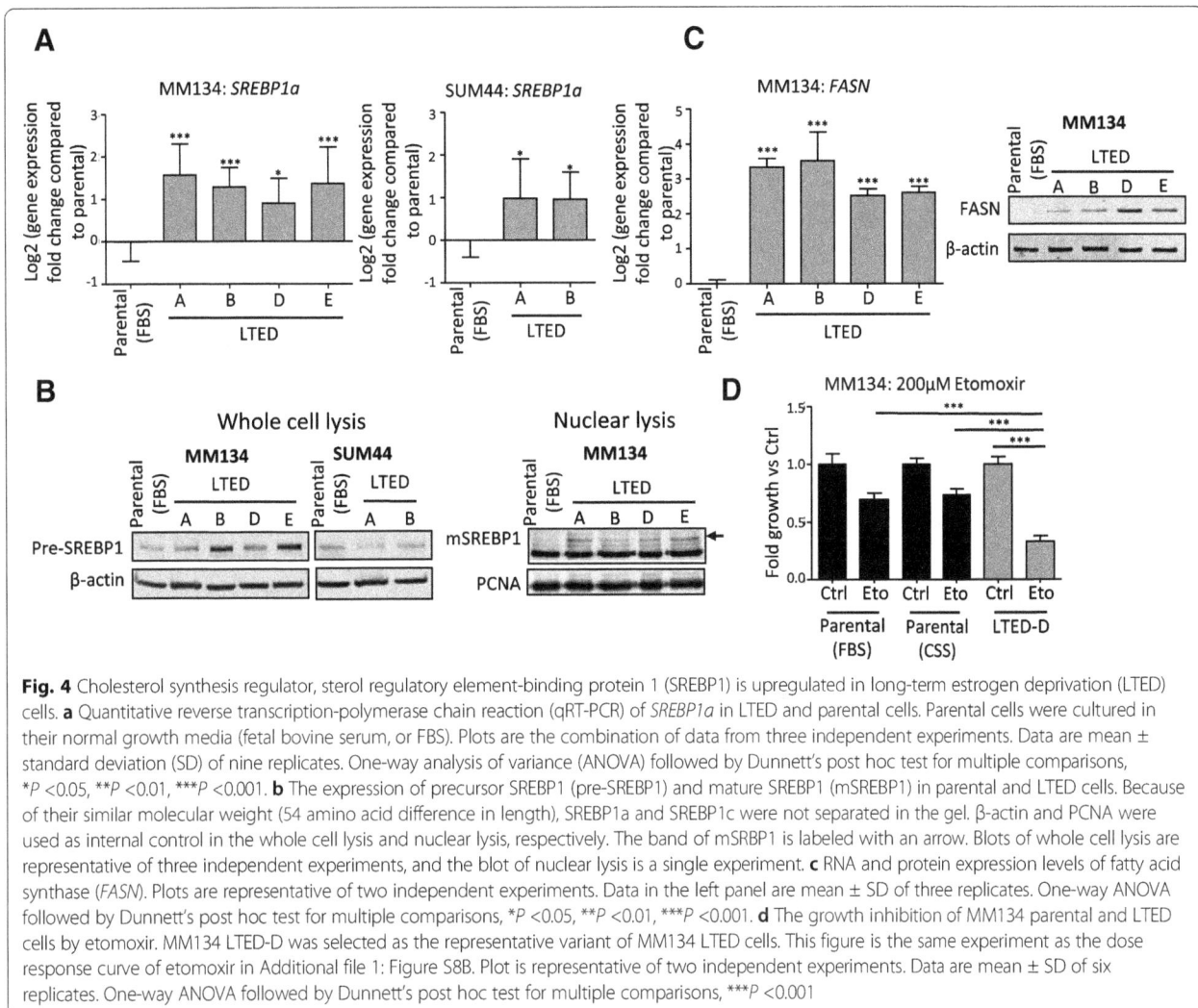

Fig. 4 Cholesterol synthesis regulator, sterol regulatory element-binding protein 1 (SREBP1) is upregulated in long-term estrogen deprivation (LTED) cells. **a** Quantitative reverse transcription-polymerase chain reaction (qRT-PCR) of *SREBP1a* in LTED and parental cells. Parental cells were cultured in their normal growth media (fetal bovine serum, or FBS). Plots are the combination of data from three independent experiments. Data are mean ± standard deviation (SD) of nine replicates. One-way analysis of variance (ANOVA) followed by Dunnett's post hoc test for multiple comparisons, *P <0.05, **P <0.01, ***P <0.001. **b** The expression of precursor SREBP1 (pre-SREBP1) and mature SREBP1 (mSREBP1) in parental and LTED cells. Because of their similar molecular weight (54 amino acid difference in length), SREBP1a and SREBP1c were not separated in the gel. β-actin and PCNA were used as internal control in the whole cell lysis and nuclear lysis, respectively. The band of mSRBP1 is labeled with an arrow. Blots of whole cell lysis are representative of three independent experiments, and the blot of nuclear lysis is a single experiment. **c** RNA and protein expression levels of fatty acid synthase (*FASN*). Plots are representative of two independent experiments. Data in the left panel are mean ± SD of three replicates. One-way ANOVA followed by Dunnett's post hoc test for multiple comparisons, *P <0.05, **P <0.01, ***P <0.001. **d** The growth inhibition of MM134 parental and LTED cells by etomoxir. MM134 LTED-D was selected as the representative variant of MM134 LTED cells. This figure is the same experiment as the dose response curve of etomoxir in Additional file 1: Figure S8B. Plot is representative of two independent experiments. Data are mean ± SD of six replicates. One-way ANOVA followed by Dunnett's post hoc test for multiple comparisons, ***P <0.001

cell lines activate and induce a number of enzymes critical in fatty acid and cholesterol metabolism for energy production.

Role for SREBPs in endocrine-resistant cell lines and in clinical samples

Next, we set out to directly assess the role of SREBP family members in the growth of the LTED cells. We selected two siRNA pools that target both genes (*SREBP1* and *SREBP2*) simultaneously, thereby inhibiting potential compensatory mechanisms. Successful knockdown was confirmed by quantitative reverse transcription-polymerase chain reaction (q-RT-PCR), which also showed that SREBP knockdown resulted in decreased levels of the target gene *FASN*, as expected (Fig. 5a). Decreased SREBP levels significantly inhibited the proliferation of MM134 LTED cells by more than 50% without having an effect in MM134 parental cells (Fig. 5b, Additional file 1: Figure S9C). MM134 LTED cells were also significantly more sensitive than their parental cells to PF429242 (Fig. 5c), an inhibitor of SREBP

maturation. Similar siRNA knockdown studies were performed in SUM44 cells, which showed decreased growth in both parental and LTED cells (Additional file 1: Figure S9A–C). When treated with PF429242, the SUM44 LTED cells were more sensitive than their parental cells (Fig. 5d), although the effect is less pronounced compared with MM134 cells. Fatostatin, a drug preventing SCAP-mediated escort of SREBP and thus interfering with downstream transcriptional effects, also inhibited growth of MM134 LTED cells (Fig. 5e), with minimal effects in SUM44 LTED cells (Additional file 1: Figure S9D).

Finally, to assess potential clinical relevance of SREBPs in endocrine resistance, we measured *SREBP1* and *SREBP2* expression in breast tumors following estrogen deprivation therapy. Specifically, we performed *in silico* gene expression analysis in 50 primary ER+ breast cancers before treatment ("pre") and after 3 months of treatment ("post") with the AI letrozole [23]. Tumors with reduction greater than 50% or less than 50% in volume were classified as letrozole responders (*n* = 36) and non-responders

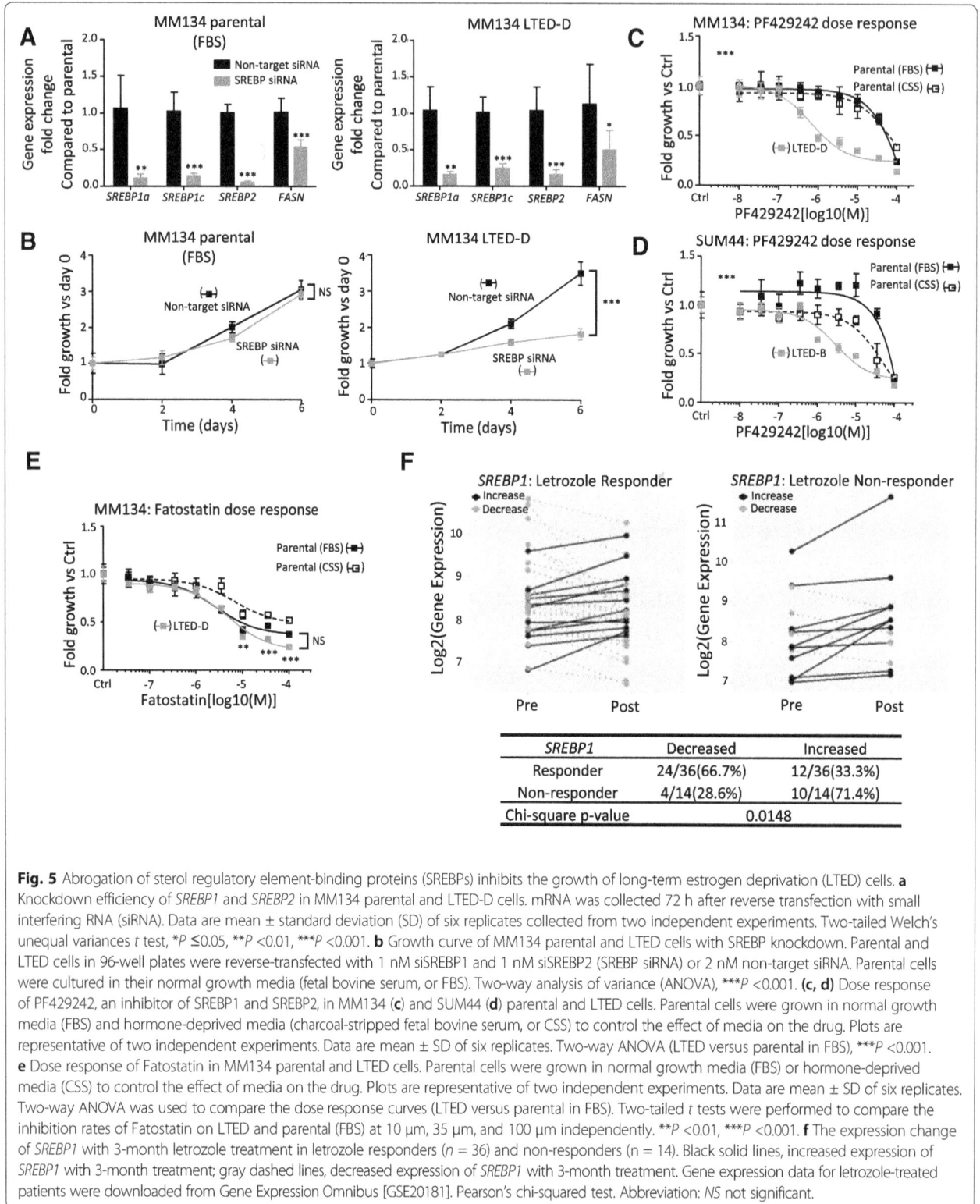

Fig. 5 Abrogation of sterol regulatory element-binding proteins (SREBPs) inhibits the growth of long-term estrogen deprivation (LTED) cells. **a** Knockdown efficiency of *SREBP1* and *SREBP2* in MM134 parental and LTED-D cells. mRNA was collected 72 h after reverse transfection with small interfering RNA (siRNA). Data are mean ± standard deviation (SD) of six replicates collected from two independent experiments. Two-tailed Welch's unequal variances t test, *$P \leq 0.05$, **$P < 0.01$, ***$P < 0.001$. **b** Growth curve of MM134 parental and LTED cells with SREBP knockdown. Parental and LTED cells in 96-well plates were reverse-transfected with 1 nM siSREBP1 and 1 nM siSREBP2 (SREBP siRNA) or 2 nM non-target siRNA. Parental cells were cultured in their normal growth media (fetal bovine serum, or FBS). Two-way analysis of variance (ANOVA), ***$P < 0.001$. **(c, d)** Dose response of PF429242, an inhibitor of SREBP1 and SREBP2, in MM134 (**c**) and SUM44 (**d**) parental and LTED cells. Parental cells were grown in normal growth media (FBS) and hormone-deprived media (charcoal-stripped fetal bovine serum, or CSS) to control the effect of media on the drug. Plots are representative of two independent experiments. Data are mean ± SD of six replicates. Two-way ANOVA (LTED versus parental in FBS), ***$P < 0.001$. **e** Dose response of Fatostatin in MM134 parental and LTED cells. Parental cells were grown in normal growth media (FBS) or hormone-deprived media (CSS) to control the effect of media on the drug. Plots are representative of two independent experiments. Data are mean ± SD of six replicates. Two-way ANOVA was used to compare the dose response curves (LTED versus parental in FBS). Two-tailed t tests were performed to compare the inhibition rates of Fatostatin on LTED and parental (FBS) at 10 μm, 35 μm, and 100 μm independently. **$P < 0.01$, ***$P < 0.001$. **f** The expression change of *SREBP1* with 3-month letrozole treatment in letrozole responders ($n = 36$) and non-responders ($n = 14$). Black solid lines, increased expression of *SREBP1* with 3-month treatment; gray dashed lines, decreased expression of *SREBP1* with 3-month treatment. Gene expression data for letrozole-treated patients were downloaded from Gene Expression Omnibus [GSE20181]. Pearson's chi-squared test. Abbreviation: *NS* not significant.

($n = 14$), respectively. Following the 3-month regimen, non-responders had a higher incidence of increased expression of *SREBP1* (Fig. 5f) compared with letrozole responders (10/14, 71.4% versus 12/36, 33.3%; Pearson's chi-squared test, P value = 0.0148). *SREBP2* upregulation was not significantly different between letrozole responders and non-responders (Additional file 1: Figure S10). These data suggest that SREBP1 induction is associated with the development of resistance to estrogen deprivation therapy.

Discussion

Resistance to endocrine therapy is a major limitation in the treatment of ER$^+$ breast cancers. Although there is the increasing realization that ILC is a disease distinct from IDC in many features [1, 2, 4, 5, 39, 40], only a few studies have investigated endocrine resistance with ILC models [13, 18, 24, 41]. In this study, we comprehensively characterized a total of six ILC LTED variants from MM134 and SUM44PE (SUM44F), the two most commonly used ER$^+$ ILC cell lines. To the best of our knowledge, we are the first group to generate endocrine-resistant cell models with MM134, a cell line that shows *de novo* tamoxifen resistance [15]. Of note, MM134 LTED cells are also resistant to ICI 182,780 (fulvestrant), which makes them a unique model to investigate ER-independent mechanisms of acquired endocrine resistance.

We found that MM134 and SUM44 LTED cells acquired some shared but also unique adaptive mechanisms of resistance to estrogen deprivation. SUM44 LTED cells showed activated E2F signaling, a pathway that was previously reported to be upregulated in endocrine-resistant IDC [24, 42]. This pathway was not activated in MM134 LTED cells that showed minimal ER expression, and had lost hormone response. Given the recent success of targeting the CDK-RB-E2F signaling pathway [43], SUM44 LTED cells might represent an excellent model for the study of CDK4/6 inhibitors in ER$^+$ endocrine-resistant ILC, which we will test in future studies.

An adaptive mechanism of resistance that was shared between the two ILC LTED models was the activation of fatty acid and cholesterol metabolism pathways. High cholesterol level was reported to be a risk factor of the early recurrence in breast cancers [44]. The BIG 1-98 study [45] showed that cholesterol-lowering medication was related to improved clinical outcomes in early-stage hormone receptor–positive breast cancers, suggesting a potential role of cholesterol in causing endocrine resistance. Recent studies by Simigdala et al. [28] and Nguyen et al. [29] showed upregulation of cholesterol biosynthesis in AI-resistant breast cancer. In addition, Martin et al. [41] recently reported that SUM44 LTED cells have higher fatty acid dependency than their parental cells, which was hypothesized to be due to increased expression of fatty acid metabolism genes as a result of an *ESR1* mutation in this set of LTED cells. Of note, *ESR1* is not mutated in any of our ILC cell line models [41]. Although (at least in part owing to technical limitations) we were unable to detect higher levels of cholesterol, cholesterol esters, and oxysterols, we did observe an increased sensitivity of SUM44 LTED cells to 25-HC, which was not seen in MM134 LTED. These results are in

line with the previously reported findings that oxysterols can directly bind to and activate ER [28, 46] and that, in the absence of estrogen, oxysterols can activate growth in an ER-dependent manner [28, 29]. However, oxysterols can also bind to other nuclear receptors such as farnesoid X receptor (FXR), liver X receptor (LXR), retinoic acid receptor-related orphan receptor (ROR), peroxisome proliferator-activated receptors (PPAR), and pregnane X receptor (PXR) [47, 48], and thus further studies are required to fully define the expression and action of oxysterols in the LTED cells.

A series of enzymes critically involved in fatty acid synthesis were induced in our ILC LTED models, especially FASN, which is known to be highly expressed in many human epithelial cancers and their pre-neoplastic lesions [38]. The upregulation of FASN has been linked to the acquisition of resistance to chemotherapy in breast and ovarian cancers [49–52]; however, there is limited information about an association between FASN and endocrine resistance. And whereas one study showed that FASN inhibition could reverse anti-estrogen resistance in MCF7 cells [53], others showed that FASN blockade increased the sensitivity of ER to E2 [54, 55] and thus there might be context-dependent effects that need to be elucidated further. Interestingly, two studies [56, 57] recently reported that endocrine therapy increases the risk of newly developed fatty liver, but it is not clear whether and how this might be linked to FASN expression in this setting. Of note, we did not observe increased sensitivity to fatty acid synthesis inhibitors, which might be due to the increased ability to use exogenous fatty acids when the *de novo* synthesis pathway is inhibited [58–60]. This has been reported in prostate cancer cells, which could be inhibited only by C75 and SB204990, inhibitors of FASN and ACLY, respectively, in the absence of lipoprotein, the transporter of exogenous fatty acid and cholesterol [61].

The ILC LTED cells showed increased sensitivity to genetic and pharmacologic inhibition of SREBP, and consistently stronger effects were seen in MM134 LTED cells. Similarly, gene expression changes were more pronounced in MM134 LTED cells. These data suggest that activation of lipid-metabolic pathways might not be related to activation of ligand-independent ER signaling but could drive fatty acid oxidation (FAO), membrane synthesis, or other processes (Fig. 6). In support of increased FAO, we found that LTED cells were more sensitive to etomoxir, an inhibitor of CPT-1, the rate-limiting enzyme in β-oxidation of fatty acids. However, these results need to be interpreted with caution, as etomoxir can elicit off-target effects, especially at higher doses such as those used in our studies [62]. In addition, the well-described inverse relationship between fatty acid synthesis and oxidation argues against increased FAO in LTED cells [63, 64].

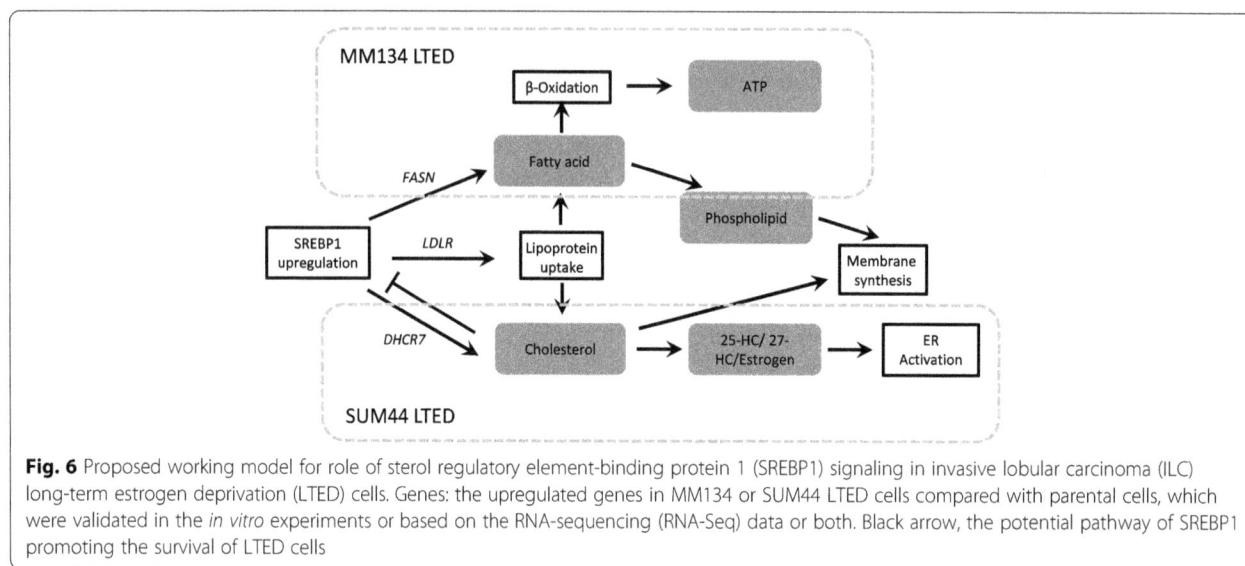

Fig. 6 Proposed working model for role of sterol regulatory element-binding protein 1 (SREBP1) signaling in invasive lobular carcinoma (ILC) long-term estrogen deprivation (LTED) cells. Genes: the upregulated genes in MM134 or SUM44 LTED cells compared with parental cells, which were validated in the *in vitro* experiments or based on the RNA-sequencing (RNA-Seq) data or both. Black arrow, the potential pathway of SREBP1 promoting the survival of LTED cells

A recent elegant study by Chen et al. [65] showed that activation of an SREBP-dependent lipogenic program promoted treatment resistance and metastasis in patients with prostate cancer. Of note, SREBPs were reported to regulate a number of other biological pathways such as cell proliferation and differentiation, insulin signaling, and immune response [66–70]. Further studies are required to determine how SREBPs contribute to endocrine resistance in ILC and whether inhibition of SREBP1 would resensitize our LTED models to endocrine therapy.

A potential limitation of our studies is that the generation of LTED cells depends on incubating the cells in CSS, in which the charcoal-stripping removes not only estradiol but also other lipophilic compounds. One could argue that the upregulation of fatty acid and cholesterol metabolism pathways might be a result of decreased lipid levels in CSS. Although this cannot be totally ruled out, we think it is unlikely since *SREBP1* levels were also upregulated in SUM44 TamR cells, which were kept in the same media as their parental cells (serum-free media with supplement of hormones) [13]. Also, our RNA-Seq analysis was performed by using RNA from parental cells kept in CSS for 3 days, thereby removing the potential effect of medium difference between parental and LTED cells on DE gene calling. Thus, we propose that the upregulation of *SREBP1* in LTED cells, and potentially the activation of lipid metabolism, is not caused by the culturing the cells in CSS but instead a mechanism of resistance to estrogen deprivation. Another limitation of our study is that the confirmation in clinical samples was performed using data from a trial that included both patients with IDC and patients with ILC. Currently, there are no gene expression data available from a neoadjuvant trial with sufficiently large numbers of patients with ILC and treatment response data (for example, Ki67) to perform such analyses.

An elegant study by Arthur et al. [69] analyzed gene expression in ILC compared with IDC tumors in the neoadjuvant setting; however, the study was limited to responders and thus does not allow comparison of SREBP levels between sensitive and resistant tumors. Finally, our cell line studies were limited to *in vitro* studies at this point in time, and future studies should include mouse models, which would further solidify our findings.

Conclusions

Our studies provide novel and potentially clinically relevant data on overexpression of and dependency on key enzymes in the fatty acid/cholesterol pathways that collectively suggest a lipogenic reprogramming of metabolism in endocrine-resistant ILC cells. We propose those key enzymes like SREBP1 and FASN as novel targets that deserve future study for the prevention and treatment of endocrine resistance for patients with ILC.

Additional files

Additional file 1: Figure S1. Procedures of generating long-term estrogen deprivation (LTED) cell models. **Figure S2.** Two-dimensional (2D) and three-dimensional (3D) growth of long-term estrogen deprivation (LTED) cells. **Figure S3** Differential expressed (DE) genes in long-term estrogen deprivation (LTED) cells. **Figure S4.** The level of intracellular free cholesterol and cholesterol esters in parental and long-term estrogen deprivation (LTED) cells. **Figure S5.** The expression of sterol regulatory element-binding protein 1c (*SREBP1c*) and *SREBP2* in long-term estrogen deprivation (LTED) cells. **Figure S6.** The maturation processes of sterol regulatory element-binding proteins (SREBPs). **Figure S7.** The expression of enzymes involved in fatty acid synthesis in long-term estrogen deprivation (LTED) cells. **Figure S8.** Dose response of fatty acid synthesis and β-oxidation inhibitors in long-term estrogen deprivation (LTED) cells. **Figure S9.** The abrogation of sterol regulatory element-binding proteins (SREBPs) in SUM44 long-term estrogen deprivation (LTED) cells. **Figure S10.** Expression of sterol regulatory element-binding proteins (*SREBPs*) in clinical samples.

Additional file 2: Table S1. Sequences of primers and small interfering RNAs (siRNAs). (XLSX 9 kb)

Additional file 3: Table S2. Mapping rate of Salmon. (XLSX 9 kb)

Additional file 4: Table S3. Differentially expressed genes in MM134 and SUM44 long-term estrogen deprivation (LTED) cells and SUM44 tamoxifen-resistant cell (SUM44 TamR) cells. (XLSX 3466 kb)

Additional file 5: Table S4. Differentially regulated pathways in MM134 and SUM44 long-term estrogen deprivation (LTED) cells. (XLSX 135 kb)

Abbreviations

2D: Two-dimensional; 25-HC: 25-hydroxycholesterol; 27-HC: 27-hydroxycholesterol; AI: Aromatase inhibitor; ATCC: American Type Culture Collection; CPT-1: Carnitine palmitoyltransferase 1; CSS: Charcoal-stripped fetal bovine serum; DE: Differential expression; DMEM: Dulbecco's modified Eagle's medium; E2: 17β-estradiol; ER: Estrogen receptor; FAO: Fatty acid oxidation; FASN: Fatty acid synthase; FBS: Fetal bovine serum; GEO: Gene Expression Omnibus; GSEA: Gene set enrichment analysis; ICI: ICI 182,780, fulvestrant; IDC: Invasive ductal carcinoma; ILC: Invasive lobular carcinoma; IMEM: Improved minimal essential medium; IPA: Ingenuity Pathway Analysis; LTED: Long-term estrogen deprivation; MM134: MDA-MB-134-VI; mSREBP1: Mature sterol regulatory element-binding protein 1; PBS: Phosphate-buffered saline; PCR: Polymerase chain reaction; Pre-SREBP1: Precursor sterol regulatory element-binding protein 1; RNA-Seq: RNA-sequencing; RXR: Retinoid X receptor; siRNA: Small interfering RNA; SREBP: Sterol regulatory element-binding protein; SUM44 TamR: SUM44 tamoxifen-resistant cell; TPM: Transcript per million

Acknowledgments

We thank Beth Knapick, Jian Chen, Sonia Salvatore, and Vera Y. Roginskaya for outstanding technical support and Adrian Lee for constructive comments on the manuscript.

Funding

The work is in part funded by the Breast Cancer Research Foundation (SO), a Susan G Komen leadership award to SO, a Pathway to Independence Award K99 CA193734 (MJS) from the National Institutes of Health, Fashion Footwear Association of New York, and P30CA047904. TD is supported by a China Scholarship Council award through the Tsinghua School of Medicine (Beijing, China). NT is supported by a Department of Defense Breakthrough Fellowship Award (BC160764). KML is supported by NIH F30 Predoctoral (CA203154) Fellow Awards.

Authors' contributions

TD, MJS, and SO contributed to conception and design. TD, MJS, BVH, and SO contributed to development of methodology. TD, MJS, RBR, SGW, BVH, and SO contributed to acquisition of data (including performing experiments, acquiring RNA-Seq data, generating models, and providing facilities). TD, KML, MJS, and NT contributed to analysis and interpretation of data (for example, statistical analysis, biostatistics, computational analysis, and interpretation). TD, MJS, KML, NT, RBR, SGW, and SO contributed to writing, review and/or revision of the manuscript. SO contributed to study supervision. All authors read and approved the final manuscript.

Competing interests

The authors declare that they have no competing interests.

Author details

[1]Women's Cancer Research Center, UPMC Hillman Cancer Institute, Magee Womens Research Institute, 204 Craft Avenue, Pittsburgh, PA 15213, USA. [2]School of Medicine, Tsinghua University, Beijing 100084, China. [3]Department of Pathology, University of Colorado Anschutz Medical Campus, Aurora, CO 80045, USA. [4]Department of Pathology, University of Pittsburgh, Pittsburgh, PA 15213, USA. [5]Department of Pharmacology and Chemical Biology, University of Pittsburgh, Pittsburgh, PA 15213, USA. [6]Department of Oncology, Georgetown-Lombardi Comprehensive Cancer Center, Georgetown University Medical Center, Washington, DC 20057, USA.

References

1. Reed AEM, Kutasovic JR, Lakhani SR, Simpson PT. Invasive lobular carcinoma of the breast: morphology, biomarkers and'omics. Breast Cancer Res. 2015;17:12.
2. Sikora MJ, Jankowitz RC, Dabbs DJ, Oesterreich S. Invasive lobular carcinoma of the breast: patient response to systemic endocrine therapy and hormone response in model systems. Steroids. 2013;78:568–75.
3. Ciriello G, Gatza ML, Beck AH, Wilkerson MD, Rhie SK, Pastore A, et al. Comprehensive molecular portraits of invasive lobular breast cancer. Cell. 2015;163:506–19.
4. Du T, Zhu L, Levine KM, Tasdemir N, Lee AV, Vignali DA, et al. Invasive lobular and ductal breast carcinoma differ in immune response, protein translation efficiency and metabolism. Sci Rep. 20188:7205.
5. Pestalozzi BC, Zahrieh D, Mallon E, Gusterson BA, Price KN, Gelber RD, et al. Distinct clinical and prognostic features of infiltrating lobular carcinoma of the breast: combined results of 15 international breast Cancer study group clinical trials. J Clin Oncol. 2008;26:3006–14.
6. Engstrøm MJ, Opdahl S, Vatten LJ, Haugen OA, Bofin AM. Invasive lobular breast cancer: the prognostic impact of histopathological grade, E-cadherin and molecular subtypes. Histopathology. 2015;66:409–19.
7. Adachi Y, Ishiguro J, Kotani H, Hisada T, Ichikawa M, Gondo N, et al. Comparison of clinical outcomes between luminal invasive ductal carcinoma and luminal invasive lobular carcinoma. BMC Cancer. 2016;16:248.
8. Metzger Filho O, Giobbie-Hurder A, Mallon E, Gusterson B, Viale G, Winer EP, et al. Relative effectiveness of letrozole compared with tamoxifen for patients with lobular carcinoma in the BIG 1-98 trial. J Clin Oncol. 2015;33:2772–9.
9. Knauer M, Gruber C, Dietze O, Greil R, Stöger H, Rudas M, et al. Abstract S2-06: survival advantage of anastrozol compared to tamoxifen for lobular breast cancer in the ABCSG-8 study. Cancer Res. 2015;75(9 Supplement):S2–06. S02–06
10. Osborne CK, Schiff R. Mechanisms of endocrine resistance in breast cancer. Annu Rev Med. 2011;62:233–47.
11. Musgrove EA, Sutherland RL. Biological determinants of endocrine resistance in breast cancer. Nat Rev Cancer. 2009;9:631.
12. Murphy CG, Dickler MN. Endocrine resistance in hormone-responsive breast cancer: mechanisms and therapeutic strategies. Endocr Relat Cancer. 2016;23:R337–52.
13. Riggins RB, Lan JP, Klimach U, Zwart A, Cavalli LR, Haddad BR, et al. ERRγ mediates tamoxifen resistance in novel models of invasive lobular breast cancer. Cancer Res. 2008;68:8908–17.
14. Huang B, Omoto Y, Iwase H, Yamashita H, Toyama T, Coombes RC, et al. Differential expression of estrogen receptor α, β1, and β2 in lobular and ductal breast cancer. Proc Natl Acad Sci. 2014;111:1933–8.
15. Sikora MJ, Cooper KL, Bahreini A, Luthra S, Wang G, Chandran UR, et al. Invasive lobular carcinoma cell lines are characterized by unique estrogen-mediated gene expression patterns and altered tamoxifen response. Cancer Res. 2014;74:1463–74.
16. Turner N, Pearson A, Sharpe R, Lambros M, Geyer F, Lopezgarcia MA, et al. FGFR1 amplification drives endocrine therapy resistance and is a therapeutic target in breast cancer. Cancer Res. 2010;70:2085.
17. Stires H, Heckler MM, Fu X, Li Z, Grasso CS, Quist MJ, et al. Integrated molecular analysis of Tamoxifen-resistant invasive lobular breast cancer cells identifies MAPK and GRM/mGluR signaling as therapeutic vulnerabilities. Mol Cell Endocrinol. 2018;471:105–17.
18. Sikora MJ, Jacobsen BM, Levine K, Chen J, Davidson NE, Lee AV, et al. WNT4 mediates estrogen receptor signaling and endocrine resistance in invasive lobular carcinoma cell lines. Breast Cancer Res. 2016;18:92.

19. Sikora MJ, Johnson MD, Lee AV, Oesterreich S. Endocrine response phenotypes are altered by charcoal-stripped serum variability. Endocrinology. 2016;157:3760–6.

20. Patro R, Duggal G, Love MI, Irizarry RA, Kingsford C. Salmon provides fast and bias-aware quantification of transcript expression. Nature Methods. 2017;14(4):417.

21. Love MI, Huber W, Anders S. Moderated estimation of fold change and dispersion for RNA-seq data with DESeq2. Genome Biol. 2014;15:550.

22. Ritchie ME, Phipson B, Wu D, Hu Y, Law CW, Shi W, et al. Limma powers differential expression analyses for RNA-sequencing and microarray studies. Nucleic Acids Res. 2015;43:e47.

23. Miller WR, Larionov A. Changes in expression of oestrogen regulated and proliferation genes with neoadjuvant treatment highlight heterogeneity of clinical resistance to the aromatase inhibitor, letrozole. Breast Cancer Res. 2010;12:R52.

24. Miller TW, Balko JM, Fox EM, Ghazoui Z, Dunbier A, Anderson H, et al. ERα-dependent E2F transcription can mediate resistance to estrogen deprivation in human breast cancer. Cancer Discov. 2011;1:338–51.

25. McPherson PAC, McEneny J. The biochemistry of ketogenesis and its role in weight management, neurological disease and oxidative stress. J Physiol Biochem. 2012;68:141–51.

26. Calkin AC, Tontonoz P. Liver x receptor signaling pathways and atherosclerosis. Arterioscler Thromb Vasc Biol. 2010;30:1513–8.

27. Werner A, Kuipers F, Verkade HJ. Fat absorption and lipid metabolism in cholestasis. Mol Pathogenesis Cholestasis. 2004:314–28.

28. Simigdala N, Gao Q, Pancholi S, Roberg-Larsen H, Zvelebil M, Ribas R, et al. Cholesterol biosynthesis pathway as a novel mechanism of resistance to estrogen deprivation in estrogen receptor-positive breast cancer. Breast Cancer Res. 2016;18:58.

29. Nguyen VT, Barozzi I, Faronato M, Lombardo Y, Steel JH, Patel N, et al. Differential epigenetic reprogramming in response to specific endocrine therapies promotes cholesterol biosynthesis and cellular invasion. Nat Commun. 2015;6:10044.

30. Horton JD, Goldstein JL, Brown MS. SREBPs: activators of the complete program of cholesterol and fatty acid synthesis in the liver. J Clin Invest. 2002;109:1125.

31. Ye J, DeBose-Boyd RA. Regulation of cholesterol and fatty acid synthesis. Cold Spring Harb Perspect Biol. 2011;3:a004754.

32. Li X, Wu JB, Li Q, Shigemura K, Chung LW, Huang W-C. SREBP-2 promotes stem cell-like properties and metastasis by transcriptional activation of c-Myc in prostate cancer. Oncotarget. 2016;7:12869.

33. Bao J, Zhu L, Zhu Q, Su J, Liu M, Huang W. SREBP-1 is an independent prognostic marker and promotes invasion and migration in breast cancer. Oncol Lett. 2016;12:2409–16.

34. Kim RS, Avivar-Valderas A, Estrada Y, Bragado P, Sosa MS, Aguirre-Ghiso JA, et al. Dormancy signatures and metastasis in estrogen receptor positive and negative breast cancer. PLoS One. 2012;7:e35569.

35. Amemiya-Kudo M, Shimano H, Hasty AH, Yahagi N, Yoshikawa T, Matsuzaka T, et al. Transcriptional activities of nuclear SREBP-1a,-1c, and-2 to different target promoters of lipogenic and cholesterogenic genes. J Lipid Res. 2002;43:1220–35.

36. Eberlé D, Hegarty B, Bossard P, Ferré P, Foufelle F. SREBP transcription factors: master regulators of lipid homeostasis. Biochimie. 2004;86:839–48.

37. Kuhajda FP. Fatty acid synthase and cancer: new application of an old pathway. Cancer Res. 2006;66:5977–80.

38. Menendez JA, Lupu R. Fatty acid synthase and the lipogenic phenotype in cancer pathogenesis. Nat Rev Cancer. 2007;7:763–77.

39. Desmedt C, Zoppoli G, Gundem G, Pruneri G, Larsimont D, Fornili M, et al. Genomic characterization of primary invasive lobular breast cancer. J Clin Oncol. 2016;34:1872–81.

40. Michaut M, Chin S-F, Majewski I, Severson TM, Bismeijer T, de Koning L, et al. Integration of genomic, transcriptomic and proteomic data identifies two biologically distinct subtypes of invasive lobular breast cancer. Sci Rep. 2016;6:18517.

41. Martin L-A, Ribas R, Simigdala N, Schuster E, Pancholi S, Tenev T, et al. Discovery of naturally occurring ESR1 mutations in breast cancer cell lines modelling endocrine resistance. Nat Commun. 2017;8:1865.

42. Guerrero-Zotano A, Stricker T, Formisano L, Hutchinson KE, Stover DG, K-m L, et al. ER+ breast cancers resistant to prolonged neoadjuvant letrozole exhibit an E2F4 transcriptional program sensitive to CDK4/6 inhibitors. Clin Cancer Res. 2018;24:2517–29.

43. Johnson J, Thijssen B, McDermott U, Garnett M, Wessels LF, Bernards R. Targeting the RB-E2F pathway in breast cancer. Oncogene. 2016;35:4829–35.

44. Bahl M, Ennis M, Tannock IF, Hux JE, Pritchard KI, Koo J, et al. Serum lipids and outcome of early-stage breast Cancer: results of a prospective cohort study. Breast Cancer Res Treat. 2005;94:135–44.

45. Borgquist S, Giobbie-Hurder A, Ahern TP, Garber JE, Colleoni M, Láng I, et al. Cholesterol, cholesterol-lowering medication use, and breast cancer outcome in the BIG 1-98 study. J Clin Oncol. 2017;35:1179–88.

46. DuSell CD, Umetani M, Shaul PW, Mangelsdorf DJ, McDonnell DP. 27-hydroxycholesterol is an endogenous selective estrogen receptor modulator. Mol Endocrinol. 2008;22:65–77.

47. Olkkonen VM, Béaslas O, Nissilä E. Oxysterols and their cellular effectors. Biomolecules. 2012;2:76–103.

48. De Boussac H, Alioui A, Viennois E, Dufour J, Trousson A, Vega A, et al. Oxysterol receptors and their therapeutic applications in cancer conditions. Expert Opin Ther Targets. 2013;17:1029–38.

49. Liu H, Liu Y, Zhang J-T. A new mechanism of drug resistance in breast cancer cells: fatty acid synthase overexpression-mediated palmitate overproduction. Mol Cancer Ther. 2008;7:263–70.

50. Vazquez-Martin A, Colomer R, Brunet J, Menendez JA. Pharmacological blockade of fatty acid synthase (FASN) reverses acquired autoresistance to trastuzumab (Herceptin™) by transcriptionally inhibiting 'HER2 super-expression'occurring in high-dose trastuzumab-conditioned SKBR3/Tzb100 breast cancer cells. Int J Oncol. 2007;31:769–76.

51. Vazquez-Martin A, Ropero S, Brunet J, Colomer R, Menendez JA. Inhibition of fatty acid synthase (FASN) synergistically enhances the efficacy of 5-fluorouracil in breast carcinoma cells. Oncol Rep. 2007;18:973–80.

52. Papaevangelou E, Almeida GS, Box C, deSouza NM, Chung YL. The effect of FASN inhibition on the growth and metabolism of a cisplatin-resistant ovarian carcinoma model. Int J Cancer. 2018;143:992–1002.

53. Menendez JA, Vellon L, Espinoza I, Lupu R. The metastasis inducer CCN1 (CYR61) activates the fatty acid synthase (FASN)-driven lipogenic phenotype in breast cancer cells. Oncoscience. 2016;3:242–57.

54. Lupu R, Menendez JA. Targeting fatty acid synthase in breast and endometrial cancer: an alternative to selective estrogen receptor modulators? Endocrinology. 2006;147:4056–66.

55. Menendez J, Lupu R. Fatty acid synthase regulates estrogen receptor-α signaling in breast cancer cells. Oncogenesis. 2017;6:e299.

56. Hong N, Yoon HG, Seo DH, Park S, Kim SI, Sohn JH, et al. Different patterns in the risk of newly developed fatty liver and lipid changes with tamoxifen versus aromatase inhibitors in postmenopausal women with early breast cancer: a propensity score–matched cohort study. Eur J Cancer. 2017;82:103–14.

57. Pan H-J, Chang H-T, Lee C-H. Association between tamoxifen treatment and the development of different stages of nonalcoholic fatty liver disease among breast cancer patients. J Formos Med Assoc. 2016;115:411–7.

58. Röhrig F, Schulze A. The multifaceted roles of fatty acid synthesis in cancer. Nat Rev Cancer. 2016;16:732–49.

59. Mashima T, Seimiya H, Tsuruo T. De novo fatty-acid synthesis and related pathways as molecular targets for cancer therapy. Br J Cancer. 2009;100:1369–72.

60. Currie E, Schulze A, Zechner R, Walther TC, Farese RV. Cellular fatty acid metabolism and cancer. Cell Metab. 2013;18:153–61.

61. Ros S, Santos CR, Moco S, Baenke F, Kelly G, Howell M, et al. Functional metabolic screen identifies 6-phosphofructo-2-kinase/fructose-2, 6-biphosphatase 4 as an important regulator of prostate cancer cell survival. Cancer Discov. 2012;2:328–43.

62. Yao C-H, Liu G-Y, Wang R, Moon SH, Gross RW, Patti GJ. Identifying off-target effects of etomoxir reveals that carnitine palmitoyltransferase I is essential for cancer cell proliferation independent of β-oxidation. PLoS Biol. 2018;16:e2003782.

63. Foster DW. Malonyl-CoA: the regulator of fatty acid synthesis and oxidation. J Clin Invest. 2012;122:1958–9.

64. Wen Y-A, Xiong X, Zaytseva YY, Napier DL, Vallee E, Li AT, et al. Downregulation of SREBP inhibits tumor growth and initiation by altering cellular metabolism in colon cancer. Cell Death Dis. 2018;9:265.

65. Chen M, Zhang J, Sampieri K, Clohessy JG, Mendez L, Gonzalez-Billalabeitia E, et al. An aberrant SREBP-dependent lipogenic program promotes metastatic prostate cancer. Nat Genet. 2018;50:206–18.

66. Shao W, Espenshade PJ. Expanding roles for SREBP in metabolism. Cell Metab. 2012;16:414–9.

67. Seo Y-K, Chong HK, Infante AM, Im S-S, Xie X, Osborne TF. Genome-wide analysis of SREBP-1 binding in mouse liver chromatin reveals a preference for promoter proximal binding to a new motif. Proc Natl Acad Sci. 2009;106:13765–9.

68. Reed BD, Charos AE, Szekely AM, Weissman SM, Snyder M. Genome-wide occupancy of SREBP1 and its partners NFY and SP1 reveals novel functional roles and combinatorial regulation of distinct classes of genes. PLoS Genet. 2008;4:e1000133.

69. Arthur LM, Turnbull AK, Webber VL, Larionov AA, Renshaw L, Kay C, et al. Molecular changes in lobular breast cancers in response to endocrine therapy. Cancer Res. 2014;74:5371–6.

70. Wang M, Zhao Y, Zhang B. Efficient test and visualization of multi-set intersections. Sci Rep. 2015;5:16923.

3

High mammographic density in women is associated with protumor inflammation

Cecilia W. Huo[1], Prue Hill[2], Grace Chew[1], Paul J. Neeson[3,4,7], Heloise Halse[4], Elizabeth D. Williams[5,6], Michael A. Henderson[1,4], Erik W. Thompson[1,5,6†] and Kara L. Britt[4,7*†]

Abstract

Background: Epidemiological studies have consistently shown that increased mammographic density (MD) is a strong risk factor for breast cancer. We previously observed an elevated number of vimentin[+]/CD45[+] leukocytes in high MD (HMD) epithelium. In the present study, we aimed to investigate the subtypes of immune cell infiltrates in HMD and low MD (LMD) breast tissue.

Methods: Fifty-four women undergoing prophylactic mastectomy at Peter MacCallum Cancer Centre or St. Vincent's Hospital were enrolled. Upon completion of mastectomy, HMD and LMD areas were resected under radiological guidance in collaboration with BreastScreen Victoria and were subsequently fixed, processed, and sectioned. Fifteen paired HMD and LMD specimens were further selected according to their fibroglandular characteristics (reasonable amount [> 20%] of tissue per block on H&E stains) for subsequent IHC analysis of immune cell infiltration.

Results: Overall, immune cell infiltrates were predominantly present in breast ducts and lobules rather than in the stroma, with CD68[+] macrophages and CD20[+] B lymphocytes also surrounding the vasculature. Macrophages, dendritic cells (DCs), B lymphocytes, and programmed cell death protein 1 (PD-1) expression were significantly increased in HMD epithelium compared with LMD. Moreover, significantly higher levels of DCs, CD4[+] T cells, and PD-1 were also observed in HMD stroma than in LMD stroma. The increased expression of interleukin (IL)-6 and IL-4, with unaltered interferon-γ, indicate a proinflammatory microenvironment.

Conclusions: Our work indicates that the immune system may be activated very early in breast cancer development and may in part underpin the breast cancer risk associated with HMD.

Keywords: Mammographic density, Immune infiltration, Macrophages, Dendritic cells, PD-L1, B cells, T cells, Biomarker, Immunotherapy

Background

Mammographic density (MD) refers to the percentage of radio-opaque fibroglandular breast tissue on a mammogram [1]. In 1969, Wolfe et al. first proposed that an increased proportion of dense breast tissue might be associated with increased breast cancer (BC) risk [2]; however, evidence was scarce at that time to support this hypothesis. Furthermore, dense breast tissue could present a

masking effect for small tumors on mammography, making early cancer detection on mammograms challenging [3]. Hence, it was widely believed that the increased BC risk was in fact secondary to the masking effect, rather than any real difference in cancer development due to MD [4]. However, over the past 20 years, well-powered case-control and cohort studies have consistently shown that increased MD is a strong risk factor for BC, independent of any potential masking effect [5–8]. In particular, McCormack and dos Santos Silva performed a meta-analysis of 14,000 cases and 226,000 noncases from 42 studies and found that the proportion of dense area, or percent MD (PMD), was consistently associated with BC risk [9]. Subsequently,

---
* Correspondence: kara.britt@petermac.org

†Erik W. Thompson and Kara L. Britt contributed equally to this work.

[4]Peter MacCallum Cancer Centre, Melbourne, Australia

[7]The Sir Peter MacCallum Department of Oncology, University of Melbourne, Melbourne, Australia

Full list of author information is available at the end of the article

important questions raised were whether BC preferentially arose from tissue of HMD areas, and if so, what are the characteristics of HMD origin BC compared with LMD. Ursin and colleagues showed in a retrospective study that ductal carcinoma in situ (DCIS) lesions were more likely to develop from HMD than from LMD areas of the breast in 28 women, by comparing mammograms at BC diagnosis with the women's previous mammograms [10]. Other studies also found that BCs arising in HMD regions are more likely to demonstrate features that suggest poor prognosis than those that arise in LMD areas [11–13].

The significance of MD-associated BC risk was highlighted by the fact that in 1993, the American College of Radiology developed the Breast Imaging Reporting and Data System (BI-RADS) system, which divides density qualitatively into four categories [14, 15]. More recently, the Density Education National Survivors' Effort (www.areyoudense.org) in the United States led a high-profile campaign that encouraged women to ask for additional investigations if their breast tissues were reported as mammographically dense [16]. This subsequently led to bold legislation changes in 32 U.S. states to mandate physicians to inform their patients of their MD categories [17, 18].

Although the association of HMD with increased BC risk has now been well established for years, the underlying biological mechanism of this association continues to perplex researchers. Many biological and molecular studies are beginning to unravel the complexities of the biology behind HMD-associated BC risk [19–24]. Using paired HMD and LMD breast tissues from women undergoing prophylactic mastectomy, we and others have found that HMD breast tissue was associated with increased epithelium, stroma, and collagen and decreased fat percentages compared with LMD tissue; furthermore, HMD regions showed increased number of CD45$^+$ immune cells in the epithelium [25, 26]. To date, there is little data on the association of MD with immune cell infiltration; however, immune cell infiltration is observed in early-stage BC (proliferative benign disease and DCIS) as well as invasive BC, where numbers can predict prognosis [27]. In this study, we further investigated the innate and adaptive immune cell infiltration and their functional polarization in HMD and LMD normal breast tissue.

Methods

Patient accrual

This study was approved by the Peter MacCallum Human Research Ethics Committee (number 08/21) and St. Vincent's Hospital Animal Ethics Committee (number 049/09). It was conducted in accordance with the Australian National Statement on Ethical Conduct in Human Research. Between 2008 and 2015, 54 women undergoing unilateral or bilateral prophylactic mastectomy at St. Vincent's Hospital and the Peter MacCallum Cancer Centre consented to tissue collection through the Victorian Cancer Biobank (VCB 10010). The reasons for their mastectomy procedures were confirmed BRCA1/2 mutation carrier status, other confirmation mutations such as PTEN gene mutation, and a strong family or personal past history of BC. Women were excluded from the study if there was suspicion of malignant lesions on radiological investigations or if the breast that the mastectomy was performed on had been diagnosed with BC or DCIS in the past.

Selection of HMD and LMD regions within the same breast

Upon the completion of mastectomy, the resected breast was immediately sent to the pathology department on ice. Using sterile techniques, 1-cm-thick, craniocaudal breast slices were resected (breadboarding), palpated for suspicious stiffness, and a slice surplus to diagnostic needs was chosen. The breast slice was then X-rayed against a calibration strip using consistent radiological parameters by trained breast radiographers, followed by selection of high and low MD tissue regions for comparative study. The method was detailed in previous studies [19–21, 26, 28, 29]. If the breast slice imaging did not result in clear black and white regions (allowing density differences to be observed) the woman was excluded from this study. The paired HMD and LMD tissues were then fixed in neutral buffered formalin, before undergoing tissue processing, embedding and sectioning at 4 μm thickness for subsequent staining.

IHC staining

Conventional H&E staining was performed on all paired high and low MD tissues. On the basis of H&E-stained slides, 15 paired high and low MD tissues were further selected for a focused examination of immune cell influx because they showed abundance of epithelial-stromal areas that represent the characteristics of mammary specimens.

These 15 paired high and low MD tissues underwent successive IHC staining for immune cell analyses. Manual staining was performed for pan-macrophage marker CD68 (1:200, Dako clone PG-M1, code M0876; Agilent Technologies, Santa Clara, CA, USA) and B lymphocyte marker CD20cy (1:100, Dako clone L26, code M0755; Agilent Technologies). A diaminobenzidine (DAB) IHC autostainer (Ventana Medical Systems, Tucson, AZ, USA) was used for dendritic cell (DC) marker CD11c (1:25, clone 5D11; Cell Marque, Rocklin, CA, USA); programmed cell death protein 1 (PD-1) (1:100, clone NAT105; Abcam, Cambridge, MA, USA); helper CD4$^+$ T cell (1:50, AP20210 PU-N; Novus Biologicals, Littleton, CO, USA); cytotoxic CD8$^+$ T cells (1:50, orb 10325;

Biorbyt, San Francisco, CA, USA); cytokines IL-4 (1:500, AB9622; Abcam) IL-6 (1:800, AB6672; Abcam), and interferon (IFN)-γ (1:500, AB25101; Abcam), and natural killer cell (NK) marker CD56 (MRQ-42, Ventana® catalogue no. 760-2625; Cell Marque). For each staining, human benign tonsil tissue was used as a positive control, and no primary antibody was used as a technical negative control. In the case of IL-6, only nine paired samples were used because the other six pairs did not have enough tissue left following staining for the other immune cell markers.

Five-micrometer paraffin-mounted tissue sections were dewaxed and underwent antigen retrieval using either citrate buffer (CD68, CD11c, CD56, CD20cy, IL-4, and IL-6) or ethylenediaminetetraacetic acid (EDTA) (CD4, CD8, PD-1, and IFN-γ) and then incubated with the appropriate primary antibodies followed by biotinylated secondary antibodies. The VECTASTAIN Elite ABC kit (Vector Laboratories, Burlingame, CA, USA) with Dako DAB peroxidase (Agilent Technologies) used as chromogen.

For CD3 and PD1 double staining, we performed Opal multiplex imaging (PerkinElmer, Waltham, MA, USA) according to the manufacturer's instructions. In brief, 3-μm formalin-fixed, paraffin-embedded sections were deparaffinized and then stained with rabbit monoclonal anti-CD3 (clone SP7; Spring Bioscience, Pleasanton, CA, USA) and a rabbit monoclonal anti-PD1 (Bio SB, Santa Barbara, CA, USA). Antigen retrieval was performed in high-pH EDTA in a pressure cooker for the first antibody and then EDTA in the microwave for subsequent antibodies. Endogenous peroxidases were blocked using hydrogen peroxidase, and following incubation with anti-rabbit secondary antibody, the immunofluorescent signal was visualized using TSA dye 570 or 650 from the Opal™ 7 color fIHC kit (PerkinElmer). All sections were counterstained with Spectral DAPI. Slides were imaged on the Vectra® 3.0 Automated Quantitative Pathology Imaging System (PerkinElmer). Color separation, tissue and cell segmentation, and phenotyping were performed using inForm® software version 2.2 (Perkin Elmer) to extract image data.

Histological review and digital image analysis

All slides were examined using digital microscopy (AxioVision photomicroscope; Carl Zeiss Microscopy, Thornwood, NY, USA) for punctate brown cytoplasmic staining of each individual immune cell marker. Four random glandular-stromal areas within each tissue sample were photographed at × 40 magnification. The number of positively stained immune cells and the total number of cells within each histological compartment (epithelial and stromal regions) were manually counted for each image. Thus, for the immune cell counts in the epithelial area, the total number of epithelial cell nuclei was counted on the

selected region, and then the number of positively stained cells was counted. The number of positive cells was then presented as a percentage of total epithelial cells. Scoring was performed in a blinded manner. The percentage of positive staining was calculated as an average value derived from results of all four images for each tissue sample. For stroma, only cells with elongated nuclei and positive cytoplasmic brown staining were counted as positive stains.

Statistical analysis

For each immune cell marker staining, the data were first assessed for equal variance using a normality test. If data passed the normality test, a paired t test was used to analyze the percentage of positive immune cell staining in the epithelium and the stroma, respectively. When data were not normally distributed, a nonparametric Wilcoxon matched-pairs rank test was used. Outliers were identified using Grubbs' test. A conventional two-tailed alpha level of 0.05 was used to define statistical significance.

Results

Characteristics of the study population and tissue samples

The mean age of the 15 selected women was 46 years. The majority had borne children and were premenopausal

Table 1 Demographic characteristics of study participants

Selected characteristics	Number or mean
Age at surgery date	Mean 46 years (range, 31–64 years)
BI-RADS category	
4	3
3	4
2	5
1	3
Risk factors (some women had > 1 risk factor)	
Strong family history	11
BRCA1+	3
BRCA 2+	5
Past history of BC or DCIS	10
Menopausal status	
Premenopausal	9
Perimenopausal	1
Postmenopausal	5
Parity	
Parous	11
Nulliparous	4

Abbreviations: BI-RADS Breast Imaging Reporting and Data System, BC Breast cancer, DCIS Ductal carcinoma in situ
BI-RADS score 1 = predominantly fat, 2 = scattered fibroglandular densities, 3 = heterogeneously dense, 4 = extremely dense

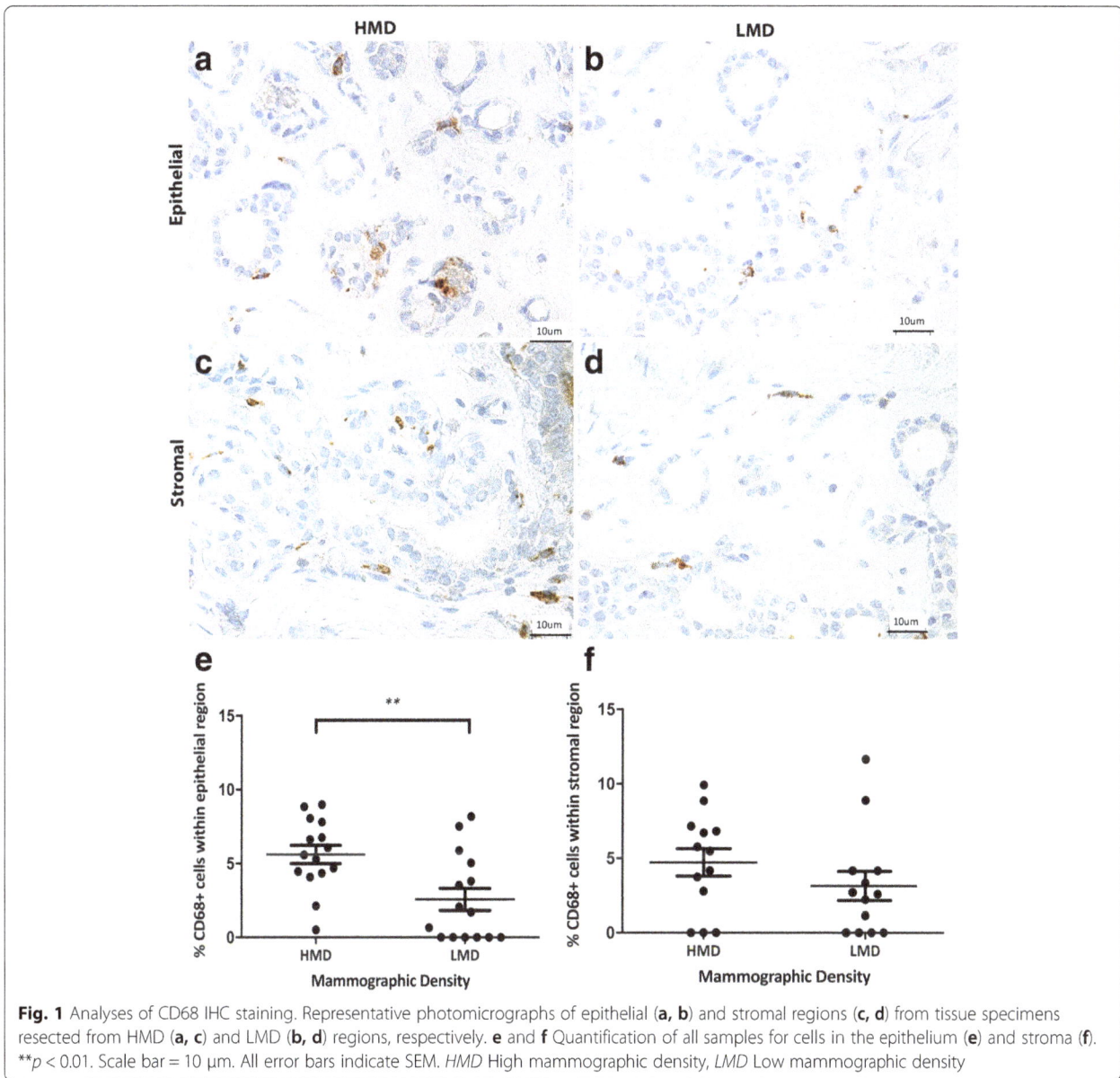

Fig. 1 Analyses of CD68 IHC staining. Representative photomicrographs of epithelial (**a, b**) and stromal regions (**c, d**) from tissue specimens resected from HMD (**a, c**) and LMD (**b, d**) regions, respectively. **e** and **f** Quantification of all samples for cells in the epithelium (**e**) and stroma (**f**). ******$p < 0.01$. Scale bar = 10 μm. All error bars indicate SEM. *HMD* High mammographic density, *LMD* Low mammographic density

(9 of 15). Over half (8 of 15) had confirmed *BRCA1/2* mutation carrier status, with or without strong past or family history of BC. Their BI-RADS scores were evenly spread across the four categories. Their characteristics are summarized in Table 1 and are representative of the entire cohort of 54 patients accrued. Of the 54 women, 14 had a BI-RADS score of 3, and 10 had a score of 4, giving an overall 44.0% of patients with heterogeneously or extremely dense breasts. For the 15 women included in our study, 3 of 15 had a BI-RADS score of 4, and 4 of 15 had a BIRADS score of 3. Thus, 46% of patients had heterogeneously or extremely dense breasts, representative of the entire cohort.

HMD breast tissue has an increased infiltration of innate and adaptive immune cells

Having shown previously that CD45$^+$ immune cells were more frequent in HMD than in LMD samples [26], in the present study we assessed which innate and adaptive immune cells were increased. The innate immune cells assessed included macrophages, DC, and NK cells. CD68$^+$ macrophages were observed in both epithelial and stromal areas in high and low MD tissue with approximately equal numbers in each cellular compartment. The parenchymal macrophages were present in both lobules and ducts, and they were scattered in both basal and luminal layers of the epithelium. In the epithelium, there were significantly more CD68[+] cells in HMD regions than in LMD regions ($p = 0.004$) (Fig. 1). CD11c[+] DC were present in the breast epithelium (lobules and ducts) as well as stroma (Fig. 2). The percentage of DC was significantly higher in HMD than in LMD regions ($p < 0.05$) in the epithelium and stroma (Fig. 2). CD56[+] NK cells were present in the breast epithelium and stroma, with approximately twofold higher levels in the former. There was no significant difference in NK cell numbers between HMD and LMD tissue in either epithelial or stromal areas (Fig. 3).

Adaptive immune cells assessed included B cells and T-cell subsets (CD4[+] and CD8[+]). We observed a trend for increased CD4[+] T cells in the epithelium ($p = 0.057$) of HMD tissues and significantly more CD4[+] T cells in the HMD stroma than in LMD areas ($p < 0.05$) (Fig. 4). The percentage of CD8[+] cytotoxic T cells was similar in the epithelium and stroma of HMD and LMD tissues (Fig. 5). The mean CD4/CD8 ratio in the stroma of HMD was 10:1, and in LMD it was 9.7:1, which was not significantly different ($p = 0.76$). Within the epithelium, the CD4/CD8 ratio was 3:1 in the HMD and 5:1 in LMD and again was not significantly different ($p = 0.52$). CD20cy[+] B cells were present in the epithelium and stroma (Fig. 6). Within the

epithelium, the number of B cells in HMD tissue was significantly higher than in LMD tissue ($p = 0.004$). In the stroma, there was a modest but nonsignificant trend for increased CD20cy[+] B-cell infiltration in HMD compared with LMD tissue.

HMD environment shows immune activation and protumor cytokines

To explore whether the T cells present were activated, we examined PD-1 expression. The number of PD-1[+] cells (1–2%) that we observed was low; however, the numbers of PD-1[+] cells in the epithelium and stroma were significantly higher in HMD than in LMD tissue ($p < 0.05$) (Fig. 7). Further staining using Opal multiplex imaging revealed that the PD-1-positive cells were CD3[+] T cells (Additional file 1: Figure S1).

We next examined immune cell functional polarization by examining signature cytokines for inflammation (IL-6) and either a Th1 (IFN-γ) or Th2 (IL-4) response. In the breast, the percentage of IL-6[+] cells ranged from a mean of 18–24% in the epithelium and 11–21% in the stroma (Fig. 8). In the epithelium and stroma, IL-6[+] cells were significantly increased in HMD areas compared with LMD areas ($p < 0.05$ and $p < 0.01$, respectively). IL-4[+] cells ranged from a mean of 16–24% in the epithelium and 1–4% in the

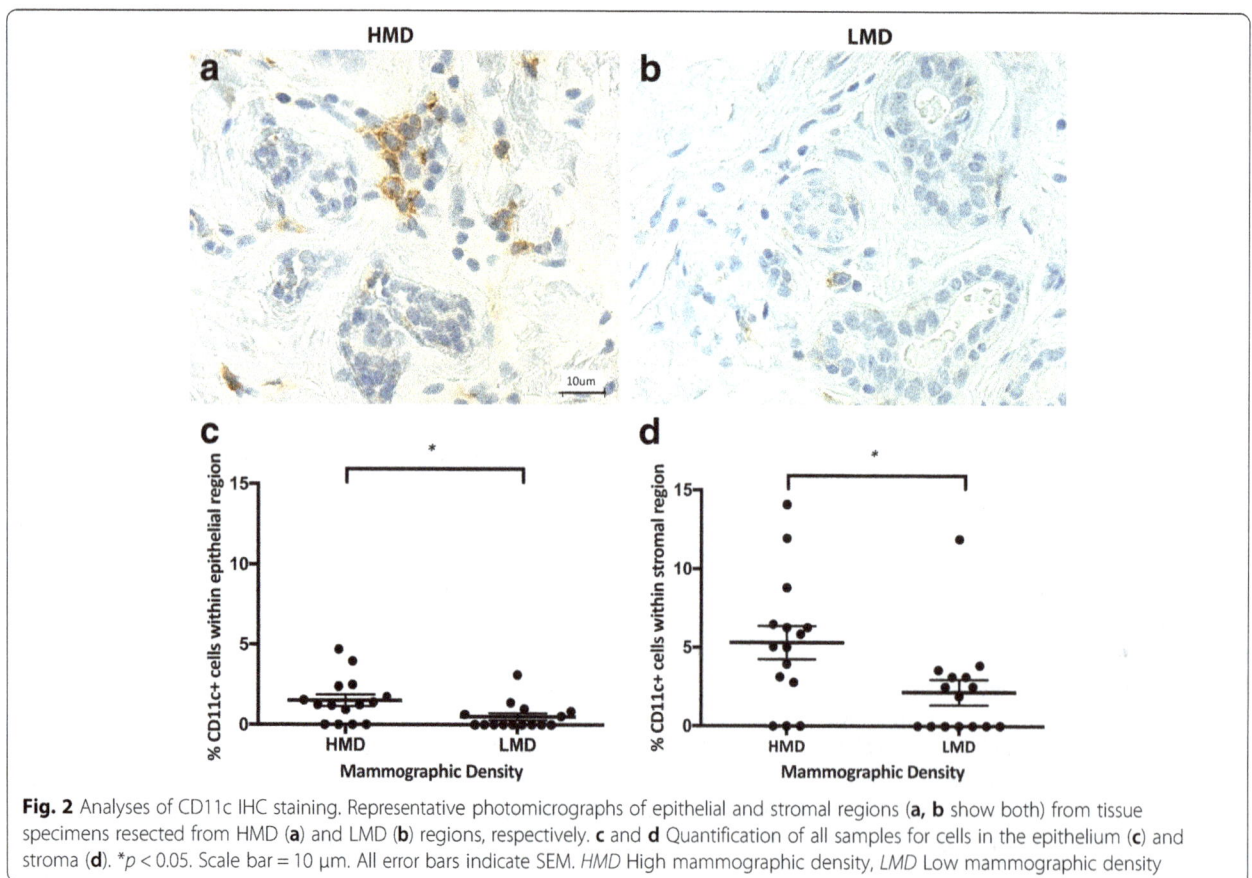

Fig. 2 Analyses of CD11c IHC staining. Representative photomicrographs of epithelial and stromal regions (**a, b** show both) from tissue specimens resected from HMD (**a**) and LMD (**b**) regions, respectively. **c** and **d** Quantification of all samples for cells in the epithelium (**c**) and stroma (**d**). *$p < 0.05$. Scale bar = 10 μm. All error bars indicate SEM. *HMD* High mammographic density, *LMD* Low mammographic density

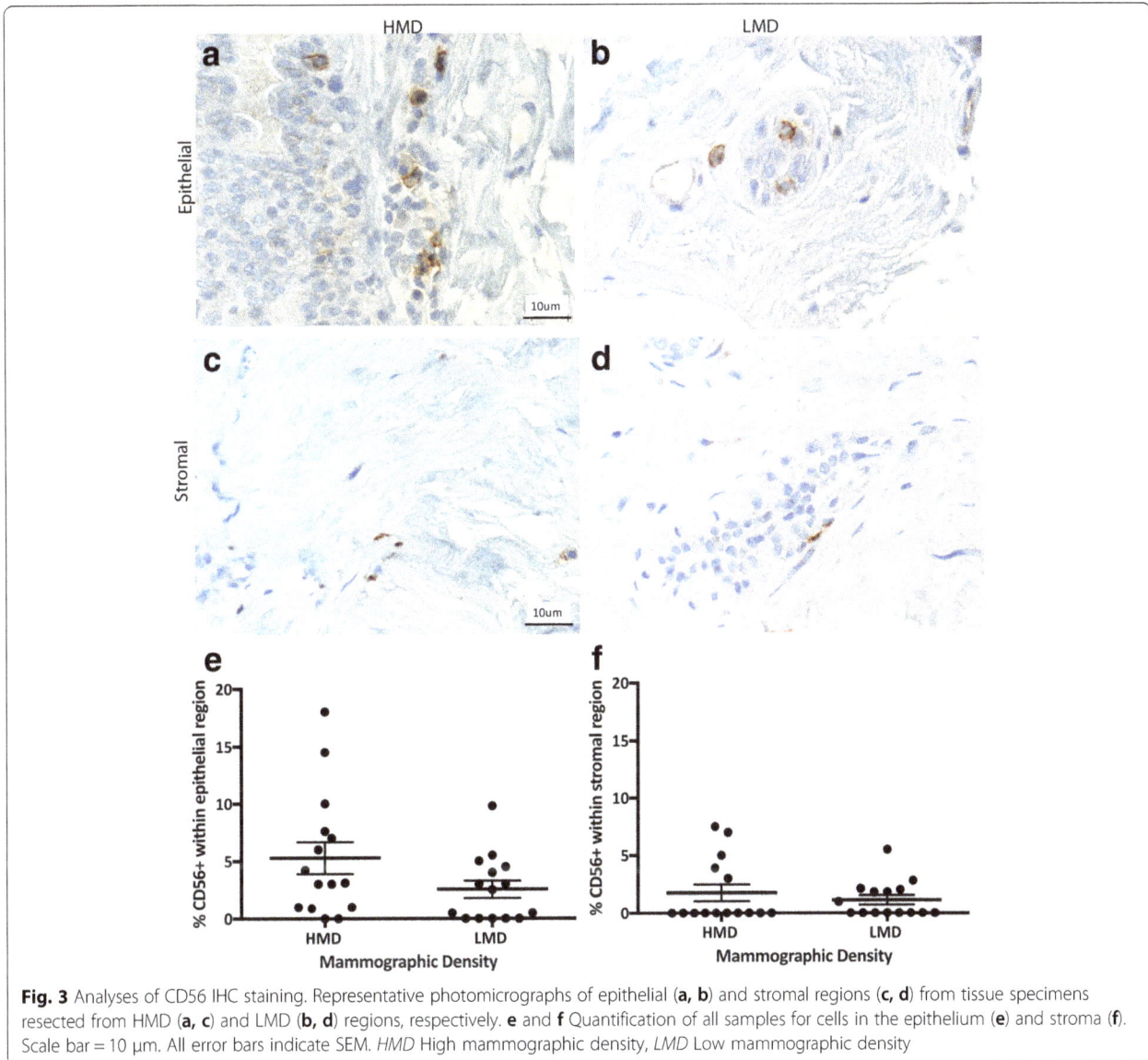

Fig. 3 Analyses of CD56 IHC staining. Representative photomicrographs of epithelial (**a, b**) and stromal regions (**c, d**) from tissue specimens resected from HMD (**a, c**) and LMD (**b, d**) regions, respectively. **e** and **f** Quantification of all samples for cells in the epithelium (**e**) and stroma (**f**). Scale bar = 10 μm. All error bars indicate SEM. *HMD* High mammographic density, *LMD* Low mammographic density

stroma (Fig. 9); however, there was no significant difference in IL-4$^+$ cell numbers between HMD and LMD. In the stroma, the percentage of IL-4$^+$ cells was significantly higher in HMD than in LMD tissue ($p < 0.05$) (Fig. 9). Of note, some epithelial cells appeared to be positive for IL-4 and IL-6, which concurs with the Human Protein Atlas databank (www.proteinatlas.org). The percentage of IFN-γ$^+$ cells in the breast was 2–4% in the epithelium and 0.67–1.41% in the stroma (Fig. 10). In the breast epithelium, there was a nonsignificant trend ($p = 0.06$) for an increase in IFN-γ$^+$ cells in HMD compared with LMD; however, there was no difference in the stroma (Fig. 10).

IFN-γ signaling is known to enable activation of the PD-1 signaling axis [30], so we assessed whether the expression of IFN-γ in our MD samples correlated with

PD-1 expression in the same samples. There was a moderate positive correlation between IFN-γ and PD-1 ($r = 0.476$, $p = 0.004$) (Additional file 2: Figure S2).

Recently, benign breast disease tissue has been shown to have higher densities of multiple immune cell types, especially macrophages and DC, compared with normal breast tissues [31]. To determine if the increased immune cell infiltration in HMD tissue was due to the presence of benign breast lesions, we scored all sections for evidence of nonproliferative disease, proliferative disease without atypia, or the presence of atypical hyperplasia (atypical ductal hyperplasia or atypical lobular hyperplasia). We found no evidence of any of these lesions. In addition to this, we assessed columnar cell hyperplasia, flat epithelial atypia, sclerosing adenosis,

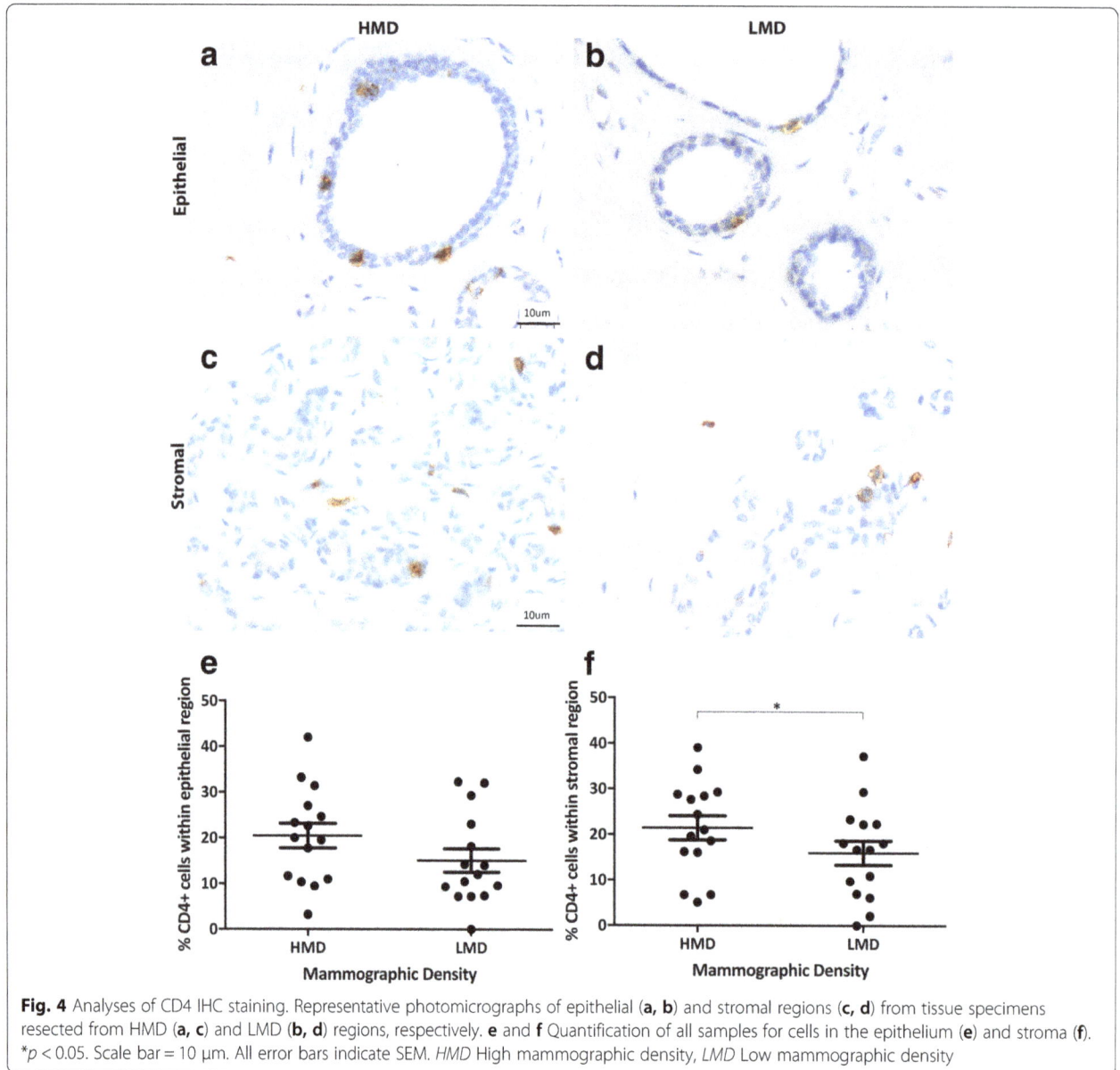

Fig. 4 Analyses of CD4 IHC staining. Representative photomicrographs of epithelial (**a, b**) and stromal regions (**c, d**) from tissue specimens resected from HMD (**a, c**) and LMD (**b, d**) regions, respectively. **e** and **f** Quantification of all samples for cells in the epithelium (**e**) and stroma (**f**). *p < 0.05. Scale bar = 10 μm. All error bars indicate SEM. *HMD* High mammographic density, *LMD* Low mammographic density

cysts, unusual ductal hyperplasia, calcification or fibroadenoma, and duct ectasia. We observed only one HMD sample with evidence of a small amount of sclerosing adenoma, and its matching LMD had a very small focal region of columnar cell change. We identified one other HMD sample with a small amount of sclerosing adenosis. Another HMD sample with a very focal amount of columnar cell change was also observed (Additional file 3: Table S1). Because there was only a very small amount of benign change present in a minority of samples, and because those samples did not harbor the strongest increase in immune cells, we concluded that benign features do not account for the increase in immune cells in HMD tissue.

Because our tissues were obtained from prophylactic mastectomies and a significant proportion of our patients had germline mutations in known predisposition genes (*BRCA1/2*), we assessed whether the immune changes differed in those with *BRCA1/2* mutations compared with those without. Although our study was not appropriately powered for such an analysis, we found that the trend was similar in both nonmutation carriers and *BRCA1* mutation carriers. In many cases, the changes were more evident in the nonmutation carriers. *BRCA2* carriers shared similar changes according to density with the nonmutation carriers and *BRCA1*, but not for all immune cells (Additional file 4: Figure S3).

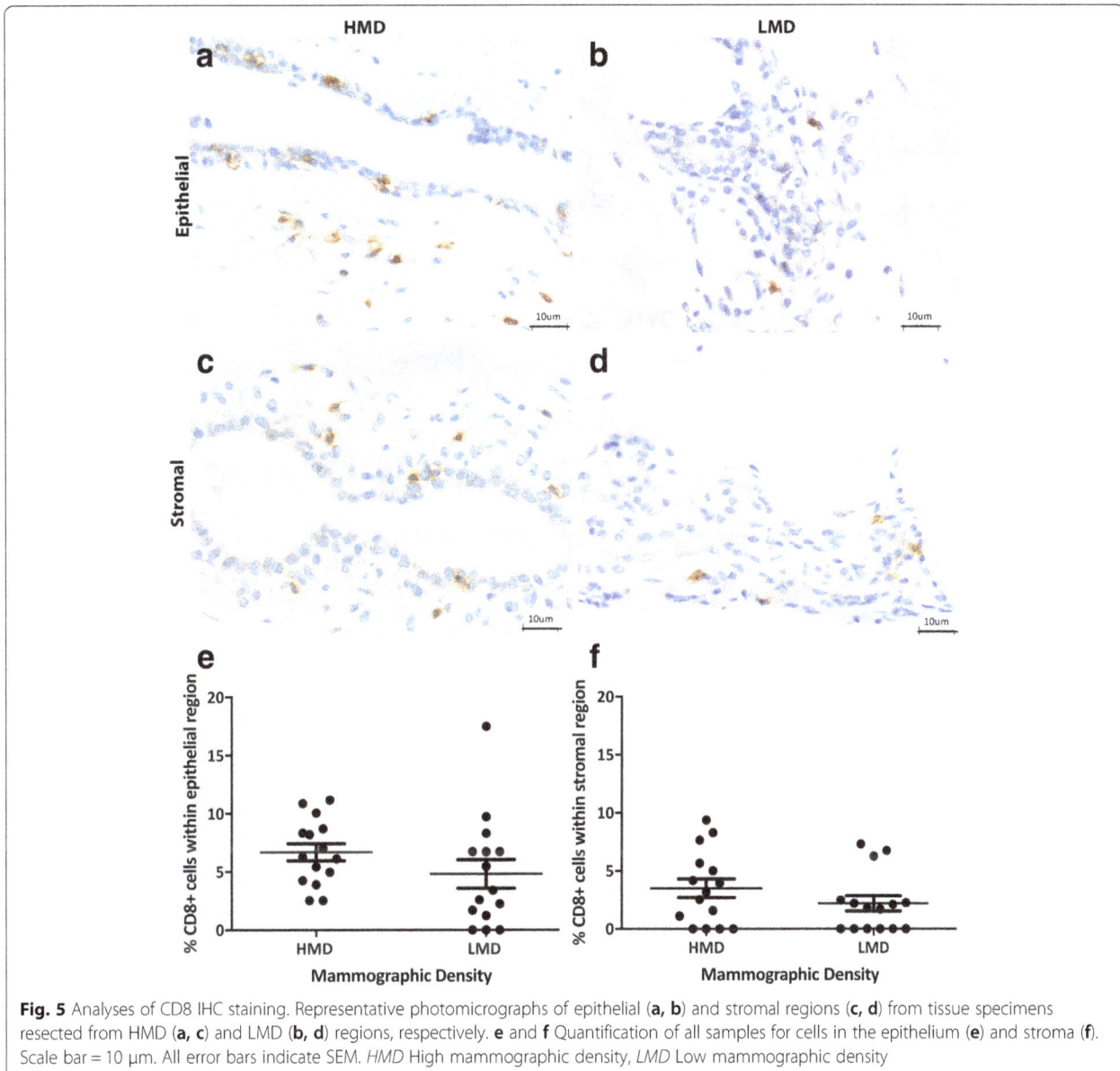

Fig. 5 Analyses of CD8 IHC staining. Representative photomicrographs of epithelial (**a, b**) and stromal regions (**c, d**) from tissue specimens resected from HMD (**a, c**) and LMD (**b, d**) regions, respectively. **e** and **f** Quantification of all samples for cells in the epithelium (**e**) and stroma (**f**). Scale bar = 10 μm. All error bars indicate SEM. *HMD* High mammographic density, *LMD* Low mammographic density

Discussion

Following our work identifying an increase in the immune cells (CD45$^+$vimentin$^+$cytokeratin$^-$ cells) within the epithelial region of dense breast tissue [26], in the present study we show dense breast tissue has increased parenchymal macrophages, DC, and B cells, but not NK cells. HMD tissue also has a trend for increased CD4$^+$ T cells and a significant increase in expression of the checkpoint inhibitor PD-1, confirming that the T cells present are activated. IL-6 was increased in the epithelial regions, and both IL-6 and IL4 were increased in the stromal regions of HMD samples, but not IFN-γ. This suggests that the preneoplastic breast tissue of women with high breast density has increased numbers of innate

and adaptive immune cells, with a proinflammatory functional polarization consistent with the increased risk of developing BC that has been associated with HMD.

BC has largely not been considered immunogenic, because incidence is not increased in patients who are immune-suppressed; however, there are now irrefutable data demonstrating that the immune cell infiltrate of a breast tumor affects its growth and metastasis [27]. In addition, progression from normal to preinvasive and invasive BC has been associated with increases in T cells, B cells, and macrophages [32, 33]. Degnim and colleagues assessed 11 normal breast samples and found increased T- and B-cell numbers in breast lobules with lobulitis and found that immune cells were present

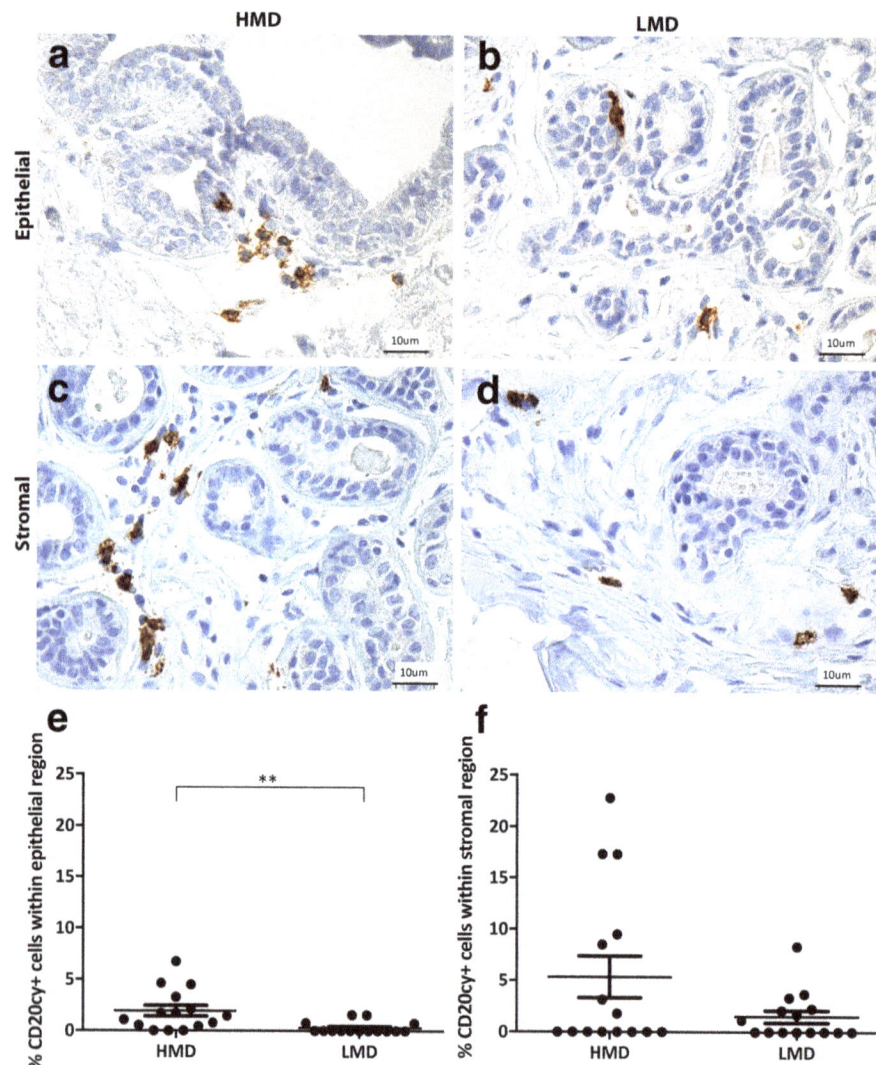

Fig. 6 Analyses of CD20cy IHC staining. Representative photomicrographs of epithelial (**a, b**) and stromal regions (**c, d**) from tissue specimens resected from HMD (**a, c**) and LMD (**b, d**) regions, respectively. **e** and **f** Quantification of all samples for cells in the epithelium (**e**) and stroma (**f**). ******$p < 0.01$. Scale bar = 10 μm. All error bars indicate SEM. *HMD* High mammographic density, *LMD* Low mammographic density

mainly in breast lobules rather than in the stroma and that cytotoxic T cells and DC were integrated within the epithelium [34]. We also found macrophages, DC, NK cells, B cells, and T cells in normal breast tissue. Furthermore, we showed the expression of PD-1 and secretion of IL-6, IL-4, and IFN-γ in glands and stroma of normal breast, suggesting that there is a dynamic breast immune surveillance system. Similarly, Degnim and colleagues assessed benign breast disease tissue and found that this tissue had higher densities of multiple immune cell types, especially macrophages and DC, compared with normal breast tissues [31]. Although our HMD tissue did not show signs of benign breast disease, we also found increased levels of these two innate immune cells,

indicating that they may be important for the early immune response to breast changes that may, in some cases, develop into lesions.

We found that the number of innate immune cells was increased in HMD samples compared with LMD samples. Macrophages are phagocytic cells that act to maintain immune surveillance within tissues and constantly survey their surroundings for signs of tissue damage or invading organisms. They stimulate lymphocytes and other immune cells to respond when danger signals are phagocytosed and/or detected by cell surface receptors [35]. In the present study, we show that macrophages were increased in the epithelial regions of HMD samples. Previously, we reported that epithelial

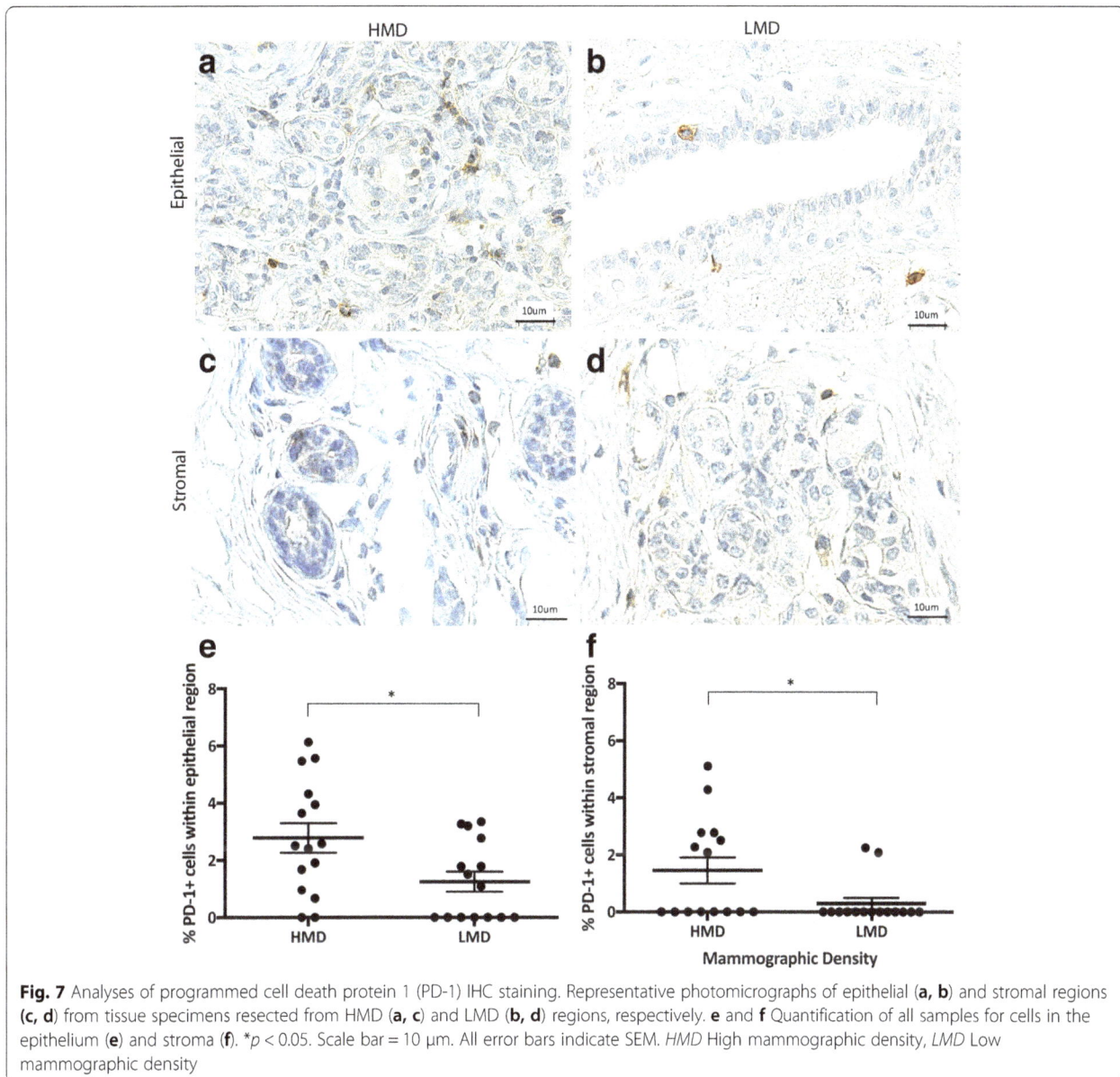

Fig. 7 Analyses of programmed cell death protein 1 (PD-1) IHC staining. Representative photomicrographs of epithelial (**a, b**) and stromal regions (**c, d**) from tissue specimens resected from HMD (**a, c**) and LMD (**b, d**) regions, respectively. **e** and **f** Quantification of all samples for cells in the epithelium (**e**) and stroma (**f**). *$p < 0.05$. Scale bar = 10 μm. All error bars indicate SEM. *HMD* High mammographic density, *LMD* Low mammographic density

macrophage numbers were not altered with density [26]; however, only nine women and three random areas of each section were assessed. The larger sample sizes and increased areas used in the present study allowed significant macrophage changes to be revealed. The increased epithelial macrophages support our recent finding that chemokine ligand 2 (CCL2) or monocyte chemoattractant protein 1 (MCP-1) is significantly increased in HMD epithelium [36]. CCL2 recruits macrophages but also stimulates protumorigenic M2 macrophage polarization [36, 37], which is supported by the increased epithelial IL-6 expression that we report here, as well as its role in M2 orientation [38].

DC are powerful antigen-presenting cells [39] with molecular sensors enabling them to sense danger and to transmit this to lymphocytes to initiate the T-cell immune response [40] and aid in tumor cell death. We found increased DC in HMD epithelial and stromal compartments compared with LMD, suggesting increased antigen presentation and hence potentially enhanced immune surveillance. Because the generation of tumor-specific T cells relies on the ability of mature DCs to cross-present tumor antigens, future studies will need to assess the functional status of DC to fully understand the implications of increased DC. NK cells are tumor cell- and virus-killing innate immune cells that do not need to match with a major histocompatibility complex (MHC) subclass, the way CD8[+] T cells do [41]. NK cell dysfunction has been associated with BC progression [42]. We found no significant difference in the

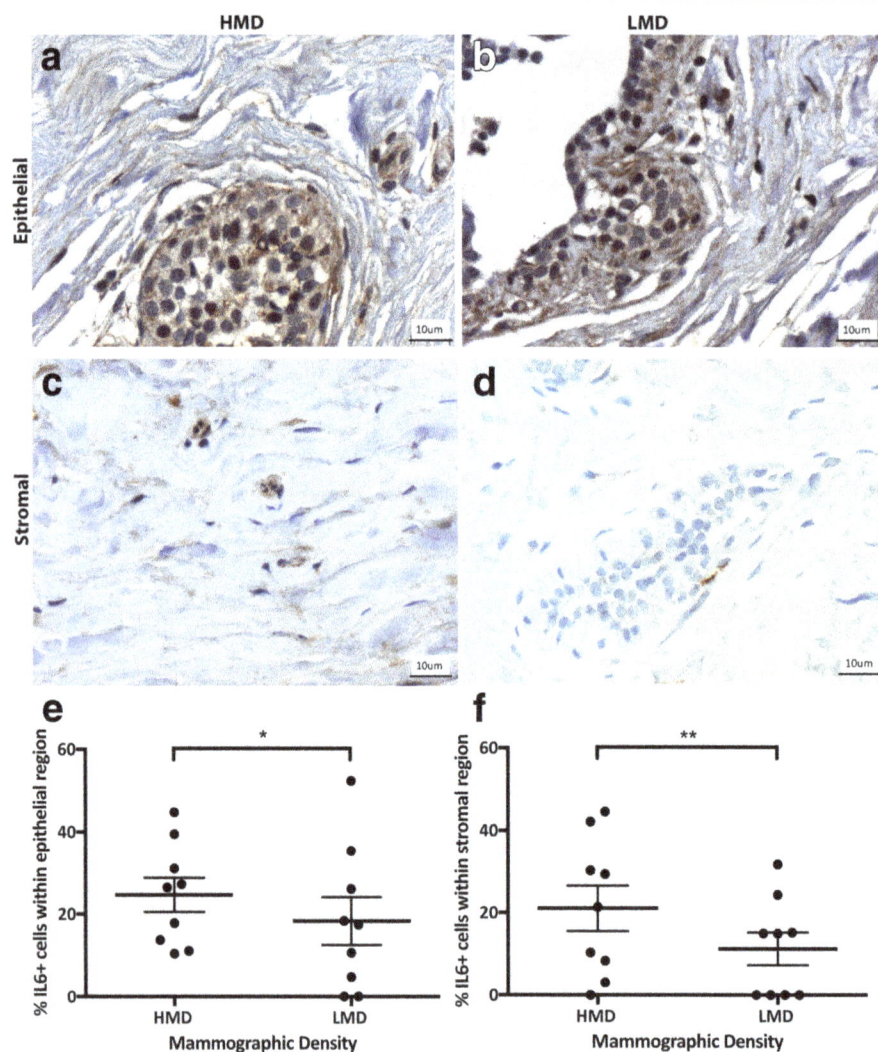

Fig. 8 Analyses of interleukin (IL)-6 IHC staining. Representative photomicrographs of epithelial (**a, b**) and stromal regions (**c, d**) from tissue specimens resected from HMD (**a, c**) and LMD (**b, d**) regions, respectively. **e** and **f** Quantification of all samples for cells in the epithelium (**e**) and stroma (**f**). *$p < 0.05$, **$p < 0.01$. Scale bar = 10 μm. All error bars indicate SEM. *HMD* High mammographic density, *LMD* Low mammographic density

percentage of NK cells between high and low MD, suggesting that NK cells do not play a key role in the inflammatory microenvironment of high breast density.

In addition to the changes in the innate immune cells, we found changes in the adaptive immune cells within high-density breast tissue. The percentage of B lymphocytes was significantly increased in HMD epithelium. B cells secrete antibodies and inflammatory cytokines and can recognize antigens, regulate antigen processing and presentation, and mount and modulate T-cell and innate immune responses. B-cell infiltration was been associated with worse outcome in patients with metastatic ovarian cancer and progression of orthotopic tumors in mice [43], and their numbers increase with the

progression of normal breast and benign proliferative disease through to DCIS and invasive ductal carcinoma [33]. We postulate that the increased number of B cells in HMD may reflect changes in the breast immune surveillance and possibly increased differentiation of B regulatory cells, which themselves can drive T-regulatory differentiation of CD4+ T cells.

The CD4+ T lymphocytes were markedly increased in the HMD stroma, whereas no significant difference was observed in terms of CD8+ T cells in either compartment. CD4+ T cells carry out multiple functions, including activation of innate immune cells, B lymphocytes, and cytotoxic T cells, as well as nonimmune cells. They also play a critical role in the suppression of immune reaction. CD4+

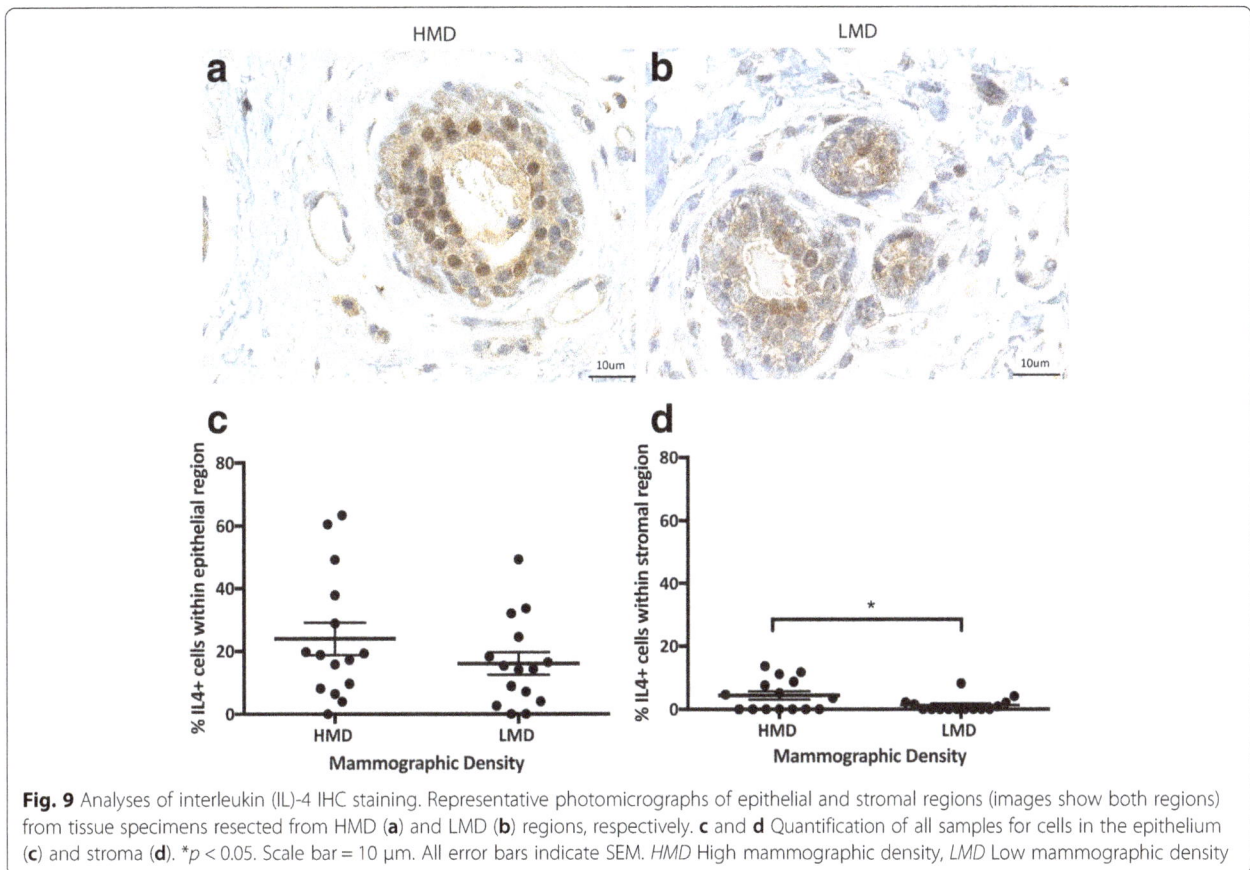

Fig. 9 Analyses of interleukin (IL)-4 IHC staining. Representative photomicrographs of epithelial and stromal regions (images show both regions) from tissue specimens resected from HMD (**a**) and LMD (**b**) regions, respectively. **c** and **d** Quantification of all samples for cells in the epithelium (**c**) and stroma (**d**). *$p < 0.05$. Scale bar = 10 μm. All error bars indicate SEM. *HMD* High mammographic density, *LMD* Low mammographic density

T cells can be either T-helper cells (Th) or regulatory T cells (Treg), and they are activated through two signals: T-cell receptor on the T cell and an antigenic peptide presented by MHC class II on the antigen-presenting cell requiring a second costimulatory signal [44, 45]. Within the Th cell population, there are a number of subtypes, including Th1, Th2, Th9, Th17, Th22, and ThFH (Follicular T helper), that differ in their functions, signature cytokine profiles, and cell targets [46]. Due to the increased levels of IL-6 and IL-4 in HMD breast tissue (but steady state of IFN-γ), we postulate that the increased CD4$^+$ T cells are Th2-oriented because IL-6 drives Th2 differentiation [47, 48] and IL-4 production is enhanced by IL-6. IL-6 has already been associated with breast density in genome-wide association studies on cancer-free breast tissue, where genetic variations in nine tagging single-nucleotide polymorphisms in the IL-6 gene were significantly associated with HMD [49]. Higher transcript expression of IL-6 has also been reported in HMD epithelial areas compared with LMD in BC [50].

The PD-1/PD-L1 pathway is an inhibitory immune check point pathway that is upregulated within the tumor microenvironment [51, 52], and PD-1/PDL-1 checkpoint inhibitors are showing unprecedented clinical efficacy in certain cancer types, especially melanoma and lung [53]. Its normal biological role lies in preventing overstimulation of the immune responses and helping maintain immune tolerance to self-antigens [54, 55]. PD-1 is expressed on activated T cells but also on other immune cells, including activated B cells and NK cells [56] and Tregs [57]. We show that PD-1 expression was increased within the epithelial and stromal regions of HMD samples compared with LMD, suggesting an increased immune self-tolerance in the HMD. The levels of PD-1 in normal human breast (0.29–2.79%) (*see* Table 2) are much lower than in BC, where expression ranges from 19% to 59% [58, 59]. In murine BC studies, tumor-induced CD8$^+$ T cells that express a high level of PD-1 were found to be ineffective in controlling tumor growth [60]. Thus, the increased level of PD-1 protein in HMD compared with LMD regions suggests that the function of T cells may be impaired, which may contribute to the increased BC risk that occurs in HMD.

Conclusions

Although BC is not classically considered to be immunoresponsive, we are among the first to report a detailed

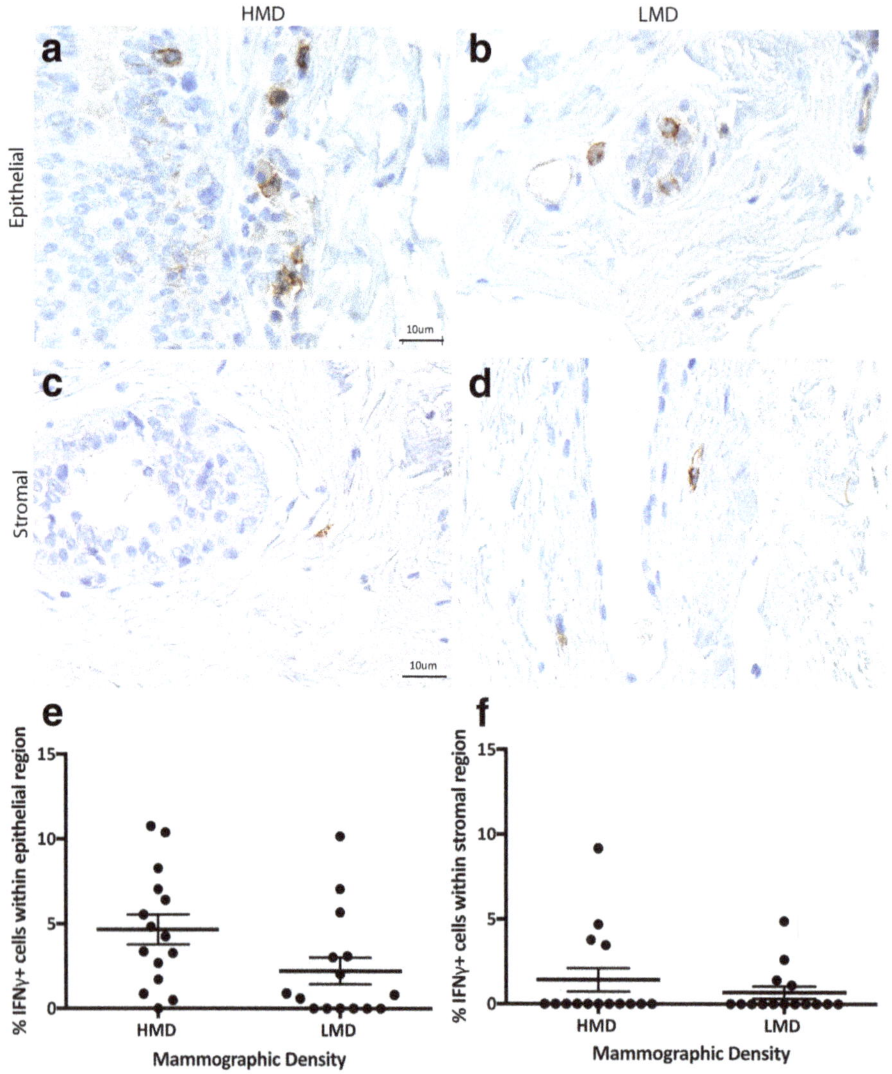

Fig. 10 Analyses of interferon (IFN)-γ IHC staining. Representative photomicrographs of epithelial (**a, b**) and stromal regions (**c, d**) from tissue specimens resected from HMD (**a, c**) and LMD (**b, d**) regions, respectively. **e** and **f** Quantification of all samples for cells in the epithelium (**e**) and stroma (**f**). Scale bar = 10 μm. All error bars indicate standard error of the mean (SEM. *HMD* High mammographic density, *LMD* Low mammographic density

study on the dynamic breast immune environment where HMD tissue is associated with increased infiltration of innate immune cells (macrophages, DC), adaptive immune cells (B cells, CD4 T cells), as well as activated T cells (PD-1 expression) and protumor Th2 polarization (elevated IL-6 and IL4 secretion). This protumorigenic microenvironment may assist an escape from immune regulation for early tumor cell variants.

In the future, assessing the tumor cell-killing function of T cells using in vitro assays and T-cell exhaustion by flow cytometry, as well as exploring DC of different origins using distinct staining markers, may permit further insights into the significance of immune cells associated with HMD. Understanding the interplay of immune cells and their effects on breast epithelium and stroma will provide a novel avenue for BC prevention and treatment that is focused on modulating the immune microenvironment. Future studies will also explore the potential of nonsteroidal anti-inflammatory drugs (NSAIDs) such as aspirin in modulating breast density by normalizing the immune environment. Aspirin is being considered for large-scale prevention studies due to strong data showing a reduced risk of BC occurrence and recurrence [61]. Although there is no evidence to date that NSAIDs can reduce breast density, the existing studies are complicated by the use of varied NSAIDs and the low baseline MD readings of the patients. Tamoxifen has its largest chemopreventative effects in the IBIS-1 (International Breast Cancer Intervention

Table 2 Overview of all immune cell analyses between high (HMD) and low (LMD) density breast samples

Marker	Epithelium		Difference (p value)	Stroma		Difference (p value)
	HMD	LMD		HMD	LMD	
CD68	5.61 (0.61)	2.56 (0.75)	**p=0.004**	4.72 (0.9)	3.14 (0.98)	p=0.15
CD11c	1.53 (0.36)	0.5 (0.22)	**p=0.02**	5.30 (1.06)	2.16 (0.80)	**p=0.03**
CD56	5.30 (1.41)	2.29 (0.73)	p=0.07	1.81 (0.74)	0.92 (0.36)	p=0.31
CD20	1.93 (0.52)	0.31 (0.15)	**p=0.0039**	5.35 (2.03)	1.50 (0.59)	p=0.28
CD4	20.47 (2.69)	15.07 (2.55)	p=0.05	21.42 (2.63)	15.95 (2.64)	**p=0.04**
CD8	6.69 (1.43)	4.82 (1.75)	p=0.22	3.49 (0.83)	2.18 (0.66)	p=0.15
PD1	2.79 (0.52)	1.25 (0.35)	**p=0.02**	1.45 (0.46)	0.29 (0.20)	**p=0.04**
IL-6	24.68 (4.13)	18.34 (5.80)	**p=0.03**	21.07 (5.53)	11.24 (3.98)	**p=0.006**
IL-4	23.94 (5.19)	16.04 (3.60)	p=0.09	4.41 (1.29)	1.28 (0.59)	**p=0.04**
IFNγ	4.66 (0.88)	2.22 (0.80)	p=0.06	1.41 (0.69)	0.67 (0.36)	p=0.56

Data are presented as the Mean+/- (SEM) percentage of immune + cells (ie: CD68) as a function of total epithelial cell nuclei counted in 4 random areas within each tissue sample. Data with significant differences $p<0.05$ are highlighted bold. N=10-15 women

Study I) clinical trials in those women with the largest decrease in breast density, which tended to occur in women with higher baseline levels. Future well-powered clinical studies with women in the highest BI-RADS categories will allow researchers to determine if aspirin can be of benefit to women with high breast density.

Abbreviations

BC: Breast cancer; BI-RADS: Breast Imaging Reporting and Data System; CD4: T helper cells; CD8: Cytotoxic T cells; DCs: Dendritic cells; DCIS: Ductal carcinoma in situ; EDTA: Ethylenediaminetetraacetic acid; HMD: High mammographic density; IFN-γ: Interferon-γ; IL: Interleukin; LMD: Low mammographic density; MD: Mammographic density; MHC: Major histocompatibility complex; NK: Natural killer cells; NSAIDs: Nonsteroidal anti-inflammatory drugs; PD-1: Programmed cell death protein 1; PMD: Percent mammographic density; Treg: T helper regulatory cell

Acknowledgements

We thank St. Vincent's BreastScreen, St. Vincent's Hospital, for help with radiography and tissue sampling and Victorian Cancer Biobank and St. Vincent's Department of Pathology for assistance with tissue accrual, processing, and staining.

Funding

This work was supported in part by the Victorian Breast Cancer Research Consortium, the St. Vincent's Hospital (Melbourne) Research Endowment Fund, the National Breast Cancer Foundation (NBCF), the University of Melbourne Research Grant Support Scheme (MRGSS), and the Princess Alexandra Hospital Foundation. CWH was supported by the Australian Postgraduate Awards scholarship. KB was supported by an NBCF Early Career Fellowship. EDW was supported by funding from the Australian Government Department of Health and the Movember Foundation and Prostate Cancer Foundation of Australia through a Movember Revolutionary Team Award. EWT was supported in part by the NBCF through a National Collaborative Research Network award (CG-10-04). This study benefited from support provided by the Victorian Government's Operational Infrastructure Support Program to St. Vincent's Institute and to the Peter MacCallum Cancer Institute. The Translational Research Institute is supported by a grant from the Australian Government.

Authors' contributions

CWH carried out the majority of the experimental work, including collecting, processing, embedding, and staining tissues; performed data analyses and imaging; and drafted the manuscript. PH participated in histological results review and revised the manuscript. GC helped with some of the tissue sample accruals and revised the manuscript. PJN assisted with study design and interpretation of the data and revised the manuscript. HH assisted with study design and IHC staining and revised the manuscript. EDW performed some of the IHC staining and revised the manuscript. MAH assisted with study design, interpreted the data, and revised the manuscript. EWT helped with study design and interpretation of the data and revised the manuscript. KB led the study design, assisted with IHC staining and analysis of the data and revised the manuscript. All authors read and approved the final manuscript.

Competing interests

The authors declare that they have no competing interests.

Author details

[1]Department of Surgery, St. Vincent's Hospital, University of Melbourne, Melbourne, Australia. [2]Department of Pathology, St Vincent's Hospital, Melbourne, Australia. [3]Pathology Department, University of Melbourne, Melbourne, Australia. [4]Peter MacCallum Cancer Centre, Melbourne, Australia. [5]Institute of Health and Biomedical Innovation and School of Biomedical Sciences, Queensland University of Technology, Brisbane, Australia. [6]Translational Research Institute, Brisbane, Australia. [7]The Sir Peter MacCallum Department of Oncology, University of Melbourne, Melbourne, Australia.

References

1. Tice JA, O'Meara ES, Weaver DL, Vachon C, Ballard-Barbash R, Kerlikowske K. Benign breast disease, mammographic breast density, and the risk of breast cancer. J Natl Cancer Inst. 2013;105(14):1043–9.
2. Wolfe JN. The prominent duct pattern as an indicator of cancer risk. Oncology. 1969;23(2):149–58.
3. Egan RL, Mosteller RC. Breast cancer mammography patterns. Cancer. 1977; 40(5):2087–90.
4. Eriksson L, Czene K, Rosenberg L, Humphreys K, Hall P. Possible influence of mammographic density on local and locoregional recurrence of breast cancer. Breast Cancer Res. 2013;15(4):R56.
5. Cecchini RS, Costantino JP, Cauley JA, Cronin WM, Wickerham DL, Bandos H, Weissfeld JL, Wolmark N. Baseline mammographic breast density and the risk of invasive breast cancer in postmenopausal women participating in the NSABP study of tamoxifen and raloxifene (STAR). Cancer Prev Res (Phila). 2012;5(11):1321–9.

6. Linton L, Martin LJ, Li Q, Huszti E, Minkin S, John EM, Rommens J, Paterson AD, Boyd NF. Mammographic density and breast cancer: a comparison of related and unrelated controls in the Breast Cancer Family Registry. Breast Cancer Res. 2013;15(3):R43.

7. Yaghjyan L, Colditz GA, Collins LC, Schnitt SJ, Rosner B, Vachon C, Tamimi RM. Mammographic breast density and subsequent risk of breast cancer in postmenopausal women according to tumor characteristics. J Natl Cancer Inst. 2011;103(15):1179–89.

8. Yaghjyan L, Colditz GA, Rosner B, Tamimi RM. Mammographic breast density and subsequent risk of breast cancer in postmenopausal women according to the time since the mammogram. Cancer Epidemiol Biomarkers Prev. 2013;22(6):1110–7.

9. McCormack VA, dos Santos Silva I. Breast density and parenchymal patterns as markers of breast cancer risk: a meta-analysis. Cancer Epidemiol Biomarkers Prev. 2006;15(6):1159–69.

10. Ursin G, Hovanessian-Larsen L, Parisky YR, Pike MC, Wu AH. Greatly increased occurrence of breast cancers in areas of mammographically dense tissue. Breast Cancer Res. 2005;7(5):R605–8.

11. Ding J, Warren R, Girling A, Thompson D, Easton D. Mammographic density, estrogen receptor status and other breast cancer tumor characteristics. Breast J. 2010;16(3):279–89.

12. Kerlikowske K, Cook AJ, Buist DS, Cummings SR, Vachon C, Vacek P, Miglioretti DL. Breast cancer risk by breast density, menopause, and postmenopausal hormone therapy use. J Clin Oncol. 2010;28(24):3830–7.

13. Sala E, Solomon L, Warren R, McCann J, Duffy S, Luben R, Day N. Size, node status and grade of breast tumours: association with mammographic parenchymal patterns. Eur Radiol. 2000;10(1):157–61.

14. Buist DS, Porter PL, Lehman C, Taplin SH, White E. Factors contributing to mammography failure in women aged 40-49 years. J Natl Cancer Inst. 2004; 96(19):1432–40.

15. Carney PA, Miglioretti DL, Yankaskas BC, Kerlikowske K, Rosenberg R, Rutter CM, Geller BM, Abraham LA, Taplin SH, Dignan M, et al. Individual and combined effects of age, breast density, and hormone replacement therapy use on the accuracy of screening mammography. Ann Intern Med. 2003; 138(3):168–75.

16. Mason C, Yokubaitis K, Howard E, Shah Z, Wang J. Impact of Henda's law on the utilization of screening breast magnetic resonance imaging. Proc (Bayl Univ Med Cent). 2015;28(1):7–9.

17. Gur D, Klym AH, King JL, Bandos AI, Sumkin JH. Impact of the new density reporting laws: radiologist perceptions and actual behavior. Acad Radiol. 2015;22(6):679–83.

18. Sprague BL, Conant EF, Onega T, Garcia MP, Beaber EF, Herschorn SD, Lehman CD, Tosteson AN, Lacson R, Schnall MD, et al. Variation in mammographic breast density assessments among radiologists in clinical practice: a multicenter observational study. Ann Intern Med. 2016;165(7):457–64.

19. Chew GL, Huang D, Huo CW, Blick T, Hill P, Cawson J, Frazer H, Southey MD, Hopper JL, Henderson MA, et al. Dynamic changes in high and low mammographic density human breast tissues maintained in murine tissue engineering chambers during various murine peripartum states and over time. Breast Cancer Res Treat. 2013;140(2):285–97.

20. Chew GL, Huang D, Lin SJ, Huo C, Blick T, Henderson MA, Hill P, Cawson J, Morrison WA, Campbell IG, et al. High and low mammographic density human breast tissues maintain histological differential in murine tissue engineering chambers. Breast Cancer Res Treat. 2012;135(1):177–87.

21. Chew GL, Huo CW, Huang D, Blick T, Hill P, Cawson J, Frazer H, Southey MC, Hopper JL, Britt K, et al. Effects of tamoxifen and oestrogen on histology and radiographic density in high and low mammographic density human breast tissues maintained in murine tissue engineering chambers. Breast Cancer Res Treat. 2014;148(2):303–14.

22. Heusinger K, Jud SM, Haberle L, Hack CC, Adamietz BR, Meier-Meitinger M, Lux MP, Wittenberg T, Wagner F, Loehberg CR, et al. Association of mammographic density with hormone receptors in invasive breast cancers: results from a case-only study. Int J Cancer. 2012;131(11):2643–9.

23. Heusinger K, Jud SM, Haberle L, Hack CC, Fasching PA, Meier-Meitinger M, Lux MP, Hagenbeck C, Loehberg CR, Wittenberg T, et al. Association of mammographic density with the proliferation marker Ki-67 in a cohort of patients with invasive breast cancer. Breast Cancer Res Treat. 2012;135(3):885–92.

24. Vachon CM, Scott CG, Fasching PA, Hall P, Tamimi RM, Li J, Stone J, Apicella C, Odefrey F, Gierach GL, et al. Common breast cancer susceptibility variants in LSP1 and RAD51L1 are associated with mammographic density measures that predict breast cancer risk. Cancer Epidemiol Biomarkers Prev. 2012; 21(7):1156–66.

25. Ghosh K, Brandt KR, Reynolds C, Scott CG, Pankratz VS, Riehle DL, Lingle WL, Odogwu T, Radisky DC, Visscher DW, et al. Tissue composition of mammographically dense and non-dense breast tissue. Breast Cancer Res Treat. 2012;131(1):267–75.

26. Huo CW, Chew G, Hill P, Huang D, Ingman W, Hodson L, Brown KA, Magenau A, Allam AH, McGhee E, et al. High mammographic density is associated with an increase in stromal collagen and immune cells within the mammary epithelium. Breast Cancer Res. 2015;17:79.

27. Unsworth A, Anderson R, Britt K. Stromal fibroblasts and the immune microenvironment: partners in mammary gland biology and pathology? J Mammary Gland Biol Neoplasia. 2014;19(2):169–82.

28. Chew GL, Huo CW, Huang D, Hill P, Cawson J, Frazer H, Hopper JL, Haviv I, Henderson MA, Britt K, et al. Increased COX-2 expression in epithelial and stromal cells of high mammographic density tissues and in a xenograft model of mammographic density. Breast Cancer Res Treat. 2015;153(1):89–99.

29. Lin SJ, Cawson J, Hill P, Haviv I, Jenkins M, Hopper JL, Southey MC, Campbell IG, Thompson EW. Image-guided sampling reveals increased stroma and lower glandular complexity in mammographically dense breast tissue. Breast Cancer Res Treat. 2011;128(2):505–16.

30. Liang SC, Latchman YE, Buhlmann JE, Tomczak MF, Horwitz BH, Freeman GJ, Sharpe AH. Regulation of PD-1, PD-L1, and PD-L2 expression during normal and autoimmune responses. Eur J Immunol. 2003;33(10):2706–16.

31. Degnim AC, Hoskin TL, Arshad M, Frost MH, Winham SJ, Brahmbhatt RA, Pena A, Carter JM, Stallings-Mann ML, Murphy LM, et al. Alterations in the immune cell composition in premalignant breast tissue that precede breast Cancer development. Clin Cancer Res. 2017;23(14):3945–52.

32. DeNardo DG, Coussens LM. Inflammation and breast cancer. Balancing immune response: crosstalk between adaptive and innate immune cells during breast cancer progression. Breast Cancer Res. 2007;9(4):212.

33. Hussein MR, Hassan HI. Analysis of the mononuclear inflammatory cell infiltrate in the normal breast, benign proliferative breast disease, in situ and infiltrating ductal breast carcinomas: preliminary observations. J Clin Pathol. 2006;59(9):972–7.

34. Degnim AC, Brahmbhatt RD, Radisky DC, Hoskin TL, Stallings-Mann M, Laudenschlager M, Mansfield A, Frost MH, Murphy L, Knutson K, et al. Immune cell quantitation in normal breast tissue lobules with and without lobulitis. Breast Cancer Res Treat. 2014;144(3):539–49.

35. Murray PJ, Wynn TA. Protective and pathogenic functions of macrophage subsets. Nat Rev Immunol. 2011;11(11):723–37.

36. Sun X, Glynn DJ, Hodson LJ, Huo C, Britt K, Thompson EW, Woolford L, Evdokiou A, Pollard JW, Robertson SA, et al. CCL2-driven inflammation increases mammary gland stromal density and cancer susceptibility in a transgenic mouse model. Breast Cancer Res. 2017;19(1):4.

37. Sierra-Filardi E, Nieto C, Dominguez-Soto A, Barroso R, Sanchez-Mateos P, Puig-Kroger A, Lopez-Bravo M, Joven J, Ardavin C, Rodriguez-Fernandez JL, et al. CCL2 shapes macrophage polarization by GM-CSF and M-CSF: identification of CCL2/CCR2-dependent gene expression profile. J Immunol. 2014;192(8):3858–67.

38. Mauer J, Chaurasia B, Goldau J, Vogt MC, Ruud J, Nguyen KD, Theurich S, Hausen AC, Schmitz J, Bronneke HS, et al. Signaling by IL-6 promotes alternative activation of macrophages to limit endotoxemia and obesity-associated resistance to insulin. Nat Immunol. 2014;15(5):423–30.

39. Brown JA, Dorfman DM, Ma FR, Sullivan EL, Munoz O, Wood CR, Greenfield EA, Freeman GJ. Blockade of programmed death-1 ligands on dendritic cells enhances T cell activation and cytokine production. J Immunol. 2003;170(3): 1257–66.

40. Banchereau J, Steinman RM. Dendritic cells and the control of immunity. Nature. 1998;392(6673):245–52.

41. Waldhauer I, Steinle A. NK cells and cancer immunosurveillance. Oncogene. 2008;27(45):5932–43.

42. Mamessier E, Sylvain A, Thibult ML, Houvenaeghel G, Jacquemier J, Castellano R, Goncalves A, Andre P, Romagne F, Thibault G, et al. Human breast cancer cells enhance self tolerance by promoting evasion from NK cell antitumor immunity. J Clin Invest. 2011;121(9):3609–22.

43. Dong HP, Elstrand MB, Holth A, Silins I, Berner A, Trope CG, Davidson B,

Risberg B. NK- and B-cell infiltration correlates with worse outcome in metastatic ovarian carcinoma. Am J Clin Pathol. 2006;125(3):451–8.

44. Ledbetter JA, Gilliland LK, Schieven GL. The interaction of CD4 with CD3/Ti regulates tyrosine phosphorylation of substrates during T cell activation. Semin Immunol. 1990;2(2):99–106.

45. Pardoll DM. Immunology beats cancer: a blueprint for successful translation. Nat Immunol. 2012;13(12):1129–32.

46. Zhu J, Yamane H, Paul WE. Differentiation of effector CD4 T cell populations. Annu Rev Immunol. 2010;28:445–89.

47. Diehl S, Anguita J, Hoffmeyer A, Zapton T, Ihle JN, Fikrig E, Rincon M. Inhibition of Th1 differentiation by IL-6 is mediated by SOCS1. Immunity. 2000;13(6):805–15.

48. Diehl S, Rincon M. The two faces of IL-6 on Th1/Th2 differentiation. Mol Immunol. 2002;39(9):531–6.

49. Ozhand A, Lee E, Wu AH, Ellingjord-Dale M, Akslen LA, McKean-Cowdin R, Ursin G. Variation in inflammatory cytokine/growth-factor genes and mammographic density in premenopausal women aged 50-55. PLoS One. 2013;8(6):e65313.

50. Hanna M, Dumas I, Orain M, Jacob S, Tetu B, Sanschagrin F, Bureau A, Poirier B, Diorio C. Association between local inflammation and breast tissue age-related lobular involution among premenopausal and postmenopausal breast cancer patients. PLoS One. 2017;12(8):e0183579.

51. Nishimura H, Honjo T. PD-1: an inhibitory immunoreceptor involved in peripheral tolerance. Trends Immunol. 2001;22(5):265–8.

52. Okazaki T, Maeda A, Nishimura H, Kurosaki T, Honjo T. PD-1 immunoreceptor inhibits B cell receptor-mediated signaling by recruiting Src homology 2-domain-containing tyrosine phosphatase 2 to phosphotyrosine. Proc Natl Acad Sci U S A. 2001;98(24):13866–71.

53. Hamanishi J, Mandai M, Matsumura N, Abiko K, Baba T, Konishi I. PD-1/PD-L1 blockade in cancer treatment: perspectives and issues. Int J Clin Oncol. 2016; 21(3):462–73.

54. Freeman GJ, Long AJ, Iwai Y, Bourque K, Chernova T, Nishimura H, Fitz LJ, Malenkovich N, Okazaki T, Byrne MC, et al. Engagement of the PD-1 immunoinhibitory receptor by a novel B7 family member leads to negative regulation of lymphocyte activation. J Exp Med. 2000;192(7):1027–34.

55. Keir ME, Liang SC, Guleria I, Latchman YE, Qipo A, Albacker LA, Koulmanda M, Freeman GJ, Sayegh MH, Sharpe AH. Tissue expression of PD-L1 mediates peripheral T cell tolerance. J Exp Med. 2006;203(4):883–95.

56. Terme M, Ullrich E, Aymeric L, Meinhardt K, Desbois M, Delahaye N, Viaud S, Ryffel B, Yagita H, Kaplanski G, et al. IL-18 induces PD-1-dependent immunosuppression in cancer. Cancer Res. 2011;71(16):5393–9.

57. Francisco LM, Salinas VH, Brown KE, Vanguri VK, Freeman GJ, Kuchroo VK, Sharpe AH. PD-L1 regulates the development, maintenance, and function of induced regulatory T cells. J Exp Med. 2009;206(13):3015–29.

58. Chawla A, Philips AV, Alatrash G, Mittendorf E. Immune checkpoints: a therapeutic target in triple negative breast cancer. Oncoimmunology. 2014; 3(3):e28325.

59. Gatalica Z, Snyder C, Maney T, Ghazalpour A, Holterman DA, Xiao N, Overberg P, Rose I, Basu GD, Vranic S, et al. Programmed cell death 1 (PD-1) and its ligand (PD-L1) in common cancers and their correlation with molecular cancer type. Cancer Epidemiol Biomarkers Prev. 2014;23(12):2965–70.

60. Liu X, Gibbons RM, Harrington SM, Krco CJ, Markovic SN, Kwon ED, Dong H. Endogenous tumor-reactive CD8[+] T cells are differentiated effector cells expressing high levels of CD11a and PD-1 but are unable to control tumor growth. Oncoimmunology. 2013;2(6):e23972.

61. Moris D, Kontos M, Spartalis E, Fentiman IS. The role of NSAIDs in breast Cancer prevention and relapse: current evidence and future perspectives. Breast Care (Basel). 2016;11(5):339–44.

4

Polyfunctional anti-human epidermal growth factor receptor 3 (anti-HER3) antibodies induced by HER3 vaccines have multiple mechanisms of antitumor activity against therapy resistant and triple negative breast cancers

Takuya Osada[1], Zachary C. Hartman[1], Junping Wei[1], Gangjun Lei[1], Amy C. Hobeika[1], William R. Gwin[2], Marcio A. Diniz[3], Neil Spector[4], Timothy M. Clay[5,7], Wei Chen[6], Michael A. Morse[4] and H. Kim Lyerly[1]* (iD)

Abstract

Background: Upregulation of human epidermal growth factor receptor 3 (HER3) is a major mechanism of acquired resistance to therapies targeting its heterodimerization partners epidermal growth factor receptor (EGFR) and human epidermal growth factor receptor 2 (HER2), but also exposes HER3 as a target for immune attack. We generated an adenovirus encoding full length human HER3 (Ad-HER3) to serve as a cancer vaccine. Previously we reported the anti-tumor efficacy and function of the T cell response to this vaccine. We now provide a detailed assessment of the antitumor efficacy and functional mechanisms of the HER3 vaccine-induced antibodies (HER3-VIAs) in serum from mice immunized with Ad-HER3.

Methods: Serum containing HER3-VIA was tested in complement-dependent cytotoxicity (CDC) and antibody-dependent cellular cytotoxicity (ADCC) assays and for its effect on HER3 internalization and degradation, downstream signaling of HER3 heterodimers and growth of metastatic HER2+ (BT474M1), HER2 therapy-resistant (rBT474), and triple negative (MDA-MB-468) breast cancers.

Results: HER3-VIAs mediated CDC and ADCC, HER3 internalization, interruption of HER3 heterodimer-driven tumor signaling pathways, and anti-proliferative effects against HER2+ tumor cells in vitro and significant antitumor effects against metastatic HER2+ BT474M1, treatment refractory HER2+ rBT474 and triple negative MDA-MB-468 in vivo.

Conclusions: In addition to the T cell anti-tumor response induced by Ad-HER3, the HER3-VIAs provide additional functions to eliminate tumors in which HER3 signaling mediates aggressive behavior or acquired resistance to HER2-targeted therapy. These data support clinical studies of vaccination against HER3 prior to or concomitantly with other therapies to prevent outgrowth of therapy-resistant HER2+ and triple negative clones.

Keywords: HER3, HER2, Immunotherapy, Adenovirus, Polyclonal antibodies, ErbB3

* Correspondence: lyerl001@mc.duke.edu
[1]Division of Surgical Sciences, Department of Surgery, Duke University Medical Center, MSRB Research Drive, Box 2714, Durham, NC 27710, USA
Full list of author information is available at the end of the article

Background

Cancer vaccines targeting well-established tumor antigens have demonstrated modest activity in clinical trials performed in the era predating effective immune checkpoint blockade. Even with more potent vaccine strategies, tumor escape may occur due to downregulation or loss of targeted antigens, as such antigens, not critical for tumor survival and proliferation, may be subject to immune editing without affecting the malignant phenotype [1]. In contrast, targeting "driver" antigens that are critical components of cellular proliferation, survival, or resistance mechanisms is an attractive strategy, as these "driver" antigens cannot be downregulated or lost due to their requirement for maintenance of the malignant phenotype. Nonetheless, the adaptive immune response against chronically overexpressed tumor antigens is often minimized or diminished due to immune tolerance and/or immunoregulation [2]. We hypothesize that a novel therapeutic strategy would be to target proteins associated with the malignant phenotype or acquired therapeutic resistance that are initially sequestered from the immune system but may become upregulated upon the initiation of therapy or tumor progression. One such upregulated mediator of therapeutic resistance is the human epidermal growth factor receptor (HER) family member HER3, associated with poor prognosis in several epithelial malignancies including breast cancer.

Although having reduced catalytic kinase activity [1–4], HER3 is thought to function as a signaling substrate for other HER proteins with which it heterodimerizes [5] thus promoting tumor proliferation and survival [6]. Importantly, it is a co-receptor for epidermal growth factor receptor (EGFR) and HER2 with which it is synergistically co-transforming [7] and rate-limiting for transformed growth [8]. Treatment of HER2-amplified breast cancers with HER2-targeting tyrosine kinase inhibitors (TKIs) promotes an increase in HER3 plasma membrane localization and downstream signaling, which can lead to resistance to the HER2-targeted therapies [9–11]. HER3 expression has been associated with poor clinical outcomes including central nervous system (CNS) metastasis in both the triple negative (TNBC) and HER2 subtypes of breast cancer [12, 13].

The pivotal role of HER3 as a hub for HER family signaling has made it an attractive therapeutic target, but its reduced kinase activity has limited the development of small molecule inhibitors. One proven method has been to disrupt the HER2-HER3 heterodimer formation. The HER2-specific monoclonal antibody pertuzumab effectively disrupts heregulin-induced HER2-HER3 dimerization and signaling [14] and has proven clinical benefit. Nonetheless, it is less effective at disrupting the elevated basal state of ligand-independent HER2-HER3 interaction and signaling in HER2-overexpressing tumor cells [15]. Alternatively, HER3 may be targeted directly, specifically with antibodies having diverse functional consequences depending on their binding site [16]. For example, HER3-specific monoclonal antibodies inhibit ligand-induced activation of the receptor [17], inhibiting downstream signaling; however, none are currently commercially available.

As an alternative to monoclonal antibodies, we and others have demonstrated that polyclonal antibodies induced by vaccination against receptors such as HER2 can recognize the cell-expressed receptor, suppress its phosphorylation, mediate profound receptor internalization and degradation, and retard the growth of established receptor-dependent tumor xenografts [18, 19]. Further, rather than repeated administration of antibodies, vaccination induces long-term anti-tumor immune responses that can be periodically boosted. Therefore, we sought to generate a vaccine capable of inducing potent anti-HER3 antibody responses.

We recently reported generation of a recombinant adenoviral vector expressing human HER3 (Ad-HER3) and demonstrated that it induced HER3-specific T cell responses and had antitumor activity [20]. However, we are aware tumor antigen-specific T cell responses may be ineffective in some patients with advanced malignancies expressing the target tumor antigen and sought evidence of alternative antitumor mechanisms. Therefore, we examined whether Ad-HER3 vaccine-induced multifunctional antibody responses, including complement-dependent cytotoxicity (CDC) and antibody-dependent cellular cytotoxicity (ADCC), may mediate antitumor responses. In addition to the expected immune-mediated functions, we also wished to demonstrate whether serum containing anti-HER3 antibody (subsequently referred to as HER3-VIA) could have a direct effect on HER3 biology, specifically mediating HER3 internalization and degradation, as well as inhibiting the downstream signaling of HER3 heterodimers. Finally, we sought to demonstrate in vivo that HER3-specific polyclonal anti-HER3 serum alone, when transferred to tumor-bearing animals, retards growth of both HER2 therapy-resistant tumors and TNBC.

Methods

Cell lines and cell culture

The human breast cancer cell lines BT474, MCF-7, MDA-MB-231, MDA-MB-468, SKBR3, and T47D (obtained from the American Type Culture Collection (ATCC), Manassas, VA, USA) were grown in the recommended medium. The BT474M1 human breast tumor cell line (kind gift from Dr. Mien-Chie Hung at The University of Texas M. D. Anderson Cancer Center, Houston, TX, USA) was grown in DMEM/F12 with 10% FBS. Lapatinib-resistant BT474 (rBT474) was generated as previously described [21]. Frozen stocks of these cell lines were made at earlier passages, and after thawing, cells were cultured no longer than 8 weeks for the experiments. Cells were authenticated by morphology and growth curve analysis and were routinely tested for the absence of mycoplasma by PCR. All mycoplasma tests performed during this study were negative. For tumor challenge, cell lines were tested for rodent pathogens (IMPACT Profile III) and proven to be negative before the injection to mice.

Reagents

Trastuzumab (Herceptin™, Genentech, San Francisco, CA, USA) and cetuximab (Erbitux®, Bristol-Myers Squibb, New York, NY, USA) were purchased from the Duke University Medical Center Pharmacy. Lapatinib was purchased from Sigma-Aldrich (CDS022971, St. Louis, MO, USA). Heregulin (377-HB/CF), heregulin with a C-terminal 6-His tag (5898-NR) and allophycocyanin (APC)-conjugated anti-His Tag antibody (IC050A) were purchased from R&D Systems (Minneapolis, MN, USA).

Adenovirus vector preparation

The human HER3 complementary DNA (cDNA) was excised from a pCMVsport6-HER3-HsIMAGE6147464 plasmid (cDNA clone MGC:88033/IMAGE:6147464 obtained from ATCC). Construction of a first-generation (E1-, E3-) Ad vector containing human full length HER3 under control of human cytomegalovirus (CMV) promoter/enhancer elements was performed using the pAdEasy system (Agilent technologies, Santa Clara, CA, USA) as previously described [22–24]. Similar Ad-vectors containing the green fluorescence protein (GFP) or lacZ rather than HER3 was similarly generated to serve as controls.

Mice

BALB/c and NOD.CB17-$Prkdc^{scid}$/J mice were purchased from Jackson Labs (Bar Harbor, ME, USA). All mice were maintained under specific pathogen-free conditions, and all work was conducted in accordance with Duke Institutional Animal Care and Use Committee (IACUC)-approved protocols.

Production of vaccine-induced antibodies (VIA)

BALB/c mice were vaccinated on day 0 and day 14 by footpad injection of Ad-GFP (control), or Ad-HER3 vectors (2.6×10^{10} particles/ mouse). At 14 days after the second vaccination, mice were euthanized and serum was collected, pooled from every 20 vaccinated mice, and 1-mL aliquots were made and stored at – 80 °C until use. Approximately 80 mice for HER3-VIA and 80 mice for control VIA were vaccinated to collect and pool serum (24 mL for both VIAs) for this study.

Cell-based ELISA

The 4 T1 cells were transduced with the HER3 gene by lentiviral vectors (4 T1-HER3 cell): 4 T1 and 4 T1-HER3 cells were incubated overnight at 37 °C in 96-well plates (3×10^4 cells/well). Mouse serum (HER3-VIA, LacZ-VIA, GFP-VIA) was diluted (final titrations 1:50 ~ 1:6400), added to the wells (50 μL/well), and incubated for 1 h on ice. The plates were washed with PBS twice, and then cells were fixed with diluted formalin (1:10 dilution).Then, near infrared (nIR) dye-conjugated anti-mouse IgG (IRDye 800CW, LI-COR Biosciences, Lincoln, NE, USA) was added (1:2000 dilution, 30 min, room temperature). After washing with PBS, the nIR signal was detected by a LI-COR Odyssey Imager (LI-COR) at 800 nm channel.

Analysis of anti-HER3 antibody binding by flow cytometry

HER3 vaccine-induced antibodies in vaccinated mouse serum were measured by flow cytometry as reported [25]. Briefly, 3×10^5 human breast cancer cells were incubated with diluted (1:100 to 1:51200) mouse, post-vaccine serum (HER3-VIA or GFP-VIA) for 1 h at 4 °C and then washed with 1% BSA-PBS. The cells were further stained with phycoerythrin (PE)-conjugated anti-mouse IgG (Dako, catalog number R0480) for 30 min at 4 °C and washed again. Samples were analyzed on a BD LSRII flow cytometer (Becton Dickenson, San Jose, CA, USA) and mean fluorescence intensity (MFI) reported. For the analysis of HER family expression on tumor cells, PE-conjugated anti-EGFR, anti-HER2 (BD Biosciences), and anti-HER3 antibody (BioLegend) were used as in the manufacturer's instructions.

Detection of HER3 epitopes bound by vaccine-induced antibody

Epitopes were mapped using spotted peptide arrays of 15-mer peptides overlapping by four amino acids representing the full length of the human HER3 protein. HER3 peptides were coated onto cellulose membranes using a Spot Robot ASP 222 (AbiMed) and HER3-VIA (1:100 dilution in saline) epitopes were mapped as described [26].

Heregulin binding assay

BT474 cells (HER3+) were incubated with medium containing no serum at 37 °C for 24 h. At 30 min before the assay, the culture plates were placed at 4 °C to avoid internalization of HER3 receptor. The following procedures were performed on ice. Cells were pre-incubated with heregulin (final concentrations: 0, 10, 100 nM) or GFP-VIA/HER3-VIA (final dilution: 1:100) for 10 min, then heregulin-His Tag (final concentration: 100 nM) was added and further incubated for 10 min. After washing three times with cold PBS, cells were incubated with APC-conjugated anti-His Tag antibody for 30 min. Cells were washed with cold PBS three times, harvested from the flask, and analyzed using the LSRII flow cytometer.

MTT assay to detect cell proliferation

The effect of HER3-VIA on the proliferation of human breast cancer cell lines was measured as previously described [27]. Briefly, 5000 cells per well were cultured in a 96-well plate with HER3-VIA (1:33 dilution), GFP-VIA (1:33 dilution) or trastuzumab 20 µg/ml for 3 days and proliferation was assessed by a 3-(4,5-dimethylthiazol-2-yl)-2.5-diphenyltetrazolium bromide (MTT) assay.

Assessment of HER3 internalization

Human HER3+ breast cancer cells (SKBR3, BT474M1 and MDA-MB-468) were incubated with 1:100 HER3-VIA or GFP-VIA at 37 °C for 60 min (SKBR3, BT474M1) or 3 h (MDA-MB-468). After washing, fixation with 4% paraformaldehyde (PFA), and application of permeabilizing solution 2 (Becton Dickenson), nonspecific binding was blocked with 2.5% goat serum at 37 °C for 30 min. Cells were incubated with 1:100 Red™-conjugated anti-mouse IgG (H + L) (Jackson ImmunoResearch Laboratories Inc. West Grove, PA, USA) in a dark chamber for 1 h at room temperature and washed with PBS. For the detection of EGFR, MDA-MB-468 cells were incubated with HER3-VIA for 3 h, then fixed and permeabilized. Cells were then labeled with cetuximab (40 µg/mL) for 10 min, followed by staining with Cy2-conjugated anti-human IgG antibody (ab97169, Abcam, Cambridge, MA, USA). For the detection of HER2, SKBR3 cells were labeled with trastuzumab (40 µg/mL) for 10 min, washed with medium, and then incubated with HER3-VIA for 3 h. Then, cells were fixed and permeabilized, and stained with Cy2-conjugated anti-human IgG antibody. Slides were mounted in VectaShield containing 4′,6-diamidino-2-phenylindole (DAPI) (Vector Laboratories, Burlingame, CA, USA) and images were acquired using a Zeiss Axio Observer wide-field fluorescence microscope (Carl Zeiss, München--Hallbergmoos, Germany).

Complement-dependent cytotoxicity assay

We performed complement-dependent cytotoxicity assays using our previously published protocol [27]. Briefly, target cells were incubated with rabbit serum (1:100) as a source of complement and the HER3-VIA or GFP-VIA in serum from mice immunized as above diluted (1:100), or trastuzumab (20 µg/mL) at 37 °C for 2 h. After incubation, cytotoxicity was measured using the CytoTox 96 Nonradioactive Cytotoxicity Assay (Promega; per manufacturer's instructions) to measure lactate dehydrogenase (LDH) release in the culture medim as evidence of cytotoxicity.

Antibody-dependent cell-mediated cytotoxicity assay

Antibody-dependent cell-mediated cytotoxicity was measured against HER3-expressing JC-HER3 cells and parental JC cells (HER3-negative) using mFcγRIV ADCC Reporter Bioassay (Promega, catalog number M1211). Target cells (25,000 or 10,000 cells/well) were seeded into 96-well plates, incubated overnight, and pre-incubated with 1:10 dilution of HER3-VIA or GFP-VIA for 30 min at room temperature. Then, effector cells were applied per manufacturer's instructions. Two different effector-target ratios (3:1, 7.5:1) were tested. After 6 h of co-incubation, Bio-Glo™ Reagent was added, and luminescence was measured. Luminescence of JC cells was subtracted from luminescence of JC-HER3 cells for each VIA.

Treatment of established HER3+ human breast tumor xenografts by passive transfer of vaccine-induced antibodies

BT474M1 cells, lapatinib-resistant rBT474 cells, or MDA-MB-468 cells (5×10^6, 1×10^6, 1×10^6 cells/mouse, respectively) were implanted in the mammary fat pads of 8–10-week-old NOD.CB17-$Prkdc^{scid}$/J mice. At 2 days prior to tumor implantation, 17-beta-estradiol pellets (0.72 mg 60-day continuous release pellets; Innovative Research of American, Sarasota, FL, USA) were subcutaneously implanted in the backs of the mice, except for the experiment with MDA-MB-468 cells. Tumors were allowed to develop for 14 days (BT474M1), 2 months (rBT474), or 12 days (MDA-MB-468), to reach the volume of approximately 50–100 mm^3, and then mice were randomized to receive intravenous injection of either GFP-VIA or HER3-VIA. VIA (100–150 µL) was injected at 2–3-day intervals for a total of 10 administrations. Tumor growth was measured in two dimensions using calipers and tumor volume was determined using the formula:

$$\text{Volume} = \tfrac{1}{2}\left[(\text{Width})^2 \text{x (Length)}\right].$$

Western blotting to analyze pathway inhibition

Tumors were isolated from euthanized, VIA-treated mice and immediately flash frozen. Tissue extracts were prepared as previously described [27]. Equal amounts of proteins (50 µg) were resolved by 4–15% gradient SDS PAGE. After transfer, membranes were probed with specific antibodies recognizing target proteins: pTyr (Sigma), ErbB2, ErbB3, Akt, pAkt473, Erk 1/2, pErk1/2 (Cell Signaling, Beverly, MA, USA), survivin, actin (Sigma, St. Louis, MO, USA), 4EBP-1, p4EBP-1, s6, ps6 (Santa Cruz Biotech, Santa Cruz, CA, USA), and then with IRDye 800 conjugated anti-rabbit or mouse IgG or Alexa Fluor 680 anti-rabbit IgG, and were visualized using the Odyssey

Infrared Imaging System (LI-COR, Lincoln, NE, USA) as previously described [27].

Immunohistochemical analysis of HER3 expression in tumor tissue

BT474M1 or rBT474 tumors were collected when mice were sacrificed, fixed with 10% neutral-buffered formalin, and embedded to paraffin. Tissue sections of 4 μm thick were deparaffinized, and heat-induced antigen retrieval was performed in sodium citrate buffer for 20 min. After blocking endogenous peroxidase activity with 3% H_2O_2, 10% normal horse serum was applied for the blocking of nonspecific binding sites. Anti-HER3 antibody (Santa Cruz) was put on the sections and incubated overnight at 4 °C. After washing with PBS, biotinylated secondary antibody (Bio-Rad) was applied for 30 min, followed by an VECTASTAIN ABC kit (Vector Lab) and then the color was developed using the DAB Peroxidase substrate kit (Vector Lab). Counterstaining was performed with hematoxylin.

Statistical analysis

Tumor volume over time was standardized by the baseline tumor volume. Area under the tumor growth curve was calculated under spline interpolation [28] and adaptive quadrature. Groups were compared based on the Kruskal-Wallis test [29] followed by multiple comparisons performed by the non-parametric Tukey test [30]. If only two groups were compared then the Mann-Whitney test [31] was applied. Normality assumption was verified by the Shapiro-Francia test [32] and homogeneity of variances by the Levene test [33]. Difference in luminescence intensity in the ADCC assay was analyzed by Fisher's exact test. All tests of hypotheses were two-sided, with a significance level of 0.05. Calculations were performed using R, version 3.2.5 [34].

Results

Ad-HER3 activates anti-HER3 antibody responses

We first assessed the antibody response to the Ad-HER3 vaccine. We vaccinated BALB/c mice twice at a 14-day interval with a recombinant E1-, E3- adenovirus serotype 5 vector expressing full length human HER3 (Ad-HER3) and 14 days later collected the serum for analysis. To detect HER3-specific antibodies that could recognize membrane-associated HER3, binding of vaccine-induced antibodies (VIA) in mouse serum was first tested using a cell-based ELISA against a murine triple negative breast cancer cell line (4 T1) transduced to express HER3 (4 T1-HER3) (Fig. 1a). Mice vaccinated with Ad-HER3 had serum titers > 1:800 against the 4 T1-HER3 cells, in contrast to the mice receiving control Ad-LacZ and Ad-GFP vaccines, which only displayed background levels of binding (Fig. 1a). We then tested HER3-VIA for binding to a series of human HER3-expressing breast tumor cell lines, including the high HER3-expressing BT474M1 and BT474, the moderately HER3-expressing SKBR3 and T47D, and the HER3 low/negative, triple negative MDA-MB-231 tumor cell lines (Fig. 1b). Serum from Ad-HER3-vaccinated mice demonstrated titers > 1/ 800 against the human high HER3-expressing cell lines and there was no binding to the HER3 low/negative cell lines (Fig. 1b). The apparent titer correlated with the extent of HER3 expression in the cell lines (Additional file 1: Figure S1).

To confirm the binding of the HER3 vaccine-induced antibodies (HER3-VIA), we also performed flow cytometric analysis of HER3-expressing BT474 exposed to the HER3-VIA serum followed by a secondary antibody to detect the presence of HER3 bound antibody (Fig. 1c): 99% of the BT474 cells stained positively with the HER3-VIA, similar to that seen with a commercially available monoclonal antibody. These data demonstrate that antibodies within the HER3-VIA bind to endogenous HER3-expressed on human breast cancer cell lines.

To demonstrate that the HER3-VIA response was polyclonal, and to confirm that multiple HER3 epitopes could be recognized, we tested pooled HER3-VIA for binding to a series of HER3 peptides displayed as peptide arrays. The HER3-VIA recognized at least 18 epitopes in both the intracellular and extracellular domain of HER3 (Additional file 2: Table S1). Surprisingly none of these epitopes included the reported heregulin binding site [35]. It should be noted that peptide arrays do not recapitulate conformationally correct protein structures. Therefore, we wished to confirm that HER3-VIA did not block the binding of the ligand, heregulin, to HER3. To detect the binding of heregulin we used His-tagged heregulin, which could be detected by fluorescently conjugated anti-His Tag antibody. We confirmed that the His-tagged heregulin could occupy the heregulin binding site on HER3 by demonstrating that it could compete with untagged heregulin in a concentration-dependent fashion in BT474 cells (Fig. 1d). His-tagged heregulin binding to HER3 on BT474 cells was not affected by HER3-VIA when the assay was performed on ice to maintain the receptor on the cell surface (Fig. 1d). Taken together, these data demonstrate that the polyclonal HER3-VIA binds to multiple sites on HER3, but not the heregulin binding site.

HER3-VIA mediates complement-dependent cytotoxicity

Having demonstrated that the HER3-VIA contains antibodies with multiple specificities, we were interested to determine whether this resulted in multiple different functions. Because direct antibody-mediated tumor cell binding and killing is an established mechanism of action of antibodies induced by vaccination, we evaluated the capacity of HER3-VIA to mediate complement-dependent

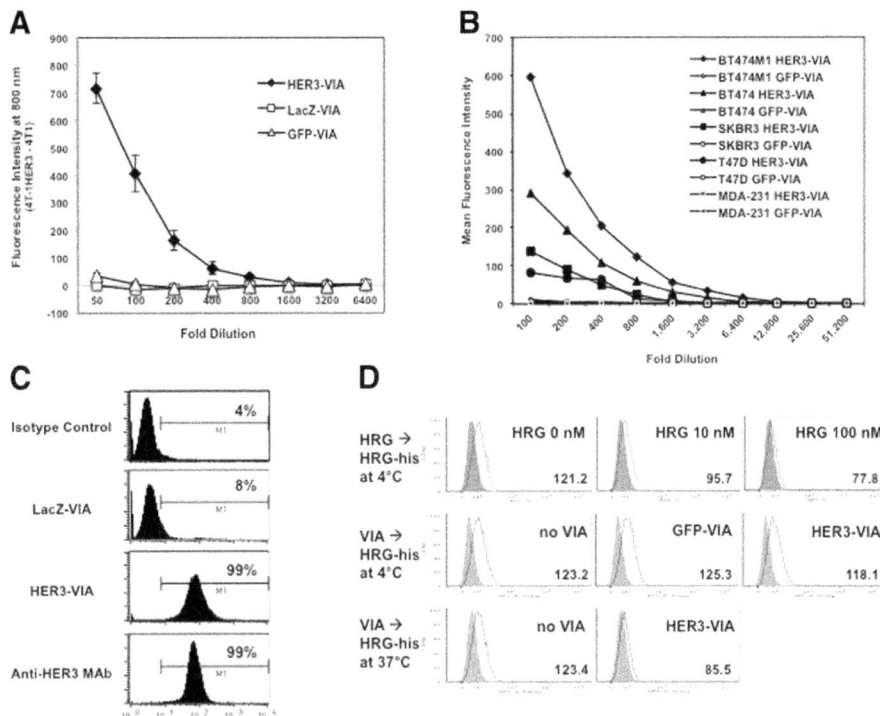

Fig. 1 Human epidermal growth factor receptor 3 (HER3)-specific antibody responses are induced by adenovirus encoding full length human HER3 (Ad-HER3) in vivo. **a** Binding of vaccine-induced antibody (VIA) in serum from mice immunized with Ad-HER3 (HER3-VIA), Ad-lacZ (lacZ-VIA), and Ad-green fluorescence protein (GFP-VIA). Serum at dilutions presented were mixed with the HER3-4 T1 cell line or wild-type 4 T1 and binding of antibody was identified with near infrared (nIR) dye-conjugated anti-mouse IgG and detected by a LI-COR Odyssey Imager. The difference in fluorescence intensity between HER3-4 T1 and 4 T1 is graphed. **b** Binding of HER3-VIA to breast cancer cell lines: a panel of human breast cancer cell lines were incubated with dilutions of the HER3-VIA, washed, and then mixed with a phycoerythrin (PE)-conjugated secondary antibody. HER3-VIA binding was analyzed based on fluorescence activated cell sorting analysis and mean fluorescence intensity was reported. **c** Flow cytometric analysis was used to identify percentage of BT474 cells able to bind HER3-VIA (1:100 dilution). **d** Binding of His-tagged heregulin to HER3 receptor was measured by pre-incubating BT474 cells with heregulin (0, 10, 100 nM), or HER3-VIA (1:100) for 10 min on ice, followed by incubation with His-tagged heregulin (100 nM) for 10 min. Receptor-bound His-tagged heregulin was visualized by staining with PE-conjugated anti-His Tag antibody. Mean fluorescence intensity is shown in each histogram

cytotoxicity (CDC). HER3-VIA exhibited significant CDC against a number of HER3-expressing human breast tumor cells but not the HER3-negative MDA-MB-231 cell line, while control LacZ-VIA did not mediate CDC (Fig. 2a). There was lower but detectable CDC against the HER3+ triple negative cell line MDA-MB-468. Further, HER3-VIA mediated similar levels of CDC against BT474 and its metastatic variant BT474-M1. As previously observed, trastuzumab did not mediate CDC. These data demonstrate immune-mediated anti-tumor activity for HER3-VIA.

HER3-VIA induces antibody-dependent cell-mediated cytotoxicity (ADCC)

We tested the ability of Ad-HER3 VIA to mediate ADCC against HER3-expressing tumor cells. ADCC activity was measured through the detection of mFcγRIV-mediated signaling in a reporter bioassay. With a 1:10 dilution of HER3-VIA and GFP-VIA, there was significantly stronger activation of the mFcγRIV-mediated signaling pathway

when HER3-VIA was co-incubated with effector and target cells, suggesting that HER3-VIA can mediate killing of HER3-expressing cells through ADCC (Fig. 2b).

Anti-proliferative effects of HER3-VIA in vitro

Although immunization with Ad-HER3 did induce antibodies with expected immune function (CDC and ADCC), we also wished to determine whether the induced antibodies could inhibit tumor cell proliferation through effects on signaling pathways governed by HER3. We found that when human breast cancer cells highly expressing HER3 (such as BT474 and highly metastatic variant BT474M1) were cultured with HER3-VIA, their proliferation was significantly inhibited compared with cells cultured with control LacZ-VIA (Fig. 2c). Of interest, the HER2/HER3 expressing tumor cells were similarly responsive to the growth inhibitory effect of the HER3-VIA as they were to the anti-HER2 antibody trastuzumab. The MDA-MB-468 cells moderately expressing HER3 and the HER3-negative MDA-MB-231 cells

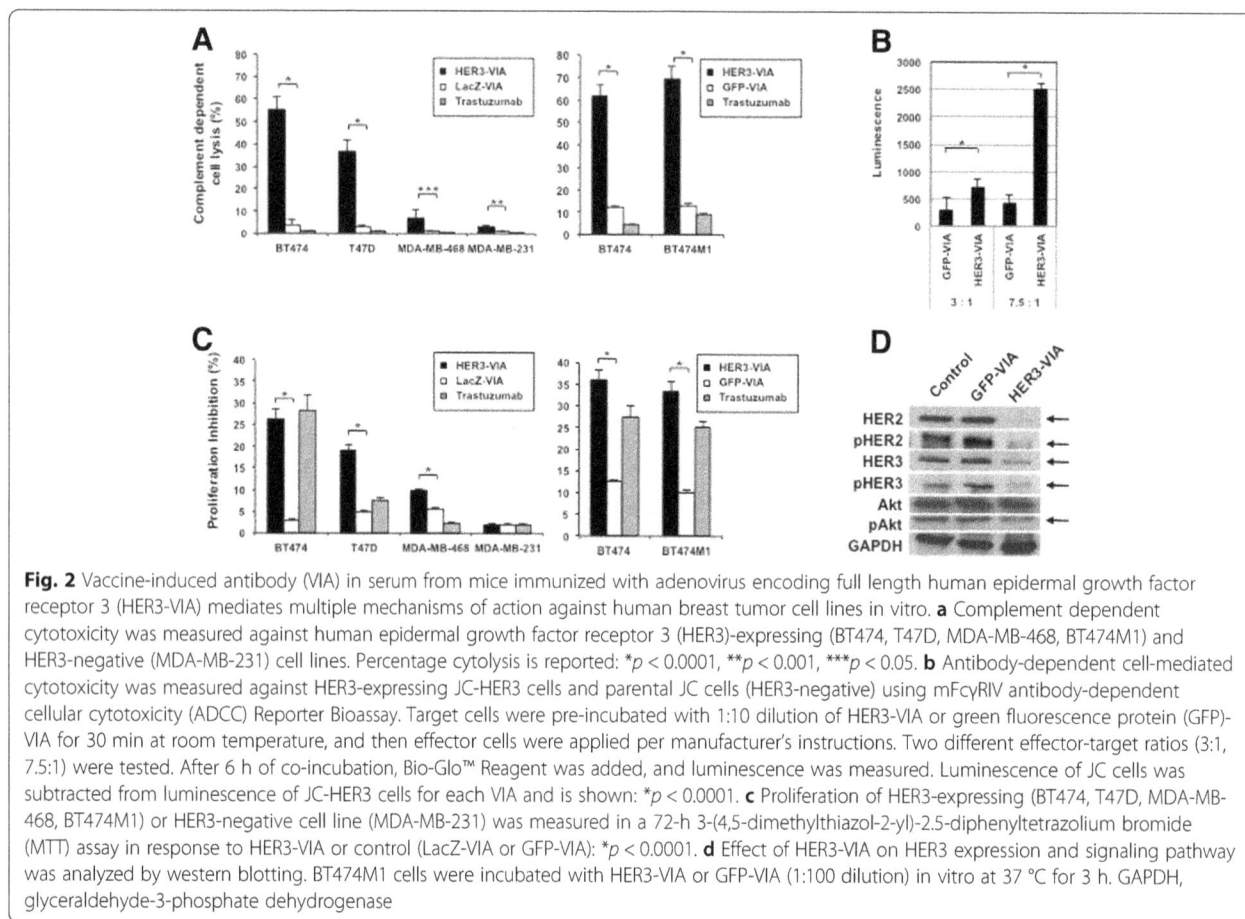

Fig. 2 Vaccine-induced antibody (VIA) in serum from mice immunized with adenovirus encoding full length human epidermal growth factor receptor 3 (HER3-VIA) mediates multiple mechanisms of action against human breast tumor cell lines in vitro. **a** Complement dependent cytotoxicity was measured against human epidermal growth factor receptor 3 (HER3)-expressing (BT474, T47D, MDA-MB-468, BT474M1) and HER3-negative (MDA-MB-231) cell lines. Percentage cytolysis is reported: *$p < 0.0001$, **$p < 0.001$, ***$p < 0.05$. **b** Antibody-dependent cell-mediated cytotoxicity was measured against HER3-expressing JC-HER3 cells and parental JC cells (HER3-negative) using mFcγRIV antibody-dependent cellular cytotoxicity (ADCC) Reporter Bioassay. Target cells were pre-incubated with 1:10 dilution of HER3-VIA or green fluorescence protein (GFP)-VIA for 30 min at room temperature, and then effector cells were applied per manufacturer's instructions. Two different effector-target ratios (3:1, 7.5:1) were tested. After 6 h of co-incubation, Bio-Glo™ Reagent was added, and luminescence was measured. Luminescence of JC cells was subtracted from luminescence of JC-HER3 cells for each VIA and is shown: *$p < 0.0001$. **c** Proliferation of HER3-expressing (BT474, T47D, MDA-MB-468, BT474M1) or HER3-negative cell line (MDA-MB-231) was measured in a 72-h 3-(4,5-dimethylthiazol-2-yl)-2,5-diphenyltetrazolium bromide (MTT) assay in response to HER3-VIA or control (LacZ-VIA or GFP-VIA): *$p < 0.0001$. **d** Effect of HER3-VIA on HER3 expression and signaling pathway was analyzed by western blotting. BT474M1 cells were incubated with HER3-VIA or GFP-VIA (1:100 dilution) in vitro at 37 °C for 3 h. GAPDH, glyceraldehyde-3-phosphate dehydrogenase

had only slight (~ 10%) and no growth inhibition by HER3-VIA, respectively, suggesting that the growth inhibitory effect of the HER3-VIA was correlated with HER3 expression. These data demonstrate that the HER3-VIA has anti-tumor functionality beyond the expected immune-mediated cell killing.

Downregulation of HER3 expression and signaling inhibition by HER3-VIA

Growth factor receptor downregulation by internalization and degradation has been proposed as a mechanism for the inhibition of tumor growth mediated by monoclonal antibodies. BT474M1 cells exposed in vitro to HER3-VIA demonstrated downregulation of HER3 and HER2 expression and inhibition of pHER3 and pAkt signaling (Fig. 2d). To ascertain whether receptor downregulation was caused by HER3-VIA and was a consequence of receptor internalization, we visualized cell membrane-associated HER3 on SKBR3 and BT474M1 tumor cells. When exposed to serum containing either HER3-VIA or GFP-VIA, the HER3-VIA exposure resulted in dramatic internalization and aggregation of the receptor within 1 h after exposure to HER3-VIA, but this was not observed with exposure to control GFP-VIA (Fig. 3a). Similar results were observed

for the HER3-expressing, TNBC cell line MDA-MB-468 when exposed to the HER3-VIA (Fig. 3b). These data demonstrate that the HER3-activated polyclonal antibodies are able to mediate HER3 internalization in both HER2-positive and TNBC cells.

There are two consequences of the downregulation of HER3; one is the lack of sites for ligand binding and the other is the loss of a heterodimer partner for EGFR or HER2. Indeed, we observed that when BT474 cells were pre-incubated with HER3-VIA for 3 h at 37 °C, the amount of bound His-tagged heregulin was much smaller, suggesting that HER3 was downregulated by VIA-induced internalization (Fig. 1d). These data suggest that the mechanism of action for the anti-proliferative effect of HER3-VIA is not interference with ligand binding but rather cell surface receptor loss interfering with signaling.

Receptor tyrosine kinases of the EGFR family are known to form homodimers or heterodimers. Therefore, we tested the effect of HER3-VIA on HER2 and EGFR expression using fluorescence microscopy (Fig. 3c, c). For some cancer cell lines, such as BT474M1, HER2 was slightly downregulated after 3 h incubation with HER3-VIA (Fig. 2d), but the trend was not clear in other cell lines. The inconsistency may derive from the different environments, such as

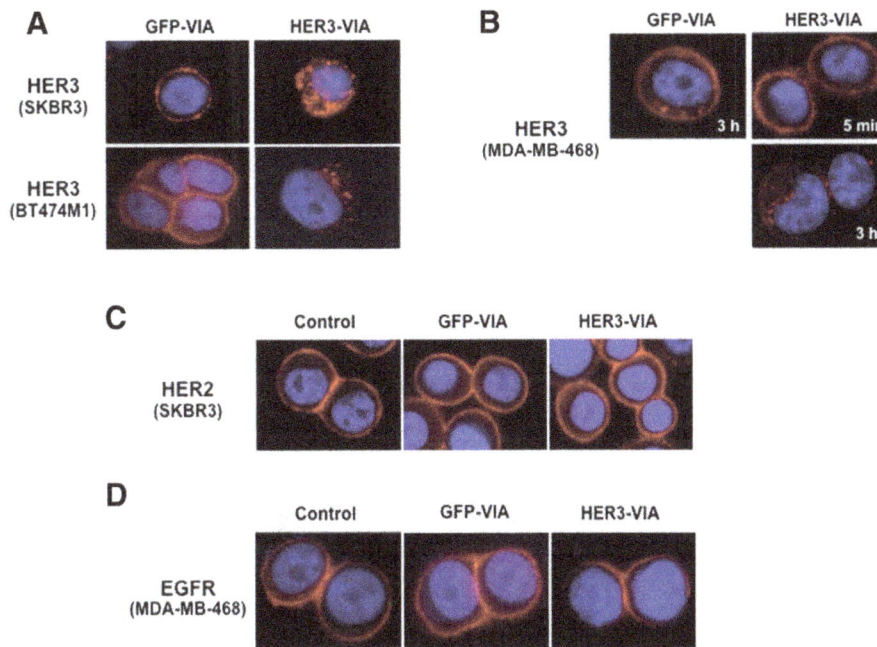

Fig. 3 Vaccine-induced antibody (VIA) in serum from mice immunized with adenovirus encoding full length human 3 epidermal growth factor receptor (HER3-VIA) induces receptor internalization and downregulation of human epidermal growth factor receptor 3 (HER3), but not epidermal growth factor receptor (EGFR) nor HER2. SKBR3, BT474-M1 (**a**) and MDA-MB-468 (**b**) were incubated with 1:100 HER3-VIA or green fluorescence protein (GFP)-VIA at 37 °C for 1 or 3 h, respectively. After washing and permeabilization, RedTM-conjugated anti-mouse IgG (H + L) was used to visualize internalization of the VIA-bound proteins with a fluorescence microscope. SKBR3 cells (**c**) or MDA-MB-468 cells (**d**) were incubated with 1:100 HER3-VIA or GFP-VIA at 37 °C for 3 h. Cells were fixed, permeabilized and stained with anti-HER2 antibody (trastuzumab, 40 μg/mL) (**c**) or anti-EGFR antibody (cetuximab, 40 μg/mL) (**d**), followed by Cy2-conjugated anti-human IgG antibody

production of heregulin by cancer cells, because heregulin will induce the heterodimerization of HER2/HER3. For SKBR3 cells, HER2 internalization was not evident (Fig. 3c). We did not find any significant effect for the EGFR expression on cell surface by exposure to HER3-VIA (Fig. 3d). Other monoclonal antibodies (trastuzumab, cetuximab) and small molecule inhibitor (lapatinib) as well as GFP-VIA/HER3-VIA were examined for their effect on cell surface expression of EGFR, HER2 and HER3 by flow cytometry (Additional file 3: Figure S2). Trastuzumab and Cetuximab did not decrease the surface expression of their target HER receptors, while HER3-VIA substantially decreased the surface expression of HER3. Lapatinib induced slight decrease of EGFR expression, and gradually enhanced HER2 and HER3 expression on the cell surface by the 24 h time point. Thus, the downregulation of cell surface HER3 was specific with HER3-VIA treatment.

Inhibition of HER2+/HER3+ tumor growth by HER3-VIA in vivo

After finding that HER3-specific antibodies inhibited HER3+ tumor cell proliferation in vitro, we sought to demonstrate the effects of HER3-VIA in vivo against the metastatic human xenograft model BT474M1 that expresses both HER2 and HER3 (Fig. 4a). The mouse model

that allowed engraftment of human tumor cells lack functional T and B cells, but also lack complement and ADCC effector cells, so these studies should focus on the direct antitumor functions of HER3 VIA. Systemically administered HER3-VIA prevented the growth of the established BT474M1 ($p < 0.001$) when compared to the control GFP-VIA-treated mice (Fig. 4b). Further, residual tumor in mice treated with HER3-VIA had decreased levels of HER3, indicating either downregulation of HER3 or elimination of tumor cells expressing HER3 (Fig. 4c). The decrease in HER3 expression following HER3-VIA administration was associated with a decrease in pHER2 (pTyr) and pAKT (Fig. 4d). These data demonstrate that the polyfunctional anti-HER3 antibodies downregulate HER3 expression and signaling in tumors overexpressing HER2/HER3.

Inhibition of therapy-resistant tumor growth by HER3-VIA in vivo

Having demonstrated anti-tumor activity for HER3-VIA in parental breast cancer cells lines, we extended our work to evaluate whether anti-tumor activity could be demonstrated against resistant variants, specifically tumor cells resistant to HER2-targeting therapies. Therefore, we tested the effects of HER3-VIA using a lapatinib-resistant cell

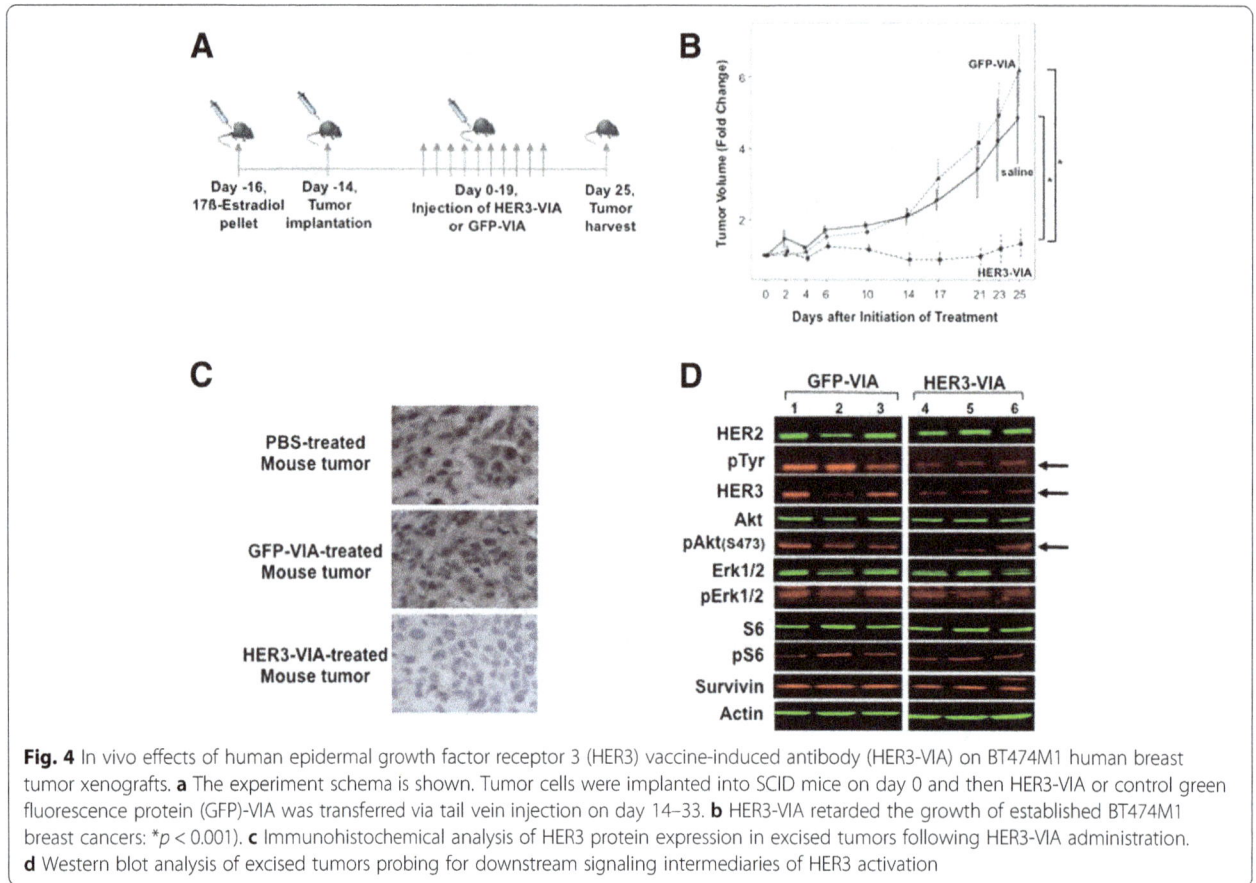

Fig. 4 In vivo effects of human epidermal growth factor receptor 3 (HER3) vaccine-induced antibody (HER3-VIA) on BT474M1 human breast tumor xenografts. **a** The experiment schema is shown. Tumor cells were implanted into SCID mice on day 0 and then HER3-VIA or control green fluorescence protein (GFP)-VIA was transferred via tail vein injection on day 14–33. **b** HER3-VIA retarded the growth of established BT474M1 breast cancers: *$p < 0.001$. **c** Immunohistochemical analysis of HER3 protein expression in excised tumors following HER3-VIA administration. **d** Western blot analysis of excised tumors probing for downstream signaling intermediaries of HER3 activation

line (rBT474), which we confirmed expresses HER2 and HER3 at similar levels to the BT474 tumor line (Fig. 5a), derived as previously reported [20]. The HER3-VIA retarded the growth of the established lapatinib-resistant tumors ($p < 0.01$) (Fig. 5b). As observed for the parental cell line, the residual laptinib-resistant tumor had decreased expression of HER3 (Fig. 5c). Decreased HER2:-HER3 signaling following HER3-VIA was demonstrated by the deceased pTyr, pAkt473(S473), pErk1/2, p4EBP1, survivin and pS6, relative to the control GFP-VIA-treated tumors. These data demonstrate that the HER3-VIA antibody response to Ad-HER3 immunization has therapeutic potential against treatment-resistant cell lines.

Inhibition of TNBC growth by HER3-VIA in vivo

Because a subset of TNBC express HER3, we wished to determine if the antitumor activity observed for HER3-VIA in HER2-expressing cell lines would also be observed in TNBC cell lines. EGFR is known to heterodimerize with HER3 on triple negative MDA-MB-468 cells. We confirmed the expression of EGFR and HER3 on MDA-MB-468 cells, and binding of HER3-VIA to the cells by flow cytometry (Fig. 6a). We also tested the effect of HER3-VIA treatment on the signaling pathway in MDA-MB-468 cells in vitro. In this study, cells were

incubated with HER3-VIA (1:100 dilution in the culture medium) at 37 °C for the indicated time. Decreased expression of HER3 and pAkt was observed after either 1-h or 3-h incubation, suggesting an effect on signal transduction by HER3-VIA treatment (Fig. 6b). In NOD.CB17-*Prkdc*[scid]/J mice bearing MDA-MB-468, HER3-VIA slowed tumor growth (Fig. 6c) when compared to controls ($p < 0.001$). We also analyzed HER3 expression and signaling in the MDA-MB-468 tumors treated with HER3-VIA. Again, HER3-VIA treatment was associated with a decrease in HER3 and pHER3 expression as analyzed by western blot (Fig. 6d). These data confirm that the HER3-VIA downregulates HER3 expression in both HER2+ and TNBC. However, there was no clear decrease in pAkt (S473) or pErk1/2. These data suggest a complex effect of the polyclonal antibodies on downstream signaling from the HER3 receptor, which may differ depending on the tumor subtype targeted.

Discussion

Although EGFR and HER2-targeted therapy has substantial activity in EGFR and HER2-overexpressing malignancies, respectively, therapeutic resistance and progression eventually develops in responders with metastatic disease

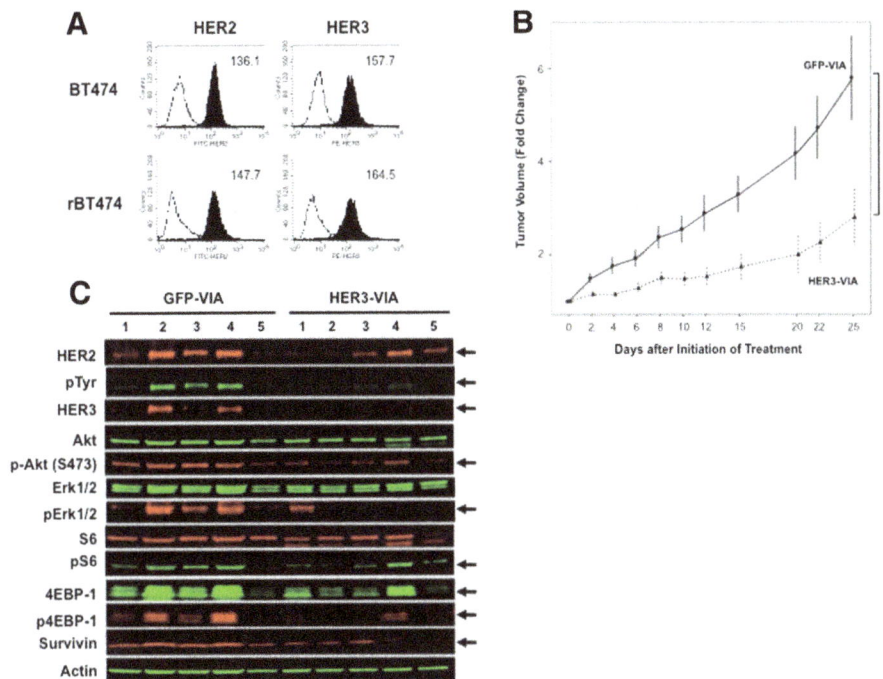

Fig. 5 In vivo effects of human epidermal growth factor receptor 3 (HER3) vaccine-induced antibody (HER3-VIA) in lapatinib-refractory rBT474 SCID tumor xenografts. **a** Flow cytometry analysis of HER2/HER3 expression (filled histograms) by BT474 and rBT474 cells. Mean fluorescence intensities are shown in each histogram. **b** The lapatinib-refractory cell line rBT474 was implanted into SCID mice and HER3-VIA was administered and tumor size was measured every 2-3 days : *$p < 0.01$. **c** Western blot analysis of excised tumors probing for downstream signaling intermediaries of HER3 activation. GFP, green fluorescence protein

who remain on therapy. Significant data implicate HER3 and more specifically, EGFR:HER3 and HER2:HER3 heterodimers as mediators of this resistance [36]. Monoclonal antibodies would be one mechanism for inhibiting HER family heterodimerization, but trastuzumab is ineffective against HER2:HER3 heterodimers [37], resistance develops to trastuzumab/pertuzumab combinations, there are no pertuzumab equivalents for EGFR, and anti-HER3 monoclonal antibodies are thus far not commercially available [38]. Our overall goal has been to develop an immunologic strategy to target HER3-expressing malignancies, reasoning that immune responses will be adaptive, pleiotropic, and persistent. Previously, we generated an Ad-HER3 vaccine and demonstrated that it induced potent HER3-specific T cell responses with anti-tumor activity [20]. In that study, we also observed preliminary evidence of the induction of HER3-VIA polyclonal serum in Ad-HER3-vaccinated mice, which suggested that further characterization of the antibody response was warranted thus leading to the experiments presented herein. We believe that while the T cell response is often regarded as the primary anti-tumor effector mechanism, antibody responses are also important as major histocompatibility complex (MHC) downregulation and epitope loss, observed in some tumors, would render them resistant to T cell-mediated cell death [39].

Vaccine-induced antibodies by virtue of their polyclonality should have the capacity to bind to multiple different epitopes and have multiple different functions, including commonly ascribed immune activities such as ADCC and CDC. Indeed, in the current study we observed immune-mediated anti-tumor activity mediated by Ad-HER3-induced antibodies (CDC and ADCC against HER3-expressing HER2+ and TNBC cells).

Additional anti-tumor activities that may be mediated by antibodies include internalization and signaling inhibition of the target-surface-expressed molecule [40–42]. Indeed, we observed that the anti-proliferative effects of HER3-VIA were likely due to internalization and signaling inhibition rather than inhibition of heregulin binding of HER3. These findings are consistent with our previously reported ability to generate polyclonal antibodies against the HER family member HER2, where we observed that these antibodies mediated HER2 receptor internalization and degradation in both mouse and human studies [19].

An important implication of HER3 downregulation is inhibition of signaling through HER3 heterodimers. Interestingly, treatment of lapatinib-sensitive and lapatinib-resistant BT474 cells with HER3-VIA led to decreased HER3, pHER3 and pERK1/2 as expected, but only treatment of the resistant BT474 cell led to a decrease in HER2, pAkt(S473), pS6,

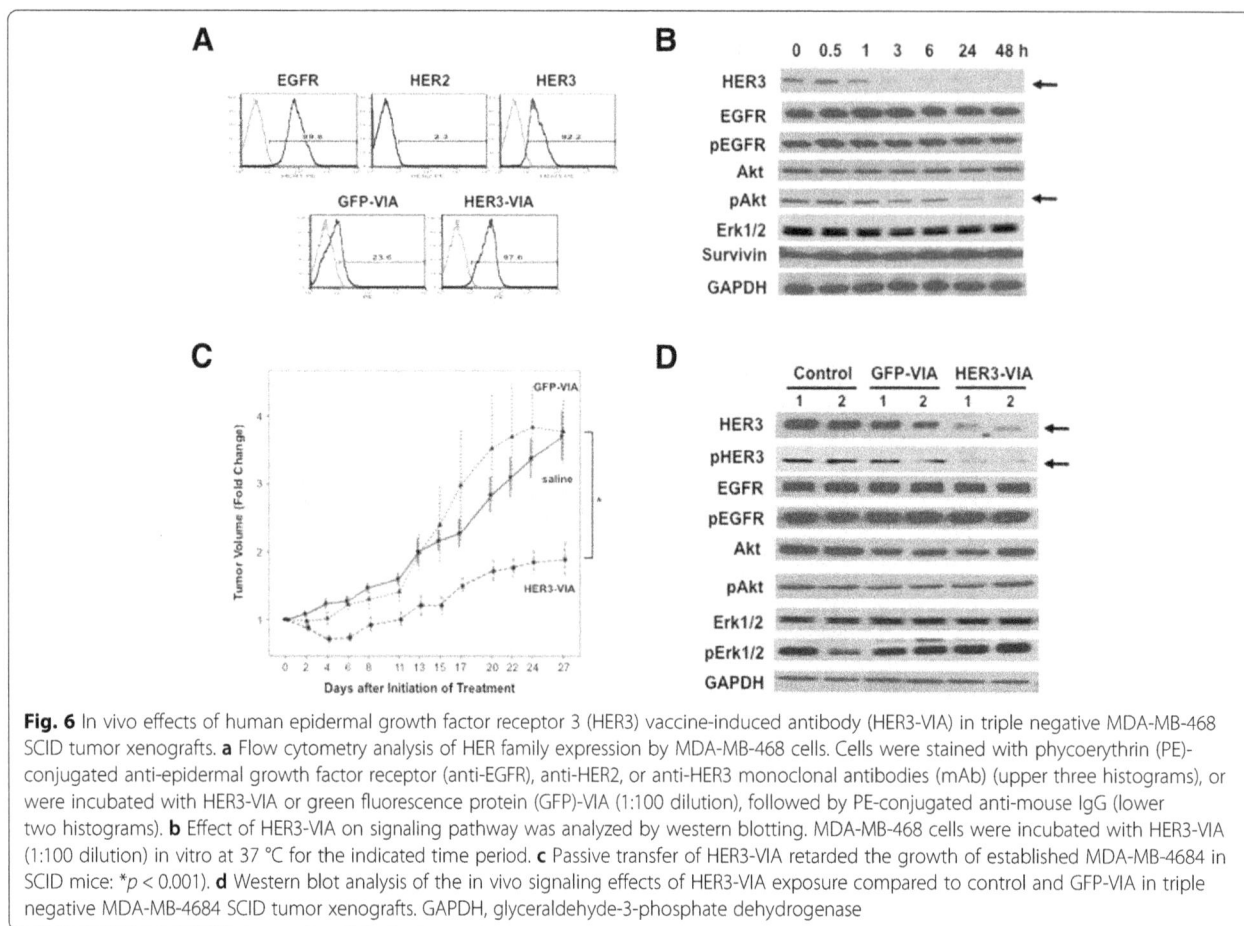

Fig. 6 In vivo effects of human epidermal growth factor receptor 3 (HER3) vaccine-induced antibody (HER3-VIA) in triple negative MDA-MB-468 SCID tumor xenografts. **a** Flow cytometry analysis of HER family expression by MDA-MB-468 cells. Cells were stained with phycoerythrin (PE)-conjugated anti-epidermal growth factor receptor (anti-EGFR), anti-HER2, or anti-HER3 monoclonal antibodies (mAb) (upper three histograms), or were incubated with HER3-VIA or green fluorescence protein (GFP)-VIA (1:100 dilution), followed by PE-conjugated anti-mouse IgG (lower two histograms). **b** Effect of HER3-VIA on signaling pathway was analyzed by western blotting. MDA-MB-468 cells were incubated with HER3-VIA (1:100 dilution) in vitro at 37 °C for the indicated time period. **c** Passive transfer of HER3-VIA retarded the growth of established MDA-MB-4684 in SCID mice: *$p < 0.001$. **d** Western blot analysis of the in vivo signaling effects of HER3-VIA exposure compared to control and GFP-VIA in triple negative MDA-MB-4684 SCID tumor xenografts. GAPDH, glyceraldehyde-3-phosphate dehydrogenase

p4EPB1, and survivin expression. The decrease in the protein survivin, an inhibitor of apoptosis, suggests that there is also an increase in apoptotic cells after Ad-HER3 treatment. In a previous study [43], when the partially trastuzumab-resistant 4 T1-HER2-expressing tumors were treated with lapatinib or HER2-VIA alone, we observed no change in survivin expression, but when these tumors were treated with a combination of lapatinib and HER2-VIA, we observed a decrease in survivin expression [27] implying that complete HER2 signaling blockade decreased survivin expression [43]. In an analogous fashion, our current findings suggest that complete blockade of HER2:HER3 signaling in lapatinib-refractory tumors is accomplished by treatment with HER3-VIA, resulting in the decreased expression of survivin.

An important observation was that the growth in vitro and in vivo of more aggressive breast cancer subtypes such as HER2+ breast cancer and TNBC, and of lapatinib-refractory (HER2 small molecule inhibitor-refractory) tumors was slowed by HER3-VIA. We believe our findings lay a framework for an immune-mediated strategy for treating aggressive breast cancer subtypes (TNBC and HER2+ breast cancer), by

co-administration of Ad-HER3 with HER2-targeted or EGFR-targeted therapies. Also, HER3 may play a role in therapeutic resistance to anti-estrogen therapies in estrogen receptor (ER)-positive breast cancers [44–47], and the development of castration resistance in prostate cancers [48]. Therefore, our findings also suggest a role for immunization with Ad-HER3 to induce HER3-VIA prior to the development of therapeutic resistance. Clinical trials of these approaches are in development.

Conclusions

In this study, we revealed that polyclonal antibodies induced by Ad-HER3 vaccine (HER3-VIAs) are multifunctional, including induction of CDC, ADCC, anti-proliferative effect, HER3 internalization, and interruption of HER3 heterodimer-driven tumor signaling pathways. In addition to the T cell anti-tumor response induced by Ad-HER3, the HER3-VIAs provide additional functions to eliminate tumors in which HER3 signaling mediates aggressive behavior or acquired resistance to HER2-targeted therapy. These data support clinical studies of vaccination against HER3 prior to or concomitantly with other therapies to prevent outgrowth of therapy-resistant HER2+ and triple negative clones.

Additional files

Additional file 1: Figure S1. Flow cytometric detection of HER3 on human breast cancer cell lines with anti-HER3 monoclonal antibodies (mAb) and HER3-VIA. To detect HER3-specific antibodies that could recognize membrane-associated HER3, binding of HER3-VIA in mouse serum was tested by flow cytometry against a series of human HER3-expressing breast tumor cell lines as targets, including the high HER3-expressing BT474, BT474M1, SKBR3, and T47D, and the HER3 negative, triple negative MDA-MB-231 tumor cell lines. Upper histograms: cells were stained with commercially available PE-conjugated anti-HER3 mAb (filled histogram), or PE-conjugate isotype control IgG as a negative staining (open histogram). Lower histograms: cells were incubated with HER3-VIA or GFP-VIA (1:100 dilution in medium), followed by staining with PE-conjugated anti-mouse IgG mAb. Filled histogram, HER3-VIA; open histogram, GFP-VIA. Percentage of staining positive cells and median fluorescence intensity are shown in each histogram. (PDF 119 kb)

Additional file 2: Table S1. Epitope mapping of HER3-VIA using spotted 15-mer peptide arrays. Epitope mapping was performed using spotted peptide arrays of 15-mer peptides overlapping by four amino acids representing the full length of the human HER3 protein. HER3 peptides were coated onto cellulose membranes using a Spot Robot ASP 222 (AbiMed) and epitope mapping of HER3-VIA (1:100 dilution in saline) was performed as described [26]. (PDF 36 kb)

Additional file 3: Figure S2. Flow cytometric detection of cell surface EGFR/HER2/HER3 expression after treatment with HER3-VIA, trastuzumab, cetuximab and lapatinib. To assess the internalization of EGFR family receptors, SKBR3 cells, positive for EGFR/HER2/HER3, were incubated with HER3-VIA, GFP-VIA (1:100 dilution), trastuzumab (1 μM), cetuximab (1 μM), or lapatinib (1 μM) for 3 h or 24 h. Cells were harvested using cell-dissociation buffer and stained with PE-conjugated anti-EGFP (clone 5E10D3, Novus Biologicals), anti-HER2 (clone Neu 24.7, BD Bioscience) or anti-HER3 antibody (Clone 1B4C3, BioLegend) and acquired by LSRII flow cytometer. Isotype control mouse IgG was used as negative control staining and is shown as filled gray histograms. Experiments were performed four times for EGFR expression analysis and twice for HER2 and HER3, and representative histograms are shown. Median fluorescence intensities (MFIs) of reagent-treated cells were compared to untreated control cells and ratios (MFI of treated/MFI of untreated) were calculated in each experiment. The averages of ratios are shown in each histogram. (PDF 732 kb)

Abbreviations

ADCC: Antibody-dependent cellular cytotoxicity; Ad-HER3: Adenovirus encoding full length human HER3; APC: Allophycocyanin; BSA: Bovine serum albumin; CDC: Complement-dependent cytotoxicity; CMV: Cytomegalovirus; CNS: Central nervous system; DAPI: 4′,6-Diamidino-2-phenylindole; DMEM: Dulbecco's modified Eagle's medium; EGFR: Epidermal growth factor receptor; ELISA: Enzyme-linked immunosorbent assay; FBS: Fetal bovine serum; GFP: Green fluorescence protein; HER2: Human epidermal growth factor receptor 2; HER3: Human epidermal growth factor receptor 3; IACUC: Institutional Animal Care and Use Committee; mAb: Monoclonal antibodies; MHC: Major histocompatibility complex; MTT: 3-(4,5-Dimethylthiazol-2-yl)-2.5-diphenyltetrazolium bromide; nIR: Near infrared; PBS: Phosphate-buffered saline; PCR: Polymerase chain reaction; PE: Phycoerythrin; PFA: Paraformaldehyde; SCID: Severe combined immunodeficiency; TKI: Tyrosine kinase inhibitor; TNBC: Triple negative breast cancer; VIA: Vaccine-induced antibody

Acknowledgements

The authors thank Ms. Tao Wang for the technical assistance.

Funding

This work was supported by grants from the Department of Defense Breast Cancer Research Program Clinical Translational Research Award (BC050221 to TMC); National Cancer Institute (NCI P50 CA89496–01 and 5P50CA068438 to HKL, NCI R01 CA95447 to TMC); and Susan G. Komen Foundation Postdoctoral Fellowship Award (KG080627 to ZH).

Authors' contributions

In vitro assays and quantification were conducted by JW, GL, TO, and WC. In vivo tumor studies were conducted by GL, JW, and ZCH. Conception and design of the study was conducted by TMC, TO, and HKL. Analysis and interpretation of data was conducted by TO, WRG, MAM, ACH, NS, TMC, and HKL. Statistical analysis was conducted by MAD. The draft of the manuscript was written by TO, MAM, WRG, TMC, and HKL, with all authors providing critical intellectual input into the final manuscript. All authors have read and approved the final version of the manuscript.

Competing interests

The authors declare that they have no competing interests.

Author details

Division of Surgical Sciences, Department of Surgery, Duke University Medical Center, MSRB Research Drive, Box 2714, Durham, NC 27710, USA. [2]Division of Medical Oncology, Department of Medicine, University of Washington, Seattle, WA, USA. [3]Biostatistics and Bioinformatics Research Center, Samuel Oschin Comprehensive Cancer Institute, Cedars-Sinai Medical Center, Los Angeles, CA, USA. [4]Division of Medical Oncology, Department of Medicine, Duke University Medical Center, Durham, NC, USA. [5]Cell and Gene Therapy Discovery Research, PTS, GlaxoSmithKline, Collegeville, PA, USA. [6]Division of Gastroenterology, Department of Medicine, Duke University Medical Center, Durham, NC, USA. [7]Division of General Surgery, Department of Surgery, Duke University Medical Center, Durham, NC, USA.

References

1. Kmieciak M, Knutson KL, Dumur CI, Manjili MH. HER-2/neu antigen loss and relapse of mammary carcinoma are actively induced by T cell-mediated anti tumor immune responses. Eur J Immunol. 2007;37:675–85. PMID: 17304628. https://doi.org/10.1002/eji.200636639.

2. Ostrand-Rosenberg S. Tolerance and immune suppression in the tumor microenvironment. Cell Immunol. 2016;299:23–9. PMID: 26435343. https://doi.org/10.1016/j.cellimm.2015.09.011.

3. Jura N, Shan Y, Cao X, Shaw DE, Kuriyan J. Structural analysis of the catalytically inactive kinase domain of the human EGF receptor 3. Proc Natl Acad Sci U S A. 2009;106:21608–13. PMID: 20007378. https://doi.org/10.1073/pnas.0912101106.

4. Shi F, Telesco SE, Liu Y, Radhakrishnan R, Lemmon MA. ErbB3/HER3 intracellular domain is competent to bind ATP and catalyze autophosphorylation. Proc Natl Acad Sci U S A. 2010;107:7692–7. PMID: 20351256. https://doi.org/10.1073/pnas.1002753107.

5. Campbell MR, Amin D, Moasser MM. HER3 comes of age: new insights into its functions and role in signaling, tumor biology, and cancer therapy. Clin Cancer Res. 2010;16:1373–83. PMID: 20179223. https://doi.org/10.1158/1078-0432.CCR-09-1218.

6. Fedi P, Pierce JH, di Fiore PP, Kraus MH. Efficient coupling with phosphatidylinositol 3-kinase, but not phospholipase C gamma or GTPase-activating protein, distinguishes ErbB-3 signaling from that of other ErbB/EGFR family members. Mol Cell Biol. 1994;14:492–500. PMID: 8264617. https://doi.org/10.1128/MCB.14.1.492.

7. Alimandi M, Romano A, Curia MC, Muraro R, Fedi P, Aaronson SA, Di Fiore PP, Kraus MH. Cooperative signaling of ErbB3 and ErbB2 in neoplastic transformation and human mammary carcinomas. Oncogene. 1995;10:1813–21. PMID: 7538656

8. Lee-Hoeflich ST, Crocker L, Yao E, Pham T, Munroe X, Hoeflich KP, Sliwkowski MX, Stern HM. A central role for HER3 in HER2-amplified breast cancer: implications for targeted therapy. Cancer Res. 2008;68:5878–87. PMID: 18632642. https://doi.org/10.1158/0008-5472.CAN-08-0380.

9.   Sergina NV, Rausch M, Wang D, Blair J, Hann B, Shokat KM, Moasser MM. Escape from HER-family tyrosine kinase inhibitor therapy by the kinase-inactive HER3. Nature. 2007;445:437–41. PMID: 17206155. https://doi.org/10.1038/nature05474.

10. Amin DN, Campbell MR, Moasser MM. The role of HER3, the unpretentious member of the HER family in cancer biology and cancer therapeutics. Semin Cell Dev Biol. 2010;21:944–50. PMID: 20816829. https://doi.org/10.1016/j.semcdb.2010.08.007.

11. Xia W, Petricoin EF 3rd, Zhao S, Liu L, Osada T, Cheng Q, Wulfkuhle JD, Gwin WR, Yang X, Gallagher RI, Bacus S, Lyerly HK, Spector NL. An heregulin-EGFR-HER3 autocrine signaling axis can mediate acquired lapatinib resistance in HER2+ breast cancer models. Breast Cancer Res. 2013; 15:R85. PMID: 24044505. https://doi.org/10.1186/bcr3480.

12. Bae SY, La Choi Y, Kim S, Kim M, Kim J, Jung SP, Choi MY, Lee SK, Kil WH, Lee JE, Nam SJ. HER3 status by immunohistochemistry is correlated with poor prognosis in hormone receptor-negative breast cancer patients. Breast Cancer Res Treat. 2013;139:741–50. PMID: 23722313. https://doi.org/10.1007/s10549-013-2570-6.

13. Da Silva L, Simpson PT, Smart CE, Cocciardi S, Waddell N, Lane A, Morrison BJ, Vargas AC, Healey S, Beesley J, et al. HER3 and downstream pathways are involved in colonization of brain metastases from breast cancer. Breast Cancer Res. 2010;12:R46. PMID: 20604919. https://doi.org/10.1186/bcr2603.

14. Agus DB, Akita RW, Fox WD, Lewis GD, Higgins B, Pisacane PI, Lofgren JA, Tindell C, Evans DP, Maiese K, et al. Targeting ligand-activated ErbB2 signaling inhibits breast and prostate tumor growth. Cancer Cell. 2002;2: 127–37. PMID: 12204533. https://doi.org/10.1016/s1535-6108(02)00097-1.

15. Yamashita-Kashima Y, Iijima S, Yorozu K, Furugaki K, Kurasawa M, Ohta M, Fujimoto-Ouchi K. Pertuzumab in combination with trastuzumab shows significantly enhanced antitumor activity in HER2-positive human gastric cancer xenograft models. Clin Cancer Res. 2011;17:5060–70. PMID: 21700765. https://doi.org/10.1158/1078-0432.CCR-10-2927.

16. Cai Z, Zhang G, Zhou Z, Bembas K, Drebin JA, Greene MI, Zhang H. Differential binding patterns of monoclonal antibody 2C4 to the ErbB3-p185her2/neu and the EGFR-p185her2/neu complexes. Oncogene. 2008;27: 3870–4. PMID: 18264138. https://doi.org/10.1038/onc.2008.13.

17. Schoeberl B, Faber AC, Li D, Liang MC, Crosby K, Onsum M, Burenkova O, Pace E, Walton Z, Nie L, et al. An ErbB3 antibody, MM-121, is active in cancers with ligand-dependent activation. Cancer Res. 2010;70:2485–94. PMID: 20215504. https://doi.org/10.1158/0008-5472.CAN-09-3145.

18. Montgomery RB, Makary E, Schiffman K, Goodell V, Disis ML. Endogenous anti-HER2 antibodies block HER2 phosphorylation and signaling through extracellular signal-regulated kinase. Cancer Res. 2005;65:650–6. PMID: 15695410

19. Ren XR, Wei J, Lei G, Wang J, Lu J, Xia W, Spector N, Barak LS, Clay TM, Osada T, et al. Polyclonal HER2-specific antibodies induced by vaccination mediate receptor internalization and degradation in tumor cells. Breast Cancer Res. 2012;14:R89. PMID: 22676470. https://doi.org/10.1186/bcr3204.

20. Osada T, Morse MA, Hobeika A, Diniz MA, Gwin WR, Hartman Z, Wei J, Guo H, Yang X-Y, Liu C-X, Kaneko K, Broadwater G, Lyerly HK. Vaccination targeting human HER3 alters the phenotype of infiltrating T cells and responses to immune checkpoint inhibition. Oncoimmunology. 2017;6: e1315495. PMID:28680745. https://doi.org/10.1080/2162402X.2017.1315495.

21. Xia W, Bacus S, Hegde P, Husain I, Strum J, Liu L, Paulazzo G, Lyass L, Trusk P, Hill J, et al. A model of acquired autoresistance to a potent ErbB2 tyrosine kinase inhibitor and a therapeutic strategy to prevent its onset in breast cancer. Proc Natl Acad Sci U S A. 2006;103:7795–800. PMID: 16682622. https://doi.org/10.1073/pnas.0602468103.

22. Amalfitano A, Hauser MA, Hu H, Serra D, Begy CR, Chamberlain JS. Production and characterization of improved adenovirus vectors with the E1, E2b, and E3 genes deleted. J Virol 1998;72:926–933. PMID: 9444984.

23. Amalfitano A, Chamberlain CJ. Isolation and characterization of packaging cell lines that coexpress the adenovirus E1, DNA polymerase, and preterminal proteins: implications for gene therapy. Gene Ther. 1997;4:258–63. PMID: 9135740. https://doi.org/10.1038/sj.gt.3300378·

24. Hartman ZC, Wei J, Osada T, Glass O, Lei G, Yang XY, Peplinski S, Kim DW,

Xia W, Spector N, et al. An adenoviral vaccine encoding full-length inactivated human Her2 exhibits potent immunogenicty and enhanced therapeutic efficacy without oncogenicity. Clin Cancer Res. 2010;16:1466–77. PMID: 20179231. https://doi.org/10.1158/1078-0432.CCR-09-2549.

25. Piechocki MP, Pilon SA, Wei WZ. Quantitative measurement of anti-ErbB-2 antibody by flow cytometry and ELISA. J Immunol Methods. 2002;259:33–42. PMID: 11730839. https://doi.org/10.1016/S0022-1759(01)00487-2.

26. Frank R, Overwin H. SPOT synthesis. Epitope analysis with arrays of synthetic peptides prepared on cellulose membranes. Methods Mol Biol. 1996;66:149–69. PMID: 8959713. https://doi.org/10.1385/0-89603-375-9:149.

27. Morse MA, Wei J, Hartman Z, Xia W, Ren XR, Lei G, Barry WT, Osada T, Hobeika AC, Peplinski S, et al. Synergism from combined immunologic and pharmacologic inhibition of HER2 in vivo. Int J Cancer. 2010;126:2893–903. PMID: 19856307. https://doi.org/10.1002/ijc.24995.

28. Wang Y. Smoothing splines: methods and applications. Boca Raton: CRC Press; 2011. p. 2011.

29. Kruskal WH, Wallis WA. Use of ranks in one-criterion variance analysis. J Am Stat Assoc. 1952;47:583–621. https://doi.org/10.2307/2280779.

30. Munzel U, Hothorn LA. A unified approach to simultaneous rank tests procedures in the unbalanced one-way layout. Biom J. 2001;43:553–69. https://doi.org/10.1002/1521-4036(200109)43:5<553:AID-BIMJ553>3.0.CO;2-N.

31. Mann HB, Whitney DR. On a test of whether one of two random variables is stochastically larger than the other. Ann Math Statist. 1947;18:50–60. https://doi.org/10.1214/aoms/1177730491.

32. Shapiro SS, Francia RS. An approximate analysis of variance test or normality. J Am Stat Assoc. 1972;67:215–6. https://doi.org/10.1080/01621459. 1972. 10481232.

33. Levene H. Robust tests for equality of variances. In: Olkin I, editor. Contributions to probability and statistics: essays in honor of Harold Hotelling. Redwood City: Stanford University Press; 1961. p. 279–92.

34. R Core Team. A language and environment for statistical computing. Vienna: R Foundation for Statistical Computing; 2016.

35. Singer E, Landgraf R, Horan T, Slamon D, Eisenberg D. Identification of a heregulin binding site in HER3 extracellular domain. J Biol Chem. 2001;276: 44266–74. PMID: 11555649. https://doi.org/10.1074/jbc.M105428200.

36. Claus J, Patel G, Ng T, Parker PJ. A role for the pseudokinase HER3 in the acquired resistance against EGFR- and HER2-directed targeted therapy. Biochem Soc Trans. 2014;42:831–6. PMID: 25109965. https://doi.org/10.1042/BST20140043.

37. Wehrman TS, Raab WJ, Casipit CL, Doyonnas R, Pomerantz JH, Blau HM. A system for quantifying dynamic protein interactions defines a role for Herceptin in modulating ErbB2 interactions. Proc Natl Acad Sci U S A. 2006; 103:19063–8. PMID: 17148612. https://doi.org/10.1073/pnas.0605218103.

38. Malm M, Frejd FY, Ståhl S, Löfblom J. Targeting HER3 using mono- and bispecific antibodies or alternative scaffolds. MAbs. 2016;8:1195–209. PMID: 27532938. https://doi.org/10.1080/19420862.2016.1212147.

39. Campoli M, Chang CC, Ferrone S. HLA class I antigen loss, tumor immune escape and immune selection. Vaccine. 2002;20(Suppl 4):A40–5. PMID: 12477427. https://doi.org/10.1016/S0264-410X(02)00386-9.

40. Friedman LM, Rinon A, Schechter B, Lyass L, Lavi S, Bacus SS, Sela M, Yarden Y. Synergistic down-regulation of receptor tyrosine kinases by combinations of mAbs: implications for cancer immunotherapy. Proc Natl Acad Sci U S A. 2005; 102:1915–20. PMID: 15684082. https://doi.org/10.1073/pnas.0409610102.

41. Ben-Kasus T, Schechter B, Lavi S, Yarden Y, Sela M. Persistent elimination of ErbB-2/HER2-overexpressing tumors using combinations of monoclonal antibodies: relevance of receptor endocytosis. Proc Natl Acad Sci U S A. 2009;106:3294–9. PMID: 19218427. https://doi.org/10.1073/pnas.0812059106.

42. Pedersen MW, Jacobsen HJ, Koefoed K, Hey A, Pyke C, Haurum JS, Kragh M. Sym004: a novel synergistic anti-epidermal growth factor receptor antibody mixture with superior anticancer efficacy. Cancer Res. 2010;70:588–97. PMID: 20068188. https://doi.org/10.1158/0008-5472.CAN-09-1417.

43. Xia W, Gerard CM, Liu L, Baudson NM, Ory TL, Spector NL. Combining lapatinib (GW572016), a small molecule inhibitor of ErbB1 and ErbB2 tyrosine kinases, with therapeutic anti-ErbB2 antibodies enhances apoptosis of ErbB2-overexpressing breast cancer cells. Oncogene. 2005;24:6213–21. PMID:16091755. https://doi.org/10.1038/sj.onc. 1208774.

44. Miller TW, Pérez-Torres M, Narasanna A, Guix M, Stål O, Pérez-Tenorio G, Gonzalez-Angulo AM, Hennessy BT, Mills GB, Kennedy JP, et al. Loss of phosphatase and Tensin homologue deleted on chromosome 10 engages ErbB3 and insulin-like growth factor-I receptor signaling to promote antiestrogen resistance in breast cancer. Cancer Res. 2009;69:4192–201. PMID: 19435893. https://doi.org/10.1158/0008-5472.CAN-09-0042.

45. Frogne T, Benjaminsen RV, Sonne-Hansen K, Sorensen BS, Nexo E, Laenkholm AV, Rasmussen LM, Riese DJ 2nd, de Cremoux P, Stenvang J, et al. Activation of ErbB3, EGFR and Erk is essential for growth of human breast cancer cell lines with acquired resistance to fulvestrant. Breast Cancer Res Treat. 2009;114:263–75. PMID: 18409071. https://doi.org/10.1007/s10549-008-0011-8.

46. Liu B, Ordonez-Ercan D, Fan Z, Edgerton SM, Yang X, Thor AD. Downregulation of erbB3 abrogates erbB2-mediated tamoxifen resistance in breast cancer cells. Int J Cancer. 2007;120:1874–82. PMID: 17266042. https://doi.org/10.1002/ijc.22423.

47. Osipo C, Meeke K, Cheng D, Weichel A, Bertucci A, Liu H, Jordan VC. Role for HER2/neu and HER3 in fulvestrant-resistant breast cancer. Int J Oncol. 2007;30:509–20. PMID: 17203234. https://doi.org/10.3892/ijo.30.2.509.

48. Zhang Y, Linn D, Liu Z, Melamed J, Tavora F, Young CY, Burger AM, Hamburger AW. EBP1, an ErbB3-binding protein, is decreased in prostate cancer and implicated in hormone resistance. Mol Cancer Ther. 2008;7:3176–86. PMID: 18852121. https://doi.org/10.1158/1535-7163.MCT-08-0526.

5

Breast fibroadenomas are not associated with increased breast cancer risk in an African American contemporary cohort of women with benign breast disease

Asra N. Shaik[1], Julie J. Ruterbusch[1], Eman Abdulfatah[2], Resha Shrestha[2], M. H. D. Fayez Daaboul[2], Visakha Pardeshi[2], Daniel W. Visscher[3], Sudeshna Bandyopadhyay[4], Rouba Ali-Fehmi[2,4] and Michele L. Cote[1,4*] (ID)

Abstract

Background: Fibroadenomas are common benign breast lesions, and studies of European American women indicate a persistent, increased risk of breast cancer after diagnosing a fibroadenoma on biopsy. This association has not been independently assessed in African American women, despite reports that these women are more likely to present with fibroadenomas.

Methods: The study cohort included 3853 African American women with a breast biopsy completed between 1997 and 2010 in metropolitan Detroit. Biopsies were microscopically reviewed for benign breast lesions, including fibroadenoma, proliferative disease, and atypia. Risk of breast cancer within the cohort was estimated using relative risk ratios and 95% CIs calculated using multivariable log-binomial regression. Relative risk of breast cancer in this cohort compared with African American women in the broader metropolitan Detroit population was estimated using standardized incidence ratios (SIRs).

Results: Fibroadenomas occurred more frequently in biopsies of younger women, and other types of benign breast lesions were less likely to occur when a fibroadenoma was present ($p = 0.008$ for lobular hyperplasia; all other p values < 0.01). Unlike women with other benign lesions (SIR, 1.41; 95% CI, 1.20, 1.66), women with fibroadenomas did not have an increased risk of developing breast cancer compared with the general population (SIR, 0.94; 95% CI, 0.75, 1.18). Biopsies that indicated a fibroadenoma were associated with a reduced risk of breast cancer after adjusting for age at biopsy, proliferation, and atypia (relative risk, 0.67; 95% CI, 0.48, 0.93) compared with biopsies without a fibroadenoma.

Conclusions: These findings have important implications for breast cancer risk models and clinical assessment, particularly among African American women, in whom fibroadenomas are common.

Keywords: Benign breast disease, Breast cancer, Risk, African American

* Correspondence: cotem@karmanos.org
[1]Department of Oncology, Wayne State University School of Medicine, 4100 John R Street, MM04EP, Detroit, MI 48201, USA
[4]Barbara Ann Karmanos Cancer Institute, Detroit, MI, USA
Full list of author information is available at the end of the article

Background

Over 1.5 million breast biopsies are pathologically assessed annually in the United States, indicated by abnormal mammography findings or patient complaints [1]. Most biopsies are not malignant, but instead exhibit a number of pathological lesions that constitute benign breast disease (BBD). Biopsies that exhibit proliferative disease or cellular atypia, as defined by Dupont and Page criteria, are consistently associated with increases in breast cancer risk [2–4]. These pathologic criteria have been included in risk assessment models to identify women at high risk of developing breast cancer. Several current risk assessment models, including the frequently used Breast Cancer Risk Assessment Tool, incorporate information on the number of prior biopsies and the presence of atypia on biopsy, but they do not account for other BBD lesions that may independently increase breast cancer risk [5]. Reliable estimates of breast cancer risk associated with individual lesions can improve risk models, allowing physicians to better identify women at high risk of developing breast cancer who may benefit from additional screening or chemoprevention.

One type of BBD, fibroadenomas, are well-circumscribed benign tumors of epithelial and stromal tissue (Fig. 1) [6]. Breast fibroadenomas most frequently occur in women in their 20s [6] but can occur at any age; it is estimated that 10% of women have breast fibroadenomas [7]. A recent meta-analysis of 11 studies reported an increase in breast cancer risk by 41% (1.41; 95% CI, 1.11–1.80) for women diagnosed with a fibroadenoma compared with women without fibroadenoma on biopsy; however, significant statistical heterogeneity was also reported with this estimate [8]. Furthermore, the studies in this meta-analysis were primarily in European ancestral populations, and the majority were

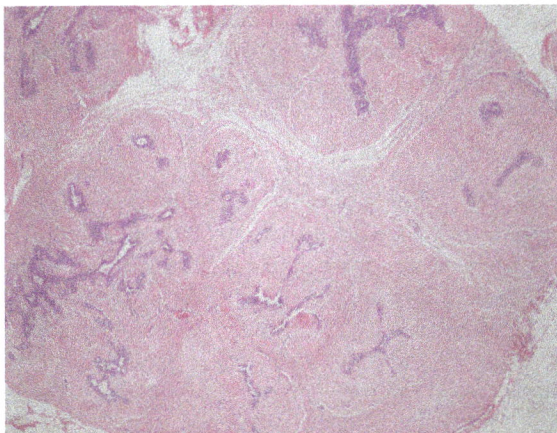

Fig. 1 Fibroadenoma. Fibroadenomas are benign tumors of stromal and epithelial tissue that are typically well-circumscribed and mobile within the tissue. The fibroadenoma shown here exhibits purple epithelial tissue surrounded by pink fibrotic stromal tissue (H&E stain; original magnification 100×)

studies done prior to the widespread use of screening mammography in the 1980s. Although African American women experience a higher incidence and recurrence of fibroadenomas at a younger age [9, 10], breast cancer risk associated with this lesion has not been independently assessed in this population of women.

African American women have a 42% higher breast cancer mortality rate than European American women [11], a burden that stems partly from differences in tumor biology. African American women are more likely to develop breast cancer at a younger age [12–14] and more likely to be diagnosed with aggressive tumors characterized by high molecular grade [15, 16] and lack of hormone receptors [13, 15, 16]. Despite this survival disparity, prior investigations on BBD and breast cancer risk focused on mostly European American cohorts. The goal of this study is to examine in a contemporary cohort whether breast cancer risk associated with fibroadenoma differs for African American women, a population more likely to present with fibroadenomas and more likely to develop aggressive breast cancers that respond poorly to treatment.

Methods

Study population

African American women with their first benign breast biopsies conducted between 1997 and 2010 were identified using University Pathology Group (UPG; Detroit, MI, USA) records. UPG provides pathology services to several hospitals in metropolitan Detroit. Women aged 18 to 84 years at the time of benign breast biopsy were eligible for this institutional review board-approved study. Exclusionary criteria included a diagnosis of invasive or in situ breast carcinoma before or within 6 months of the breast biopsy, a history of mastectomy or reduction mammoplasty, lipoma, fat necrosis, epidermal cysts, hematoma, accessory structure, phyllodes tumor, or a lymph node biopsy without breast tissue. For this type of study, the Wayne State University Institutional Review Board determined that formal consent was not required.

Histological review

Core needle and excisional benign biopsies were microscopically reviewed by blinded study pathologists (RAF, SB) using original H&E-stained slides. Slides from the first biopsy were assessed for the presence of 12 pathologic lesions, including apocrine metaplasia, calcifications, columnar alterations, cysts, duct ectasia, ductal hyperplasia, fibroadenoma, fibrosis, intraductal papilloma, lobular hyperplasia, radial scars, and sclerosing adenosis. The biopsies were additionally categorized into three groups using criteria described by Dupont and Page [2] based on the presence of proliferative disease and cellular atypia. Biopsies classified as showing atypia and a random sample of all other biopsies were reassessed by a blinded study pathologist at the Mayo Clinic (DWV). Breast biopsies that could not be assessed for fibroadenoma presence were excluded from analysis ($n = 23$).

Cancer ascertainment

Women who developed breast cancer were identified through hospital medical records and also through the use of the Metropolitan Detroit Cancer Surveillance System (MDCSS), a founding member of the National Cancer Institute's Surveillance, Epidemiology, and End Results (SEER) program. MDCSS collects cancer incidence, treatment, and survival data in the tricounty metropolitan Detroit area. Use of both data sources allowed the identification of cancers in women residing in the entire tricounty metropolitan Detroit area. Women were matched between UPG records and MDCSS using name, date of birth, and/or Social Security number; follow-up information was complete to December 31, 2015. Median length of follow-up was 13.3 years (range, 0.5–19.0 years); median time to breast cancer diagnosis was 6.6 years (range, 0.7–18.5 years).

Statistical analysis

Associations between fibroadenoma and other benign lesions were examined using chi-squared tests. Relative risks of breast cancer associated with biopsies, with or without fibroadenoma, were estimated using age-adjusted standardized incidence ratios (SIRs) calculated from SEER estimates of cancer incidence in African American women in MDCSS from 1999 to 2014. Risk of breast cancer associated with fibroadenomas relative to other nonfibroadenoma BBD was examined within the cohort by relative risk ratios and 95% CIs calculated using multivariable log-binomial regression and adjusting for age at biopsy. Regression models were further adjusted using backwards selection based on Bayesian information criteria. Models were stratified by age (below or above 50 years) to estimate risk based on likely menopausal status. Time to breast cancer diagnosis was assessed using competing risk analysis with death considered as a competing risk.

Results

Distribution of BBD features and characteristics by fibroadenoma status

A total of 3845 benign breast biopsies were assessed in this African American cohort, 1798 (47%) of which were diagnosed with fibroadenoma. Fibroadenomas showed high concordance between pathologists (86.9%; Cohen's $\kappa = 0.7022$). Women with a fibroadenoma on biopsy were more likely to be under the age of 40 years at biopsy (31.9%) than women without a fibroadenoma on biopsy (18.9%) ($p < 0.001$) (Table 1). The presence of a fibroadenoma was associated with the absence of all other benign

breast lesions assessed on biopsy ($p = 0.008$ for lobular hyperplasia; all other $p < 0.001$) (Table 1 and Additional file 1: Tables S1 and S2). Additionally, biopsies with a fibroadenoma were less likely to be classified as proliferative disease (25.0%) or proliferative disease with atypia (1.3%) than biopsies without a fibroadenoma (51.5% and 6.1%, respectively).

Breast cancer risk compared with population level risk

Overall, this cohort of women exhibited an increased incidence of approximately 20% (SIR, 1.19; 95% CI, 1.05–1.36) of breast cancer compared with the general African American population in metropolitan Detroit (Table 2). Stratifying the cohort by presence of fibroadenoma on biopsy revealed that breast cancer incidence associated with fibroadenoma was indistinguishable from population level (SIR, 0.93; 95% CI, 0.75–1.17), but the breast cancer incidence associated with the absence of fibroadenoma on biopsy was significantly higher than population level (SIR, 1.40; 95% CI, 1.19–1.65).

Breast cancer risk within the BBD cohort

Adjusting for age at biopsy alone, the presence of fibroadenoma was associated with a reduced breast cancer risk (relative risk [RR], 0.64; 95% CI, 0.45–0.85) compared with the absence of fibroadenoma within the BBD cohort (Table 3). When the model was fully adjusted for age at biopsy, proliferation, and atypia, fibroadenoma was still associated with a reduced risk (RR, 0.67; 95% CI, 0.48–0.93) of developing breast cancer. Fibroadenoma diagnosed in women under the age of 50 years was associated with a decrease in breast cancer risk after adjusting for age at biopsy, proliferation, and cellular atypia (RR, 0.58; 95% CI, 0.34–0.96). Fibroadenoma diagnosed in women aged 50 years or older also showed a reduction in breast cancer risk but failed to reach statistical significance after adjusting for age at biopsy, proliferation, and cellular atypia (RR, 0.79; 95% CI, 0.52–1.19).

Cumulative incidence of cancers in subgroups

Women with fibroadenoma on biopsy accumulated fewer breast cancers over the study period than women without fibroadenoma on biopsy (Fig. 2) ($p < 0.001$ by Fine and Gray test). Stratifying by likely menopausal status by age indicated the incidence of breast cancers was lower in women under the age of 50 years than in women aged 50 years or older (data not shown). In both strata, women with fibroadenoma on biopsy accumulated fewer cancers over the study period than women without fibroadenoma on biopsy (Fine and Gray test, $p = 0.014$ for under age 50 years and $p = 0.059$ for ages 50 years and older).

Table 1 Distribution of benign breast features and other characteristics by fibroadenoma status

Characteristic	Status, n (%)[a]		P value[b]
	No fibroadenoma 2047 (53.2)	Fibroadenoma 1798 (46.8)	
Age at benign biopsy, years			< 0.001
< 40	387 (18.9)	573 (31.9)	
40–49	692 (33.8)	582 (32.4)	
50–59	577 (28.2)	374 (20.8)	
60–69	249 (12.2)	164 (9.1)	
70+	142 (6.9)	105 (5.8)	
Biopsy type			< 0.001
Excisional	826 (40.4)	536 (30.8)	
Core needle	1221 (59.6)	1262 (70.2)	
Apocrine metaplasia			< 0.001
Absent	1202 (58.7)	1401 (82.3)	
Present	845 (41.3)	301 (17.7)	
Ductal hyperplasia			< 0.001
Absent	1272 (62.1)	1365 (80.6)	
Present	775 (37.9)	329 (19.4)	
Lobular hyperplasia			0.008
Absent	2012 (98.3)	1662 (99.3)	
Present	34 (1.7)	11 (0.7)	
Calcifications			< 0.001
Absent	1209 (59.1)	1229 (70.8)	
Present	837 (40.9)	507 (29.2)	
Cysts			< 0.001
Absent	970 (47.4)	1339 (78.9)	
Present	1076 (52.6)	359 (21.1)	
Duct ectasia			< 0.001
Absent	1652 (80.7)	1546 (91.0)	
Present	394 (19.3)	152 (9.0)	
Fibrosis			< 0.001
Absent	648 (31.7)	1031 (63.8)	
Present	1397 (68.3)	586 (36.2)	
Intraductal papilloma			< 0.001
Absent	1662 (81.2)	1629 (96.1)	
Present	385 (18.8)	66 (3.9)	
Sclerosing adenosis			< 0.001
Absent	1416 (69.2)	1404 (82.7)	
Present	630 (30.8)	294 (17.3)	
Columnar alterations			< 0.001
Absent	1302 (63.6)	1439 (84.7)	
Present	744 (30.8)	259 (15.3)	
Radial scar			< 0.001
Absent	1975 (96.5)	1665 (98.6)	
Present	71 (3.5)	23 (1.4)	

Table 1 Distribution of benign breast features and other characteristics by fibroadenoma status *(Continued)*

Characteristic	Status, n (%)[a]		P value[b]
	No fibroadenoma 2047 (53.2)	Fibroadenoma 1798 (46.8)	
Dupont and Page criteria			< 0.001
Nonproliferative disease	868 (42.4)	1325 (73.7)	
Proliferative disease without atypia	1054 (51.5)	450 (25.0)	
Proliferative disease with atypia	125 (6.1)	23 (1.3)	
Developed breast cancer			< 0.001
No	1902 (92.9)	1722 (95.8)	
Yes	145 (7.1)	76 (4.2)	

[a]Numbers may not sum to the total number of patients if features could not be assessed on biopsy
[b]χ^2 test comparing distribution of features across absence or presence of fibroadenoma on biopsy

Discussion

We report findings in a contemporary cohort of African American women who have had a breast biopsy that show those with a fibroadenoma observed on biopsy are not at increased risk of subsequent breast cancer compared with the general population of African American women. When compared with all benign biopsies, biopsies that indicated a fibroadenoma were associated with a reduced risk of breast cancer that remains significant even after adjusting for age, proliferative disease, and atypia. These findings suggest that current breast cancer risk models that incorporate benign biopsies without considering the pathological lesion overestimate risk in African American women who have fibroadenomas on biopsy. Given that fibroadenomas were identified in nearly half of all breast biopsies in this population and were the only lesion identified in 19% of all biopsies, these findings represent a significant clinical population.

Our investigation suggests that biopsies indicating fibroadenoma exhibit a reduced risk of breast cancer compared with all other BBD biopsies, contrary to most other studies' estimates of increased risk of breast cancer [8]. Discordant risk estimates between our investigation and those from other studies may reflect differences in race, age, and period of cohorts used. The Nashville group [17], which found a significant increase in breast cancer risk with fibroadenoma (SIR, 1.61; 95% CI, 1.30–2.00) compared with the Connecticut Tumor Registry, studied European American women diagnosed

with a fibroadenoma between 1950 and 1968. The Mayo Clinic BBD cohort [18] studied European American women diagnosed with fibroadenoma between 1967 and 1991 and found modest increases breast cancer risk with fibroadenoma (SIR, 1.60; 95% CI, 1.38–1.85) compared with biopsies without fibroadenoma (SIR, 1.50; 95% CI, 1.39–1.62). A BBD cohort from Henry Ford Health System (HFHS) [19], where women with fibroadenomas on biopsy had a decreased odds (OR, 0.55; 95% CI, 0.39–0.77) of developing breast cancer compared with women without fibroadenoma on biopsy, more closely approximating our risk estimates, studied a mixed cohort of European American and African American women in metropolitan Detroit diagnosed between 1981 and 1994. However, it is unlikely that the differences in risk estimates are due solely to race: the HFHS group tested an interaction factor between race and BBD and did not find statistical significance [19].

Period effects may also contribute to variation in risk estimates. Inclusion criteria for BBD studies span from 1950 to 2010; thus, differences in risk estimates may also reflect the endogenous and exogenous exposures that varied over this period. Exogenous hormone use, including hormone replacement therapy and contraceptive use, have changed in frequency, dose, and formulation. Changes in exogenous hormone use can alter total estrogen exposure, a strong breast cancer risk factor, and influence risk estimates of tissue-based markers. Environmental exposures that vary over time and/or

Table 2 Risk of breast cancer compared with population level risk

	Standardized incidence ratio[a]	95% confidence interval
Population rate	Ref	
Entire BBD cohort (N = 221 cancers)	1.19	1.05–1.36
Biopsy without fibroadenoma (N = 145 cancers)	1.40	1.19–1.65
Fibroadenoma (N = 76 cancers)	0.93	0.75–1.17

[a]Standardized incidence ratio compares the observed number of breast cancers that developed in the study to the number expected on the basis of the Detroit surveillance, epidemiology, and end results data for African American women of a similar age and calendar period

Table 3 Relative risk of breast cancer by fibroadenoma status

	Age-adjusted relative risk[a] (95% CI)	P value[b]	Fully adjusted relative risk[c] (95% CI)	P value[b]
No fibroadenoma on biopsy	Ref		Ref	
Fibroadenoma	0.64 (0.48, 0.85)[d]	0.003	0.67 (0.48, 0.93)[e]	0.017
Under age 50 years				
No fibroadenoma on biopsy	Reference		Reference	
Fibroadenoma	0.71 (0.45, 1.11)[f]	0.133	0.58 (0.34, 0.96)[g]	0.037
Age 50 years or older				
No fibroadenoma on biopsy	Reference		Reference	
Fibroadenoma	0.68 (0.46, 0.98)[h]	0.042	0.79 (0.52, 1.19)[i]	0.275

[a]Multivariable logistic regression model adjusting for age at biopsy
[b]Wald test statistic
[c]Multivariable logistic regression model adjusting for age, proliferative disease, and cellular atypia at biopsy
Number at risk: [d]3845, [e]3761, [f]2234, [g]2071, [h]1611, [i]1536

geographic areas can further add to risk estimate variation. Changes in the indication for biopsy are perhaps the most pertinent shift over these study periods: physicians are more likely to biopsy now than in the 1950s. Population uptake of mammography began in the 1970s [20], and screening technology has continued to improve since then [21, 22], leading to an increase in breast biopsy incidence. The adoption of core needle biopsies, which are less invasive than excisional biopsies, further increased the likelihood of a breast biopsy, especially in what are considered high-risk populations.

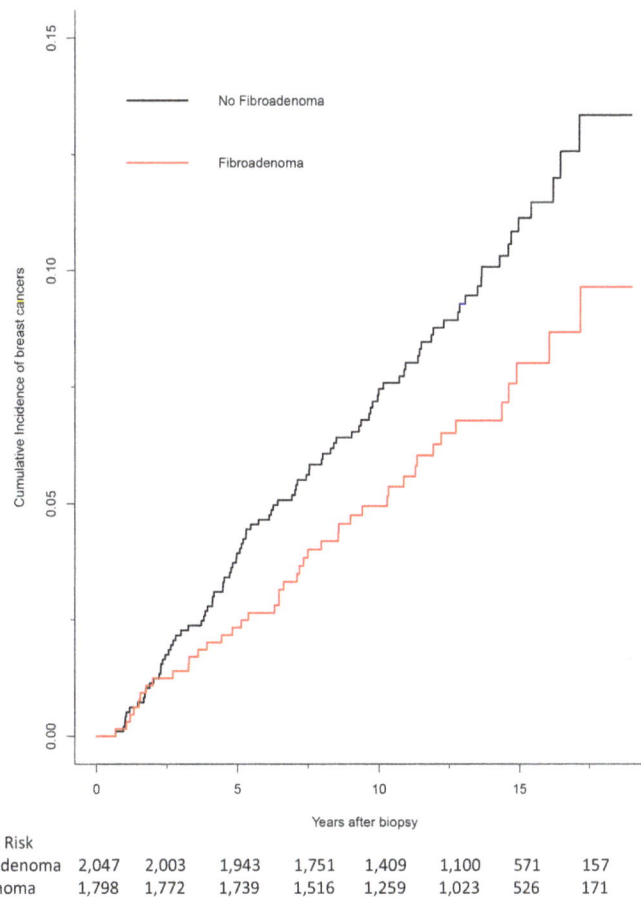

Fig. 2 Cumulative incidence of breast cancers over study period. Women with biopsies that indicated fibroadenomas accumulated fewer breast cancers over the study period than women whose biopsies did not indicate fibroadenomas. p < 0.001 by Fine and Gray test

The strengths of our study stem from the cohort study design, where all breast biopsies were reexamined for benign lesions in a centralized and standardized manner by Wayne State University pathologists, and identification of breast cancers occurred through institutional medical records and then standardized for the region through use of the population-based SEER registry. This allowed for the identification of breast cancers among women who sought care outside of the hospitals served by the UPG. It should be noted there are limitations to our study. First, the population estimates used in the SIR analysis includes women who have been diagnosed with BBD in the metropolitan Detroit area; thus, the SIR may slightly underestimate the risk associated with breast cancer. Next, our assessment was limited to the presence or absence of fibroadenomas on breast biopsy, but there may be added value in assessing whether these fibroadenomas exhibit other BBD lesions. There are conflicting reports on the breast cancer risk associated with complex fibroadenomas (fibroadenomas that exhibit cysts, calcifications, sclerosing adenosis, and/or apocrine metaplasia) [17, 18]. Because of the high prevalence of fibroadenomas in this population, breast cancer risk associated with complex fibroadenoma should also be independently reviewed in African American women.

Conclusions

Currently, a diagnosis of fibroadenoma requires no further intervention and is followed by a primary care physician or gynecologist unless the patient elects to have a mass removed, usually due to size of the tumor, recurrence, or pain [23, 24]. Because previous investigations of fibroadenoma on biopsy estimated an elevated risk of breast cancer that persists for 20 years [17], physicians may currently screen women with fibroadenomas frequently. Our study suggests that fibroadenomas do not increase risk of subsequent breast cancers. Ultimately, examining specific features of BBD will improve risk estimates used in breast cancer risk models, reduce patient anxiety, and improve management of fibroadenoma in the clinic by reducing overscreening and overtreatment of this population, both associated with potential patient harms and excessive resource allocation.

Abbreviations

BBD: Benign breast disease; FA: Fibroadenoma; HFHS: Henry Ford Health System; MDCSS: Metropolitan Detroit Cancer Surveillance System; RR: Relative risk; SEER: Surveillance, Epidemiology, and End Results program; SIR: Standardized incidence ratio; UPG: University Pathology Group

Funding

This work was supported by Susan G. Komen for the Cure (IIRG 222547 to MLC, GTDR14299438 to MLC and ANS) and the National Institutes of Health (NCI grant 1F31CA22133301 to ANS).

Authors' contributions

MLC, DWV, SB, and RAF designed the study. EA, RS, MFD, VP, and RAF performed data acquisition. ANS and JJR had full access to all study data and take responsibility for the integrity of the data, the accuracy of the data analysis, and interpretation of data. All authors were responsible for critical revisions, and all authors read and approved the final version of this work.

Competing interests

The study sponsors had no role in the design of the study; the collection, analysis, or interpretation of the data; the writing of the manuscript; or the decision to submit the manuscript for publication. The authors declare they have no competing interests.

Author details

[1]Department of Oncology, Wayne State University School of Medicine, 4100 John R Street, MM04EP, Detroit, MI 48201, USA. [2]Department of Pathology, Wayne State University School of Medicine, Detroit, MI, USA. [3]Department of Laboratory Medicine and Pathology, Mayo Clinic, Rochester, MN, USA. [4]Barbara Ann Karmanos Cancer Institute, Detroit, MI, USA.

References

1. Silverstein MJ, Recht A, Lagios MD, et al. Image-detected breast cancer: state-of-the-art diagnosis and treatment. J Am Coll Surg. 2009;209(4):504–20. https://doi.org/10.1016/j.jamcollsurg.2009.07.006.
2. Dupont WD, Page DL. Risk factors for breast cancer in women with proliferative breast disease. N Engl J Med. 1985;312(3):146–51. https://doi.org/10.1056/NEJM198501173120303.
3. Hartmann LC, Sellers TA, Frost MH, et al. Benign breast disease and the risk of breast cancer. N Engl J Med. 2005;353(3):229–37. https://doi.org/10.1056/NEJMoa044383.
4. Cote ML, Ruterbusch JJ, Alosh B, et al. Benign breast disease and the risk of subsequent breast cancer in African American women. Cancer Prev Res (Phila Pa). 2012;5(12):1375–80. https://doi.org/10.1158/1940-6207.CAPR-12-0175.
5. Gail MH, Brinton LA, Byar DP, et al. Projecting individualized probabilities of developing breast cancer for white females who are being examined annually. J Natl Cancer Inst. 1989;81(24):1879–86.
6. Kuijper A, Mommers ECM, van der Wall E, Diest V. J P. Histopathology of fibroadenoma of the breast. Am J Clin Pathol. 2001;115(5):736–42. https://doi.org/10.1309/F523-FMJV-W886-3J38.
7. Hughes LE, Mansel RE, Webster DJT, Gravelle IH. Benign disorders and diseases of the breast: concepts and clinical management. London: Baillière Tindall; 1989.
8. Dyrstad SW, Yan Y, Fowler AM, Colditz GA. Breast cancer risk associated with benign breast disease: systematic review and meta-analysis. Breast Cancer Res Treat. 2015;149(3):569–75. https://doi.org/10.1007/s10549-014-3254-6.
9. Oluwole SF, Freeman HP. Analysis of benign breast lesions in blacks. Am J Surg. 1979;137(6):786–9.
10. Organ CH, Organ BC. Fibroadenoma of the female breast: a critical clinical assessment. J Natl Med Assoc. 1983;75(7):701–4.
11. DeSantis CE, Fedewa SA, Goding Sauer A, Kramer JL, Smith RA, Jemal A. Breast cancer statistics, 2015: convergence of incidence rates between black and white women. CA Cancer J Clin. 2016;66(1):31–42. https://doi.org/10.3322/caac.21320.
12. Althuis MD, Brogan DD, Coates RJ, et al. Breast cancers among very young premenopausal women (United States). Cancer Causes Control. 2003;14(2):151–60.
13. Newman LA. Breast cancer in African-American women. Oncologist. 2005;10(1):1–14. https://doi.org/10.1634/theoncologist.10-1-1.
14. Shavers VL, Harlan LC, Stevens JL. Racial/ethnic variation in clinical presentation, treatment, and survival among breast cancer patients under age 35. Cancer. 2003;97(1):134–47. https://doi.org/10.1002/cncr.11051.
15. Earl Henson D, Chu KC, Levine PH. Histologic grade, stage, and survival in breast carcinoma. Cancer. 2003;98(5):908–17. https://doi.org/10.1002/cncr.11558.
16. Amend K, Hicks D, Ambrosone CB. Breast cancer in African-American women: differences in tumor biology from European-American women. Cancer Res. 2006;66(17):8327–30. https://doi.org/10.1158/0008-5472.CAN-06-1927.

17. Dupont WD, Page DL, Parl FF, et al. Long-term risk of breast cancer in women with fibroadenoma. N Engl J Med. 1994;331(1):10–5. https://doi.org/10.1056/NEJM199407073310103.

18. Nassar A, Visscher DW, Degnim AC, et al. Complex fibroadenoma and breast cancer risk: a Mayo Clinic benign breast disease cohort study. Breast Cancer Res Treat. 2015;153(2):397–405. https://doi.org/10.1007/s10549-015-3535-8.

19. Worsham MJ, Raju U, Lu M, et al. Risk factors for breast cancer from benign breast disease in a diverse population. Breast Cancer Res Treat. 2009;118(1): 1–7. https://doi.org/10.1007/s10549-008-0198-8.

20. Dodd GD. American Cancer Society guidelines on screening for breast cancer: an overview. CA Cancer J Clin. 1992;42(3):177–80. https://doi.org/10.3322/canjclin.42.3.177.

21. Haus AG. Historical technical developments in mammography. Technol Cancer Res Treat. 2002;1(2):119–26.

22. Yaffe MJ, Mainprize JG, Jong RA. Technical developments in mammography. Health Phys. 2008;95(5):599–611. https://doi.org/10.1097/01.HP.0000327648.42431.75.

23. Greenberg R, Skornick Y, Kaplan O. Management of breast fibroadenomas. J Gen Intern Med. 1998;13(9):640–5. https://doi.org/10.1046/j.1525-1497.1998.cr188.x.

24. Sklair-Levy M, Sella T, Alweiss T, Craciun I, Libson E, Mally B. Incidence and management of complex fibroadenomas. Am J Roentgenol. 2008;190(1): 214–8. https://doi.org/10.2214/AJR.07.2330.

6

Intra-operative spectroscopic assessment of surgical margins during breast conserving surgery

Dustin W. Shipp[1], Emad A. Rakha[2], Alexey A. Koloydenko[3], R. Douglas Macmillan[4], Ian O. Ellis[2] and Ioan Notingher[1]* ⓘ

Abstract

Background: In over 20% of breast conserving operations, postoperative pathological assessment of the excised tissue reveals positive margins, requiring additional surgery. Current techniques for intra-operative assessment of tumor margins are insufficient in accuracy or resolution to reliably detect small tumors. There is a distinct need for a fast technique to accurately identify tumors smaller than 1 mm^2 in large tissue surfaces within 30 min.

Methods: Multi-modal spectral histopathology (MSH), a multimodal imaging technique combining tissue auto-fluorescence and Raman spectroscopy was used to detect microscopic residual tumor at the surface of the excised breast tissue. New algorithms were developed to optimally utilize auto-fluorescence images to guide Raman measurements and achieve the required detection accuracy over large tissue surfaces (up to 4 × 6.5 cm^2). Algorithms were trained on 91 breast tissue samples from 65 patients.

Results: Independent tests on 121 samples from 107 patients - including 51 fresh, whole excision specimens - detected breast carcinoma on the tissue surface with 95% sensitivity and 82% specificity. One surface of each uncut excision specimen was measured in 12–24 min. The combination of high spatial-resolution auto-fluorescence with specific diagnosis by Raman spectroscopy allows reliable detection even for invasive carcinoma or ductal carcinoma in situ smaller than 1 mm^2.

Conclusions: This study provides evidence that this multimodal approach could provide an objective tool for intra-operative assessment of breast conserving surgery margins, reducing the risk for unnecessary second operations.

Keywords: Auto-fluorescence, Breast cancer, Raman spectroscopy, Intra-operative margin evaluation

Background

Breast conserving surgery (BCS), also referred to as lumpectomy or wide local excision, is currently the most widely used surgical procedure for resection of breast cancer [1]. The goal of BCS is to remove the entire tumor while leaving healthy breast tissue intact, providing better cosmetic outcome. Nevertheless, this is challenging because of the lack of tools available for intra-operative assessment of margins to indicate complete tumor excision.

Postoperatively, typically over a period of 1–2 weeks, the excised tissues are examined histologically to determine the proximity of tumor to the surface of the excision. In more than 20% of BCS procedures, positive margins are detected (i.e. tumor close to the edge) and additional operations are required to achieve complete excision [2, 3]. Nearly half of these "re-excisions" are for "on-ink" margins [3], meaning that tumor was found on the surface of the excised tissue. Guidelines from the Society of Surgical Oncology and the American Society for Radiation Oncology state that clear on-ink margins are sufficient to remove tumor and more widely clear margins did not significantly increase the risk of recurrence [4, 5].

* Correspondence: ioan.notingher@nottingham.ac.uk
[1]School of Physics and Astronomy, University of Nottingham, Nottingham NG7 2RD, UK
Full list of author information is available at the end of the article

Intra-operative resection of additional tissue (i.e. cavity shaves) has been shown to reduce the need for re-excisions [6]. However, cavity shaving can result in excessive tissue loss and poor cosmetic outcomes. Additional techniques are therefore needed to assess the margins of BCS specimens within intra-operative timescales (i.e. less than 30 min). Frozen section histopathologic assessment and cytologic imprint preparation (i.e. touch preparation) analysis can assess margins within this time [7, 8], but are often considered impractical for BCS due to the large size of the specimens, sampling errors [7, 9], and sample preparation artifacts [10] in addition to pathologist time and cost implications. The MarginProbe device, which assesses margins using radiofrequency spectroscopy, has entered operating theaters, but with 75.2% sensitivity and 46.4% specificity [11]. ClearEdge measures tissue-specific electrical properties with preliminary results indicating sensitivity of 84.3–87.3% and specificity of 81.9–75.6% [12]. Higher diagnostic accuracy has been reported for techniques with higher molecular specificity, such as fluorescence lifetime imaging (FLIm) [13] and mass spectrometry [14]. A recent preliminary study using a FLIm probe on 2×2 cm^2 cut breast tissues indicted automated classification accuracy greater than 97% [13]. For mass spectrometry handheld devices, 93.4% sensitivity and 94.9% specificity were reported, but with spatial resolution limited to approximately 4×4 mm^2 [15]. Limitations related to spatial resolution and tissue sampling coverage make hand-held technologies vulnerable to missing small tumors (e.g. ductal carcinoma in situ (DCIS) smaller than 1 mm^2), which are responsible for a disproportionate number of re-excisions [5].

Sampling errors may be overcome by optical imaging techniques that can provide diagnosis with microscopic spatial resolution [16–22]. While diagnoses with sensitivity and specificity as high as 93% have been reported, structure-based imaging diagnoses rely on specially trained pathologists and are therefore subject to inter-observer and intra-observer variability, especially if large, detailed images need to be viewed [19, 21]. Attempts to avoid subjectivity through automated diagnosis by diffuse reflectance spectroscopy (DRS) [23, 24], elastic scattering spectroscopy (ESS) [25], and spatial frequency domain imaging (SFDI) [26] have been proposed. However, DRS and SFDI have insufficient spatial resolution to detect small tumors (< 1 mm^2) and ESS was shown to have 69% sensitivity and 85% specificity [25]. Furthermore, of these imaging techniques, only light sheet microscopy using fluorescent labels [22] and SFDI [26] have been demonstrated on tissue areas approaching that of most BCS specimens (i.e. larger than 2×2 cm^2). Extending these techniques to large breast tissue surfaces (e.g. 4×6 cm^2) results in measurement times unacceptable for intra-operative use.

Raman spectroscopy is a highly sensitive optical technique that can provide a medical diagnosis based on quantitative molecular attributes of the tissue [27, 28]. Raman spectroscopy achieves molecular specificity by measuring the vibrational frequencies of tissue molecules excited by the laser. Basing the diagnosis on quantitative properties instead of human interpretation of structural images has been shown to reduce inter-observer variability [29]. Raman spectroscopy has been applied to the assessment of breast cancer with 94% sensitivity and 96% specificity [30], including hand-held fiber-probes for in vivo point-measurements [31, 32], albeit with no imaging capability and low spatial accuracy. Spatially offset Raman spectroscopy (SORS) was also proposed for tumors embedded within resected tissue [33, 34], but has thus far demonstrated only limited spatial resolution.

Spontaneous Raman spectroscopy alone is slow to image typical BCS specimens with sufficient spatial accuracy to allow accurate detection of small residual tumors that are of particular clinical interest. One approach for reducing the acquisition time is surface-enhanced Raman spectroscopy (SERS). A recent study by Wang et al. detected tumor at the excision surface with 89% sensitivity and 92% specificity by using gold nanoparticles functionalized with reporter SERS labels and monoclonal antibodies targeting biomarkers including epidermal growth factor receptor (EGFR), human epidermal growth factor receptor 2 (HER2), estrogen receptor (ER), or CD44 [35].

An alternative approach to reduce analysis time is selective-sampling Raman spectroscopy, which uses spatial information from the sample to guide Raman measurements [36–39]. This approach has the advantage that no exogenous labels are required. In a previous study, we have demonstrated the feasibility of multimodal spectral histopathology (MSH), a selective-sampling technique that combines high-resolution wide-field auto-fluorescence (AF) microscopy and Raman spectroscopy to detect ductal carcinomas in frozen breast micro-sections (5×5 mm^2) [38]. This method acquires sensitive and specific Raman measurements while preserving the spatial resolution of AF images (10–20 μm), enabling MSH to identify small tumors. However, previous MSH studies were optimized for measurements of small tissue samples (less than 0.5×0.5 cm^2) cut from surgical specimens. Extending these measurements to large breast tissue surfaces resulted in timescales unacceptable for intra-operative use (i.e. longer than 3 hours).

In this study, we have integrated an MSH instrument (combined confocal AF and Raman microscope, see Fig. 1a) and optimized the sampling and data processing algorithms combining spatial and spectral information for measuring the surface of large tissues (4×6.5 cm^2

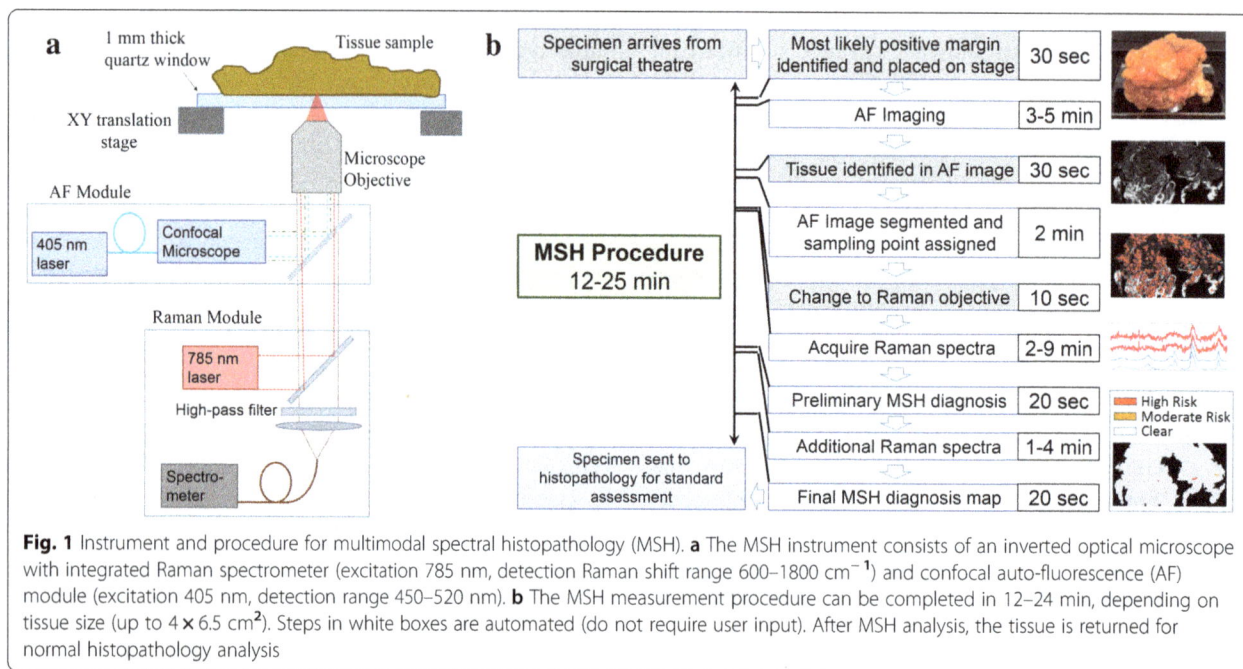

Fig. 1 Instrument and procedure for multimodal spectral histopathology (MSH). **a** The MSH instrument consists of an inverted optical microscope with integrated Raman spectrometer (excitation 785 nm, detection Raman shift range 600–1800 cm^{-1}) and confocal auto-fluorescence (AF) module (excitation 405 nm, detection range 450–520 nm). **b** The MSH measurement procedure can be completed in 12–24 min, depending on tissue size (up to 4 × 6.5 cm^2). Steps in white boxes are automated (do not require user input). After MSH analysis, the tissue is returned for normal histopathology analysis

area) such as BCS specimens. The large-scale MSH technique reduces the number of required Raman measurements and allows analysis of the radial aspect of greatest concern in 12–24 min (see Fig. 1b), a timeframe considered appropriate for intra-operative use.

New data acquisition and analysis techniques were also automated to account for patient-to-patient variations and provide reliable, user-independent diagnosis across a broad range of tumor types and sizes. The segmentation and sampling algorithms were optimized to ensure consistent, thorough sampling of tumors on the surface of tissues with varying properties. The Raman spectral classifier was trained to distinguish between malignant and healthy tissues, even for difficult cases of hypercellular tissues. These spatial and molecular measurements were integrated into a final diagnosis image showing the presence or absence of tumor on the tissue surface. Through independent tests of these algorithms and measurement protocols on breast tissue samples and real, whole BCS specimen surfaces, we show that MSH has great potential for objective, intra-operative assessment of the excision surface of BCS specimens immediately after excision without requiring any sample preparation (sectioning or labeling).

Methods
Sample collection
Two sets of breast tissue samples were used in this study. Smaller samples of breast tissue cut from mastectomy samples were used for training (91 samples from 65 patients) and validation (70 samples from 56 patients) of MSH

procedures and diagnosis algorithms. The mastectomy samples varied from 4×6 mm^2 to 32×28 mm^2 and were approximately 2–10 mm thick. These samples were frozen in liquid nitrogen and stored at -20 °C until being thawed for measurement of one tissue surface. Principal component analysis (PCA) showed no differences between Raman spectra acquired from fresh and thawed samples. Samples known to contain confounding tissue types (e.g. fibroadenoma, fibrocystic change) were preferentially included in the training set to broaden the scope of the Raman spectroscopy classifier. After measurements, the samples were submitted for histological processing and hematoxylin and eosin (H&E) sections were obtained for each measured surface. Two validation samples in which conditions not included in the training set (e.g. metaplastic carcinoma) were discovered on histopathologic assessment were excluded from analysis. Future studies will target the inclusion of these rarer tissue types in the training set.

Fresh, uncut BCS specimens from 51 patients were measured as they arrived from the operating theater, without any preparation or processing. One surface was chosen for scanning based on proximity to palpable or visible lesions and to avoid high concentrations of surgical dyes. Following measurement, the scanned surface was colored with yellow ink and the specimen was evaluated by standard histopathological processes and protocols. This included cutting the specimen in a cruciate fashion and recovering H&E sections radially from the tumor to the tissue surface. Thus, these H&E sections were perpendicular to the surface measured by MSH. Pathologists reported the presence or absence of tumor on the measured surface marked in yellow.

Multimodal MSH

A schematic of the MSH instrument and procedure is shown in Fig. 1. Tissues were placed directly onto a 5.1×7.6 cm^2 quartz window for measurement in an inverted microscope configuration. Raman spectra were measured at the corners of the window and the window level was adjusted to reduce the tilt. Quartz is a popular substrate for Raman spectroscopy as it avoids fluorescence or scattering contributions common in other substrates. Tissues were found to be malleable such that their own weight pressed with sufficient force to ensure thorough, flat surface contact with the window.

AF images were acquired by a Nikon C2 confocal microscope module (405 nm laser, emission 511 nm long-pass filter, and detected by a photomultiplier tube). The portion of the AF image containing the tissue sample was automatically detected, allowing the background to be removed by a virtual mask. The user adjusted the intensity threshold for this algorithm by visual inspection to ensure appropriate masking. Dark regions or "segments" in the AF image were identified by an unsupervised algorithm. A threshold was varied automatically across several intensity values. For each threshold value, pixels with AF intensity values below the threshold were grouped into contiguous regions. Each contiguous region was marked as a segment. The threshold was varied to maximize the segmentation parameter $A \cdot N$, where A is the area included in all segments within the image and N is the number of segments in the image. For MSH measurements, Raman measurement points were assigned within both dark segments and large regions of high AF intensity. The number and location of measurement points were determined as described in [40], with a minimum of two points per segment and a target density of one point per square millimeter.

Raman spectra were acquired by a fiber-coupled Raman spectroscopy module (785 nm excitation, 600–1800 cm^{-1} detection). The procedure for Raman spectral acquisition differed depending on the phase of the study. In the initial training set measurement phase, regions of interest were identified by eye in the AF image. Raman spectra were then acquired in a raster scanning scheme. Scanned areas ranged from 3×4 to 20×16 mm^2 with 40–100 μm step-sizes. For each scan, spectra were divided into four to eight groups based on spectral similarities by k-means cluster analysis. These groups were assigned arbitrary colors and the scan was displayed as a hyperspectral image. Under guidance of one or two trained pathologists, like-colored regions in the hyperspectral image were manually assigned to various tissue classes based on spatial correlation to AF and H&E images. Spectra within

these regions were added to the training set for the corresponding tissue type. These tissue assignments are described in "Quantitative diagnosis based on Raman spectra".

MSH-sampled measurements were generated from the raster scan using the nearest acquired spectra to the generated sampling points. These MSH measurements were limited to the raster-scanned area. For test set samples (both mastectomy tissue and whole BCS specimens), Raman measurement points were identified automatically by the segmentation and sampling procedure described above. For both of these schemes, the acquisition time was set to 0.3 s. All spectra were processed, analyzed, and classified individually.

Raman spectra were processed by standard algorithms including cosmic ray removal, wavenumber calibration, throughput correction, background subtraction [41], and smoothing [42]. Spectra with poor signal to noise ratio (SNR) were withheld from analysis (see Additional file 1 for details), removing approximately 2% of spectra from the training set. Raman raster scans from 91 breast tissue samples in the training set (28 with tumor, 63 without tumor, > 1000 spectra per sample, > 100,000 spectra total) were annotated and used to train a linear discriminant analysis (LDA) classification model as subsequently described.

Using this model, segments in the AF image were assigned class labels based on the Raman spectra acquired from the corresponding area. For samples included in the training set, spectral diagnoses were performed using a new classification model trained excluding the sample under evaluation (leave-one-out cross-validation). If the classification of spectra within a segment was not unanimous, the segment was split into smaller segments, each containing spectra with homogeneous diagnosis. Tissue regions diagnosed as tumor were assigned a second round of Raman measurements. Second round measurements were acquired with higher sampling density and doubled acquisition time per spectrum (0.6 s). In MSH measurements generated from raster scans, second round measurements averaged spectra from neighboring raster scan points.

First-round and second-round Raman spectra were used to create a final diagnosis image. For each segment, a tumor score (TS) ranging from 1 to 10 was calculated from the class probabilities returned by the LDA model for spectra within that segment. The TS for MSH measurements of training samples (see Additional file 1: Figures S3A and S4A) guided the creation of thresholds into "clear," "moderate risk," and "high risk" TS. These thresholds were applied to independent test MSH measurements of mastectomy samples and whole BCS excision surfaces to create three-color

MSH diagnosis maps that could be quickly and easily interpreted in the operating theater.

Statistical evaluation

The accuracy of the LDA classifier was estimated by fivefold cross-validation in which the spectra from 80% of patients (i.e. training set) were used to train a model to evaluate the remaining spectra (i.e. validation set). This was repeated five times to include each patient in the validation set once. Results were then reported on a per spectrum basis, including up to 1000 spectra per tissue type per sample.

For statistical evaluation of MSH diagnosis, a sample was considered positive if it contained tumor anywhere in the measured area. Likewise, the MSH diagnosis was considered positive if any tumor was identified (moderate risk or high risk) in the diagnosis image. Samples

from mastectomy tissue were small enough that the MSH-identified tumor overlapped with histopathologically identified tumor in all cases where both were present. Similar correlation was not tested in BCS specimens as the H&E sections were obtained perpendicular to the MSH-measured surface per standard clinical procedure.

Results

Unsupervised segmentation of AF images

Although the absolute origin of the signal in the AF signal is not fully understood, several endogenous fluorophores can be detected by the 405 nm excitation/ 511 nm long-pass emission system, including flavin adenine dinucleotide (FAD), reduced nicotinamide adenine dinucleotide (NADH), and collagen, the last of which is most common in stromal tissue [43]. In our observations

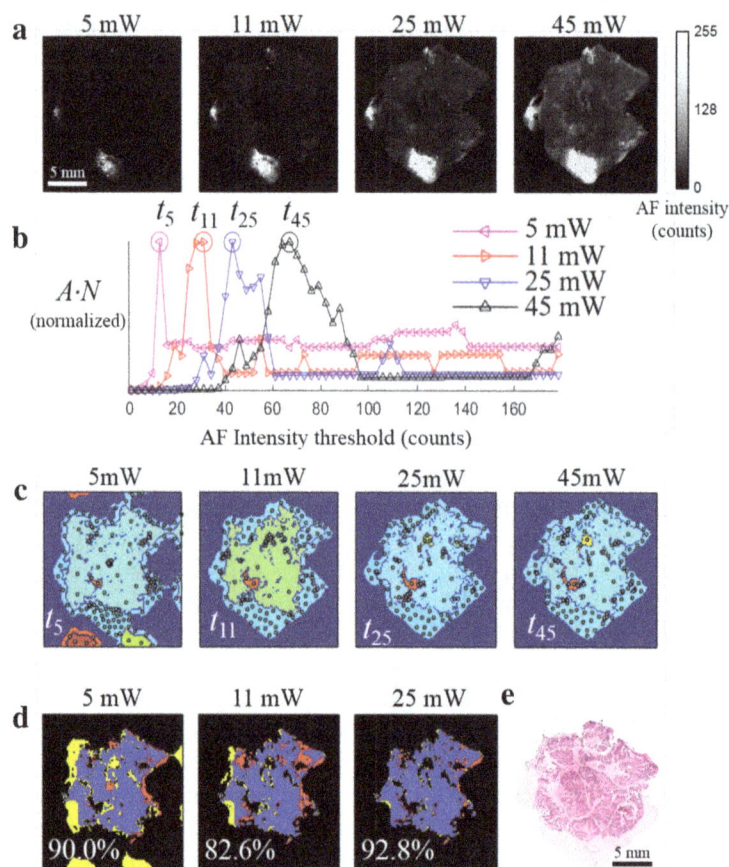

Fig. 2 Method for unsupervised segmentation of auto-fluorescence (AF) images of breast tissue. a AF intensity images of a typical breast tissue sample containing invasive carcinoma obtained at difference excitation laser powers. b Representation of the total area captured by all segments to total number of segments for each image ($A \cdot N$) versus the segmentation threshold. c Segmented AF images using the optimized intensity thresholds t_5, t_{11}, t_{25}, t_{45}; white dots indicate the sampling points for Raman spectroscopy. Each segment is assigned a unique, arbitrary color in these images. d The computed overlap with segmentation of the 45-mW image; blue, regions captured in segments in both AF images; red, regions were in segments in the 45-mW image but not in the images at lower power; yellow, regions in segments of AF image at lower laser power but not the 45-mW image. e Hematoxylin and eosin (H&E) section. The dense clusters of dark blue dots are tumor cells

within this study, dark regions in the acquired AF images generally contained tumor, benign growths (e.g. fibroadenoma), and adipose tissue (see Fig. 2). Therefore, these dark regions were identified as "segments" targeted for subsequent Raman measurements. The sampling algorithm also assigned additional Raman measurement points to bright regions in the AF image to address samples where the tumor may have higher AF intensity, i.e. samples containing only tumor and adipose tissues or with tumor cells scattered within stroma.

Automated algorithms were used to segment AF images and assign sampling points to minimize the number of Raman measurements while still acquiring spectra from any regions of tumor present on the surface of the sample. Each AF image was segmented by finding the maximum value of $A \cdot N$ (where A is the total area captured by all segments and N is the total number of segments) as a function of the segmentation intensity threshold. Maximizing N leads to the discrimination of small features while maximizing A favors larger segments, allowing faster measurements of large surfaces. The process of optimizing the segmentation and sampling algorithms toward these goals is described in "Optimization of segmentation and sampling algorithms" in Additional file 1.

The accuracy of the segmentation and sampling algorithms was ultimately evaluated by calculating the "tumor hit rate" as a figure of merit. The tumor hit rate describes the probability that a region of tumor on the surface of a sample will contain at least one Raman measurement. If the Raman spectral classifier were 100% accurate, the tumor hit rate would be equivalent to the sensitivity of the complete MSH procedure. The tumor hit rate was calculated for all 28 mastectomy samples containing tumor in the training set. For these samples, the median tumor hit rate was 100%. One sample contained approximately 5 mm^2 of low-density tumor cells scattered within stroma that went unsampled. The tumor hit rates for the other mastectomy samples ranged from 73 to 100% (see Additional file 1: Figure S2). Therefore, this new method for optimizing the segmentation threshold allowed using fewer targeted Raman measurements to detect the majority of tumor regions over large surfaces. Indeed, the algorithm was optimized for assigning sampling points to large tissue areas detects most tumors - even those smaller than 1–2 mm - with a sampling density of one point per square millimeter. These algorithms allowed even large tissue surfaces (4×6.5 cm^2) to be thoroughly analyzed by fewer than 2000 Raman measurements.

Sample to sample variations in the intensity of AF emission (depending on patient age, various tissue structures, etc.) is a key challenge when attempting to use an absolute intensity threshold for the segmentation of all AF intensity images. To ensure a user-independent and accurate diagnosis result, all data analysis steps were automated and designed to be invariant across the full range of samples. To evaluate the invariance of the segmentation algorithm to these conditions, we induced large AF intensity variations by imaging a set of eight breast tissue samples with four different excitation powers (5 mW, 12 mW, 25 mW, and 45 mW).

When the AF images recorded at different laser powers (Fig. 2a) were segmented using the intensity threshold values corresponding to the maximum values in Fig. 2b (t_5, t_{11}, t_{25}, t_{45}), consistent results were obtained regarding the shape and size of the dark segments and the generated locations of sampling points for Raman spectroscopy measurements (white dots) (see Fig. 2c). The percent overlap with the segments from the 45-mW image with AF images obtained at lower excitation powers ranged from 82 to 93%. Furthermore, segments identified in the image acquired at all laser powers correspond to the area of tissue containing tumor, shown by the dense clusters in the H&E image in Fig. 2e. These results indicate that the maximum value of the $A \cdot N$ function may provide a consistent, unsupervised, user-independent method for selecting an optimal intensity threshold for each AF image.

Quantitative diagnosis based on Raman spectra

After establishing a method for guiding Raman spectroscopy measurements based on AF images of breast tissue, a supervised model was developed for classification of breast tissues based on Raman spectra. Figure 3 compares the AF image (Fig. 3a), pseudo-color k-means clustering hyperspectral image from the Raman spectra (Fig. 3b), and the histopathology image obtained by H&E staining (Fig. 3c) for a typical breast sample containing invasive carcinoma, benign tissue with inflamed stroma, and fat. These images show that the k-means clustering images can accurately capture the main tissue structures, including the tumor, based solely on the molecular composition of tissue measured by the Raman spectra.

Under guidance of one or two trained breast pathologists, the k-means clustering hyperspectral images acquired from all mastectomy samples in the training set allowed for individual Raman spectra to be assigned a label corresponding to invasive carcinoma (IC), other tumor types (OT, e.g. DCIS, lobular carcinoma in situ (LCIS), malignant phyllodes (MP)), benign proliferative lesions (BG, e.g. fibroadenoma, sclerosing adenosis, epithelial hyperplasia), inflammation (IN), parenchyma (P), normal mammary stroma (S), fat (F), or a mixture of fat and stroma (F + S) (see Fig. 3e). A maximum of 1000 spectra of each tissue type was included from each sample. These eight tissue types were later relabeled into three classes based on spectral similarities: fat (including F and F + S), benign/healthy (including S, P, IN, and BG),

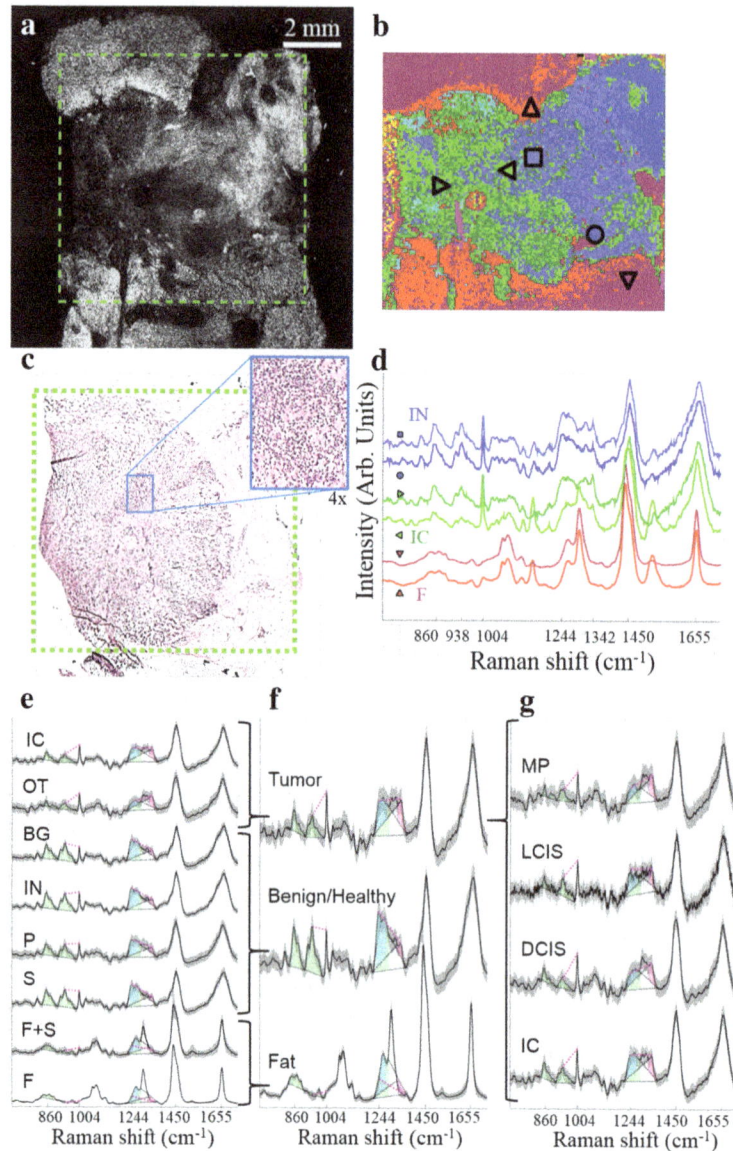

Fig. 3 Raman spectral acquisition and annotation. Tumor regions (clusters of blue dots in the H&E image in (**c**)) appear darker in the auto-fluorescence (AF) image (**a**). The region in the green box was measured by a Raman raster scan. *K*-means cluster analysis of these spectra identifies similar spectra to create a hyperspectral image (**b**). Single spectra from locations marked in **b** are shown in **d**. Based on the information in **a-d**, pre-processed spectra from green areas (horizontal triangles) are marked as tumor, blue (square/circle) as inflamed stroma, and red (vertical triangles) as fat. Other clusters (cyan, yellow, and magenta) were background or noise and were withheld from the training set. Mean and standard deviation of all spectra in the training set show that the annotated tissue types (**e**) could be simplified to three classes used by the spectral classifier (**f**). Spectral features used for classification are marked as shaded areas (peak areas) and magenta lines (peak intensity differences). These peak areas are shaded blue for lipid-associated bands, green for protein-associated bands, and magenta for nucleic acid-associated bands. These features are consistent across all tumor types (**g**). Classes: IC, invasive carcinoma; OT, other tumor types (includes ductal carcinoma in situ (DCIS), lobular carcinoma in situ (LCIS), malignant phyllodes (MP)); BG, benign growths (includes fibroadenoma, sclerosing adenosis, hyperplasia); IN, inflammation; P, parenchyma; S, healthy stroma; F, fat; F + S, mixture of fat and stroma

and tumor (including invasive carcinoma (IC), DCIS, LCIS, and malignant phyllodes (MP)) (see Fig. 3f).

The simplified classes preserve major spectral features corresponding to cancer (nucleic acids, non-collagen proteins), stroma (collagen and other proteins), and fat (lipids) (see Fig. 3f) that are consistent with previously reported Raman spectra of breast cancers, adipose tissue, and other healthy breast tissue [27, 30, 38, 43]. Spectra from various tumor types (see Fig. 3g) share the characteristic features typical of tumor: intense bands assigned to nucleic acids (788 cm^{-1}, 1098 cm^{-1}, 1342 cm^{-1}), phenylalanine (1004 cm^{-1}), and amide I vibrations (1655 cm^{-1}), less intense bands corresponding to collagen (860 cm^{-1}, 938 cm^{-1}). Although there are spectral differences between these tumor types, they are less pronounced than the differences between spectra from tumor and other tissue types. These and other features (eight features in total) were identified to reduce the dimensionality of Raman spectra for more robust classification (see Additional file 1: Table S1). Briefly, spectra from tumor tissue was distinguished from benign tissues based on higher intensities in bands assigned to nucleic acids and lower intensities in collagen-assigned and amide III-assigned bands, in agreement with previous reports [38].

The model for classifying Raman spectra was optimized over several classifier families with varied parameters, including spectral features (see "Optimization of Raman Spectral Classifier" in Additional file 1). The overall sensitivity and specificity for the best-performing model (linear discriminant analysis (LDA)), were 90.2% and 93.4%, respectively (see Additional file 1: Table S3 for breakdown by tissue type). This represents the performance of the classifier on a single Raman spectrum, not taking into account any information from the AF image or neighboring spectra.

When the classifier performance was evaluated for different sub-types of tumor, the sensitivity was greater than 99% for DCIS, LCIS and malignant phyllodes, which were always found with closely packed tumor cells. However, the sensitivity was 89% for tissues containing invasive carcinoma, which often consisted of scattered tumor cells within benign tissue.

Another significant source of misclassification was spectra from benign/healthy tissues being classified as tumor. Although this "benign/healthy" class contains many tissue types such as stroma, parenchyma, and inflammation, classification errors occurred most often (50–80% specificity by spectrum) with spectra from hypercellular tissues including epithelial hyperplasia, sclerosing adenosis, and, to a lesser degree, fibroadenoma. Although these tissues were specifically targeted for inclusion in the training set, their low prevalence (three samples with sclerosing adenosis, four samples with hyperplasia, nine samples with fibroadenoma) suggest that the classifier could be further improved by including more measurements of these tissues in the training set.

MSH tissue diagnostic model by integrating AF and Raman

The MSH diagnosis relied on both spatial information from segmented AF images and molecular information from Raman spectra. Within an AF image, the likelihood that a segment corresponded to a tumor (i.e. tumor score, TS) was calculated based on the Raman classification results of each spectrum within the segment.

To evaluate the performance of the MSH algorithm, we used leave-one-sample-out cross-validation to compare the MSH results for training set samples with the diagnoses obtained by raster-scanning Raman imaging and histopathology. An MSH diagnosis was obtained based on AF images and spectra from raster scan Raman measurements corresponding to locations assigned by the sampling algorithm. Figure 4 presents typical examples of MSH and Raman raster scan diagnoses for breast tissue samples containing the most common breast carcinomas: IC, LCIS, and DCIS. In all cases, the diagnostic images obtained by raster-scanning Raman spectroscopy and MSH were in agreement with histopathological H&E images. However, MSH dramatically reduced the acquisition time, as it required 100-fold to 200-fold fewer Raman spectra compared with raster scanning while providing similar diagnostic accuracy for breast carcinomas, even those comprising small tumors (< 1 mm^2).

Under guidance from a trained breast cancer surgeon, the MSH diagnosis images were designed for ease of interpretation in the operating theater. The MSH results from training set samples were used to set thresholds to display the maps of TS as clear, moderate risk, or high risk. Setting the thresholds for the high-risk tumor at 9.9 (targeting high specificity) resulted in estimated sensitivity and specificity of 82% and 75%, respectively. The more sensitive moderate-risk threshold at 9.4 had estimated sensitivity and specificity for MSH of 96% and 59%, respectively.

Independent test of MSH diagnosis on mastectomy samples

The first independent validation of MSH was carried out on mastectomy samples (sizes ranging from 6 × 7 to 20 × 25 mm^2) as H&E sections could be obtained from the measured surface to confirm the MSH diagnosis. Measurements for all tissue samples were performed according to the complete MSH protocol presented in Fig. 1b and lasted less than 4 min per sample. The receiver operating characteristic (ROC) curve for this test and examples of these MSH measurements are shown in Fig. 5. Tumor scores for all segments in independent mastectomy samples are shown in Additional file 1: Figure S4(B) with the maximum TS for each sample shown in Additional file 1: Figure S3(B).

Although a tumor such as DCIS may consist of many small tumor regions (0.2–1 mm), the main objective here was not to detect each individual microscopic region, rather to locate residual tumor within ~ 1 mm at the excision margin to facilitate intra-operative re-excisions. Thus,

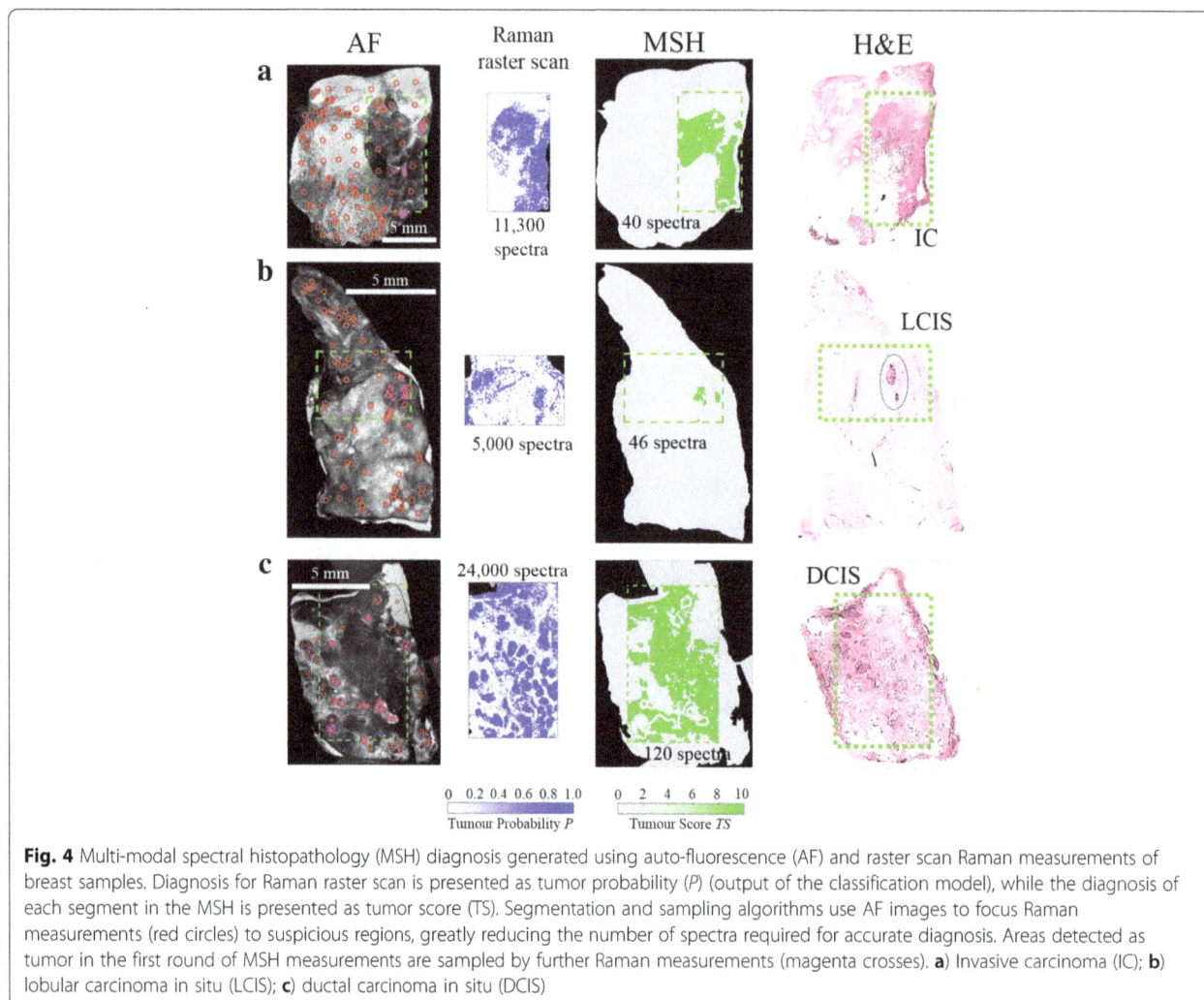

Fig. 4 Multi-modal spectral histopathology (MSH) diagnosis generated using auto-fluorescence (AF) and raster scan Raman measurements of breast samples. Diagnosis for Raman raster scan is presented as tumor probability (*P*) (output of the classification model), while the diagnosis of each segment in the MSH is presented as tumor score (*TS*). Segmentation and sampling algorithms use AF images to focus Raman measurements (red circles) to suspicious regions, greatly reducing the number of spectra required for accurate diagnosis. Areas detected as tumor in the first round of MSH measurements are sampled by further Raman measurements (magenta crosses). **a)** Invasive carcinoma (IC); **b)** lobular carcinoma in situ (LCIS); **c)** ductal carcinoma in situ (DCIS)

the sensitivity and specificity of the independent test samples was calculated by considering only the maximum TS found in the MSH measurement for the whole sample. Based on the moderate-risk TS threshold, the sensitivity and specificity were 91% and 83%, respectively. The results indicate successful detection of tumors, including DCIS consisting of tumor regions smaller than 1×1 mm^2. Using the high-risk threshold increases the specificity to 97% while decreasing the sensitivity to 64%.

Thus, a surgeon observing a region diagnosed as high risk (see Fig. 5c-e) could remove more tissue from the corresponding region with high confidence of it being tumor. The surgeon would take action on a moderate-risk diagnosis (such as Fig. 5b) taking into account other information available at the time of surgery including patient history, disease type (e.g. DCIS), radiographic appearances, and size and location of detected tumor. The higher sensitivity of the moderate-risk threshold ensures that MSH misses few tumors on the excision surface.

Proof of principle tests of MSH on whole BCS specimens in intra-operative timescales

Next, MSH measurements were acquired from 51 fresh, whole BCS specimens immediately after surgery with no sample preparation. The MSH measurements covered a surface area between 2×2 to 4×6.5 cm^2 and were completed in 12–24 min. Simulating clinical application, a single side was analyzed that the surgeon may have considered of greatest concern.

MSH detected residual tumors on the surface of 18 BCS specimens. For 10 of the BCS specimens detected positive by MSH, the histopathological examination confirmed positive on-ink margins (see Fig. 6), including small ($\sim 1 \times 1$ mm^2) pockets of DCIS (see Fig. 6d-e). MSH detected tumor in all specimens for which histopathological assessment identified positive margins (see all examples in Additional file 1: Figure S5).

For eight specimens where MSH detected tumor, histopathological assessment identified margins wider

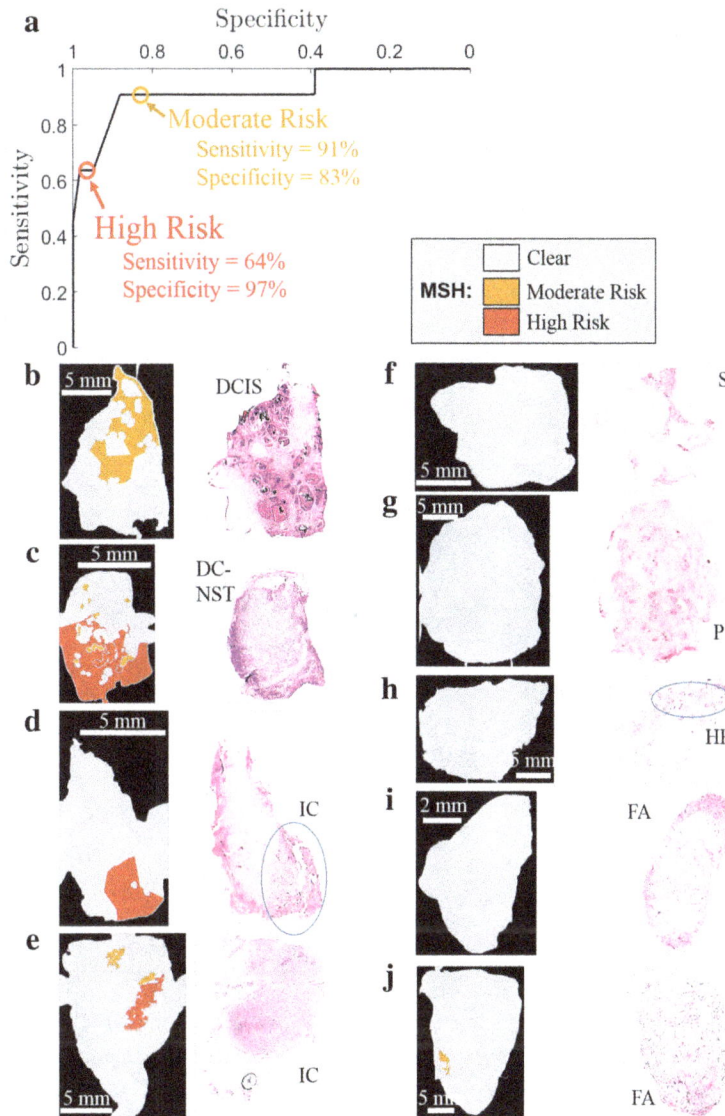

Fig. 5 Validation of multi-modal spectral histopathology (MSH) on independent mastectomy breast samples. **a** Receiver-operator curve (ROC) for independent test samples at varying tumor score thresholds. Results corresponding to the thresholds determined based on training set data are marked with circles. (**b-e**) Examples of tumor tissue detected by MSH and confirmed by histopathology. DCIS, ductal carcinoma in situ; DC-NST, ductal carcinoma of no special type; IC, invasive carcinoma. **f-i** Examples of tissue identified as clear by both MSH and histopathology. S, stroma; P, parenchyma; HP, hyperplasia; FA, fibroadenoma. **j** Example of false positive where MSH marked segments as moderate risk although histopathological assessment identified fibroadenoma

than the penetration depth of our technique. Each of these measurements are presented in Additional file 1: Figure S6. Figure 7e shows an MSH measurement that detected positive margins. Histopathological assessment of this specimen identified lactation adenoma at the margin, but no tumor within 100 μm. For BCS specimens, histopathology sections were not available for the entire surface measured by MSH, only sections perpendicular to the measured surface. Therefore, these detected tumor regions could either be false positives or true positives not detected by histopathology. If these

eight positive MSH results without confirmation by co-located histopathology sections are considered false positives, the specificity of MSH on BCS specimens is 80%, which is in agreement with the specificity for the independent test on mastectomy samples.

MSH provided a "clear" diagnosis in 33 BCS specimens (see Fig. 7a-d, all examples in Additional file 1: Figure S7). Normal histopathological assessment of these specimens detected no tumor near the measured surface. Therefore, MSH detected tumor on the surface of all specimens for which histopathological assessment later

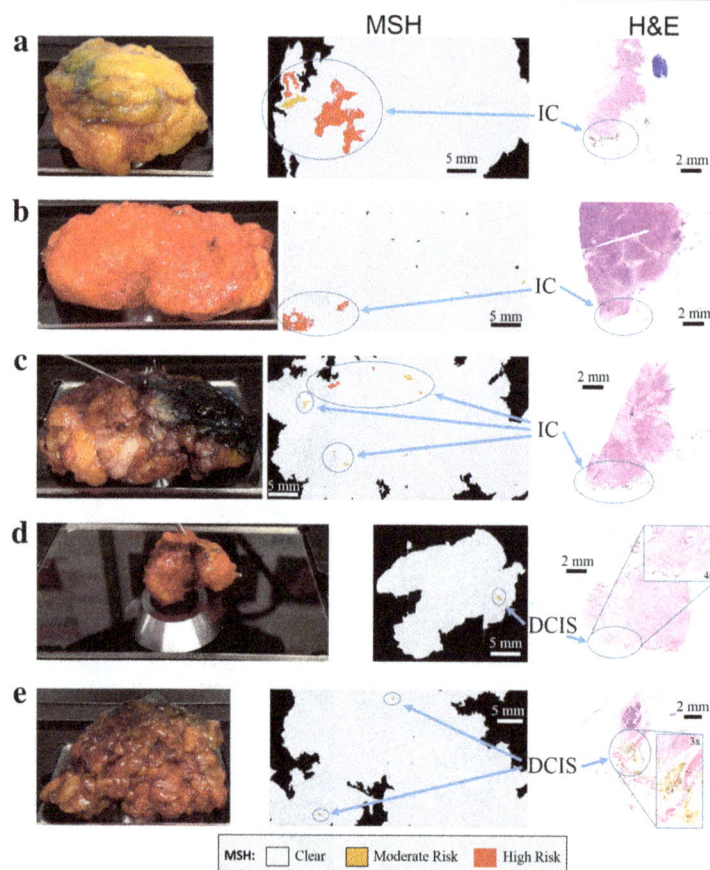

Fig. 6 Examples of multi-modal spectral histopathology (MSH) measurements of whole breast conserving surgery (BCS) specimens with positive margins confirmed by histopathological assessment. The surface measured by MSH is facing downward in the specimen images. MSH detected tumor on the surface of all specimens in 12–24 min. **a-c**) invasive carcinoma (IC); **d, e**) ductal carcinoma in situ (DCIS)

identified positive margins. For the 51 BCS surfaces measured in this independent test of MSH, the sensitivity was 100% and the specificity was at least 80%.

Discussion

The main objective of this study was to evaluate the potential of multimodal spectral histopathology (MSH) to accurately detect tumors on the surface of excised BCS specimens within timescales compatible with intra-operative use. New measurement and data analysis algorithms were developed to obtain objective diagnoses of varied, large specimens free from user variability. These algorithms were optimized to measure a large tissue surface in intra-operative timescales while maintaining the ability to detect small tumors.

We aimed to assess the surface area of the specimen in the radial margin, which will enable assessment of one tissue surface plus approximately half of the adjacent surfaces at the same time due to fatty tissue deformation. Concentrating on the margins of greatest concern (surfaces up to 4×6.5 cm^2) as informed by visual and tactile inspection of the specimen and intraoperative radiography

could allow scanning in the time frame required for an intra-operative procedure (12–24 min).

Although DCIS occurs less often than IC, it often co-exists with small tumors and frequently extends beyond the boundaries of the index tumor, making re-excisions more common [5]. Small residual foci of DCIS are difficult to detect by alternative intra-operative techniques under development because of limited spatial resolution or sampling coverage. However, MSH utilizes the high spatial resolution, speed, and sensitivity (but low specificity) of AF imaging to guide Raman spectroscopy with its high chemical specificity to detect small tumors. Indeed, MSH was able to detect residual DCIS and other small tumors (1–2 mm) on the surface of whole BCS specimens that were missed during surgery.

Mastectomy samples were chosen for developing the diagnosis model and the initial independent test because H&E sections could be obtained from the same surface measured by MSH, thus providing a reliable standard of reference. These tests estimated the sensitivity and specificity of the technique as 91% and 83%, respectively. These results included challenging

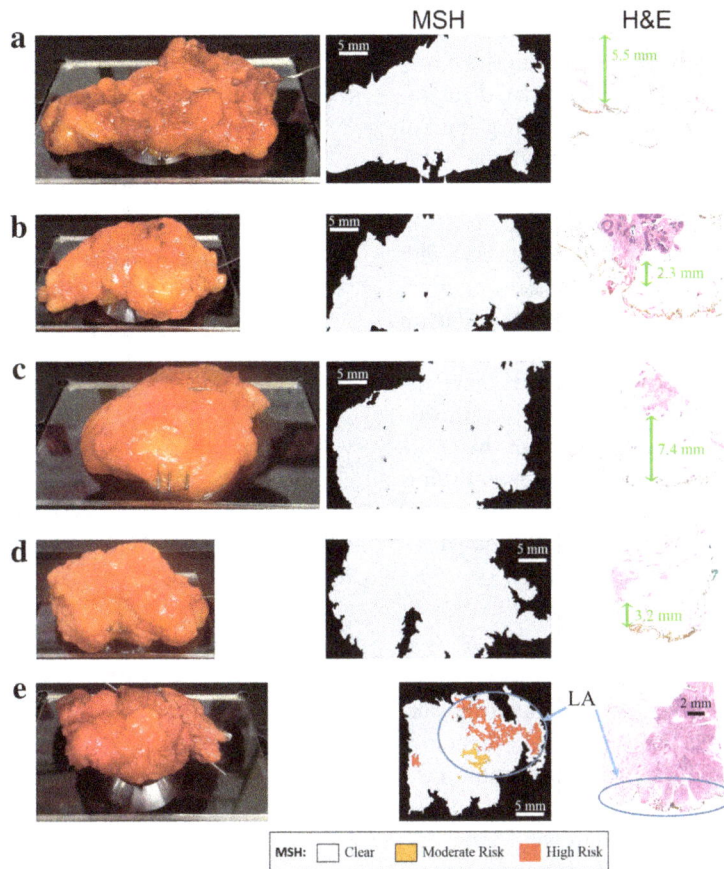

Fig. 7 Examples of multi-modal spectral histopathology (MSH) measurements of whole breast conserving surgery (BCS) specimens for which histopathological examination identified negative margins. **a-d** MSH detected no tumor on the surface of 80% of specimens declared clear by histopathological examination. Distances from the measured margin to tumor are marked with green arrows. **e** MSH detected tumor although only lactation adenoma (LA) was found within 100 μm of the measured surface in sections sampled by histopathological examination

cases (highly proliferative but non-malignant lesions) that were under-represented in the training set for the classification model. Still, MSH provided accurate detection of breast carcinomas including DCIS.

The validation of the technique using 51 whole BCS specimen surfaces (4×6.5 cm^2) measured immediately after surgery allowed demonstration of the feasibility of intra-operative use of MSH (12–24 min). MSH detected tumors in all scanned surfaces that had positive margins subsequently confirmed by histopathological assessment, including those with DCIS. Had the MSH results been available in the operating theater, the residual tumor may have been immediately removed.

As standard histopathology practice sparsely involves sectioning BCS tissue perpendicular to the surface measured by MSH, H&E sections were not available at all locations where MSH detected tumor. Although MSH provides a more comprehensive analysis of the excision surface compared to slide-based histology, histopathology obtains information such as

tumor type and progression, which is important for continuing patient care, but not urgently required during surgery. The non-destructive, non-labeling nature of MSH allows BCS specimens to be submitted for normal histopathological processing following the MSH measurement.

These results suggest that clinical use of MSH could detect 95% of residual tumors in BCS surgeries and prevent re-excisions in these cases. Positive margins remaining undetected by MSH would proceed through treatment following current protocols. Any false positives would result in cavity shaves, similar to the untargeted approach of Chagpar et al. [6]. Thus, MSH can be used with minimal risk and great potential benefit to the patient.

Our investigation confirms the extension of the MSH technique to real specimens. The quartz window (5.1×7.6 cm^2) was able to accommodate most BCS specimens. Within 12–24 min, the excision surface of greatest concern could be measured with diagnostic results displayed as three-color images, allowing surgeons to make immediate, informed decisions on further resections while incorporating additional clinical factors. Nevertheless, the analysis time can be further reduced in the future by developing a more optimized and automated instrument to eliminate the current manual steps (e.g. microscope focusing, change between AF and Raman objectives, and faster microscope translation stage [39]). In clinical use, additional information such as radiographic images of the specimens would be used to identify the surface with the highest risk, allowing prioritization of faster or more accurate measurements (e.g. by increasing the Raman acquisition time over a smaller area). Faster multi-beam Raman spectroscopy could also be used to parallelize the acquisition of the Raman spectra of tissue [44] to provide additional speed and allow the measurement of the entire specimen surface within a shorter measurement time. With such further development and integration into clinical practice, many re-excision operations may be prevented.

Conclusion

Combining the fast, high-resolution imaging of AF and the accurate molecular diagnosis of Raman spectroscopy, MSH is able to identify small residual tumors on the surface of breast excision specimens within intra-operative timescales. Measurement and diagnosis algorithms have been trained and optimized to quickly evaluate large tissue surfaces. A future fully automated system will further improve on accuracy and speed. MSH diagnosis images could guide the surgeon to remove additional tissue immediately and potentially prevent a large number of secondary operations.

Additional file

Additional file 1: Figure S1. Detailed performance of the linear discriminant analysis (LDA) Raman spectral classifier. **Figure S2.** Optimization of auto-fluorescence (AF) segmentation (A-E) and sampling (F) algorithms. **Table S1.** Molecular assignments of Raman spectral features and relative prevalence in each tissue class. **Table S2.** Performance of various classification models on Raman spectra from breast samples in the training set. **Table S3.** Confusion matrix for Raman spectral classifier based on fivefold cross-validation for breast samples in the training set. Statistics are median values for 10 re-partitions of fivefold cross-validation. **Figure S3.** Histogram of maximum tumor scores for each sample in the training set (A) and independent test set (B). Samples containing a segment with a tumor score greater than 9.0 were considered positive in this study. **Figure S4.** Tumor scores for all segments in mastectomy tissue samples from the training set (A) and independent test set (B). **Figure S5.** All BCS specimens with positive margins detected by MSH and confirmed by histopathology. **Figure S6.** All BCS specimens for which MSH detected positive margins but no tumor was found at the surface in sections sampled by histopathology. **Figure S7.** All BCS specimens for which the measured surface was diagnosed as clear by both MSH and histopathology. (DOCX 5487 kb)

Abbreviations

AF: Auto-fluorescence; BCS: Breast conserving surgery; DCIS: Ductal carcinoma in situ; DRS: Diffuse reflectance spectroscopy; ESS: Elastic scattering spectroscopy; FAD: Flavin adenine dinucleotide; FLIm: Fluorescence lifetime imaging; H&E: Hematoxylin and eosin; IC: Invasive carcinoma; LCIS: Lobular carcinoma in situ; LDA: Linear discriminant analysis; MSH: Multi-modal spectral histopathology; NADH: Reduced nicotinamide adenine dinucleotide; PCA: Principal component analysis; ROC: Receiver operating characteristic; SERS: Surface-enhanced Raman spectroscopy; SFDI: Spatial frequency domain imaging; SORS: Spatially offset Raman spectroscopy; TS: Tumor score

Acknowledgements

We gratefully acknowledge the contributions of the Nottingham Health Services Biobank and the Department of Pathology at Nottingham University Hospitals including Dr. Andrew Green, Dr. Zsolt Hodi, Irene Attenborough, Palminder Dusanjh, Andy Harwood, and Matthew Russell for their assistance in procuring and processing samples.

Funding

This work was supported by the Engineering and Physical Sciences Research Council [grant number EP/L025620/1, EP/K503800/1], the first grant through the Established Career Fellowship and the second grant through the University of Nottingham Impact Accelerator.

Authors' contributions

DS constructed the instrument, created and executed measurement protocols, and performed data analysis. AK supported the training and optimization of spectral classifiers and diagnosis maps. IN, ER, IE, and DS designed the study. ER, IE, and DM coordinated with histopathology, guided clinical applications, and interpreted pathological results. IN organized collaborative efforts and directed the research. All authors read and approved the final manuscript.

Competing interests

The authors have no competing interests to declare. IN has filed a patent application related to MSH.

Author details

[1]School of Physics and Astronomy, University of Nottingham, Nottingham NG7 2RD, UK. [2]Division of Oncology, School of Medicine, University of Nottingham, Nottingham NG5 1PB, UK. [3]Mathematics Department, Royal Holloway, University of London, Egham TW20 0EX, UK. [4]Nottingham Breast Institute, Nottingham University Hospitals NHS Trust, Nottingham NG5 1PB, UK.

References

1. Kummerow KL, Du L, Penson DF, Shyr Y, Hooks MA. Nationwide trends in mastectomy for early-stage breast cancer. JAMA Surg. 2015;150:9–16.

2. Jeevan R, Cromwell DA, Trivella M, Lawrence G, Kearins O, Pereira J, et al. Reoperation rates after breast conserving surgery for breast cancer among women in England: retrospective study of hospital episode statistics. BMJ. 2012;345:e4505.

3. Landercasper J, Whitacre E, Degnim AC, Al-Hamadani M. Reasons for re-excision after lumpectomy for breast cancer: insight from the American Society of Breast Surgeons Mastery Database. Ann Sur Oncol. 2014;21:3185–91.

4. Moran MS, Schmitt SJ, Giuliano AE, Harris JR, Khan SA, Horton J, et al. Society of Surgical Oncology – American Society for Radiation Oncology consensus guideline on margins for breast conserving surgery with whole-breast irradiation in stages I and II invasive breast cancer. Ann Surg Oncol. 2014;21:704–16.

5. Morrow M, Van Zee KJ, Solin LJ, Houssami N, Chavez-MacGregor M, Harris JR, et al. Society of Surgical Oncology – American Society for Radiation Oncology – American Society of Clinical Oncology consensus guideline on margins for breast-conserving surgery with whole-breast irradiation in ductal carcinoma in situ. J Clin Oncol. 2016;34(33):4040–6.

6. Chagpar AB, Killelea BK, Tsangaris TN, Butler M, Starvis K, Li F, et al. A randomized, controlled trial of cavity shave margins in breast cancer. NEJM. 2015;373(6):503–10.

7. Keating JJ, Fisher C, Batiste R, Singhal S. Advances in intraoperative margin assessment for breast cancer. Curr Surg Rep. 2016;4:15.

8. Jorns JM, Daignault S, Sabel MS, Wu AJ. Is intraoperative frozen section analysis of reexcision specimens of value in preventing reoperation in breast-conserving therapy? Am J Clin Pathol. 2014;142:601–8.

9. Rosenthal EL, Warram JM, Bland KI, Zinn KR. The status of contemporary image-guided modalities in oncologic surgery. Ann Surg. 2015;261(1):46.

10. Valdes EK, Boolbol SK, Ali I, Feldman SM, Cohen JM. Intraoperative touch preparation cytology for margin assessment in breast-conservation surgery: does it work for lobular carcinoma? Ann Surg Oncol. 2007;14(10):2940–5.

11. Schnabel F, Boolbol SK, Gittleman M, Karni T, Tafra L, Feldman S, et al. A randomized prospective study of lumpectomy margin assessment with use of MarginProbe in patients with nonpalpable breast malignancies. Ann Surg Oncol. 2014;21:1589–95.

12. Dixon JM, Renshaw L, Young O, Kulkarni D, Saleem T, Sarfaty M, et al. Intra-operative assessment of excised breast tumour margins using ClearEdge imaging device. Eur J Surg Oncol. 2016;42:1834–40.

13. Phipps JE, Gorpas D, Unger J, Darrow M, Bold RJ, Marcu L. Automated detection of breast cancer in resected specimens with fluorescence lifetime imaging. Phys Med Biol. 2017;63(1):015003.

14. Zhang J, Rector J, Lin JQ, Young JH, Sans M, Katta N, et al. Nondestructive tissue analysis for ex vivo and in vivo cancer diagnosis using a handheld mass spectrometry system. Sci Transl Med. 2017;9(406):eaan3968.

15. St John ER, Balog J, McKenzie JS, Rossi M, Covington A, et al. Rapid evaporative ionization mass spectrometry of electrosurgical vapours for the identification of breast pathology: towards an intelligent knife for breast cancer surgery. Breast Canc Res. 2017;19:59.

16. Assayag O, Antoine M, Sigal-Zafrani B, Riben M, Harms F, Burcheri A, et al. Large field, high resolution full-field optical coherence tomography: a pre-clinical study of human breast tissue and cancer assessment. Tech. Cancer Res Treat. 2014;13(5):455–68.

17. Kennedy BF, McLaughlin RA, Kennedy KM, Chin L, Wijesinghe P, Curatolo A, et al. Investigation of optical coherence micro-elastography as a method to visualize cancers in human breast tissue. Cancer Res. 2015;75(4):3236–45.

18. Wong TTW, Zhang R, Hai P, Zhang C, Pleitez MA, Aft RL, et al. Fast label-free multilayered histology-like imaging of human breast cancer by photoacoustic microscopy. Sci Adv. 2017;3:e1602168.

19. Brachtel EF, Johnson NB, Huck AE, Rice-Stitt TL, Vangel MG, Smith BL, et al. Spectrally encoded confocal microscopy for diagnosing breast cancer in excision and margin specimens. Lab Investig. 2016;96:459–67.

20. Tao YK, Shen D, Sheikine Y, Ahsen OO, Wang HH, Schmolze DB, et al. Assessment of breast pathologies using nonlinear microscopy. Proc Natl Acad Sci U S A. 2014;111(43):15304–9.

21. Robertson S, Azizpour H, Smith K, Hartman J. Digital image analysis in breast pathology – from image processing techniques to artificial intelligence. Transl Res. 2017;194:19–35.

22. Glaser AK, Reder NP, Chen Y, McCarty EF, Yin C, Wei L, et al. Light-sheet microscopy for slide-free non-destructive pathology of large clinical specimens. Nat Biomed Eng. 2017;1:0084.

23. de Boer LL, Molenkamp BG, Bydlon TM, Hendriks BHW, Wesseling J, Sterenborg HJCM, et al. Fat/water ratios measured with diffuse reflectance spectroscopy to detect breast tumor boundaries. Breast Cancer Res Treat. 2015;152:509–18.

24. Nichols BS, Llopis A, Palmer GM, McCachren SS III, Senlik O, Miller D, et al. Miniature spectral imaging device for wide-field quantitative functional imaging of the morphological landscape of breast tumor margins. J Biomed Opt. 2017;22(2):026007.

25. Bigio IJ, Brown SG, Briggs G, Kelley C, Lakhani S, Pickard DCO, et al. Diagnosis of breast cancer using elastic-scattering spectroscopy: preliminary clinical results. J Biomed Opt. 2000;5(2):221–8.

26. Laughney AM, Krishnaswamy V, Rizzo EJ, Schwab MC, Barth RJ Jr, Cuccia DJ, et al. Spectral discrimination of breast pathologies *in situ* using spatial frequency domain imaging. Breast Canc Res. 2013;15:R61.

27. Shipp DW, Sinjab F, Notingher I. Raman spectroscopy: techniques and applications in the life sciences. Adv Opt Photon. 2017;9(2):315–428.

28. Santos IP, Barroso EM, Bakker Schut TC, Caspers PJ, van Lanschot CGF, Choi DH, et al. Raman spectroscopy for cancer diagnostics and cancer surgery guidance: translation to the clinics. Analyst. 2017;142:3025–47.

29. Kendall C, Stone N, Shepherd N, Geboes K, Warren B, Bennett R, et al. Raman spectroscopy, a potential tool for the objective identification and classification of neoplasia in Barrett's oesophagus. J Pathol. 2003;200:602–9.

30. Haka AS, Shafer-Peltier KE, Fitzmaurice M, Crowe J, Dasari RR, Feld MS. Diagnosing breast cancer by using Raman spectroscopy. Proc Natl Acad Sci U S A. 2005;102(35):12371–6.

31. Barman I, Dingari NC, Saha A, McGee S, Galindo LH, Liu W, et al. Application of Raman spectroscopy to identify microcalcifications and underlying breast lesions at stereotactic core needle biopsy. Cancer Res. 2013;73(11):3206–15.

32. Day JCC, Stone N. A subcutaneous Raman needle probe. Appl Spec. 2013; 67(3):349–54.

33. Stone N, Baker R, Rogers K, Parker AW, Matousek P. Subsurface probing of calcifications with spatially offset Raman spectroscopy (SORS): future possibilities for the diagnosis of breast cancer. Analyst. 2007;132:899–905.

34. Keller MD, Vargis E, de Matos Granja N, Wilson RH, Mycek MA, Kelley MC, et al. Development of a spatially offset Raman spectroscopy probe for breast tumor surgical margin evaluation. J Biomed Opt. 2011;16(7):077006.

35. Wang Y, Reder NP, Kang S, Glaser AK, Yang Q, Wall MA, et al. Raman-encoded molecular imaging (REMI) with topically applied SERS nanoparticles for intraoperative guidance of lumpectomy. Cancer Res. 2017; 77(16):1–11.

36. Rowlands CJ, Varma S, Perkins W, Leach IH, Williams HC, Notingher I. Rapid acquisition of Raman spectral maps through minimal sampling: applications in tissue imaging. J Biophotonics. 2012;5(3):220–9.

37. Kong K, Rowlands CJ, Varma S, Perkins W, Leach IH, Koloydenko AA, et al. Diagnosis of tumor during tissue-conserving surgery with integrated autofluorescence and Raman scattering microscopy. Proc Natl Acad Sci U S A. 2013;110(38):15189–94.

38. Kong K, Zaabar F, Rakha EA, Ellis IO, Koloydenko AA, Notingher I. Towards intra-operative diagnosis of tumours during breast conserving surgery by selective-sampling Raman micro-spectroscopy. Phys Med Biol. 2014;59: 6141–52.

39. Boitor R, Kong K, Shipp DW, Varma S, Koloydenko AA, Kulkarni K, et al. Automated multimodal spectral histopathology for quantitative diagnosis of residual tumour during basal cell carcinoma surgery. Biomed Opt Exp.. 2017; 8(12):5749–66.

40. Takamori S, Kong K, Varma S, Leach I, Williams HC, Notingher I. Optimization of multimodal spectral imaging for assessment of resection margins during Mohs micrographic surgery for basal cell carcinoma. Biomed Opt Exp. 2014; 6(1):98–111.

41. Beier BD, Berger AJ. Method for automated background subtraction from Raman spectra containing known contaminants. Analyst. 2009;134:1198–202.

42. Savitsky A, Golay MJE. Smoothing and differentiation of data by simplified least squares procedures. Anal Chem. 1964;36(8):1627–39.

43. Tu AT. Raman spectroscopy in biology: principles and applications. New York: Wiley; 1982.

44. Sinjab F, Kong K, Gibson G, Varma S, Williams HC, Padgett M, et al. Tissue diagnosis using power-sharing multifocal Raman micro-spectroscopy and auto-fluorescence imaging. Biomed Opt Exp.. 2016;7(8):2993–3006.

7

Efficient and tumor-specific knockdown of MTDH gene attenuates paclitaxel resistance of breast cancer cells both in vivo and in vitro

Liu Yang[1†], Yanhua Tian[2†], Wei Sun Leong[3†], Heng Song[4], Wei Yang[1], Meiqi Wang[1], Xinle Wang[1], Jing Kong[3], Baoen Shan[1] and Zhengchuan Song[1*]

Abstract

Background: Drug resistance of paclitaxel (TAX), the first-line chemotherapy drug for breast cancer, was reported to develop in 90% of patients with breast cancer, especially metastatic breast cancer. Investigating the mechanism of TAX resistance of breast cancer cells and developing the strategy improving its therapeutic efficiency are crucial to breast cancer cure.

Methods and Results: We here report an elegant nanoparticle (NP)-based technique that realizes efficient breast cancer treatment of TAX. Using lentiviral vector-mediated gene knockdown, we first demonstrated that TAX therapeutic efficiency was closely correlated with metadherin (MTDH) gene expression in breast cancer cell lines. This finding was also supported by efficacy of TAX treatment in breast cancer patients from our clinical studies. Specifically, TAX treatment became more effective when MTDH expression was decreased in MCF-7 cancer cells by the blocking nuclear factor-kappa B (NF-κB) pathway. Based on these findings, we subsequently synthesized a polymeric NP that could co-deliver MTDH-small interfering RNA (MTDH–siRNA) and TAX into the breast cancer tumors in tumor-bearing mice. The NPs were composed of a cationic copolymer, which wrapped TAX in the inside and adsorbed the negatively charged siRNA on their surface with high drug-loading efficiency and good stability.

Conclusions: NP-based co-delivery approach can effectively knock down the MTDH gene both in vitro and in vivo, which dramatically inhibits breast tumor growth, achieving effective TAX chemotherapy treatment without overt side effects. This study provides a potential therapeutic strategy for the treatment of a wide range of solid tumors highly expressing MTDH.

Keywords: Breast cancer, Metadherin (MTDH) gene, Paclitaxel (TAX), Drug resistance, Nanoparticle (NP), Co-delivery

Background

The key options in breast cancer treatment so far include surgery, chemotherapy, radiotherapy, and molecular targeted therapy [1]. Out of these approaches, chemotherapy appears to be the most widely adopted. In particular, paclitaxel (TAX) was commonly used as one of the first-line chemotherapy drugs in breast cancer therapy and has shown remarkable efficacy in inhibiting tumor growth

through mitotic arrest [2–4]. Despite the excellent initial therapeutic efficacy, drug resistance of TAX develops in 90% of breast cancer patients during the disease progression [5]. The molecular mechanism of such resistance remains elusive and has become a clinical issue that requires an immediate solution.

Metadherin (MTDH), also known as LYRIC, AEG-1, or 3D3, has been expressed in multiple tumor types as an oncogene and associated with aberrant proliferation and drug resistance of tumor cells [6–10]. In particular, a recent study reported that MTDH gene promotes the cisplatin resistance of cervical cancer cells by activating

* Correspondence: songzhch@hotmail.com
†Liu Yang, Yanhua Tian and Wei Sun Leong contributed equally to this work.
1Breast Center, Fourth Hospital of Hebei Medical University, Shijiazhuang 050035, China
Full list of author information is available at the end of the article

the Erk/nuclear factor-kappa B (Erk/NF-κB) pathway and decreasing cleavage of caspase-3 [11–14]. Based on these findings, we explored the relationship between MTDH gene expression and TAX resistance in breast cancer cell lines as well as the effect of MTDH knockdown on TAX therapeutic efficiency. For in vivo therapeutic study, we employed targeted nanocarriers to specifically co-deliver anti-MTDH small interfering RNA (siRNA) (for tumor-specific silence of MTDH gene) and TAX drug.

We first explored the role of MTDH gene in the TAX therapeutic efficiency toward breast cancer cells and then investigated whether a nanoparticle (NP)-based co-delivery method can be used to address TAX resistance issue in breast cancer treatment. We hypothesized that the two drugs-loaded NPs displayed onsite gene silencing in tumor tissues, which improved drug sensitivity of TAX with good tolerability. In addition, poly(lactic-co-glycolic acid) (PLGA) polymeric molecule is approved by the US Food and Drug Administration with high biosafety; this study thus presents a promising strategy for clinical practice.

Methods

Patients and clinicopathology characteristics

This is a retrospective study that was approved by the Fourth Hospital of Hebei Medical University in Shijiazhuang, China. In this study, we selected 44 cases with breast cancer, which were proven to be breast invasive ductal carcinoma by pathological diagnosis from March to December 2010. The median follow-up time was 84 months (range of 8–90 months). The primary endpoints were disease-free survival (DFS) and overall survival (OS). We detected the samples from carcinoma of 44 patients before neoadjuvant chemotherapy. Immunohistochemistry was used to detect MTDH expression in all tissues. All the patients were recommended to use combination chemotherapy of taxol and anthracycline. Clinical benefit was evaluated by the Response Evaluation Criteria in Solid Tumors (RECIST version 1.1) and pathologic complete response (pCR) rates after neoadjuvant therapy. pCR was defined as ypT0 ypN0. All of above procedures were approved by the Fourth Hospital Ethics Committee of Hebei Medical University in Shijiazhuang, China (SCXK2009–0037).

Immunohistochemistry

All of the immunohistochemistry slides for MTDH were reviewed again by two independent pathologists. Immunohistochemistry staining of 4-μm sections of formalin-fixed paraffin-embedded tissue was rehydrated and incubated with anti-MTDH primary monoclonal antibodies (Cell Signaling Technology, Danvers, MA, USA) or phosphate-buffered saline (PBS) at 4 °C overnight, followed by

sequential incubation with MaxVision™/horseradish peroxidase (HRP) and diaminobenzidine (DAB). Then slides were counterstained with hematoxylin, dehydrated, and mounted.

The levels of MTDH expression were evaluated on the basis of the staining intensity (SI) and percentage of positively stained tumor cells (PP). SI was defined as 0 (no staining), 1 (weak staining), 2 (moderate staining), and 3 (strong staining). PP was graded according to the following criteria: 0 (no positive tumor cells), 1 (1%–20% positive tumor cells), 2 (21%–50% positive tumor cells), 3 (51%–70% positive tumor cells), and 4 (>70% positive tumor cells). The immunoreactive score (IRS) was calculated as follows: IRS = SI × PP. IRS of 0 means negative expression, IRS of 1–3 means weakly positive, IRS of 4–6 means moderately positive, and IRS of 8–12 means strong positive. Here, low expression was defined as an IRS of 3 or less. High expression was defined as an IRS of 4 and more [15].

Cell lines and reagents

The human breast cancer cell lines MCF-7 and MDA-MB-435S were purchased from the American Type Culture Collection (Manassas, VA, USA) and propagated in RPMI-1640 medium (Thermo Fisher Scientific, Waltham, MA, USA) supplemented with 10% fetal bovine serum (Biological Industries Israel Beit-Haemek Ltd., Kibbutz Beit-Haemek, Israel) and antibiotics. All cells were maintained in 5% CO_2 at 37 °C. TAX was purchased from Yangzijiang Medicine Co. Ltd. (Jiangsu, China).

Lentiviral-mediated overexpression or silencing of MTDH gene in MCF-7 cells

The plasmids containing MTDH gene or MTDH-short hairpin RNA (MTDH-shRNA) (5′-gcaattgggtagacgaag aaa-3′) were designed and amplified by transfecting into *Escherichia coli*. DH5α. Real-time polymerase chain reaction (RT-PCR) and Western blot were used to detect the expression of MTDH mRNA and protein of MTDH-shRNA to verify the effect of transfection. Plasmids enveloped in lentivirus were incubated with MCF-7 cells for 6 h according to the MOI (multiplicity of infection) value and the virus titer and subsequently placed in fresh medium. Puromycin (0.4 μg/mL) was used to screen stable transfection cell lines.

RT-PCR analysis

Total RNA from treated cells was extracted with Trizol (Takara, Dalian, China) in accordance with the instructions of the manufacturer. Total RNA was used to synthesize cDNA by using PrimeScript RT reagent Kit (Takara). Then RT-PCR was carried out using Power Up SYBR Green Master Mix (Life Technologies, Thermo Fisher Scientific). The reaction was conducted using the following parameters: 95 °C for 30 s, 95 °C for 5 s, and 60 °C for 30 s during 40 cycles. Internal control and primers for RT-PCR were obtained from the reference. RT-PCR was then employed to determine the change of MTDH mRNA in MCF-7–MTDH cell line and MCF-7–MTDH–shRNA cell line. The experiments were repeated for three times and data were analyzed using $2^{-\Delta\Delta Ct}$. The data were normalized to the geometric mean of housekeeping gene *β-actin* to control the variability in expression levels. RT-PCR primers were synthesized by SBS Genentech Co. Ltd. (Shanghai, China). The specific primers for MTDH and reference gene (β-actin) are as follows:

MTDH forward: 5′-AAATAGCCAGCCTATCAAG ACTC-3′;
MTDH reverse: 5′-TTCAGACTTGGTCTGTGAA GGAG-3′.
β-actin forward, 5′-GCTACAGCTTCACCACCACAG-3′;
β-actin reverse, 5′-GGTCTTTACGGATGTCAAC GTC-3′.

Western blot analysis
Cells were lysed and total proteins were separated by 10% SDS-PAGE and transferred (300 mA, 2 h) onto a PVDF membrane. After blotting with 5% nonfat milk, the membranes were incubated with primary antibodies (anti-MTDH 1:20000, anti-p65 1:5000, anti-p-p65 (S536) 1:1000, anti-IκBα1:1000, and β-actin 1:1000) at 4 °C overnight. Then the membranes were washed by TBS-T buffer and incubated with secondary HRP-labeled anti-rabbit antibody at room temperature for 1 h and washed with TBS-T buffer three times (10 min each time). The target proteins were visualized with a chemiluminescence system (Gene Company Ltd., Shanghai, China) and normalized to β-actin from the same membrane.

Cell apoptosis and cycle detection
Cell apoptosis was performed using an Annexin V-PE/ 7-AAD Apoptosis Detection Kit (KeyGEN BioTECH, Nanjing, China). The experiments were carried out strictly in accordance with the instructions of the manufacturer. The cells were then analyzed by Beckman Coulter Cytomics FC 500 flow cytometry (Beckman Coulter, Inc., Brea, CA, USA). The data were analyzed by EXPO32 ADC analysis software. Cell cycle analysis was performed by using the standard method with some modifications. In brief, cells were fixed with 75% ethanol at 4 °C overnight. The fixed cells were washed by PBS and suspended with 200 μL RNaseA at 37 °C for 10 min, and 250 μL PI (100 μg/mL) was added to stain the DNA of cells in the dark for 15 min. Cell cycle was analyzed with a Beckman Coulter Cytomics FC 500 flow cytometry, and the data were analyzed by Multicycle AV for Windows (version 295) software.

Cell viability assay
Cell viability was determined by a Cell Counting Kit-8 (CCK-8) assay. MCF-7, MCF-7-vector, MCF-7–MTDH, and MCF-7–MTDH–shRNA cells were seeded into 96-well plates at a density of 1×10^4/well (TAX 0 μg/mL) or 5×10^4/well (TAX 1 μg/mL) in 100 μL RPMI-1640 medium. After incubation in 5% CO_2 at 37 °C overnight, the RPMI-1640 medium in each well was replaced with a different concentration of TAX (0 and 1 μg/mL) and further incubated for 0, 24, 48, and 72 h. Afterwards, 10 μL of CCK-8 was added to each well for another 2 h at 37 °C. The absorbance at 450 nm was read by the Microliate Reader (BioTek, Winooski, VT, USA). The inhibitory rate of cell growth was calculated on the basis of the following equation: cell growth inhibition rate = (1 – experimental OD450 / control OD450) × 100%. The experiments were repeated three times.

Tumorigenicity assay
MCF-7, MCF-7-vector, MCF-7–MTDH, and MCF-7–MTDH–shRNA cells (5×10^6 in 0.1 mL) were injected subcutaneously into 4-week-old female nude mice, respectively. TAX treatment was started at the third week after cell injection. The mice were randomly assigned to an untreated group and TAX treatment groups. The dose of TAX was 10 mg/kg and administered by intraperitoneal (IP) injection once a week for a total of four injections. Tumor volume was measured every three days (volume = $0.5 \times$ length $\times$ width^2, measured with a Vernier caliper). After the last treatment, the mice were sacrificed and the tumors were removed for weight analysis.

Preparation of NPs
For poly(etherimide)-poly(lactic-co-glycolic acid) (PEI-PLGA) NP synthesis, 20 mg was dissolved in 1 mL of methylene chloride and mixed with 0.2 mL deionized water. The mixture was emulsified through sonication by using probe sonicator at 25% power for 5 min. Then 2 mL of 2% poly(vinyl alcohol) (PVA) and 0.2 mL of hydrophobic TAX (with different ratios) dissolved in methylene chloride were added into the mixture. The solution was emulsified again at 30% power for 5 min, added dropwise into 10 mL of 0.6% PVA, and stirred for 3 min. The organic solvent was removed in a rotary evaporator under reduced pressure. The core particles containing TAX were centrifuged at 12,000 revolutions per minute (rpm) for 5 min and rinsed with deionized water. For loading siRNA, different ratios of TAX were added into the solution of core NPs and stirred at a rate of 200 rpm for 20 min. The core NPs absorbed by siRNA on their surface were centrifuged at 12,000 rpm for 5 min.

Morphological characterization of NPs

The NPs were negatively stained with uranyl acetate solution (2%) and deposited on a carbon-coated copper grid. The morphology was characterized with a transmission electron microscope (TEM) (JEM-200CX; Jeol Ltd., Tokyo, Japan). Size distribution (diameter in nanometers) and surface charge (zeta potential in millivolts) of NPs were determined by using a ZetaSizer Nano series Nano-ZS (Malvern Instruments Ltd., Malvern, UK) equipped with a He-Ne Laser beam at a wavelength of 633 nm and a fixed scattering angle of 90. Determinations were performed at 25 °C for samples appropriately diluted in distilled water.

Tumor-bearing nude mouse model

Six-week-old female BALB/c nude mice were purchased from Beijing Vital River Laboratories (Beijing, China). Human breast cancer cells (MCF-7, 2.0×10^6 cells in 50 mL PBS) mixed with 50 mL of Matrigel were transplanted into the mammary fat pads of the mice and allowed to grow to a tumor size of about 100 mm^3 (volume = 0.5 × length × width^2, measured with a Vernier caliper). The mice were then randomly divided into different experimental groups. All procedures were approved by the Committee on the Ethics of Animal Experiments of the Health Science Center of Peking University (Beijing, China).

Statistical analysis

Data analyses were performed with one-way analysis of variance (ANOVA) and the least significance difference (LSD) multiple comparisons test with PASW Statistics 23. Tumor volumes were compared by using a Kruskal–Wallis test followed by the Mann–Whitney test.

Results

Association of MTDH expression with the probability of disease-free survival and overall survival and efficacy of TAX treatment in patients with breast cancer

In a cohort of 44 neoadjuvant chemotherapy breast cancer patients, 29 patients were MTDH gene positive and 15 patients were negative. Patients with high MTDH protein expression (tan or brown staining in the cell membrane or cytoplasm, Fig. 1a) had significantly worse probability of disease-free survival (DFS) and overall survival (OS) than those with low MTDH protein expression (Fig. 1c, d). Furthermore, we found that MTDH protein expression negatively correlated with the TAX-containing chemotherapy efficacy (Fig. 1b). Based on

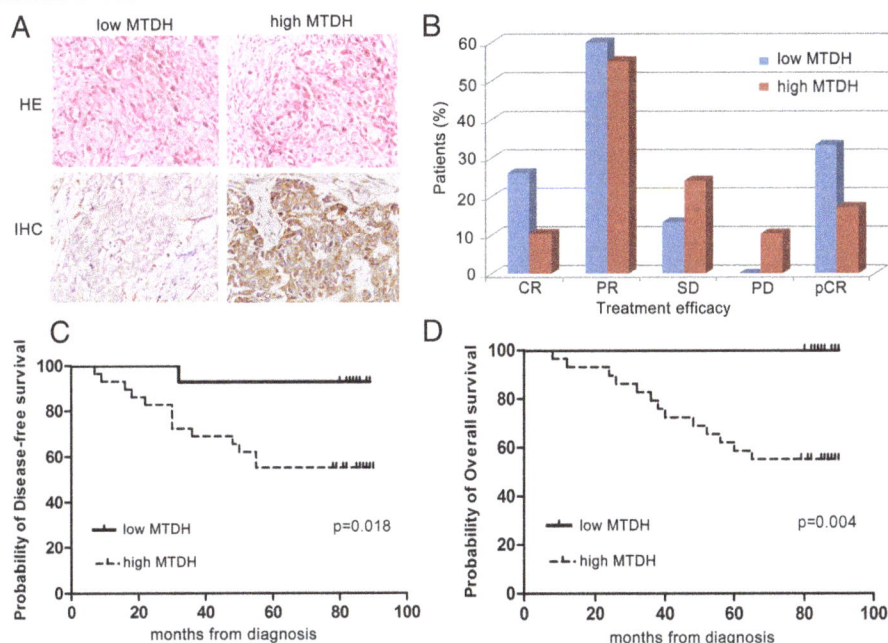

Fig. 1 Metadherin (MTDH) overexpression affects the prognosis of breast cancer patients who were treated with neoadjuvant chemotherapy. **a** Immunohistochemical staining with MTDH expression in breast cancer tissues (200×). Abbreviations: *HE* histopathology, *IHC* immunohistochemistry. **b** After neoadjuvant chemotherapy, in the MTDH low group (*n* = 15), 4 cases achieved complete response (CR), 9 cases achieved partial response (PR), 2 cases achieved stable disease (SD), and 0 case achieved progression disease (PD). In the high MTDH expression group (*n* = 29), 3 cases achieved CR, 16 cases achieved PR, 7 cases achieved SD, and 3 cases achieved PD. After surgery, the percentages of pathologic complete response (pCR) were 33.3% in the low MTDH expression group and 17.2% in the high MTDH expression group. **c** and **d** Patients with high MTDH expression had worse disease-free survival (*P* = 0.018) and overall survival (*P* = 0.004) than those with low MTDH expression

these MTDH gene-associated clinical characteristics, we conducted the subsequent study to confirm the function of MTDH gene in breast cancer and its possible relationship with TAX chemotherapy.

Effect of MTDH expression on MCF-7 breast cancer cells

To investigate the effect of MTDH expression in breast cancer cell lines, we first performed RT-PCR tests on our modified MCF-7 breast cancer cells. We constructed four groups of shRNA and one control shRNA. After transfecting, amplifying, and extracting the four groups of plasmids, we selected the optimal silent shRNA (MTDH-shRNA3: 5′-GCAATTGGGTAGACGAAGAAA-3′) via RT-PCR and Western blot (Additional file 1: Figure S1). As shown in Fig. 2a, the relative MTDH mRNA expression level in our MCF-7–MTDH cell was 2.1 times higher than the reference MCF-7 cell. On the other hand, the relative MTDH mRNA expression level in our MCF-7–MTDH–shRNA cell was only 0.3 times the MCF-7 cell

(Fig. 2b). Western blot tests were then conducted on MCF-7 cell and modified MCF-7 cells. We found that the protein level in MCF-7–MTDH cell was 2.86 times higher than the reference MCF-7 cell but in MCF-7–MTDH–shRNA cell was 90% lower than the reference cell (Fig. 2c, d). Furthermore, through CCK-8 assay, we observed that the growth rates of MCF-7–MTDH and MCF-7–MTDH–shRNA cells were higher and lower than that of the reference cell, respectively (Fig. 2e). Apart from that, through the cell apoptosis test, a test that measures the programmed cell death rate, we showed that the apoptosis percentage in an MCF-7–MTDH cell was much lower than MCF-7 cell but that of MCF-7–MTDH–shRNA was higher compared with MCF-7 cell (Fig. 2f, Additional file 1: Figure S2). In Fig. 2g and Additional file 1: Figure S4, we compared the proportion of G_0/G_1, S and G_2/M phases in MCF-7–MTDH and MCF-7–MTDH–shRNA with the reference MCF-7 cell, respectively. Compared with MCF-7 cell, the MCF-7–MTDH

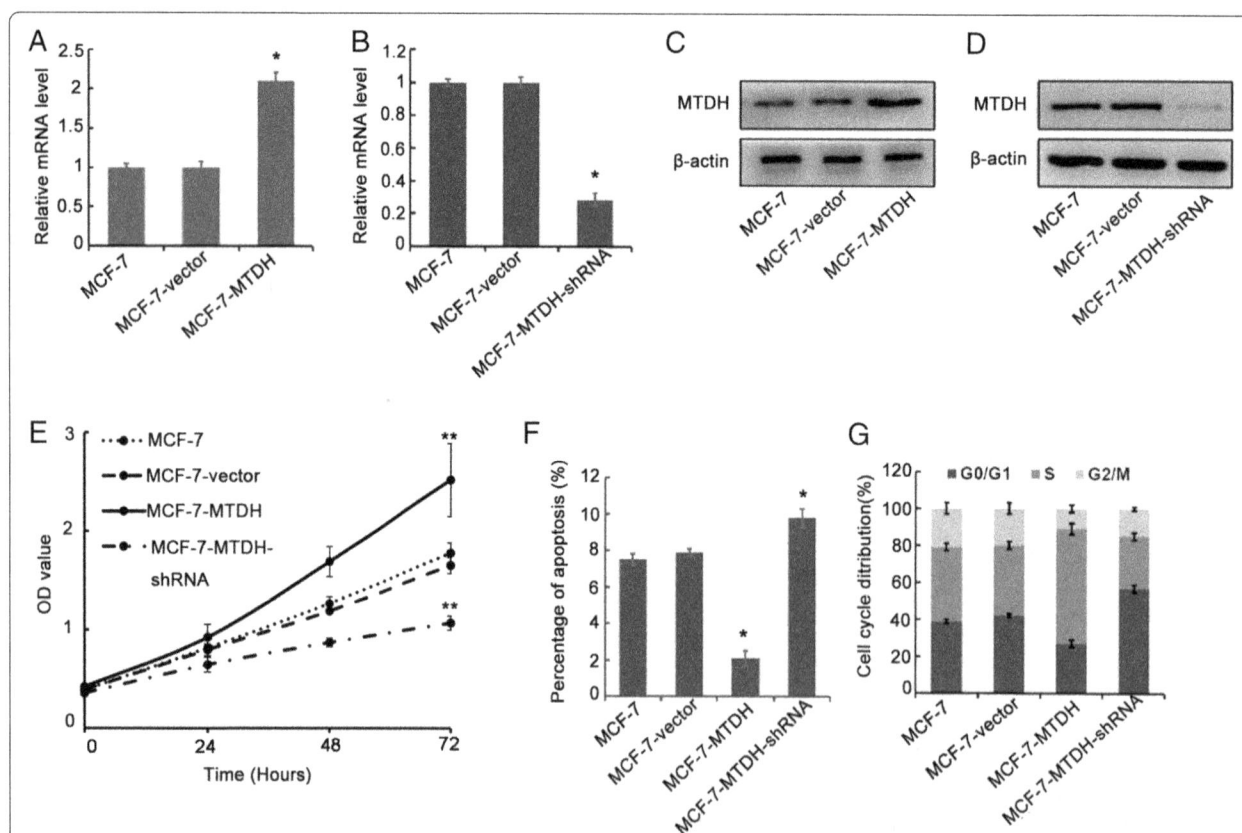

Fig. 2 Effect of metadherin (MTDH) expression in MCF-7 breast cancer cells. **a** and **c** Relative MTDH mRNA and protein expression levels after transfection of MCF-7 cells with MTDH plasmid. **b** and **d** After transfection with MTDH-short hairpin RNA (MTDH-shRNA) plasmids, the relative MTDH mRNA and protein expression levels were significantly lower than control cells. **e** Cell growth rate was evaluated by using a Cell Counting Kit-8 assay. Knockdown of MTDH inhibited MCF-7 cell proliferation, while MTDH overexpression induced cell growth. Abbreviation: *OD* optical density. **f** Flow cytometric analysis of apoptosis of the MCF-7–MTDH and MCF-7–MTDH–shRNA cells. MTDH overexpression decreased cell apoptosis, while knockdown of MTDH did the opposite. **g** Overexpression of MTDH arrested cells in S phase, while MTDH silencing increased the proportion of cells in G_0/G_1 phase. In all of these tests, the MCF-7 and MCF-7-vector cells were used as a reference sample. *P <0.05 and **P <0.01 compared with MCF-7

cell had more S phase and less G_0/G_1 and G_2/M phases while the MCF-7–MTDH–shRNA cell contained much lesser S phase and more G_0/G_1 and G_2/M phases.

Relationship between MTDH expression and TAX treatment in MCF-7 cell

We now study how the MTDH expression in MCF-7 cell affects the effectiveness of the TAX drug treatment on breast cancer. We evaluated and compared the cytotoxicity of the modified MCF-7 cell with a reference MCF-7 cell through a CCK-8 assay. In Fig. 3a and b, we can see that the inhibition rate of the MCF-7–MTDH cell ($25.89 \pm 1.33\%$) was much lower than that of the MCF-7 cell ($40.46 \pm 1.31\%$) while that of MCF-7–MTDH–shRNA cell was the highest ($64.33 \pm 2.21\%$) at 48 h. In addition, the apoptosis percentage in MCF-7–MTDH cell ($2.91 \pm 0.89\%$) was lower than MCF-7 cell ($9.31 \pm 1.04\%$) while that of MCF-7–MTDH–shRNA cell ($27.56 \pm 2.40\%$) was higher compared with MCF-7 cell after TAX treatment

(Fig. 3c, Additional file 1: Figure S3). As expected, the proportion of G_2/M phase ratio in the MCF-7–MTDH cell was significantly lower than the MCF-7 reference cell after TAX treatment (Fig. 3d, Additional file 1: Figure S5). The NF-κB pathway was closely associated with chemotherapy resistance, so we examined the expression level of p65, p-p65, and IκBα. As shown in Fig. 3e, upregulation of MTDH increased p65 and p-p65 expression but reduced the expression of IκBα (suggesting the activation of NF-κB pathway). On the contrary, silencing of MTDH reduced p65 and p-p65 and increased IκBα expression. These results suggested that MTDH was related to NF-κB and TAX sensitivity.

Overexpression of MTDH promotes MCF-7 tumor growth in vivo and diminishes TAX activity

We further examined the effect of MTDH expression on in vivo MCF-7 tumor cell growth and TAX treatment efficiency using a mouse xenograft model. Figure 4a and b

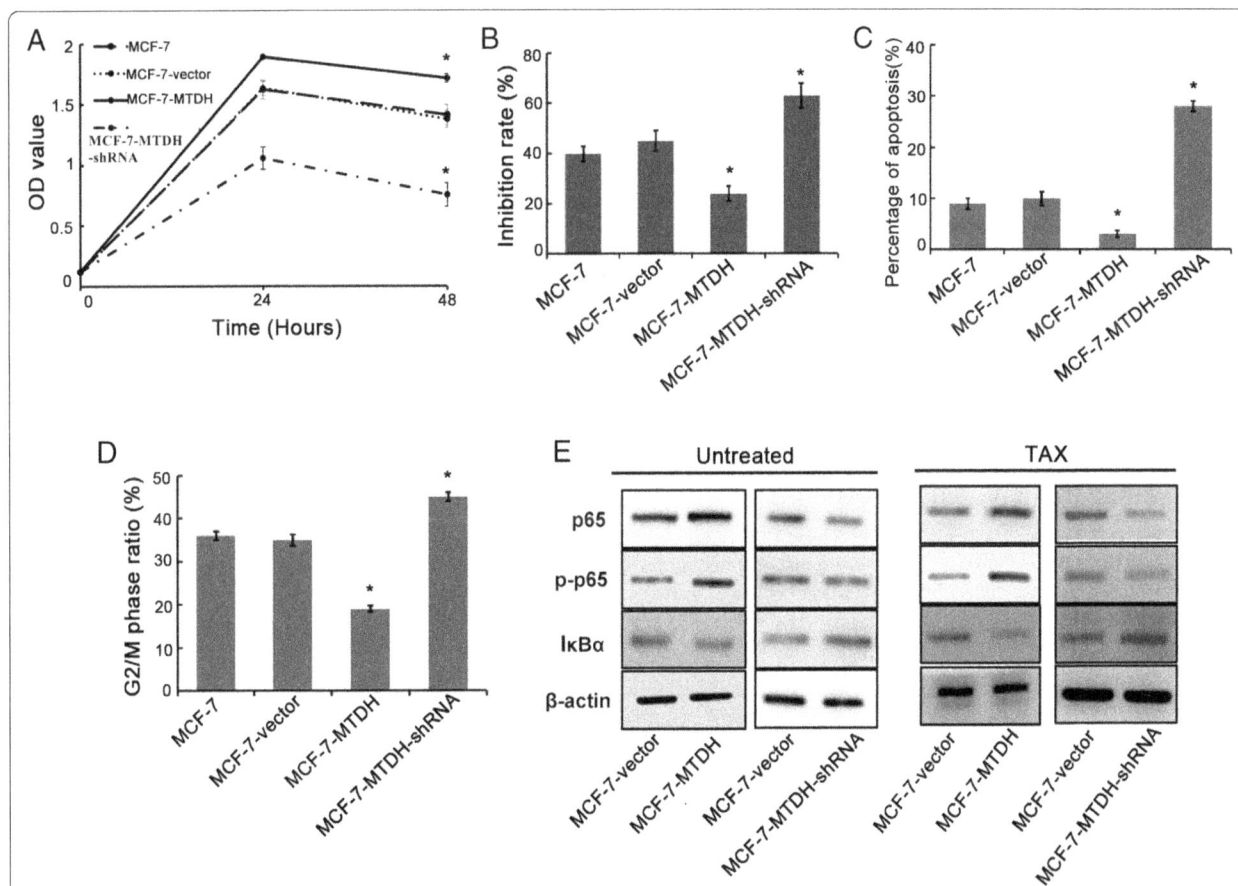

Fig. 3 Effect of metadherin (MTDH) expression on the efficacy of paclitaxel (TAX) in MCF-7 cells. **a** Cytotoxicity was evaluated by Cell Counting Kit-8 assay after treatment with TAX for 48 h. Abbreviation: *OD* optical density. **b** The inhibition rates of MCF-7–MTDH–short hairpin RNA (MCF-7–MTDH–shRNA) cells were much higher than those of MCF-7–MTDH cells. **c** MTDH suppressed cell apoptosis induced by TAX, while MTDH silencing increased the sensitivity of TAX. **d** Knockdown of MTDH increased the G_2/M phase arrest induced by TAX, while the opposite effect was found in MTDH overexpressing MCF-7 cells. **e** Western blot analysis revealed that protein expression of p65 was higher in MCF-7–MTDH cells, while IκBα was lower. On the contrary, in MCF-7–MTDH–shRNA cells, the protein expression level of p65 decreased and IκBα increased. Knockdown of MTDH could inhibit the activity of the nuclear factor-kappa B (NF-κB) pathway. *$P <0.05$ and **$P <0.01$ compared with MCF-7

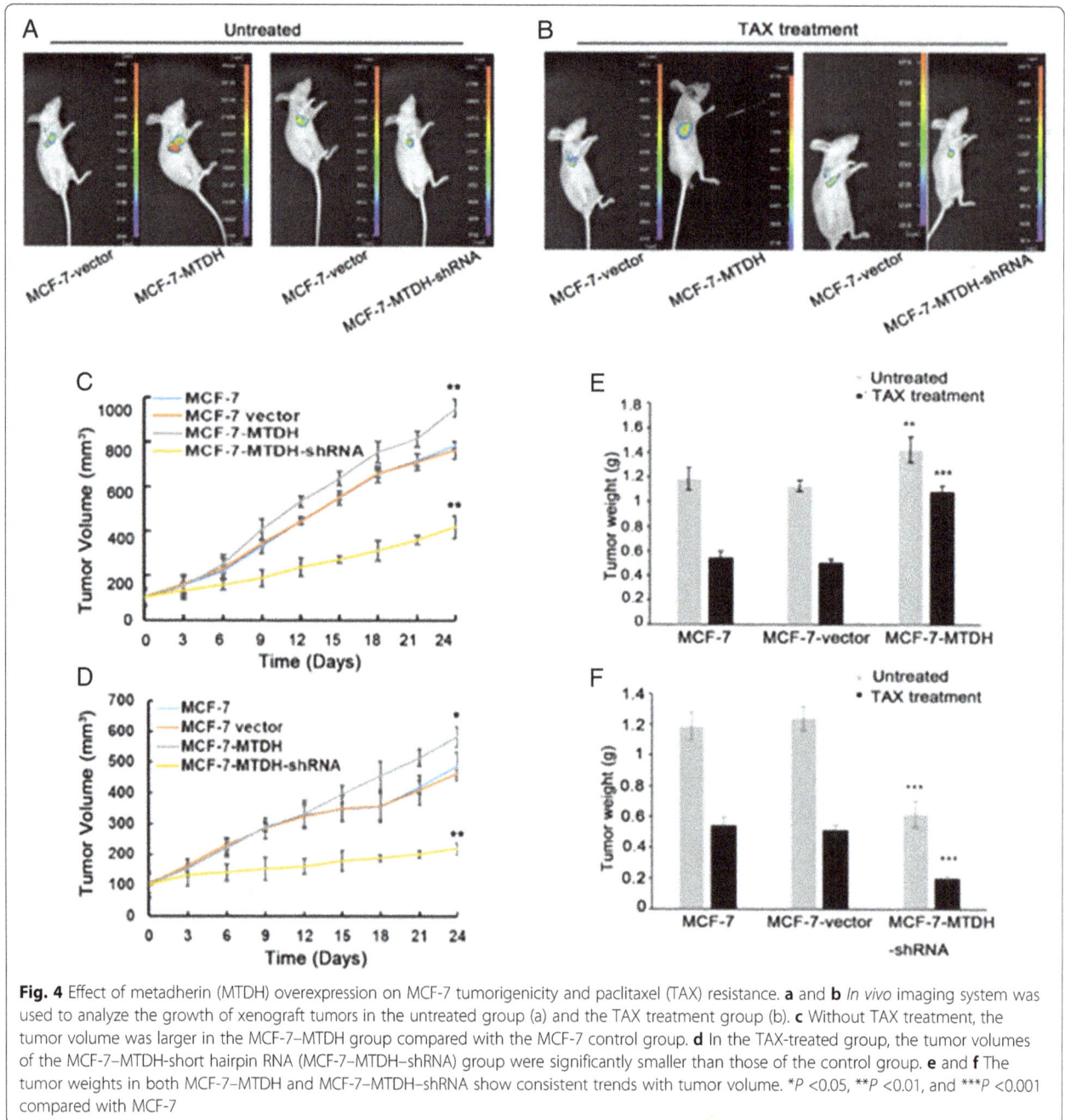

Fig. 4 Effect of metadherin (MTDH) overexpression on MCF-7 tumorigenicity and paclitaxel (TAX) resistance. **a** and **b** *In vivo* imaging system was used to analyze the growth of xenograft tumors in the untreated group (a) and the TAX treatment group (b). **c** Without TAX treatment, the tumor volume was larger in the MCF-7–MTDH group compared with the MCF-7 control group. **d** In the TAX-treated group, the tumor volumes of the MCF-7–MTDH–short hairpin RNA (MCF-7–MTDH–shRNA) group were significantly smaller than those of the control group. **e** and **f** The tumor weights in both MCF-7–MTDH and MCF-7–MTDH–shRNA show consistent trends with tumor volume. *P <0.05, **P <0.01, and ***P <0.001 compared with MCF-7

compared the in vivo images of xenograft tumors in untreated mice (MCF-7) and TAX-treated mice (MCF-7–MTDH and MCF-7–MTDH–shRNA). As can be seen, the tumor was significantly larger in the MCF-7–MTDH group but was smaller in the MCF-7–MTDH–shRNA group after subcutaneous injection of cells for 14 days. Mice were then treated with TAX by IP injection once a week for a total of four injections. The tumor in the MCF-7–MTDH–shRNA group was dramatically smaller than MCF-7–MTDH group as well as both controls (Fig. 4b), confirming that the knockdown of MTDH

enhanced cell sensitivity to TAX exposure. Tumor volume measurement results also supported these observations (Fig. 4c, d). In addition, the tumor weight in the MCF-7–MTDH–shRNA group with or without TAX treatment was lower than that of the MCF-7–MTDH group or control group (Fig. 4e, f).

Development of MTDH–siRNA and TAX co-delivery technique

Based on the findings above, we have developed a new technique (amphiphilic copolymer PEI-PLGA) that allows both MTDH–siRNA and TAX to be concurrently delivered into breast cancer cells to effectively control the breast cancer condition. After emulsification twice, the TAX was loaded into the hydrophobic layer and the MTDH–siRNA was bound at the NP surface after addition through electrostatic interactions. Figure 5 shows the TEM images of blank NPs, TAX-encapsulated NPs (NP-TAX), and NP-TAX–siRNA. As can be seen, all NPs were dispersed with a well-defined spherical core shell structure. Dynamic light scattering (DLS) measurement suggested that the average hydrodynamic diameters of blank NPs, NP-TAX, and NP-TAX–siRNA were 218.5 ± 13.3 nm, 220.1 ± 9.1 nm, and 228.5 ± 10.4 nm, respectively (Fig. 5b, c). The zeta potentials of the blank NPs, NP-TAX, and NP-TAX–siRNA were 33.2 ± 0.6 mV, 42.4 ± 0.8 mV, and −22.5 ± 0.3 mV, respectively (Fig. 5c). When siRNA was mixed with NP-TAX, the zeta potential of NP-TAX–siRNA changed from 42.4 to −22.5 mV, indicating the successful and a large capacity of absorption of negatively charged nucleic acids on the NP surface. We also investigated the release profile of TAX at different pHs over time (Additional file 1: Figure S6). At pH 7.4, no significant release of TAX was observed in the first 10 h; however, TAX was released at a fast rate at pH 4.4, and a release ratio of around 40% was reached in the first 10 h.

Therefore, the polymeric core is expected to show a pH-dependent drug release, which facilitates complete drug release in lysosomes after cellular uptake.

Cellular uptake and gene silencing of NP-TAX–siRNA

Two prerequisites for efficient siRNA-mediated gene silencing effect are high siRNA uptake levels and successful release of siRNA to cytoplasm. To study cellular uptake of NPs, we labeled NP-TAX–siRNA with near-infrared fluorescent dye Cy5. After incubation of MCF-7 cells with NP-TAX–Cy5–siRNA for 6 h, obvious red fluorescence appeared in the cytoplasm (Fig. 6a, upper panel). In contrast, there was barely red fluorescence in cells treated with free Cy5–siRNA (Fig. 6a, lower panel) and this was probably due to their high molecular weight, hydrophilic nature, and high density of charge. The knockdown efficiency of MTDH–siRNA encapsulated in NPs was then tested in MCF-7 cells by using RT-PCR and Western blot analysis. The downregulation of MTDH mRNA and protein expression in cells was observed after the NP-TAX–siRNA treatment, indicating the successful release of siRNA from lysosomes to cytoplasm (Fig. 6b, c). In addition, we examined the cytotoxicity of NP-TAX–siRNA to breast cancer cells in vitro. The MCF-7 cells were incubated with saline, blank NPs, free TAX, free

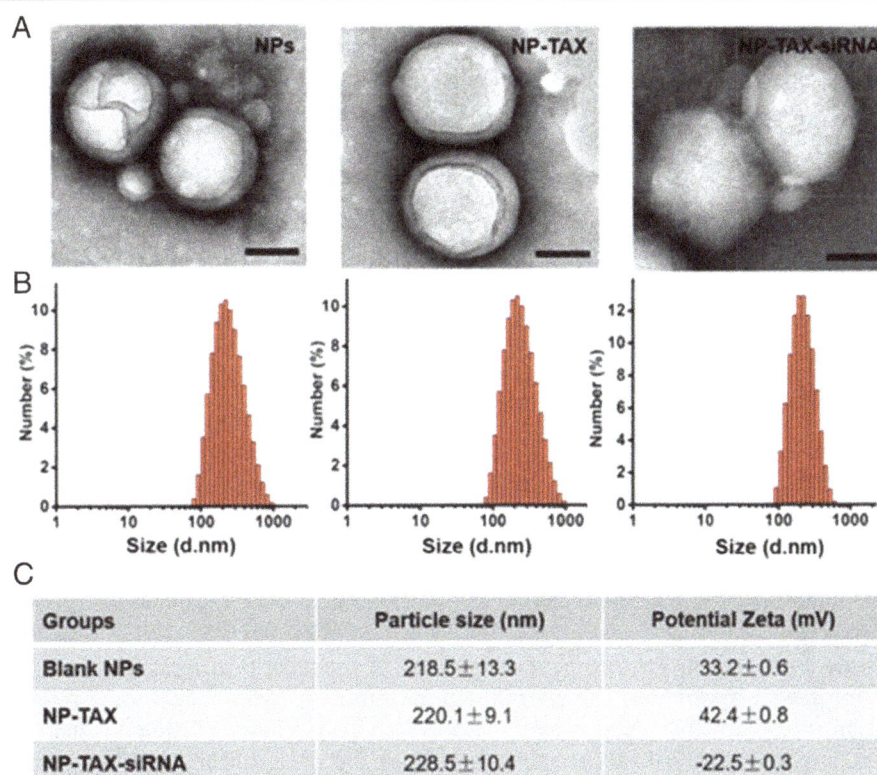

Fig. 5 Morphology, size, and surface charge characterization of drug-loaded nanoparticles (NPs). a Blank NPs (NPs), NP-TAX, and NP-TAX–siRNA. Scale bars = 100 nm. b Size distribution of blank NPs, NP-TAX, and NP-TAX–siRNA. c Particle size and potential zeta of NPs

Groups	Particle size (nm)	Potential Zeta (mV)
Blank NPs	218.5 ± 13.3	33.2 ± 0.6
NP-TAX	220.1 ± 9.1	42.4 ± 0.8
NP-TAX-siRNA	228.5 ± 10.4	-22.5 ± 0.3

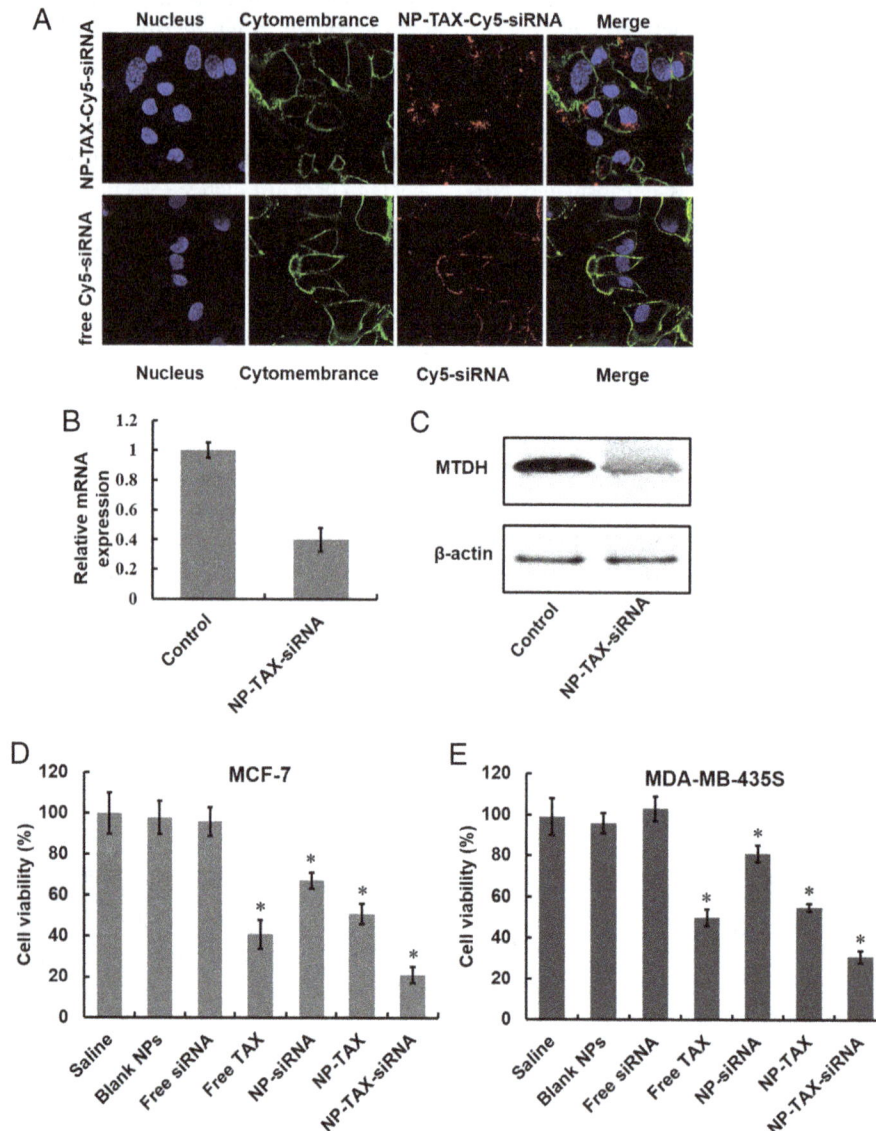

Fig. 6 Cellular uptake, intracellular distribution, and cytotoxicity of nanoparticle-paclitaxel–small interfering RNA (NP-TAX–siRNA). **a** Cellular uptake of NP-TAX–siRNA. Confocal microscopic images of MCF-7 cells treated with NP-TAX–siRNA for 6 h. Cell nucleuses (blue) were stained by DAPI, cytomembrane was labeled with DiO green fluorescence, and siRNA was labeled with Cy5 red fluorescence. **b** and **c** Gene silencing ability of NP-TAX–siRNA. MCF-7 cells were treated with free metadherin (MTDH)-siRNA and NP-TAX–siRNA in serum-free media for 6 h. After 48 h, the mRNA levels of MTDH were measured by real-time polymerase chain reaction (RT-PCR) (**b**). The expression of MTDH protein was analyzed by Western blot (**c**). **d** and **e** Cell viability of MCF-7 (**d**) and MDA-MB-435S (**e**) breast cancer cells was measured by using Cell Counting Kit (CCK) assay. Cells were incubated with different drug formulations (Saline, Blank NPs, Free siRNA, Free TAX, NP-siRNA, NP-TAX, and NP-TAX–siRNA) at 37 °C for 48 h. The cell viability of saline was set as 100%. Each bar represents the mean ± standard deviation of three replicates. *P <0.05

siRNA, NP-TAX, NP-siRNA, or NP-TAX–siRNA for 48 h, followed by quantification of cell viability using a CCK-8 cell proliferation assay. As shown in Fig. 6d, compared with the saline group, free siRNA did not show significant inhibition in tumor cell growth. A possible reason for this phenomenon is that free siRNA cannot be taken up by cells easily. In contrast, the siRNA encapsulated in NPs (NP-siRNA) exhibits effective inhibition of cell growth, indicating successful delivery of siRNA into cells. Free TAX was more toxic than TAX encapsulated in NPs, while the inhibitory effect of NP-TAX–siRNA on cell growth outperformed all other groups. In addition, no cytotoxicity was observed in the blank NP-treated group, suggesting that the polymers are non-toxic. To confirm the inhibition effect of NP-TAX–siRNA on cell growth, we also tested cell proliferation after NP-TAX–siRNA treatment by using another human breast tumor cell line MDA-MB-435S (Fig. 6e), which has been demonstrated to express MTDH. Comparable results were observed.

In vivo biodistribution and antitumor activity of NP-TAX–siRNA

The MCF-7 cells were injected subcutaneously into BALB/c nude mice. When the tumors reached a size of about 100 mm^3, Cy5.5-labeled NP-TAX–siRNA were injected by the tail vein. In vivo imaging results showed that the NPs gradually accumulated in tumor sites as a function of time (Additional file 1: Figure S7). Ten hours after the administration, we observe maximal fluorescence intensity in tumors, and at 24 h, the NPs were excreted from the mice body except for the tumor tissues, which is one of the desired characteristics of nanomaterials for in vivo application. In contrast, no special fluorescence was detected over time for the Cy5.5-labeled free siRNA treated group. We further performed ex vivo imaging assay. The mice were sacrificed after 10 h of administration, and the tumors and major organs (liver, heart, lung, spleen, and kidney) were collected. As can be seen in Fig. 7a, NP-TAX–siRNA accumulates mainly in the tumor tissues, and there is little accumulation in the liver and kidney and barely any in the heart, lung, and spleen.

Apart from that, we evaluated the antitumor activity of NP-TAX–siRNA using MCF-7 tumor-bearing mice. We randomly divided mice bearing about 100 mm^3 tumors into seven groups: saline, blank NPs, free TAX, free siRNA, NP-TAX, NP-siRNA, and NP-TAX–siRNA. Mice were treated with different vehicles via the tail vein every two days for a total of 21 days. In the saline and blank NPs groups, the tumors grew fast and the mice were sacrificed two days after the last injection because of having large tumor size (~800 mm^3) (Fig. 7b). Treatment with free siRNA or NP-siRNA has no significant inhibition effect on tumor growth. Although free TAX and NP-TAX slow down the tumor growth to a certain extent, their inhibitory effects are far lesser than the NP-TAX–siRNA.

To confirm the role of MTDH knockdown in the interference of tumor growth, we sectioned tumors and analyzed the levels of MTDH protein. Figure 7c shows that the MTDH expression level was dramatically suppressed by the NP-siRNA and NP-TAX–siRNA treatments compared with that in the saline group. Nevertheless, the free siRNA does not decrease the MTDH expression in tumor tissues. In the blank NP, free TAX, or NP-TAX–treated group, MTDH expression is similar to that in the saline group. In brief, the results suggest that siRNA is capable of effectively diminishing the MTDH gene expression in vivo only when delivered into the tumors by NPs and thus increasing the TAX antitumor effect.

Discussion

MTDH was identified as an oncogene that functions in both drug resistance and metastasis [16]. Upregulation of the MTDH gene could promote the proliferation of a variety of tumor cells, such as esophageal cancer, gastric cancer, glioma, and breast cancer [17–20]. Previous study showed that overexpression of MTDH induces estrogen-independent growth of MCF-7 breast cancer cells and mediates tamoxifen resistance [21]. Similarly, in our previous studies, overexpression of MTDH enhances the resistance of MDA-MB-231 cells to doxorubicin [9]. In contrast, downregulation of MTDH could inhibit tumor cell growth, induce apoptosis, and increase the sensitivity of tumor cells to chemotherapeutic drugs. In gastric cancer, studies showed that knockdown of MTDH by siRNA in SGC790 cells could apparently inhibit cell proliferation by blocking cell cycle in G_0/G_1 phase [18].

In our study cohort of 44 patients with breast cancer, we found that MTDH expression was negatively correlated with the probability of DFS and efficacy of TAX treatment, which should be further confirmed in a large population of patients with breast cancer. At cellular level study, we tested the cell proliferation of MCF-7–MTDH and MCF-7–MTDH–shRNA cells by CCK-8 assay and found that MTDH knockdown inhibits cell growth. The results of flow cytometry demonstrated that knockdown of MTDH resulted in an increase of G_0/G_1 phase cells and reduction of S and G_2/M phase cells but that MTDH overexpression induced cell cycle arrest in S phase. Additionally, knockdown of MTDH inhibits the growth of xenograft tumor in vivo. Taken together, our results suggest that MTDH expression plays a crucial role in the MCF-7 breast cancer cell proliferation and is potentially useful for breast cancer treatment.

As one of the most important anticancer drugs, TAX has been widely used for chemotherapy in various malignant tumors for about 40 years [22] and is the first-line chemotherapy drug in breast cancer therapy [23]. By stabilizing the microtubule polymer and preventing microtubules from disassembly, TAX arrests the cell cycle in the G_2/M phase and induces cell apoptosis [23–25]. However, the chemotherapy resistance is a major limitation of its effect and impacts the prognosis of patients with breast cancer. In the present work, we determined the sensitivity of wild type of MCF-7 (MCF-7–MTDH) and MTDH silencing cell (MCF-7–MTDH–shRNA) to TAX treatment. The results suggested that MCF-7–MTDH–shRNA was inhibited by TAX with a much higher rate than MCF-7–MTDH. We further examined the cell apoptosis rate and found that the apoptosis induced by TAX in MCF-7–MTDH–shRNA cells was higher than that in MCF-7–MTDH cells. Furthermore, the percentage of G_2/M phase in MCF-7–MTDH–shRNA treated with TAX was significantly higher than that

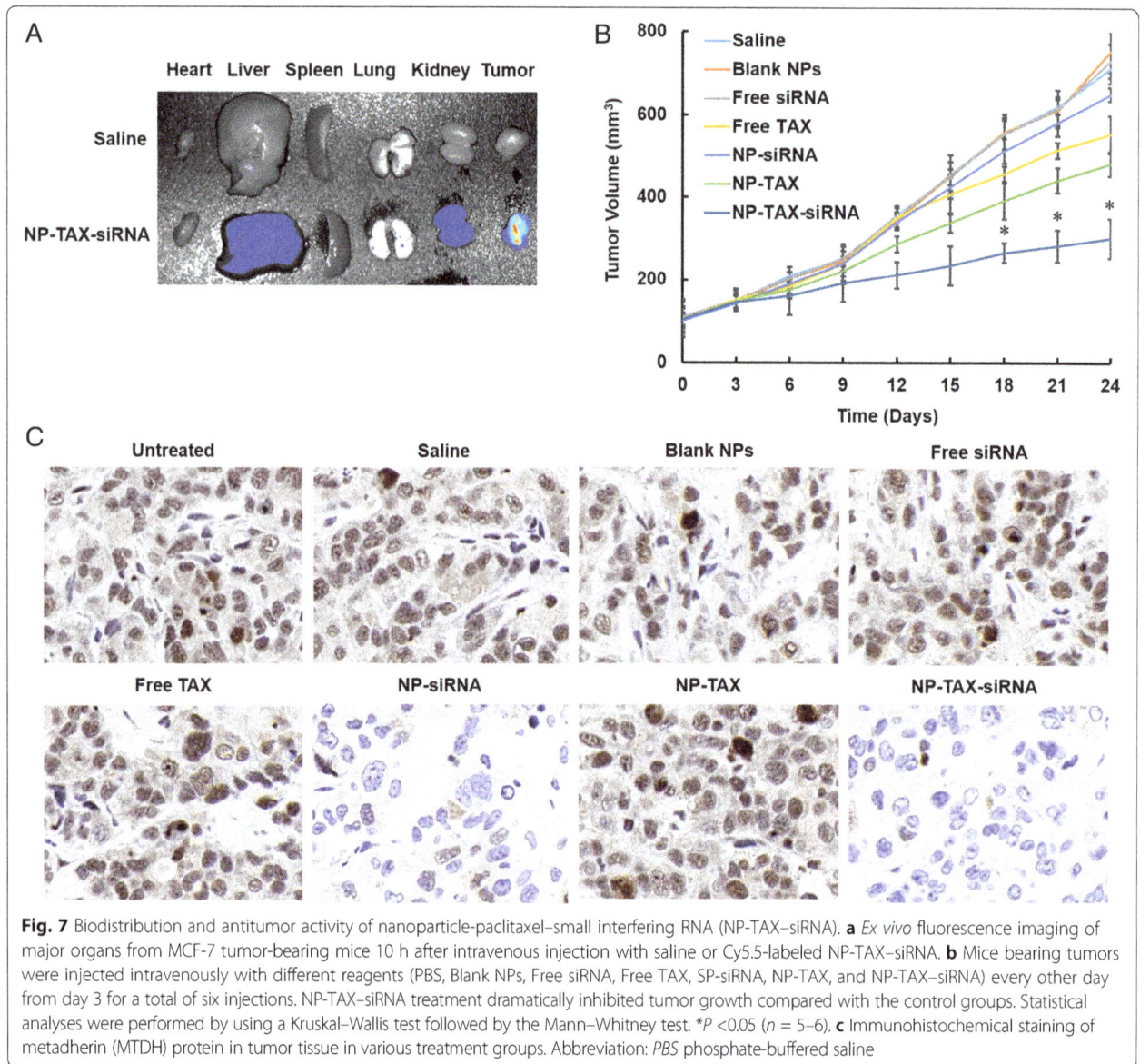

Fig. 7 Biodistribution and antitumor activity of nanoparticle-paclitaxel–small interfering RNA (NP-TAX–siRNA). **a** *Ex vivo* fluorescence imaging of major organs from MCF-7 tumor-bearing mice 10 h after intravenous injection with saline or Cy5.5-labeled NP-TAX–siRNA. **b** Mice bearing tumors were injected intravenously with different reagents (PBS, Blank NPs, Free siRNA, Free TAX, SP-siRNA, NP-TAX, and NP-TAX–siRNA) every other day from day 3 for a total of six injections. NP-TAX–siRNA treatment dramatically inhibited tumor growth compared with the control groups. Statistical analyses were performed by using a Kruskal–Wallis test followed by the Mann–Whitney test. *$P < 0.05$ ($n = 5$–6). **c** Immunohistochemical staining of metadherin (MTDH) protein in tumor tissue in various treatment groups. Abbreviation: *PBS* phosphate-buffered saline

in the control and MCF-7–MTDH groups. In in vivo experiments, compared with the MCF-7–MTDH and control groups, the volume of MCF-7–MTDH–shRNA xenograft tumors treated with TAX was significantly smaller. These data together suggest that overexpression of MTDH resisted TAX but that MTDH knockdown increased the sensitivity of MCF-7 cells to TAX treatment. In addition, MTDH plays a key role in the activation of diverse signaling pathways, including PI3K/Akt, NF-κB, and Wnt/β-catenin pathways [3, 26]. The activation of NF-κB is critical to the resistance of tumor cells to cytotoxic agents and microtubule-disrupting agents [27, 28]. We also examined the protein expression level of p65 and IκBα in various MCF-7 cells and showed that MTDH overexpression was correlated with chemoresistance to TAX but that MTDH knockdown increased the

sensitivity of TAX by inhibiting the NF-κB/IκBα pathway. This implies that one can increase the effectiveness of TAX treatment on breast cancer by lowering MTDH expression in tumor cells.

Chemoresistance is currently the major cause for breast cancer treatment failure, especially for metastatic breast cancer. Numerous siRNAs have been demonstrated to be effective for in vivo tumor growth modulations [29], but the delivery of siRNAs in vivo has been challenging for antitumor therapy because of their instability in physiological conditions, improper cellular distribution, and low bioactivity [30]. Naked siRNA has a short half-life in the bloodstream because of rapid degradation by nucleases in plasma or excreted by kidney [31]. Moreover, owing to high molecular weight, hydrophilic properties, and high density of charge, naked siRNA hardly penetrates across cell membranes [32]. Using NPs, especially the biodegradable polymer NPs to load siRNA can realize controlled and targeted drug delivery with high efficacy and low side effects [33, 34]. Also, the polymeric NPs readily realize the co-delivery of siRNA with hydrophobic or hydrophilic drugs [35]. In order to reverse drug resistance and improve the utilization of drug effectively, researchers have developed multiple nanocarriers and different dosage forms, such as NP albumin-bound TAX [36]. In this study, for tumor-specific MTDH knockdown, we constructed an amphiphilic PLGA-based copolymer NP for co-delivery of anti-MTDH siRNA and TAX into tumors. In vivo imaging results showed that the two drugs-loaded NPs (NP-TAX–siRNA) accumulated mainly in the tumor tissues, because of the passive targeting ability from the enhanced penetration and retention (EPR) effect of tumor vessels [37, 38], and inhibited tumor growth dramatically, further confirming that MTDH silencing effectively enhances the TAX therapeutic efficiency. In addition, throughout the whole therapeutic experiment, neither weight loss nor tissue damage was observed in the NP-TAX–siRNA–treated mice, indicating the biosafety of NP-TAX–siRNA for tumor treatment.

Conclusions

In summary, we have revealed, for the first time, that overexpression of MTDH in breast cancer cells is related to TAX chemotherapeutic drug resistance. To achieve in vivo therapeutic assessment by tumor-specific knockdown of MTDH, we have devised a polymer-based nanocarrier to co-deliver anti-MTDH siRNA and TAX into tumor tissues. The designed NPs were composed of a cationic copolymer, which wrapped TAX in the inside and adsorbed the negatively charged siRNA on their surface. After systemic administration, the NPs had good tumor-targeting ability based on the EPR effect of tumor vasculatures and displayed effective antitumor activity without overt side effects. Based on our study, we provide a new strategy for reversing TAX resistance in breast cancer treatment, especially for those with high MTDH protein level.

Additional file

Additional file 1: Table S1. Characteristics of 44 breast cancer patients with neoadjuvant chemotherapy. **Figure S1**. The MTDH mRNA and protein expressions level in different groups after transfecting. We constructed four groups of shRNA and one control shRNA. Then we selected the optimal silent shRNA via real-time PCR and western blot. **Figure S2**. Annexin V-PE/7-AAD assay for determination of apoptosis of cells overexpressing or knocking down metadherin (MTDH) with a flow cytometer. Annexin-positive cells are presented in gate 4. **Figure S3**. Annexin V-PE/7-AAD assay for the determination of apoptosis of different cells after paclitaxel (TAX) treatment. The apoptosis rate of MCF-7–metadherin–short hairpin RNA (MCF-7–MTDH–shRNA) cells was significantly enhanced. **Figure S4**. Flow cytometry was adopted to analyze cell cycle after cells overexpressing or knocking-downing MTDH. Compared to MCF-7 cell, the MCF-7-MTDH cell had more S phase

and less G0/G1 and G2/M phases, while knockdown of MTDH did the opposite. **Figure S5**. Cell cycle assay for different cells after paclitaxel (TAX) treatment. Compared with MCF-7 and MCF-7-vector, the G2/M phase rate of MCF-7–metadherin–short hairpin RNA (MCF-7–MTDH–shRNA) cells was significantly enhanced. While overexpression of MTDH did the opposite. **Figure S6**. Paclitaxel (TAX) release from the polymer nanoparticles (NPs). The NPs showed a faster release rate for TAX over time in PBS at pH 4.4 than at pH 7.4. Each bar represents the mean ± standard deviation of three replicates. **Figure S7**. In vivo tumor targeting of nanoparticles (NPs). Nude mice bearing MCF-7 tumors (~100 mm3) were given a single intravenous injection of Cy5.5-labeled free small interfering RNA (siRNA) or NP-TAX–siRNA by the tail vein. In vivo fluorescence signals were recorded by using a Maestro2.10.0 imaging system for up to 24 h post-injection. Abbreviation: TAX paclitaxel. (DOC 2597 kb)

Abbreviations

CCK-8: Cell Counting Kit-8; DFS: Disease-free survival; EPR: Enhanced penetration and retention; HRP: Horseradish peroxidase; IP: Intraperitoneal; IRS: Immunoreactive score; MTDH: Metadherin; NF-κB: Nuclear factor-kappa B; NP: Nanoparticle; OS: Overall survival; PBS: Phosphate-buffered saline; pCR: Pathologic complete response; PEI: Poly(etheriamide); PLGA: Poly(lactic-co-glycolic acid); PP: Percentage of positively stained tumor cells; PVA: Poly(vinyl alcohol); rpm: Revolutions per minute; RT-PCR: Real-time polymerase chain reaction; SI: Staining intensity; siRNA: Small interfering RNA; TAX: Paclitaxel

Acknowledgments

We thank L.Z. Xu (Medical and Health Analysis Center of Peking University) for animal imaging as well as technical and methodological assistance. We thank Suping Li (CAS Key Laboratory for Biomedical Effects of Nanomaterials & Nanosafety, CAS Center for Excellence in Nanoscience, National Center for Nanoscience and Technology, Beijing, China) for our nanoparticle experiment and her useful suggestions on the manuscript.

Funding

This study is supported by the Hebei Province Natural Science Foundation (H2012206169), the Hebei Province Science and Technology Foundation (162777114D), and the Wu Jieping Medical Foundation for Clinical Scientific Research (320.6750.13295). The funding body had no role in the design or execution of the study.

Authors' contributions

ZS conceived and designed the study. LY, WY, HS, MW, and BS conducted experiments. XW performed sample collection. YT drafted the manuscript. WL and JK revised the manuscript. All authors contributed to data analysis or interpretation (or both) and read and approved the final manuscript.

Competing interests

The authors declare that they have no competing interests.

Author details

[1]Breast Center, Fourth Hospital of Hebei Medical University, Shijiazhuang 050035, China. [2]Peking-Tsinghua Center for Life Sciences, Academy for

Advanced Interdisciplinary Studies, Peking University, Beijing 100871, China. [3]Department of Electrical Engineering and Computer Science, Massachusetts Institute of Technology, Cambridge, MA 02139, USA. [4]Laboratory of Experimental Pathology, Hebei Medical University, Shijiazhuang, China.

References

1. Siegel RL, Miller KD, Jemal A. Cancer statistics. CA Cancer J Clin. 2016;66:7–30.
2. Gradishar WJ, Anderson BO, Balassanian R, Blair SL, Burstein HJ, Cyr A, et al. NCCN guidelines in sights breast cancer, version 1.2016. J Natl Compr Cancer Netw. 2015;13:1475–85.
3. Quispe-Soto ET, Calaf GM. Effect of curcumin and paclitaxel on breast carcinogenesis. Int J Oncol. 2016;49:2569–77.
4. Kim YM, Tsoyi K, Jang HJ, Park EJ, Park SW, Kim HJ, et al. CKD712, a synthetic isoquinoline alkaloid, enhances the anti-cancer effects of paclitaxel in MDA-MB-231 cells through regulation of PTEN. Life Sci. 2014;112:49–58.
5. Murray S, Briasoulis E, Linardou H, Bafaloukos D, Papadimitriou C. Taxane resistance in breast cancer: mechanisms, predictive biomarkers and circumvention strategies. Cancer Treat Rev. 2012;38:890–903.
6. Huang Y, Li LP. Progress of cancer research on astrocyte elevated gene-1/Metadherin (review). Oncol Lett. 2014;8:493–501.
7. Meng X, Thiel KW, Leslie KK. Drug resistance mediated by AEG-1/MTDH/LYRIC. Adv Cancer Res. 2013;120:135–57.
8. Shi X, Wang X. The role of MTDH/AEG-1 in the progression of cancer. Int J Clin Exp Med. 2015;8:4795–807.
9. Song Z, Wang Y, Li C, Zhang D, Wang X. Molecular modification of Metadherin/MTDH impacts the sensitivity of breast Cancer to doxorubicin. PLoS One. 2015;10:e0127599.
10. Kong X, Moran MS, Zhao Y, Yang Q. Inhibition of metadherin sensitizes breast cancer cells to AZD6244. Cancer Biol Ther. 2014;13:43–9.
11. Zhao N, Wang R, Zhou L, Zhu Y, Gong J, Zhuang SM. MicroRNA-26b suppresses the NF-kappaB signaling and enhances the chemosensitivity of hepatocellular carcinoma cells by targeting TAK1 and TAB3. Mol Cancer. 2014;13:35.
12. Zhang J, Zhang Y, Liu S, Zhang Q, Wang Y, Tong L. Metadherin confers chemoresistance of cervical cancer cells by inducing autophagy and activating ERK/NF-kappaB pathway. Tumour Biol. 2013;34:2433–40.
13. Jain SK, Utreja P, Tiwary AK, Mahajan M, Kumar N, Roy P. Anti-cancer, pharmacokinetic and biodistribution studies of cremophorel free alternative paclitaxel formulation. Curr Drug Saf. 2014;9:145–55.
14. Nehate C, Jain S, Saneja A, Khare V, Alam N, Dubey RD, et al. Paclitaxel formulations: challenges and novel delivery options. Curr Drug Deliv. 2014;11:666–86.
15. Du C, Han T, Liu ZZ, Ding ZY, Zheng ZD, Piao Y, et al. MTDH mediates trastuzumab resistance in HER2 positive breast cancer by decreasing PTEN expression through an NFkB-dependent pathway. MBC Cancer. 2014;14:869.
16. Su ZZ, Kang DC, Chen Y, Pekarskaya O, Chao W, Volsky DJ, et al. Identification and cloning of human astrocyte genes displaying elevated expression after infection with HIV-1 or exposure to HIV-1 envelope glycoprotein by rapid subtraction hybridization, RaSH. Oncogene. 2002;21:3592–602.
17. Yu C, Chen K, Zheng H, Guo X, Jia W, Li M, et al. Overexpression of astrocyte elevated gene-1(AEG-1) is associated with esophageal squamous cellcarcinoma (ESCC) progression and pathogenesis. Carcinogenesis. 2009;30:894–901.
18. Jian-bo X, Hui W, Yu-long H, Chang-hua Z, Long-juan Z, Shi-rong C, et al. Astrocyte-elevated gene-I overexpression is associated with poor prognosis in gastric cancer. Med Oncol. 2011;28:455–62.
19. Lee SG, Jeon HY, Su ZZ, Richards JE, Vozhilla N, Sarkar D, et al. Astrocyte elevated gene-1contributes to the pathogenesis of neuroblastoma. Oncogene. 2009;28:2476–84.
20. Li J, Yang L, Song L, Xiong H, Wang L, Yan X, et al. Astrocyte elevated gene-1 is a proliferation promoter in breast cancer via suppressing transcriptional factor FOXO1. Oncogene. 2009;28:3188–96.
21. Xu C, Kong X, Wang H, Zhang N, Kong X, Ding X, et al. MTDH mediates estrogen-independent growth and tamoxifen resistance by down-regulating PTEN in MCF-7 breast Cancer cells. Cell Physiol Biochem. 2014;33:1557–67.
22. Wall ME, Wani MC, Taylor H. Plant antitumor agents, 27. Isolation, structure, and structure activity relationships of alkaloids from Fagara macrophylla. J Nat Prod. 1987;50:1095–9.
23. Wen G, Qu XX, Wang D, Chen XX, Tai XC, Gao F, et al. Recent advances in design, synthesis and bioactivity of paclitaxel-mimics. Fitoterapia. 2016;110:26–37.
24. Bharadwaj R, Yu H. The spindle checkpoint, aneuploidy, and cancer. Oncogene. 2004;23:2016–27.
25. Brito DA, Yang Z, Rieder CL. Microtubules do not promote mitotic slippage when the spindle assembly checkpoint cannot be satisfied. J Cell Biol. 2008;182:623–9.
26. Emdad L, Das SK, Dasgupta S, Hu B, Sarkar D, Fisher PB. AEG-1/MTDH/LYRIC: signaling pathways, downstream genes, interacting proteins, and regulation of tumor angiogenesis. Adv Cancer Res. 2013;120:75–111.
27. Jeong YJ, Kang JS, Lee SI, So DM, Yun J, Baek JY, et al. Breast cancer cells evade paclitaxel-induced cell death by developing resistance to dasatinib. Oncol Lett. 2016;12:2153–8.
28. Li F, Sethi G. Targeting transcription factor NF-kappaB to overcome chemoresistance and radioresistance in cancer therapy. Biochim Biophys Acta. 2010;1805:167–80.
29. Rao DD, Vorhies JS, Senzer N, Nemunaitis J. siRNA vs. shRNA: similarities and differences. Adv Drug Deliv Rev. 2009;61:746–59.
30. Malhotra M, Tomaro-Duchesneau C, Saha S, Prakash S. Systemic siRNA delivery via peptide-tagged polymeric nanoparyocles, targeting PLK1 gene in a mouse xenograft model of colorectal Cancer. Int J Biomater. 2013;2013:252531.
31. Kanasty R, Dorkin JR, Vegas A, Anderson D. Delivery materials for siRNA therapeutics. Nat Mater. 2013;12:967–77.
32. Li CX, Parker A, Menocal E, Xiang S, Borodyansky L, Fruehauf JH. Delivery of RNA interference. Cell Cycle. 2006;18:2103–9.
33. Oh YK, Park TG. siRNA delivery systems for cancer treatment. Adv Drug Deliv Rev. 2004;61:850–62.
34. Li J, Huang L. Targeted delivery of RNAi therapeutics for cancer therapy. Nanomedicine (London). 2010;5:1483–6.
35. Wang H, Wu Y, Zhao R, Nie G. Engineering the assemblies of biomaterial nanocarriers for delivery of multiple theranostic agents with enhanced antitumor efficacy. Adv Mater. 2013;25:1616–22.
36. Gardner ER, Dahut WL, Scripture CD, Jones J, Aragon-Ching JB, Desai N, et al. Randomized crossover pharmacokinetic study of solvent-based paclitaxel and nab-paclitaxel. Clin Cancer Res. 2008;14:4200–5.
37. Zhao X, Li F, Li Y, Wang H, Ren H, Chen J, et al. Co-delivery of HIF1alpha siRNA and gemcitabine via biocompatible lipid-polymer hybrid NPs for effective treatment of pancreatic cancer. Biomaterials. 2015;46:13–25.
38. Su S, Tian Y, Li Y, Ding Y, Ji T, Wu M, et al. "Triple-punch" strategy for triple negative breast cancer therapy with minimized drug dosage and improved antitumor efficacy. ACS Nano. 2015;9:1367–78.

8

TNFAIP3 is required for FGFR1 activation-promoted proliferation and tumorigenesis of premalignant DCIS.COM human mammary epithelial cells

Mao Yang[1†], Xiaobin Yu[2†], Xuesen Li[1], Bo Luo[1], Wenli Yang[1], Yan Lin[1], Dabing Li[1], Zhonglin Gan[1], Jianming Xu[2*] ⓘ and Tao He[1*]

Abstract

Background: Although ductal carcinoma in situ (DCIS) is a non-invasive breast cancer, many DCIS lesions may progress to invasive cancer and the genes and pathways responsible for its progression are largely unknown. FGFR1 plays an important role in cell proliferation, differentiation and carcinogenesis. The purpose of this study is to examine the roles of FGFR1 signaling in gene expression, cell proliferation, tumor growth and progression in a non-invasive DCIS model.

Methods: DCIS.COM cells were transfected with an empty vector to generate DCIS-Ctrl cells. DCIS-iFGFR1 cells were transfected with an AP20187-inducible iFGFR1 vector to generate DCIS-iFGFR1 cells. iFGFR1 consists of the v-Src myristoylation membrane-targeting sequence, FGFR1 cytoplasmic domain and the AP20187-inducible FKBP12 dimerization domain, which simulates FGFR1 signaling. The CRISPR/Cas9 system was employed to knockout *ERK1*, *ERK2* or *TNFAIP3* in DCIS-iFGFR1 cells. Established cell lines were treated with/without AP20187 and with/without FGFR1, MEK, or ERK1/2 inhibitor. The effects of these treatments were determined by Western blot, RNA-Seq, real-time RT-PCR, cell proliferation, mammosphere growth, xenograft tumor growth, and tumor histopathological assays.

Results: Activation of iFGFR1 signaling in DCIS-iFGFR1 cells enhanced ERK1/2 activities, induced partial epithelial-to-mesenchymal transition (EMT) and increased cell proliferation. Activation of iFGFR1 signaling promoted DCIS growth and progression to invasive cancer derived from DCIS-iFGFR1 cells in mice. Activation of iFGFR1 signaling also altered expression levels of 946 genes involved in cell proliferation, migration, cancer pathways, and other molecular and cellular functions. TNFAIP3, a ubiquitin-editing enzyme, is upregulated by iFGFR1 signaling in a FGFR1 kinase activity and in an ERK2-dependent manner. Importantly, TNFAIP3 knockout not only inhibited the AP20187-induced proliferation and tumor growth of DCIS-iFGFR1 cells, but also further reduced baseline proliferation and tumor growth of DCIS-iFGFR1 cells without AP20187 treatment.

Conclusions: Activation of iFGFR1 promotes ERK1/2 activity, EMT, cell proliferation, tumor growth, DCIS progression to invasive cancer, and altered the gene expression profile of DCIS-iFGFR1 cells. Activation of iFGFR1 upregulated TNFAIP3 in an ERK2-dependent manner and TNFAIP3 is required for iFGFR1 activation-promoted DCIS.COM cell proliferation, mammosphere growth, tumor growth and progression. These results suggest that TNFAIP3 may be a potential target for inhibiting DCIS growth and progression promoted by FGFR1 signaling.

Keywords: Breast cancer, FGFR1, Gene regulation, TNFAIP3, Cell proliferation, Tumor growth

* Correspondence: jxu@bcm.edu; hetao198@163.com
†Mao Yang and Xiaobin Yu contributed equally to this work.
²Department of Molecular and Cellular Biology, Baylor College of Medicine, Houston, TX 77030, USA
¹Institute for Cancer Medicine and School of Basic Medical Sciences, Southwest Medical University, Luzhou Sichuan, 646000, China

Background

The high incidence of breast cancer is a severe threat to woman's health [1]. Ductal carcinoma in situ (DCIS) is the earliest detectable form of breast cancer, which represents 20–25% of newly diagnosed breast cancers [2, 3]. Although DCIS contains malignant tumor cells confined within the basement membrane and is non-lethal, about 14–50% of DCIS cases are estimated to progress to invasive cancer over time if left untreated [4]. To date, there are still no histopathological classification or conventional biomarkers that can accurately predict whether a DCIS lesion will progress to invasive and metastatic breast cancer. The molecular mechanisms responsible for DCIS progression are also largely unclear. The cell lines derived from the MCF10A normal human breast epithelial cells exhibit different grades of malignancy, which have been used as cellular models for studying breast cancer progression, including DCIS progression. Specifically, MCF10AT cells were derived from MCF10A cells transfected with mutated T24 Ha-ras that carries a G12D mutation [5]. The original transplants of MCF10AT cells in mice mainly generated differentiated ducts lined by simple or hyperplastic epithelium. Serial passages of the MCF10AT xenografts produced different grades of lesions that recapitulated the human proliferative breast disease in most mice, as well as DCIS and invasive cancer in a small subset of mice [6, 7]. DCIS.COM is a clonal breast cancer cell line derived from a passaged MCF10AT xenograft with DCIS morphology [8]. Injection of DCIS.COM cells into SCID mice produces rapidly growing lesions that are predominantly comedo DCIS [8]. This DCIS.COM model has been successfully used for studying DCIS progression in vivo [8, 9]. In this study, we utilize the DCIS.COM model to study the impact of fibroblast growth factor receptor 1 (FGFR1) signaling on DCIS growth and progression.

The FGFR tyrosine kinase family with FGFR1/2/3/4 plays important roles in cancer [10]. Whole genome sequencing data of multiple types of human cancers showed that amplifications, mutations and rearrangements of FGFR1/2/3/4 were detected in 3.5%, 1.5%, 2.0%, and 0.5%, respectively [11]. Importantly, the frequency of these genetic aberrations of FGFR1 was found to be particularly high in breast cancers, which reached 18% of the breast tumor samples examined [11]. FGFRs and their ligands, fibroblast growth factors (FGFs), also promote breast cancer resistance to endocrine therapy and chemotherapy [12–14]. Therefore, it is important to understand how FGF and FGFR signaling pathways promote breast cancer growth and progression.

There are 22 FGFs in human, and 18 of these FGFs can bind to the extracellular domains of one or more FGFRs in the presence of heparan sulfate and/or Klotho co-receptors [15–18]. In addition to their extracellular ligand-binding domain, FGFRs also contain transmembrane and intracellular tyrosine kinase domains. Upon FGF binding, FGFR dimerizes and transphosphorylates specific tyrosine residues in each intracellular domain of the dimer, resulting in activation of downstream signaling pathways via direct or indirect interactions with FGFR substrate 2α (FRS2α), PLCγ and/or STAT1/3/5. The FGFR-phosphorylated FRS2α further relays the signal to activate the Ras-Raf-MEK-ERK1/2 pathway [17, 19]. The FGF-FGFR signaling pathways play crucial roles in cell growth, cell differentiation, embryonic development, and many physiological processes [10]. Their activities are subjected to precise temporal and spatial regulatory mechanisms, while their deregulations may cause many severe developmental and physiological health problems [20].

Abnormal activation of FGF/FGFR signaling pathways can increase cell proliferation, induce epithelial-to-mesenchymal transition (EMT), cell motility and invasiveness, promote carcinogenesis, and make cancer cell resistant to drug treatment [10]. For example, although activation of the FGF signaling in the estrogen receptor-positive (ER+) MCF7 breast cancer cells is unable to enhance cell proliferation [21], activation of FGFR1 in the ER-negative (ER-) human mammary epithelial cells increases cell proliferation, and knockdown of FGFR1 in the ER- mouse breast cancer cells also inhibits cell proliferation [22, 23]. Deregulated FGFR1 signaling also causes epithelial hyperplasia or adenocarcinoma and synergizes with the Wnt1-signaling pathway or PTEN loss-activated PI3K-AKT signaling to drive carcinogenesis and metastasis in mouse models of breast or prostate cancers [24, 25]. FGFR1 amplification and overexpression in certain breast cancer cells increases MAPK and PI3K-AKT activities [26]. In ER+/human epidermal growth factor receptor 2-negative (HER2-) breast cancers, FGFR gene amplification is more frequent in endocrine therapy-resistant cases versus endocrine therapy-sensitive cases [12]. Human breast tumors with FGFR1 overexpression possess higher cell proliferation rates and have poor prognosis [26]. It has also been shown that HER2 expression in breast cancer cells upregulates FGF2 and FGFR1, which promotes EMT and resistance to Lapatinib [14]. Moreover, certain cancer cells resistant to paclitaxel or EGFR, Met and VEGFR inhibitors can regain sensitivity to these drugs after blocking the FGF/FGFR signaling [27–30]. Finally, although clinical trials with FGFR inhibitors are currently underway, it is possible that FGFR mutation, gene fusion, alternative kinase activation or MAPK/Akt reactivation may make the cancer cells resistant to these inhibitors [31–34]. Given all these detrimental roles of FGF/FGFR signaling pathways in promoting carcinogenesis and possible resistance of cancer cells to FGFR inhibitors, it is important to find alternative molecular targets of the FGF/FGFR signaling through identifying their regulated genes important for this signaling pathway-promoted carcinogenesis.

Based on molecular mechanisms of FGFR1 activation by FGF, a ligand-inducible chimeric FGFR1 (iFGFR1) fusion protein has been created to mimic the FGF/FGFR1 signaling system [35, 36]. This fusion protein consists of the v-Src myristoylation membrane-targeting sequence, the cytoplasmic domain of FGFR1 for signaling and two repeats of the AP20187-inducible FKBP12 dimerization domain. AP20187-induced dimerization of this iFGFR1 fusion protein faithfully activates the FGFR1 signaling pathway [35, 36]. In the current study, we have generated iFGFR1-expressing DCIS.COM cell lines and used these cell lines as a model to study the impact of FGFR1 signaling on the growth, progression and gene expression of breast DCIS tumor cells. We show that the AP20187-activated iFGFR1 enhances extracellular-signal regulated kinases 1/2 (ERK1/2) MAPK activities, increases DCIS.COM cell proliferation in culture and promotes DCIS progression to invasive cancer in mice. Activation of iFGFR1 in DCIS.COM cells altered the expression levels of many genes involved in cancer and other cellular functions. Among the iFGFR1-upregulated genes, we are particularly interested in TNFAIP3. TNFAIP3 is a ubiquitin-editing enzyme with both deubiquitylase and E3 ubiquitin ligase activity [37]. Multiple studies have reported tumor suppressor roles for TNFAIP3 in inhibiting NF-κB in chronic myeloid leukemia [38], suppressing EMT, cell migration and invasion in nasopharyngeal carcinoma [39], and inhibiting liver inflammation, hepatocellular carcinoma proliferation, and metastasis through inhibition of *Twist1* expression and TNFα-induced cell motility [40]. However, other studies have reported the cancer-promoting roles for TNFAIP3 in conferring tamoxifen resistance in ER+ breast cancers [41], promoting EMT and metastasis of basal-like breast cancers by mono-ubiquitination of SNAIL1 [42], and preventing adult T-cell leukemia cells from apoptosis [43]. TNFAIP3 has also been found to be overexpressed in metastatic cholangiocarcinomas and esophageal squamous cell carcinomas [44, 45]. In the current study, we found that iFGFR1 activation upregulates TNFAIP3 expression through activating ERK2 MAPK in DCIS.COM cells. We also demonstrate that knockout (KO) of TNFAIP3 blocks FGFR1 signaling-promoted DCIS cell proliferation and progression, suggesting that TNFAIP3 is required for FGFR1 signaling-promoted DCIS growth and progression.

Methods

Plasmids, cell lines and cell culture
pSH1/M-FGFR1-Fv-Fvls-E plasmid for iFGFR1 expression was provided by Dr. David M. Spencer [25]. The iFGFR1 DNA sequence in this plasmid was subcloned into the pRevTRE plasmid to generate the pRevTRE-iFGFR1 plasmid. DCIS.COM cells were cultured in DMEM/F12 (1:1) medium with 5% horse serum, 29 mM sodium bicarbonate, 10 mM HEPES, 100 IU/ml penicillin and 100 μg/ml penicillin/streptomycin (PS) as described previously [9].

PT67 cells were cultured in DMEM with 10% fetal bovine serum (FBS) and PS. All cells were cultured at 37 °C in an incubator supplied with 5% CO_2.

Generation of iFGFR1-expressing cell lines
PT67 cells (2×10^6) were cultured overnight and then transfected with 5 μg of pRevTRE or pRevTRE-iFGFR1 plasmids using Lipofectamine 3000 Reagent (Invitrogen, Waltham, MA, USA). The transfected cells were cultured in the medium containing 400 μg/ml of hygromycin for 2 weeks. The conditioned medium of the transfected PT67 cells containing retrovirus particles was filtered through a 0.45 μm membrane, and then used to transduce DCIS.COM cells for 24 h in the presence of 4 μg/ml polybrene. These cells were growth-selected in medium containing 400 μg/ml of hygromycin for 2 weeks. Surviving clones were picked up and expanded for immunoblotting using an HA antibody to detect the iFGFR1 C-terminal HA tag. Clones expressing iFGFR1 were designated as DCIS-iFGFR1 cell lines. Clones transduced by pRevTRE empty virus served as DCIS control (DCIS-Ctrl) cells.

Cell growth assay
DCIS-Ctrl, DCIS-iFGFR1, and TNFAIP3 KO DCIS-iFGFR1 cells were seeded in 96- or 6-well plate at 2×10^3 or 10^5 cells/well, cultured overnight, and treated with 0.02% DMSO (vehicle) or 100 nM AP20187 for different time periods. CellTiter method was used to measure cell viability. In this assay, 20 μl of CellTiter 96 Aqueous One Solution (Promega, Madison, Wi, USA) was added to each well and the plate was incubated at 37 °C for 2 h. The absorbance was measured at 490 nm using a Synergy HT plate reader (BioTek, Winooski, VT, USA). Cell number was also directly counted under a phase-contrast microscope by using a blood cell counting chamber as needed.

Immunoblotting
Vehicle or AP20187-treated cells were lysed using RIPA buffer containing 25 mM Tris HCl (pH 7.6), 150 mM NaCl, 1% sodium deoxycholate, 0.1% SDS and the protease inhibitor cocktail (Roche, Basel, Switzerland). Cell extracts with 5–20 μg of total protein were subjected to immunoblotting assays using primary antibodies against HA (3724, Cell Signaling Technology, Danvers, MA, USA), TNFAIP3 (sc-166,692, Santa Cruz Biotechnology, Dallas, TX, USA), E-cadherin (610,181, BD Biosciences, San Jose, CA, USA), N-cadherin (610,920, BD Biosciences), β-catenin (sc-7963, Santa Cruz Biotchnology), fibronectin (610,077, BD Biosciences), ERK1/2 (9102, Cell Signaling Technology), p-ERK1/2 (9101, Cell Signaling Technology), RSK1/2/3 (9355 s, Cell Signaling Technology), Phospho-p90 RSK (11,989 s, Cell Signaling Technology), GAPDH (2118 s, Cell Signaling Technology) and β-actin (A5441, Sigma-Aldrich, St., Louis, MO, USA). Appropriate horseradish peroxidase (HRP)-conjugated

or fluorescence-labeled secondary antibodies (LI-COR Biosciences, Lincoln, NE, USA) were used to detect the primary antibodies bound to their antigens on the nitrocellulose membranes. The HRP activity was detected by using the ECL substrate solution (32,106, Thermo Fisher Scientific, Waltham, MA, USA), followed by exposure to X-ray film and quantified by the Odyssey Imaging System (LI-COR).

Phalloidin staining

DCIS-iFGFR1 cells were cultured on cover slips placed in a 6-well plate, followed by AP20187 or vehicle treatment for 6 days. Cells were fixed for 15 min in 4% formaldehyde, and then washed three times in PBS. Cells were permeabilized in PBS containing 0.1% Triton X-100 for 5 min and washed 3 times with PBS. The prepared cells were stained in 1:20 dilution of Alexa Fluor® 488 Phalloidin (8878, Cell Signaling Technology) and 1:5000 dilution of DAPI in PBS for 15 min at room temperature. The stained cells were washed three times in PBS and dehydrated in serial ethanol solutions. After mounting the cover slip with stained cells onto glass slides, the stained cells were examined and imaged under a fluorescence microscope.

RT-qPCR

Total RNA was extracted from cells by using Trizol reagent (Invitrogen). cDNA was synthesized by using a reverse transcription kit (Roche). TaqMan qPCR was performed in triplicates using a 7900 Real-time PCR machine (Applied Biosystems, Foster City, CA, USA). β-actin mRNA served as an internal control for gene expression. The average of delta Ct numbers was employed to calculate relative gene expression. The 5′ primers, 3′ primers and fluorescent probes matched from the Universal Probe Library (Cat. No. 04688970001, Roche) were: 5′-tgcacactgtgtttcatcgag, 5′-ac gctgtgggactgactttc, Probe #74 for *TNFAIP3*; 5′-atcaggggcca ggttttc, 5′-gggccaagcaccatctaat, Probe #13 for *PIM1*; 5′-ccagctgacaacaggaggag, 5′-cccatgagctccttgtacagat, Probe #3 for *SERPINE1*; 5′-ggccttgtgaacagatcagc, 5′-ctccggt tcctgcacttg, Probe #69 for *FOSL1*; 5′-gtggacgggcagaatgtta, 5′-cgtggccagaatctccat, Probe #41 for *SDCBP2*; 5′-gctcc tactgtgataagtccttcc, 5′-tgtcgcctgtgtggattct, Probe #10 for *ZNF362*; and 5′-tcccacccagaatctttaggta, 5′-gccggggttgagattc at, Probe #10 for *EHF*.

RNA-Seq

DCIS-iFGFR1 cells (4.0×10^6) were cultured in 10-cm plates overnight, treated with vehicle or 100 nM AP20187 for 3 and 16 h. Total RNA was extracted with Trizol reagent (Invitrogen) and subjected to RNA-Seq using Illumian HiSeqTM 2000. Biocomputational analysis was carried out to compare differential gene expression profiles induced by iFGFR1 activation at different time points. Differentially expressed genes were further analyzed by

using the DAVID online analysis tool with the Gene Ontology (GO) and the Kyoto Encyclopedia of Genes and Genomes (KEGG) databases [46, 47]. $p < 0.05$ was used to select significant GO terms and KEGG pathways. The -log(p value) is the negative log10 of the p value.

CRISPR/Cas9-based gene KO

To KO human *ERK1*, ERK,2 and *TNFAIP3* genes, gRNAs for each gene were designed using the Optimized CRISPR Design Tool as described previously [48]. Double-strand oligo DNA for each gRNA was cloned into the BbsI site of the SpCas9-2A-GFP plasmid (PX458, Addgene, Cambridge, MA, USA) for expressing sgRNA and Cas9. DCIS-iFGFR1 cells were transfected with the expression plasmids using Lipofectamin 2000. After 48 h, GFP-positive cells were sorted by flow cytometry and seeded in 96-well plates at an opportunity of 1 cell/well. Single cell clones were marked, amplified, and tested for gene expression by immunoblotting using antibodies against ERK1/2 or TNFAIP3. DNA samples of the candidate KO clones were prepared and sequenced to confirm the gene KO. Non-KO clones were used as control cells.

Mammosphere growth assay

This assay was performed as described previously [49]. Briefly, an aliquot of 3000 cells in 100 μl of culture medium was added to each well of ultra-low attachment U bottom 96-well plates (Corning, Corning, NY, USA) to grow mammospheres. After culturing for 24 h, cells were treated with vehicle or 100 nM AP20187 for 7 days. Each treatment group had eight parallel samples. The cell spheres formed in each well were imaged and their diameters were measured using the Image Pro Plus 5.0 Software (Media Cybernetics, Rockville MD, USA).

Xenograft tumor growth

Six- to 7-week-old BALB/c-nu mice were purchased from Beijing Huafukang Biosciences Inc., Beijing, China. DCIS-iFGFR1-Ctrl or DCIS-iFGFR1-TNFAIP3 KO cells were injected into each of the fourth pair mammary gland fat pads of these mice. After 3 days, mice were treated with AP20187 (1 mg/kg, 3 times/week, i.p.) or equal volume of solvent (< 50 μl). AP20187 was dissolved in ethanol at a stocking concentration of 10 mg/ml, and further diluted to 400 μg/ml in water solution of 10% PEG400 and 2% Tween-80 for injection. Tumor length and width were measured three times per week by using a caliper. Tumor volume was calculated by the formula: (length × width^2) × π/6. Mice were sacrificed when the biggest tumor exceeded 1.5 cm in length. Tumors were harvested and weighed immediately.

Hematoxylin and eosin (H&E) staining and immunohistochemistry

Collected xenograft tumor tissues were fixed in 4% para-formaldehyde, embedded in paraffin, and sectioned at a thickness of 5 μm. Sections were deparaffinized in xylene and rehydrated by going through ethanol series and water. Some sections were stained with H&E and used for histo-pathological examination. Other sections were soaked in 10 mM sodium citrate (pH 6.0) and heat-treated in a high-pressure cooker for 4 min. The section slides were washed in PBS and blocked in 5% bovine serum albumin (BSA) for 1 h. The prepared sections were incubated over-night at 4 °C with p-ERK1/2 antibody (4370 s, Cell Signal-ing Technology) at 1:400 dilution in PBS containing 5% BSA. After washing and incubation with biotinylated anti-rabbit IgG, the immunostaining signal was visualized with DAB kit (8059S, Cell Signaling Technology). The sec-tions were counterstained with Harris Modified Hematoxylin, dehydrated and mounted with Permount for microscopy and imaging.

Results

Activation of iFGFR1 signaling in DCIS-iFGFR1 cells induces ERK1/2 phosphorylation, partial EMT, and cell proliferation

To study the mechanism of FGFR1 signaling in human breast cancer progression, we generated DCIS-Ctrl control cell lines containing an empty vector and DCIS-iFGFR1 cell lines expressing the C-terminally HA-tagged iFGFR1 fusion protein (Fig. 1a). It has been shown that AP20187-induced dimerization of iFGFR1 resulted in the activation of the FGFR1 signaling [25, 35, 36]. After treatment with AP20187, both total ERK1/2 and p-ERK1/2 showed no changes in DCIS-Ctrl cells, while the levels of pERK1/2 were signifi-cantly increased in DCIS-iFGFR1 cell lines although total ERK1/2 levels remained the same (Fig. 1b). The high levels of p-ERK1/2 in DCIS-iFGFR1 cells were significantly in-duced by AP20187 within 1 min and could be maintained for hours (Fig. 1c and data not shown). Furthermore, the majority (89% ± 1.5%) of vehicle-treated DCIS-iFGFR1 cells formed epithelial colonies with tight cell-cell interactions, while only 20% ± 0.4% of AP20187-treated DCIS-iFGFR1 cells retained epithelial colony morphology and 80% ± 0.9% of these cells exhibited fibroblast cell morphology (Fig. 1d and data now shown). In the AP20187-treated cells, the epithelial markers E-cadherin, cytokeratin 8 (K8), and β-catenin were significantly reduced and the mesenchymal markers including vimentin, fibronectin, and N-cadherin were increased (Fig. 1e). Moreover, AP20187 treatment had no effect on DCIS-Ctrl cells but significantly increased the proliferation rates of DCIS-iFGFR1 cells (Fig. 1f). These re-sults demonstrate that the AP20187-activated iFGFR1 is fully functional in terms of ERK1/2 activation, EMT induction, and cell proliferation.

Activation of iFGFR1 signaling pathway changes the expression levels of important genes for regulating gene expression, cell proliferation, and cancer

To identify the genes regulated by the iFGFR1-signaling, we performed RNA-Seq analyses with nine RNA samples pre-pared from DCIS-iFGFR1 cells treated with vehicle (n = 3), AP20187 for 3 h (n = 3) or AP20187 for 16 h (n = 3). In general, more than 15,000 mRNA transcripts were detected in all three groups, and the expression levels of 6–7% of these transcripts were changed by AP20187 treatment (Fig. 2a). Specifically, when compared with vehicle treatment, AP20187 treatment for 3 h upreg-ulated and downregulated mRNA expression of 259 and 314 genes, respectively (Fig. 2b and Additional file 1), and AP20187 treatment for 16 h upregulated and downregu-lated mRNA expression of 201 and 195 genes, respectively (Fig. 2b and Additional file 2). When compared between cells treated with AP20187 for 16- and 3-h, there were 211 upregulated and 184 downregulated genes (Fig. 2b and Additional file 3). After the overlapping mRNAs changed during 3 and 16 h of AP29187 treatment were fil-tered out, there were a total of 946 mRNAs that were ei-ther upregulated or downregulated (Fig. 2b). Eighty and 68 of the 946 mRNAs were consecutively upregulated and downregulated, respectively, at both 3- and 16-h time points of AP20187 treatment when compared with the vehicle-treated group (Fig. 2b and c). The remaining mRNAs were either upregulated at the 3-h time point and then downregulated at the 16-h time point or vice versa (Fig. 2b). RT-qPCR analysis validated all of the six selected mRNAs upregulated by AP20187 and two of the three se-lected mRNAs downregulated by AP20187 in DCIS-iFGFR1 cells. The remaining one showed a downregula-tion trend without reaching a significant level because of the larger expression variations in one group of samples (Fig. 2d). These results suggest that activation of the FGFR1-signaling pathway temporally regulates a subset of genes, which may reflect the functional complexity of the interactive networks involving the gene products regulated directly and indirectly by the FGFR1 signaling.

GO analysis of the differentially expressed 946 mRNAs upon AP20187 treatment revealed their enrichment in multiple biological processes such as inflammatory re-sponses, angiogenesis, cell proliferation/migration/adhe-sion and gene regulation, and in multiple molecular functions including DNA binding, gene transcription, signaling protein-protein interaction, and Ras signaling (Fig. 3a and b). KEGG pathway analysis also indicates that the FGFR1-regulated genes are involved in pathways important for regulating stem cells, inflammation such as the TNF and NF-κB pathways, cancer growth and metastasis such as the NF-κB, hippo, PI3K-Akt, p53, and Ras pathways (Fig. 3c). These results suggest that the FGFR1 signaling pathway can promote EMT, cell growth, and

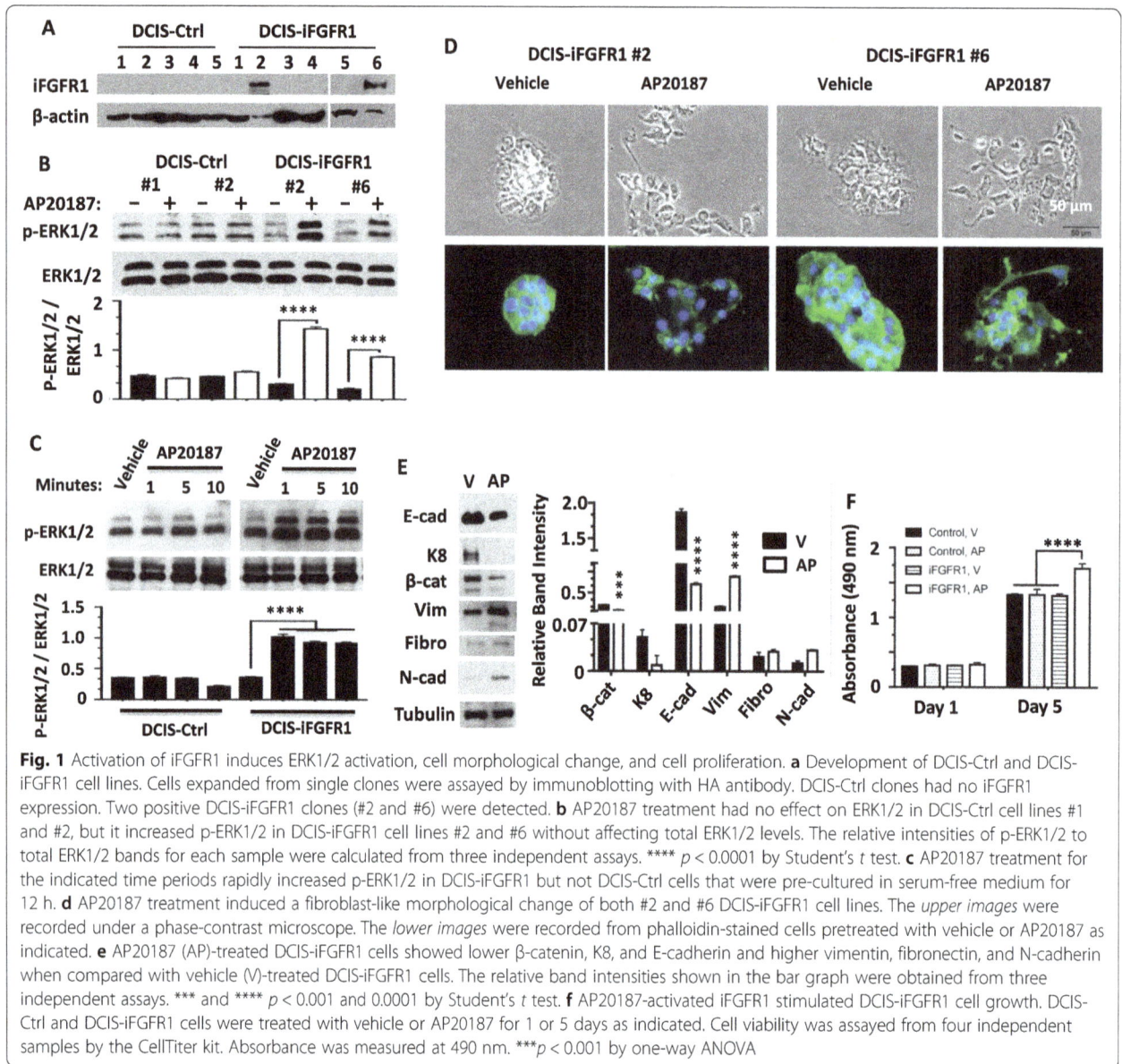

Fig. 1 Activation of iFGFR1 induces ERK1/2 activation, cell morphological change, and cell proliferation. **a** Development of DCIS-Ctrl and DCIS-iFGFR1 cell lines. Cells expanded from single clones were assayed by immunoblotting with HA antibody. DCIS-Ctrl clones had no iFGFR1 expression. Two positive DCIS-iFGFR1 clones (#2 and #6) were detected. **b** AP20187 treatment had no effect on ERK1/2 in DCIS-Ctrl cell lines #1 and #2, but it increased p-ERK1/2 in DCIS-iFGFR1 cell lines #2 and #6 without affecting total ERK1/2 levels. The relative intensities of p-ERK1/2 to total ERK1/2 bands for each sample were calculated from three independent assays. **** $p < 0.0001$ by Student's t test. **c** AP20187 treatment for the indicated time periods rapidly increased p-ERK1/2 in DCIS-iFGFR1 but not DCIS-Ctrl cells that were pre-cultured in serum-free medium for 12 h. **d** AP20187 treatment induced a fibroblast-like morphological change of both #2 and #6 DCIS-iFGFR1 cell lines. The *upper images* were recorded under a phase-contrast microscope. The *lower images* were recorded from phalloidin-stained cells pretreated with vehicle or AP20187 as indicated. **e** AP20187 (AP)-treated DCIS-iFGFR1 cells showed lower β-catenin, K8, and E-cadherin and higher vimentin, fibronectin, and N-cadherin when compared with vehicle (V)-treated DCIS-iFGFR1 cells. The relative band intensities shown in the bar graph were obtained from three independent assays. *** and **** $p < 0.001$ and 0.0001 by Student's t test. **f** AP20187-activated iFGFR1 stimulated DCIS-iFGFR1 cell growth. DCIS-Ctrl and DCIS-iFGFR1 cells were treated with vehicle or AP20187 for 1 or 5 days as indicated. Cell viability was assayed from four independent samples by the CellTiter kit. Absorbance was measured at 490 nm. ***$p < 0.001$ by one-way ANOVA

carcinogenesis through regulating different genes involving multiple biological events and molecular signaling pathways.

Activation of iFGFR1 signaling upregulates TNFAIP3 expression

Among the genes consecutively upregulated by AP20187-activated iFGFR1, we were particularly interested in understanding how FGFR1 signaling regulates TNFAIP3 expression, since it plays an important role in NF-κB regulation but its role in breast cancer is unknown [37, 50]. AP20187-activated iFGFR1 robustly increased the expression of TNFAIP3 mRNA in DCIS-iFGFR1 cells, while this increase could be completely blocked by treating cells with FGFR inhibitors LY2874455 [51] and AZD4547 [52] (Fig. 4a).

Accordingly, the TNFAIP3 and p-ERK1/2 protein levels were similar in DCIS-Ctrl cells treated with AP20187 or FGFR inhibitors, while the TNFAIP3 and p-ERK1/2 protein levels in DCIS-iFGFR1 cells were increased by AP20187 treatment and these increases were abolished by LY2874455 or AZD4547 treatment (Fig. 4b). Furthermore, the AP20187-induced TNFAIP3 mRNA and protein were positively associated with the increases in the phosphorylated active forms of ERK1/2 and/or p90-RSK. Inhibition of ERK1/2 activities by either ERK1/2 inhibitor GDC0994 or MEK inhibitor PD0325901 that prevents ERK1/2 activation abolished ERK1/2-mediated p90-RSK phosphorylation (activation), which also significantly reduced the basal and AP20187-induced levels of TNFAIP3 mRNA and protein

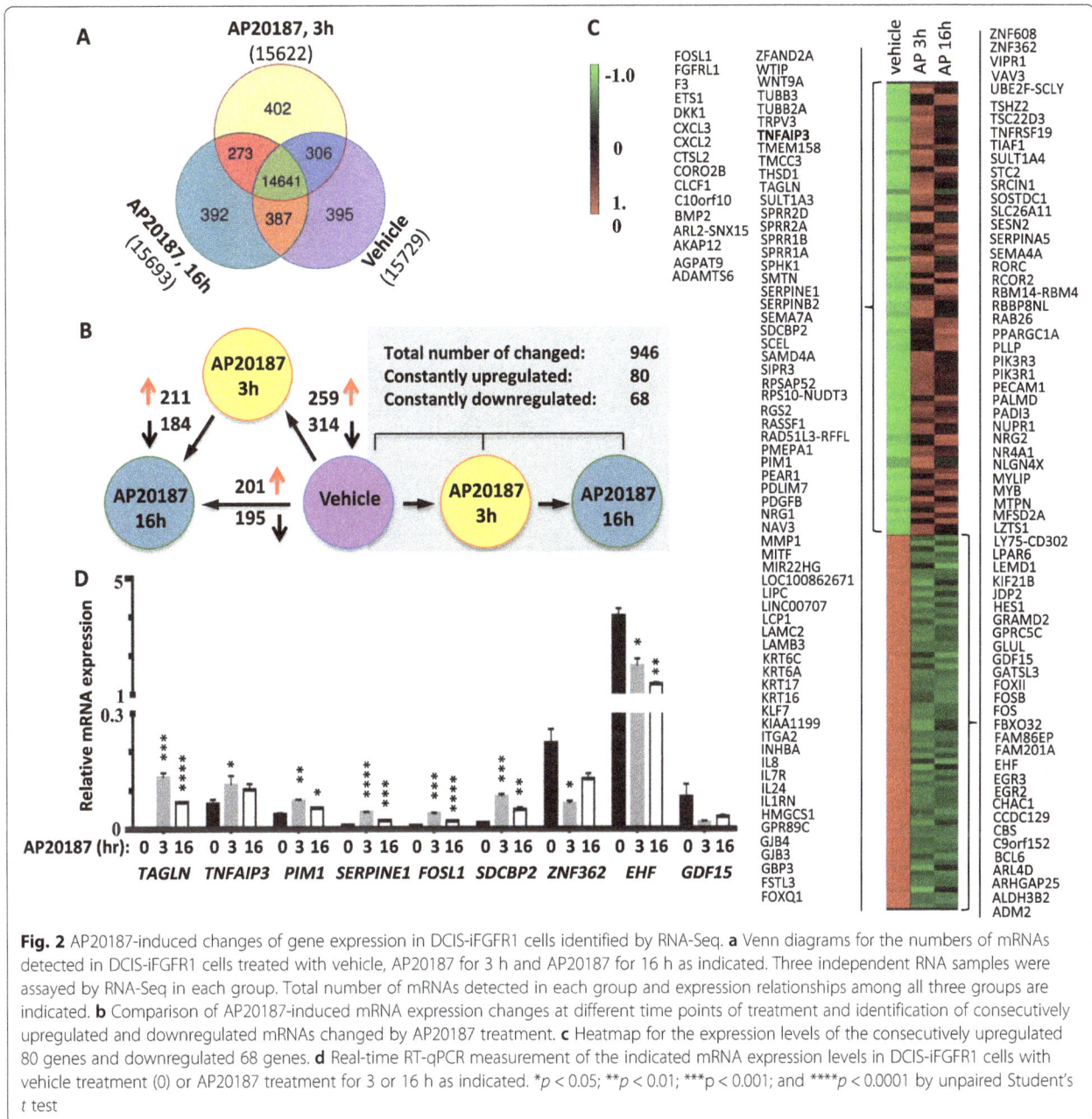

Fig. 2 AP20187-induced changes of gene expression in DCIS-iFGFR1 cells identified by RNA-Seq. **a** Venn diagrams for the numbers of mRNAs detected in DCIS-iFGFR1 cells treated with vehicle, AP20187 for 3 h and AP20187 for 16 h as indicated. Three independent RNA samples were assayed by RNA-Seq in each group. Total number of mRNAs detected in each group and expression relationships among all three groups are indicated. **b** Comparison of AP20187-induced mRNA expression changes at different time points of treatment and identification of consecutively upregulated and downregulated mRNAs changed by AP20187 treatment. **c** Heatmap for the expression levels of the consecutively upregulated 80 genes and downregulated 68 genes. **d** Real-time RT-qPCR measurement of the indicated mRNA expression levels in DCIS-iFGFR1 cells with vehicle treatment (0) or AP20187 treatment for 3 or 16 h as indicated. *$p < 0.05$; **$p < 0.01$; ***$p < 0.001$; and ****$p < 0.0001$ by unpaired Student's t test

(Fig. 4c and d). These results demonstrate that activation of the FGFR1 signaling pathway upregulates TNFAIP3 expression in an ERK1/2 activation-dependent manner.

Upregulation of TNFAIP3 by iFGFR1 signaling is mainly dependent on ERK2 in DCIS-iFGFR1 cells

Although ERK1 and ERK2 share redundant functions, their specific roles have also been reported [53]. To define the specific roles of ERK1 and ERK2 in FGFR1-mediated TNFAIP3 expression, we co-expressed Cas9 with the sgRNA that specifically targets exon 2 of the human *ERK1* gene or the sgRNA that specifically targets exon 2 of the human *ERK2* gene in DCIS-iFGFR1 cells. Multiple KO cell

lines for each gene were identified by screening individually isolated clones by PCR, followed by DNA sequencing (data not shown). Immunoblotting analysis confirmed the absence of the p44 ERK1 protein and the presence of the p42 ERK2 protein in the ERK1 KO cell lines and vice versa in the ERK2 KO cell lines (Fig. 5a and b). As indicated by the immunoblotting results of multiple experiments, KO of ERK1 or ERK2 did not change or only marginally increased the level of ERK2 or ERK1 (Fig. 5a–c). These KO cell lines showed normal growth in culture.

Again, AP20187 treatment induced TNFAIP3 protein expression in DCIS-iFGFR1 cells. Interestingly, AP20187 treatment also upregulated TNFAIP3 protein in two

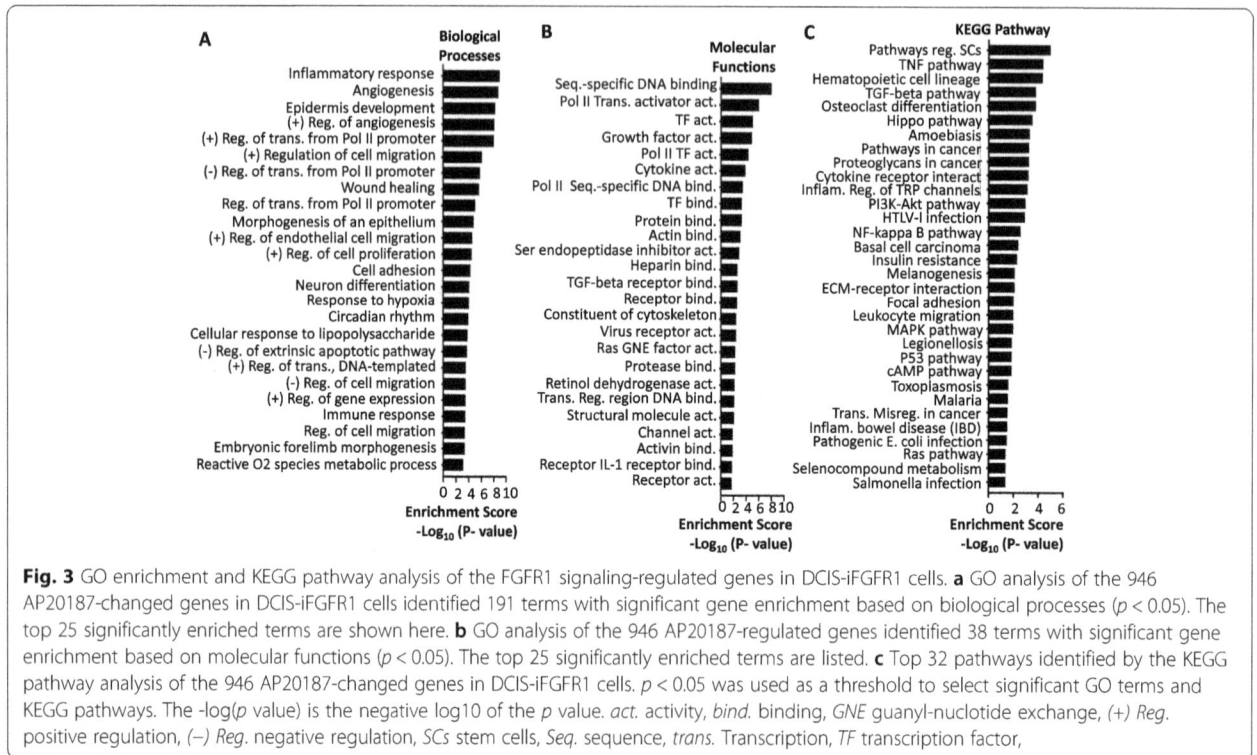

Fig. 3 GO enrichment and KEGG pathway analysis of the FGFR1 signaling-regulated genes in DCIS-iFGFR1 cells. **a** GO analysis of the 946 AP20187-changed genes in DCIS-iFGFR1 cells identified 191 terms with significant gene enrichment based on biological processes ($p < 0.05$). The top 25 significantly enriched terms are shown here. **b** GO analysis of the 946 AP20187-regulated genes identified 38 terms with significant gene enrichment based on molecular functions ($p < 0.05$). The top 25 significantly enriched terms are listed. **c** Top 32 pathways identified by the KEGG pathway analysis of the 946 AP20187-changed genes in DCIS-iFGFR1 cells. $p < 0.05$ was used as a threshold to select significant GO terms and KEGG pathways. The -log(p value) is the negative log10 of the p value. *act.* activity, *bind.* binding, *GNE* guanyl-nuclotide exchange, *(+) Reg.* positive regulation, *(−) Reg.* negative regulation, *SCs* stem cells, *Seq.* sequence, *trans.* Transcription, *TF* transcription factor,

DCIS-iFGFR1 cell lines with ERK1 KO as it did in DCIS-iFGFR1 control cells with wild-type ERK1/2. However, AP20187 treatment failed to induce TNFAIP3 protein in two DCIS-iFGFR1 cell lines with ERK2 KO. Accordingly, AP20187 induced a more dramatic increase in ERK2 phosphorylation in ERK1 KO cells than ERK1 phosphorylation in ERK2 KO cells (Fig. 5c). These results demonstrate that TNFAIP3 expression stimulated by FGFR1 signaling is largely dependent on the activation of ERK2.

TNFAIP3 is required for iFGFR1-mediated cell proliferation
To address whether TNFAIP3 is required for FGFR1-mediated cell proliferation, we co-expressed Cas9 with the sgRNA that targets the second exon of the human *TNFAIP3* gene. Our screening identified several KO clones and we used two of these clones for experiments (Fig. 6a). As expected, AP20187 treatment significantly increased the proliferation rate of the DCIS-iFGFR1 #2 parent control cells. Interestingly, TNFAIP3 KO cells derived from the DCIS-iFGFR1 parent cells failed to respond to AP20187 treatment in terms of cell proliferation, indicating that TNFAIP3 is required for iFGFR1-mediated cell proliferation. Furthermore, KO of TNFAIP3 inhibited cell proliferation when compared with their parent control cells in the absence of AP20187 treatment, suggesting that TNFAIP3 may also be required for the endogenous FGFR1-mediated cell growth or involved in other cell

growth pathways. (Fig. 6b). Consistent results were also obtained from assaying the growth of three-dimensional (3D) mammospheres. DCIS-Ctrl cells formed medium-sized spheres that were insensitive to AP20187 treatment. The DCIS-iFGFR1 #2 parent control cells formed medium-sized spheres in the absence of AP20187, while AP20187 treatment significantly increased the sphere sizes formed from these cells. However, both #3 and #4 lines of the TNFAIP3 KO DCIS-iFGFR1 cells only developed small spheres and AP20187 treatment was unable to enhance their growth (Fig. 6c). These results indicate that TNFAIP3 is essential for FGFR1 signaling-stimulated cell proliferation and mammosphere growth.

TNFAIP3 is required for the iFGFR1 signaling pathway-promoted tumor growth in mice
To investigate the role of TNFAIP3 in FGFR1-promoted breast tumor growth in vivo, we injected DCIS-iFGFR1 #2 parent control cells and TNFAIP3 KO DCIS-iFGFR1 cells into the fat pads of nude mouse mammary glands. DCIS-iFGFR1 cells formed tumors and the average tumor weight reached about 0.25 g in 14 days. AP20187 treatment of mice markedly accelerated tumor growth, which increased the average tumor weight to about 0.5 g in 14 days. Interestingly, TNFAIP3 KO DCIS-iFGFR1 cells only grew very small tumors either with or without AP20187 treatment. Their average tumor weight was less than 0.08 g on day 14 after the same number of cells

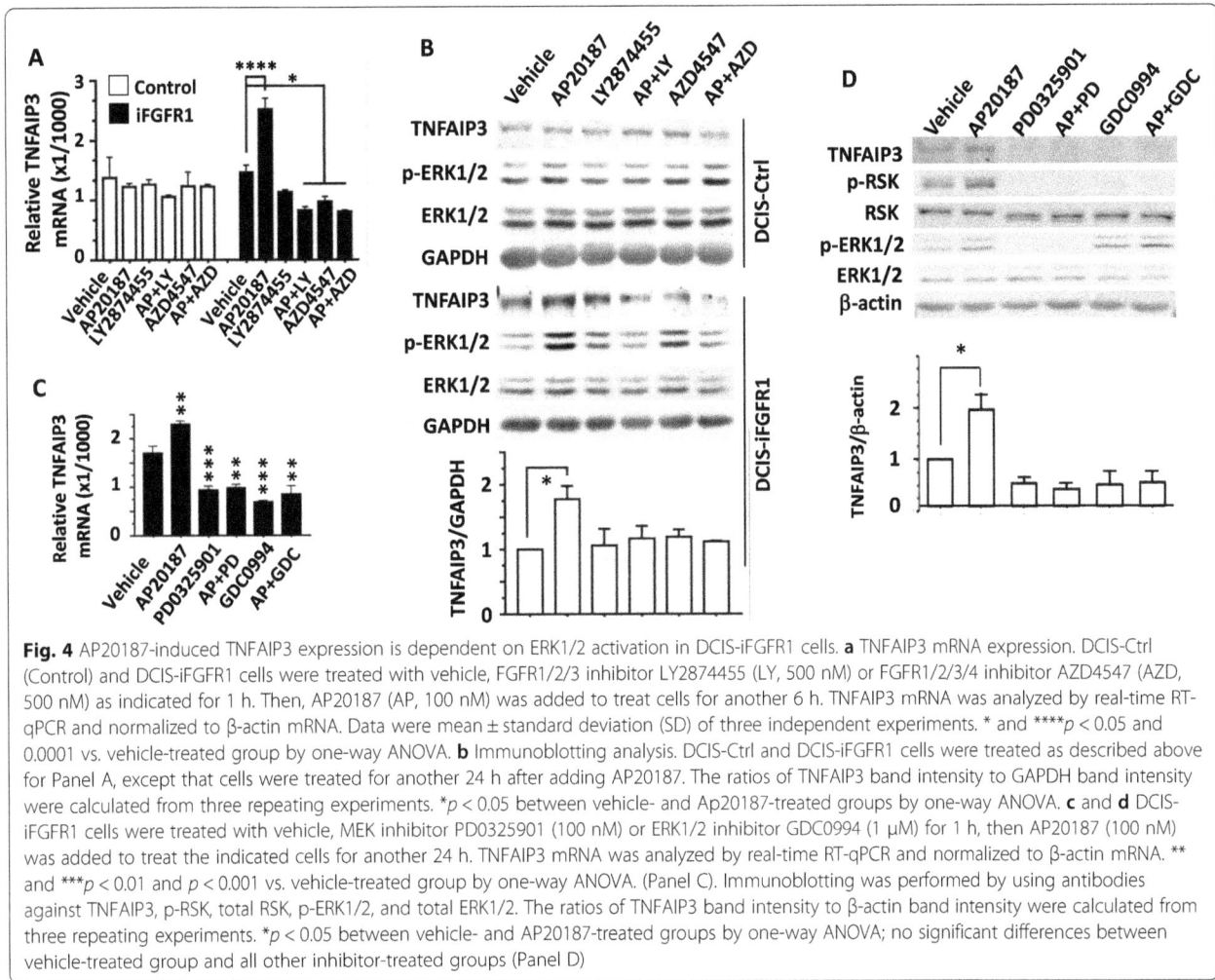

Fig. 4 AP20187-induced TNFAIP3 expression is dependent on ERK1/2 activation in DCIS-iFGFR1 cells. **a** TNFAIP3 mRNA expression. DCIS-Ctrl (Control) and DCIS-iFGFR1 cells were treated with vehicle, FGFR1/2/3 inhibitor LY2874455 (LY, 500 nM) or FGFR1/2/3/4 inhibitor AZD4547 (AZD, 500 nM) as indicated for 1 h. Then, AP20187 (AP, 100 nM) was added to treat cells for another 6 h. TNFAIP3 mRNA was analyzed by real-time RT-qPCR and normalized to β-actin mRNA. Data were mean ± standard deviation (SD) of three independent experiments. * and ****$p < 0.05$ and 0.0001 vs. vehicle-treated group by one-way ANOVA. **b** Immunoblotting analysis. DCIS-Ctrl and DCIS-iFGFR1 cells were treated as described above for Panel A, except that cells were treated for another 24 h after adding AP20187. The ratios of TNFAIP3 band intensity to GAPDH band intensity were calculated from three repeating experiments. *$p < 0.05$ between vehicle- and Ap20187-treated groups by one-way ANOVA. **c** and **d** DCIS-iFGFR1 cells were treated with vehicle, MEK inhibitor PD0325901 (100 nM) or ERK1/2 inhibitor GDC0994 (1 μM) for 1 h, then AP20187 (100 nM) was added to treat the indicated cells for another 24 h. TNFAIP3 mRNA was analyzed by real-time RT-qPCR and normalized to β-actin mRNA. ** and ***$p < 0.01$ and $p < 0.001$ vs. vehicle-treated group by one-way ANOVA. (Panel C). Immunoblotting was performed by using antibodies against TNFAIP3, p-RSK, total RSK, p-ERK1/2, and total ERK1/2. The ratios of TNFAIP3 band intensity to β-actin band intensity were calculated from three repeating experiments. *$p < 0.05$ between vehicle- and AP20187-treated groups by one-way ANOVA; no significant differences between vehicle-treated group and all other inhibitor-treated groups (Panel D)

was injected into the mammary fat pads of nude mice (Fig. 7a–c). In both vehicle-treated DCIS-iFGFR1 and TNFAIP3 KO xenograft tumors, p-ERK1/2 signals were only detected in a subset of tumor cells and these immunostaining signals were relatively weak. In contrast, in both AP20187-treated DCIS-iFGFR1 and TNFAIP3 xenograft tumors, p-ERK1/2 immunostaining signals were detected in almost all of the tumor cells at stronger levels (Fig. 7d). In both types of vehicle-treated tumors, the tumor cells grew in clusters and each cell cluster was surrounded by multiple layers of stromal cells, which simulates the DCIS lesion morphologies. However, in AP20187-treated DCIS-iFGFR1 tumors, the tumor cell morphology exhibited much higher degrees of heterogeneity and invasiveness. Some tumor cells had invaded the skeletal muscle tissue. In the AP20187-treated TNFAIP3 KO tumors, most tumor areas displayed similar morphologies observed in the vehicle-treated TNFAIP3 KO tumors. In certain areas, highly differentiated DCIS-like structures were also observed (Fig. 7e). These results demonstrate that TNFAIP3 is not required

for iFGFR1-mediated ERK1/2 activation, but it is essential for iFGFR1-induced DCIS-iFGFR1 tumor growth and progression in vivo.

Discussion

FGFR1 signaling is known to activate ERK1/2 MAPKs to regulate cell growth, differentiation and transformation [54]. Although FGFR1 signaling pathways have been well studied, some key questions remain unaddressed. For example, it is not easy to discern the functional specificity of ERK1 from ERK2 in mediating the FGFR1 signaling to the downstream signaling components because of their significant functional redundancy. In addition, the FGFR1 signaling-regulated genes important for cell proliferation and carcinogenesis are still largely undefined. In this study, we established DCIS-iFGFR1 cell lines in which iFGFR1 activation is induced by AP20187 treatment. We demonstrated that activated iFGFR1 activates ERK1/2, induces partial EMT, and increases cell proliferation, which is consistent with the results reported previously [25, 35, 36].

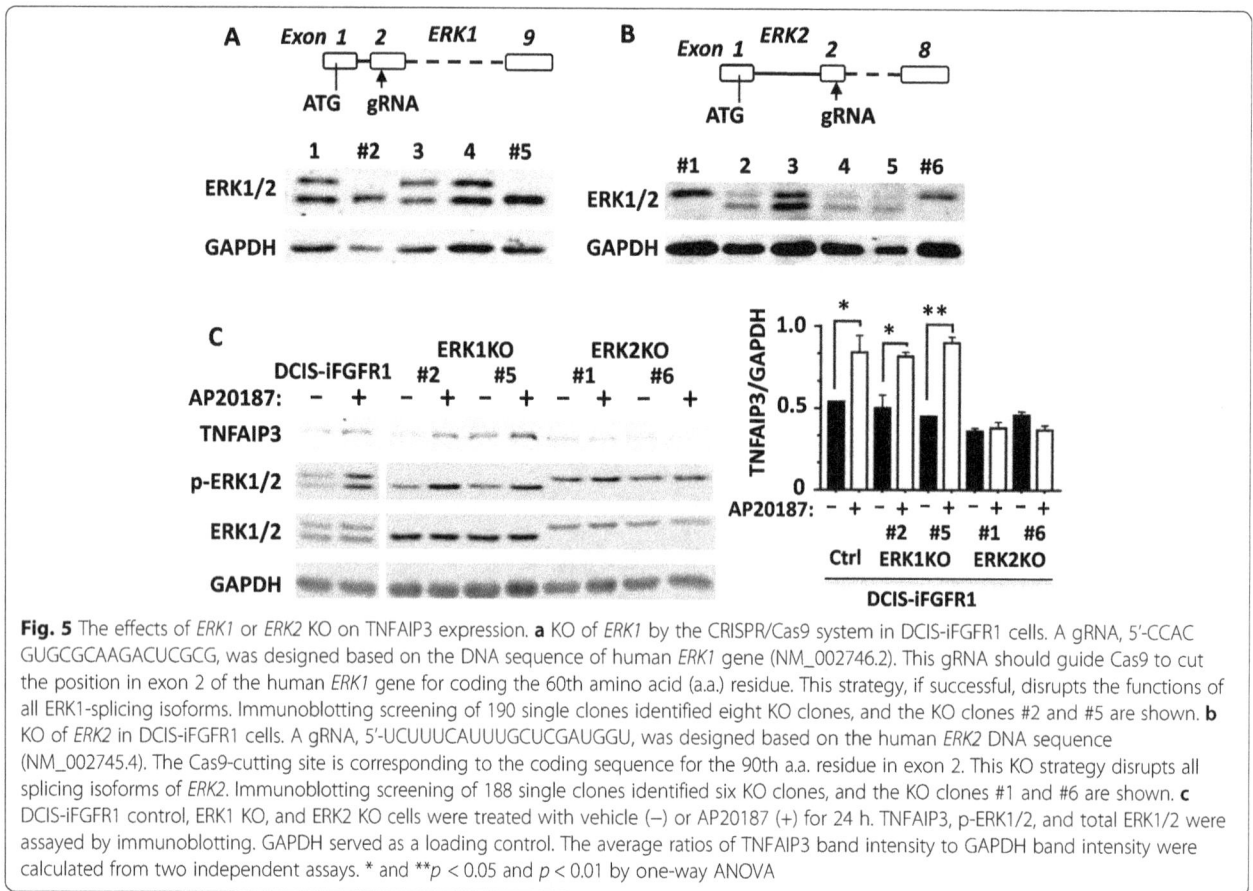

Fig. 5 The effects of *ERK1* or *ERK2* KO on TNFAIP3 expression. **a** KO of *ERK1* by the CRISPR/Cas9 system in DCIS-iFGFR1 cells. A gRNA, 5'-CCAC GUGCGCAAGACUCGCG, was designed based on the DNA sequence of human *ERK1* gene (NM_002746.2). This gRNA should guide Cas9 to cut the position in exon 2 of the human *ERK1* gene for coding the 60th amino acid (a.a.) residue. This strategy, if successful, disrupts the functions of all ERK1-splicing isoforms. Immunoblotting screening of 190 single clones identified eight KO clones, and the KO clones #2 and #5 are shown. **b** KO of *ERK2* in DCIS-iFGFR1 cells. A gRNA, 5'-UCUUUCAUUUGCUCGAUGGU, was designed based on the human *ERK2* DNA sequence (NM_002745.4). The Cas9-cutting site is corresponding to the coding sequence for the 90th a.a. residue in exon 2. This KO strategy disrupts all splicing isoforms of *ERK2*. Immunoblotting screening of 188 single clones identified six KO clones, and the KO clones #1 and #6 are shown. **c** DCIS-iFGFR1 control, ERK1 KO, and ERK2 KO cells were treated with vehicle (−) or AP20187 (+) for 24 h. TNFAIP3, p-ERK1/2, and total ERK1/2 were assayed by immunoblotting. GAPDH served as a loading control. The average ratios of TNFAIP3 band intensity to GAPDH band intensity were calculated from two independent assays. * and **$p < 0.05$ and $p < 0.01$ by one-way ANOVA

Using this cell system, we characterized the genes regulated by FGFR1 signaling. We found that activation of iFGFR1 changed the expression levels of 946 genes. These genes exhibited several expression patterns: the expression levels of 80 genes were consecutively increased while the expression levels of 68 genes were consecutively decreased during both short-time (3 h) and long-time (16 h) activation of the iFGFR1 signaling; a subset of genes were upregulated at the 3-h time point but downregulated at the 16-h time point; and another subset of these genes were downregulated at the 3-h time point but upregulated at the 16-h time point. These complex gene regulatory patterns by the activated iFGFR1 signaling suggest that the FGFR1 signaling pathway can directly activate and suppress gene expression, as well as, potentially regulate the expression of many other genes through its directly regulated gene products. Understanding this FGFR1-regulated gene network will help to identify downstream targets of the FGFR1 signaling pathway.

In agreement with the role of FGFR1 in promoting cell proliferation and carcinogenesis, a number of iFGFR1-upregulated genes are cancer-driving genes such as ETS1, PIM1, NRG1, MMP1, and FOXQ1, while some iFGFR1-downregulated genes are tumor suppressors

such as NR4A1 and GDF15. However, it is currently unclear why the activated FGFR1 signaling also downregulates some growth-promoting genes such as EGR2/3, MYB, and PIK3R1/3 (Fig. 2c). Bioinformatic analysis of the FGFR1 signaling-regulated genes revealed that these genes are involved in many biological processes, molecular functions, and signaling pathways, including cell proliferation, adhesion and migration, gene regulation, basal cell carcinogenesis, as well as general cancer-promoting pathways such as MAPK, Hippo, PI3K-AKT, Ras, p53, and NF-κB pathways (Fig. 3). These results suggest that the downstream molecular mechanisms responsible for mediating FGFR1 function are through coordinating multiple signaling pathways that govern cell proliferation, behavior and differentiation.

Among the iFGFR1-upregulated genes, we further studied the role of TNFAIP3 in FGFR1 signaling-promoted DCIS.COM cell growth. We demonstrated that activation of iFGFR1 robustly upregulates TNFAIP3 mRNA and protein in DCIS-iFGFR1 cells and this upregulation can be completely blocked by either FGFR inhibitors or ERK1/2 inhibitors. Furthermore, KO of ERK2 completely abolished the FGFR1 signaling-induced TNFAIP3 upregulation, while KO of ERK1 showed little effect on

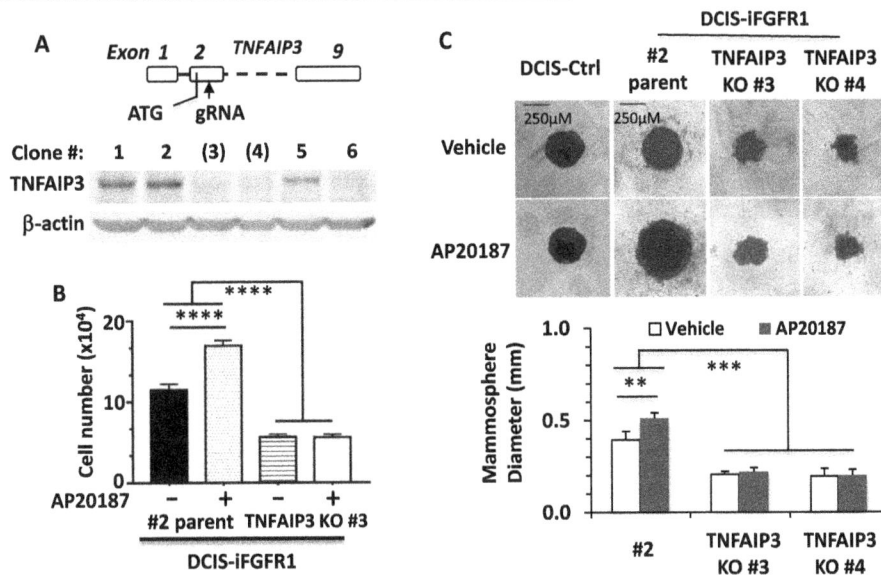

Fig. 6 TNFAIP3 is required for FGFR1 activation-induced cell growth. **a** Generation of TNFAIP3 KO cell lines by the CRISPR/Cas9 system from DCIS-iFGFR1 cells. The gRNA 5′-UGCACCGAUACACACUGG was designed based on the human TNFAIP3 DNA sequence (NM_001270508.1) to guide Cas9 to cut the coding sequence for the a.a. residue 48 in exon 2. This targeting event disrupts the function of all three splicing variants of TNFAIP3. Immunoblotting screening of 100 individual clones identified six KO clones, and three KO clones (#3, #4 and #6) are shown. **b** KO of TNFAIP3 inhibited cell proliferation. DCIS-iFGFR1 #2 parent cells and TNFAIP3 KO #3 cells derived from the DCIS-iFGFR1 #2 parent cells were cultured in 6-well plate with 50,000 cells/well and treated with vehicle (DMSO) (−) or AP20187 (+) for 3 days before cells in each well were counted. Data are presented as average ± SD of six repeat assays in two independent experiments. ****$p < 0.0001$ by one-way ANOVA. **c** KO of TNFAIP3 inhibited mammosphere growth. The indicated cell lines were cultured in the U-bottom ultra-low attachment 96-well plates and treated with vehicle or AP20187 for 7 days. The DCIS-iFGFR1-#2 cell line is the parent cell line from which the TNFAIP3 KO #3 and #4 cell lines are derived. Representative images of the spheres formed were shown. The mean of the sphere diameters for each group was calculated from eight replicates. The experiment was repeated three times. ** and ***$p < 0.01$ and $p < 0.001$ by one-way ANOVA

TNFAIP3 expression. These findings identified a gene expression-regulatory axis of FGFR1-ERK2-TNFAIP3. Our data also showed that in both 2D culture and 3D mammosphere growth assays, activation of the iFGFR1 signaling increased the growth of DCIS-iFGFR1 cells, while KO of TNFAIP3 in these cells completely diminished the iFGFR1 signaling-induced cell growth. Consistent results were also observed in the xenograft tumor growth assay in mice, where activation of the iFGFR1 signaling markedly enhanced tumor growth and KO of TNFAIP3 inhibited tumor growth derived from DCIS-iFGFR1 cells. Interestingly, KO of TNFAIP3 not only abolished cell, mammosphere, and tumor growth induced by AP29187-activated iFGFR1, but also reduced cell, mammoshpere, and tumor growth in the absence of AP29187 treatment when compared with the tumors derived from DCIS-iFGFR1 cells with wild-type *TNFAIP3*. This may be explained by the role of TNFAIP3 in mediating the cell growth function of the endogenous FGFRs and/or the additional functions of TNFAIP3 involved in other cell growth-promoting pathways. In summary, our results indicate that TNFAIP3 is essential for FGFR1 signaling-induced breast cancer cell growth in culture and tumor growth in vivo.

Histopathological examination of the xenograft tumors revealed that activation of the iFGFR1 signaling promoted

DCIS.COM tumor progression to invasive cancer. Interestingly, TNFAIP3 KO DCIS.COM xenograft tumors were insensitive to iFGFR1 activation induced by AP20187. These KO tumors exhibited mostly DCIS morphology. These results suggest that FGFR1 signaling can strongly promote DCIS progression to invasive cancer and TNFAIP3 is an essential contributing factor in this process.

The active mutants of HRAS, KRAS, and NRAS were found in a subset of breast cancers [55]. Although active Ras mutations and FGFR1 amplification and overexpression barely occur in the same breast cancer cells, FGFs are always present in the tumor microenvironment and FGFRs are expressed in breast epithelial and cancer cells. It is unknown whether FGFR1 activation can further activate downstream signaling in breast epithelial and tumor cells with an active Ras mutation to promote these cell growth and progression to a more aggressive cancer cell phenotype. MCF10AT cells are derived from mutant H-Ras transfected MCF10A normal cells and the initial transplantation of MCF10AT cells only develop differentiated ducts in mice. DCIS.COM cells are derived from passaged MCF10AT xenograft growth and DCIS.COM cells mainly form non-invasive DCIS tumors [5–8]. These findings suggest that expression of mutant H-Ras in these cells is insufficient to promote invasive

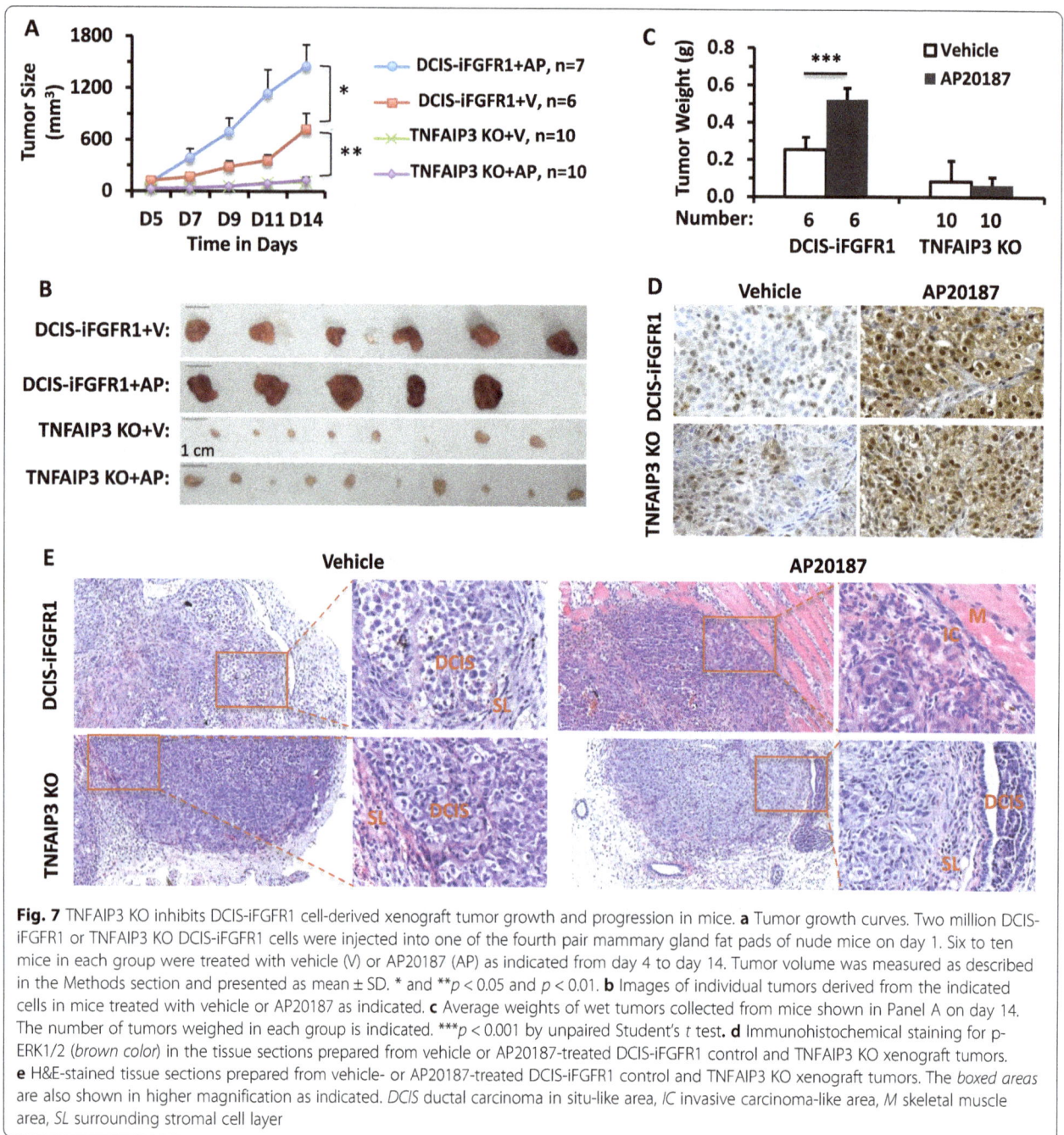

Fig. 7 TNFAIP3 KO inhibits DCIS-iFGFR1 cell-derived xenograft tumor growth and progression in mice. **a** Tumor growth curves. Two million DCIS-iFGFR1 or TNFAIP3 KO DCIS-iFGFR1 cells were injected into one of the fourth pair mammary gland fat pads of nude mice on day 1. Six to ten mice in each group were treated with vehicle (V) or AP20187 (AP) as indicated from day 4 to day 14. Tumor volume was measured as described in the Methods section and presented as mean ± SD. * and **$p < 0.05$ and $p < 0.01$. **b** Images of individual tumors derived from the indicated cells in mice treated with vehicle or AP20187 as indicated. **c** Average weights of wet tumors collected from mice shown in Panel A on day 14. The number of tumors weighed in each group is indicated. ***$p < 0.001$ by unpaired Student's t test. **d** Immunohistochemical staining for p-ERK1/2 (*brown color*) in the tissue sections prepared from vehicle or AP20187-treated DCIS-iFGFR1 control and TNFAIP3 KO xenograft tumors. **e** H&E-stained tissue sections prepared from vehicle- or AP20187-treated DCIS-iFGFR1 control and TNFAIP3 KO xenograft tumors. The *boxed areas* are also shown in higher magnification as indicated. *DCIS* ductal carcinoma in situ-like area, *IC* invasive carcinoma-like area, *M* skeletal muscle area, *SL* surrounding stromal cell layer

cancer cells. In our study, iFGFR1 activation further increases ERK1/2 activity in DCIS.COM cells, accelerates their proliferation in culture and promotes their tumor growth and progression to invasive cancer in vivo. Our results indicate that FGFR1 activation has an additive role to mutant H-Ras in promoting DCIS cell growth and progression. It has been reported that wild-type H- and N-Ras promote mutant K-ras-driven tumorigenesis [56]. It is possible that activation of FGFR1 activates the

endogenous Ras proteins in DCIS.COM cells, which cooperate with mutant H-Ras to promote breast cancer cell proliferation, and progression. Alternatively, FGFR1 activation may also work with mutant Ras to promote breast cancer cell proliferation and progression via its other signaling pathways that do not use Ras and ERK1/2. Importantly, KO of TNFAIP3 inhibited tumor growth promoted by both mutant H-Ras and FGFR1 activation, suggesting that TNFAIP3 may serve as a potential target for inhibiting ER- breast cancer with active mutant Ras and/or active FGFR1 signaling.

Conclusions

Activation of FGFR1 signaling in DCIS.COM cells induces ERK1/2 activity, EMT, and cell proliferation in culture and promotes cell-derived xenograft tumor growth and progression to invasive cancer in mice. Activation of FGFR1 signaling upregulates and downregulates many genes. FGFR1 signaling upregulates TNFAIP3 expression via activating ERK2. TNFAIP3 expression is required for FGFR1 signaling-promoted DCIS.COM cell proliferation, mammosphere growth, tumor growth and progression.

Abbreviations

DCIS: Ductal carcinoma in situ; EMT: Epithelial-to-mesenchymal transition; ERK1/2: Extracellular-signal regulated kinases 1 and 2; ER: Estrogen receptor; FGF: Fibroblast growth factor; FGFR: Fibroblast growth factor receptor; HER2: Human epidermal growth factor receptor 2; KO: Knockout

Acknowledgments

We thank Lan Liao, Suoling Zhou, Junjiang Fu, Xianyu Zhu, Ting Wu, Chen Xu, and Xuehan Wang for experimental assistance. We thank Lisa Kay Mullany and Jarrod Don Martinez for editorial assistance.

Funding

This work is supported by Chinese Natural Science Foundation grant 81572619, Department of Education of Sichuan Province (China) grants No. 18ZD0000 and No. 15TD0020, joint program grants of the Science and Technology Department of Sichuan Province (China), Luzhou City and Luzhou Medical Coll
ege No. 14ZC0022 and No. 14ZC0024, Funding of Department of Science and Technology of Sichuan Province (China) No. 2014HH0010, joint program grants of the Luzhou City and Sichuan Medical University No. 2015LZCYD-S02 and No. 2013LZLY-J29. This work is also partially supported by NIH grant CA112403, and CPRIT grants RP120732-P5 and RP150197 to J. Xu.

Authors' contributions

MY and XY performed most experiments, analyzed data, and helped draft the manuscript. XL supervised MY, BL, and YL to perform experiments and helped draft the manuscript. BL generated ERK1/2 KO cell lines. WY and DL helped establish DCIS-iFGFR1 cells and processed RNA-Seq analysis. YL analyzed mRNA expression by real-time RT-PCR and assisted xenograft tumor assay in mice. ZG performed histopathological examination of the xenograft tumors. JX and TH designed and supervised the study and wrote the manuscript. All authors read and approved the final manuscript.

Competing interests

The authors declare that they have no competing interests.

References

1. Torre LA, Bray F, Siegel RL, Ferlay J, Lortet-Tieulent J, Jemal A. Global cancer statistics, 2012. CA Cancer J Clin. 2015;65(2):87–108.
2. Donegan WL, Spratt JS. Cancer of the breast, vol. 5. Philadelphia: Saunders; 2002.
3. Ernster VL, Ballard-Barbash R, Barlow WE, Zheng Y, Weaver DL, Cutter G, Yankaskas BC, Rosenberg R, Carney PA, Kerlikowske K, et al. Detection of ductal carcinoma in situ in women undergoing screening mammography. J Natl Cancer Inst. 2002;94(20):1546–54.
4. Erbas B, Provenzano E, Armes J, Gertig D. The natural history of ductal carcinoma in situ of the breast: a review. Breast Cancer Res Treat. 2006;97(2): 135–44.
5. Santner SJ, Dawson PJ, Tait L, Soule HD, Eliason J, Mohamed AN, Wolman SR, Heppner GH, Miller FR. Malignant MCF10CA1 cell lines derived from premalignant human breast epithelial MCF10AT cells. Breast Cancer Res Treat. 2001;65(2):101–10.
6. Dawson PJ, Wolman SR, Tait L, Heppner GH, Miller FR. MCF10AT: a model for the evolution of cancer from proliferative breast disease. Am J Pathol. 1996;148(1):313–9.
7. Miller FR, Soule HD, Tait L, Pauley RJ, Wolman SR, Dawson PJ, Heppner GH. Xenograft model of progressive human proliferative breast disease. J Natl Cancer Inst. 1993;85(21):1725–32.
8. Miller FR, Santner SJ, Tait L, Dawson PJ. MCF10DCIS.com xenograft model of human comedo ductal carcinoma in situ. J Natl Cancer Inst. 2000;92(14):1185–6.
9. Behbod F, Kittrell FS, LaMarca H, Edwards D, Kerbawy S, Heestand JC, Young E, Mukhopadhyay P, Yeh HW, Allred DC, et al. An intraductal human-in-mouse transplantation model mimics the subtypes of ductal carcinoma in situ. Breast Cancer Res. 2009;11(5):R66.
10. Babina IS, Turner NC. Advances and challenges in targeting FGFR signalling in cancer. Nat Rev Cancer. 2017;17(5):318–32.
11. Helsten T, Elkin S, Arthur E, Tomson BN, Carter J, Kurzrock R. The FGFR landscape in Cancer: analysis of 4,853 tumors by next-generation sequencing. Clin Cancer Res. 2016;22(1):259–67.
12. Formisano L, Stauffer KM, Young CD, Bhola NE, Guerrero-Zotano AL, Jansen VM, Estrada MM, Hutchinson KE, Giltnane JM, Schwarz LJ, et al. Association of FGFR1 with ERalpha maintains ligand-independent ER transcription and mediates resistance to estrogen deprivation in ER(+) breast Cancer. Clin Cancer Res. 2017;23(20):6138–50.
13. Aguilar H, Sole X, Bonifaci N, Serra-Musach J, Islam A, Lopez-Bigas N, Mendez-Pertuz M, Beijersbergen RL, Lazaro C, Urruticoechea A, et al. Biological reprogramming in acquired resistance to endocrine therapy of breast cancer. Oncogene. 2010;29(45):6071–83.
14. Brown WS, Akhand SS, Wendt MK. FGFR signaling maintains a drug persistent cell population following epithelial-mesenchymal transition. Oncotarget. 2016;7(50):83424–36.
15. Itoh N, Ornitz DM. Fibroblast growth factors: from molecular evolution to roles in development, metabolism and disease. J Biochem. 2011; 149(2):121–30.
16. Goetz R, Mohammadi M. Exploring mechanisms of FGF signalling through the lens of structural biology. Nat Rev Mol Cell Biol. 2013;14(3):166–80.
17. Li X, Wang C, Xiao J, McKeehan WL, Wang F. Fibroblast growth factors, old kids on the new block. Semin Cell Dev Biol. 2016;53:155–67.
18. Kan M, Wang F, Xu J, Crabb JW, Hou J, McKeehan WL. An essential heparin-binding domain in the fibroblast growth factor receptor kinase. Science. 1993;259(5103):1918–21.
19. Ornitz DM, Itoh N. The fibroblast growth factor signaling pathway. Wiley Interdiscip Rev Dev Biol. 2015;4(3):215–66.
20. Brewer JR, Mazot P, Soriano P. Genetic insights into the mechanisms of Fgf signaling. Genes Dev. 2016;30(7):751–71.
21. Wieder R, Fenig E, Wang H, Wang Q, Paglin S, Menzel T, Gabrilove J, Fuks Z, Yahalom J. Overexpression of basic fibroblast growth factor in MCF-7 human breast cancer cells: lack of correlation between inhibition of cell growth and MAP kinase activation. J Cell Physiol. 1998;177(3):411–25.
22. Tarkkonen KM, Nilsson EM, Kahkonen TE, Dey JH, Heikkila JE, Tuomela JM, Liu Q, Hynes NE, Harkonen PL. Differential roles of fibroblast growth factor receptors (FGFR) 1, 2 and 3 in the regulation of S115 breast cancer cell growth. PLoS One. 2012;7(11):e49970.
23. Xian W, Pappas L, Pandya D, Selfors LM, Derksen PW, de Bruin M, Gray NS, Jonkers J, Rosen JM, Brugge JS. Fibroblast growth factor receptor 1-transformed mammary epithelial cells are dependent on RSK activity for growth and survival. Cancer Res. 2009;69(6):2244–51.
24. Pond AC, Herschkowitz JI, Schwertfeger KL, Welm B, Zhang Y, York B, Cardiff RD, Hilsenbeck S, Perou CM, Creighton CJ, et al. Fibroblast growth factor receptor signaling dramatically accelerates tumorigenesis and enhances oncoprotein translation in the mouse mammary tumor virus-Wnt-1 mouse model of breast cancer. Cancer Res. 2010;70(12):4868–79.

25. Acevedo VD, Gangula RD, Freeman KW, Li R, Zhang Y, Wang F, Ayala GE, Peterson LE, Ittmann M, Spencer DM. Inducible FGFR-1 activation leads to irreversible prostate adenocarcinoma and an epithelial-to-mesenchymal transition. Cancer Cell. 2007;12(6):559–71.

26. Turner N, Pearson A, Sharpe R, Lambros M, Geyer F, Lopez-Garcia MA, Natrajan R, Marchio C, Iorns E, Mackay A, et al. FGFR1 amplification drives endocrine therapy resistance and is a therapeutic target in breast cancer. Cancer Res. 2010;70(5):2085–94.

27. Kim B, Wang S, Lee JM, Jeong Y, Ahn T, Son DS, Park HW, Yoo HS, Song YJ, Lee E, et al. Synthetic lethal screening reveals FGFR as one of the combinatorial targets to overcome resistance to met-targeted therapy. Oncogene. 2015;34(9):1083–93.

28. Anreddy N, Patel A, Sodani K, Kathawala RJ, Chen EP, Wurpel JN, Chen ZS. PD173074, a selective FGFR inhibitor, reverses MRP7 (ABCC10)-mediated MDR. Acta Pharm Sin B. 2014;4(3):202–7.

29. Terai H, Soejima K, Yasuda H, Nakayama S, Hamamoto J, Arai D, Ishioka K, Ohgino K, Ikemura S, Sato T, et al. Activation of the FGF2-FGFR1 autocrine pathway: a novel mechanism of acquired resistance to gefitinib in NSCLC. Mol Cancer Res. 2013;11(7):759–67.

30. Gyanchandani R, Ortega Alves MV, Myers JN, Kim S. A proangiogenic signature is revealed in FGF-mediated bevacizumab-resistant head and neck squamous cell carcinoma. Mol Cancer Res. 2013;11(12):1585–96.

31. Lau WM, Teng E, Huang KK, Tan JW, Das K, Zang Z, Chia T, Teh M, Kono K, Yong WP, et al. Acquired resistance to FGFR inhibitor in diffuse-type gastric Cancer through an AKT-independent PKC-mediated phosphorylation of GSK3beta. Mol Cancer Ther. 2018;17(1):232–42.

32. Datta J, Damodaran S, Parks H, Ocrainiciuc C, Miya J, Yu L, Gardner EP, Samorodnitsky E, Wing MR, Bhatt D, et al. Akt activation mediates acquired resistance to fibroblast growth factor receptor inhibitor BGJ398. Mol Cancer Ther. 2017;16(4):614–24.

33. Cowell JK, Qin H, Hu T, Wu Q, Bhole A, Ren M. Mutation in the FGFR1 tyrosine kinase domain or inactivation of PTEN is associated with acquired resistance to FGFR inhibitors in FGFR1-driven leukemia/lymphomas. Int J Cancer. 2017;141(9):1822–9.

34. Malchers F, Ercanoglu M, Schutte D, Castiglione R, Tischler V, Michels S, Dahmen I, Bragelmann J, Menon R, Heuckmann JM, et al. Mechanisms of primary drug resistance in FGFR1-amplified lung Cancer. Clin Cancer Res. 2017;23(18):5527–36.

35. Freeman KW, Welm BE, Gangula RD, Rosen JM, Ittmann M, Greenberg NM, Spencer DM. Inducible prostate intraepithelial neoplasia with reversible hyperplasia in conditional FGFR1-expressing mice. Cancer Res. 2003;63(23):8256–63.

36. Freeman KW, Gangula RD, Welm BE, Ozen M, Foster BA, Rosen JM, Ittmann M, Greenberg NM, Spencer DM. Conditional activation of fibroblast growth factor receptor (FGFR) 1, but not FGFR2, in prostate cancer cells leads to increased osteopontin induction, extracellular signal-regulated kinase activation, and in vivo proliferation. Cancer Res. 2003;63(19):6237–43.

37. Ma A, Malynn BA. A20: linking a complex regulator of ubiquitylation to immunity and human disease. Nat Rev Immunol. 2012;12(11):774–85.

38. Jia Q, Sun H, Xiao F, Sai Y, Li Q, Zhang X, Yang S, Wang H, Yang Y, Wu CT, et al. miR-17-92 promotes leukemogenesis in chronic myeloid leukemia via targeting A20 and activation of NF-kappaB signaling. Biochem Biophys Res Commun. 2017;487(4):868–74.

39. Huang T, Yin L, Wu J, Gu JJ, Ding K, Zhang N, Du MY, Qian LX, Lu ZW, He X. TNFAIP3 inhibits migration and invasion in nasopharyngeal carcinoma by suppressing epithelial mesenchymal transition. Neoplasma. 2017;64(3):389–94.

40. Chen H, Hu L, Luo Z, Zhang J, Zhang C, Qiu B, Dong L, Tan Y, Ding J, Tang S, et al. A20 suppresses hepatocellular carcinoma proliferation and metastasis through inhibition of Twist1 expression. Mol Cancer. 2015;14:186.

41. Vendrell JA, Ghayad S, Ben-Larbi S, Dumontet C, Mechti N, Cohen PA. A20/TNFAIP3, a new estrogen-regulated gene that confers tamoxifen resistance in breast cancer cells. Oncogene. 2007;26(32):4656–67.

42. Lee JH, Jung SM, Yang KM, Bae E, Ahn SG, Park JS, Seo D, Kim M, Ha J, Lee J, et al. A20 promotes metastasis of aggressive basal-like breast cancers through multi-monoubiquitylation of Snail1. Nat Cell Biol. 2017;19(10):1260–73.

43. Saitoh Y, Hamano A, Mochida K, Kakeya A, Uno M, Tsuruyama E, Ichikawa H, Tokunaga F, Utsunomiya A, Watanabe T, et al. A20 targets caspase-8 and FADD to protect HTLV-I-infected cells. Leukemia. 2016;30(3):716–27.

44. Wang Y, Wan M, Zhou Q, Wang H, Wang Z, Zhong X, Zhang L, Tai S, Cui Y. The prognostic role of SOCS3 and A20 in human cholangiocarcinoma. PLoS One. 2015;10(10):e0141165.

45. Hadisaputri YE, Miyazaki T, Yokobori T, Sohda M, Sakai M, Ozawa D, Hara K, Honjo H, Kumakura Y, Kuwano H. TNFAIP3 overexpression is an independent factor for poor survival in esophageal squamous cell carcinoma. Int J Oncol. 2017;50(3):1002–10.

46. Huang da W, Sherman BT, Lempicki RA. Systematic and integrative analysis of large gene lists using DAVID bioinformatics resources. Nat Protoc. 2009;4(1):44–57.

47. Huang da W, Sherman BT, Lempicki RA. Bioinformatics enrichment tools: paths toward the comprehensive functional analysis of large gene lists. Nucleic Acids Res. 2009;37(1):1–13.

48. Ran FA, Hsu PD, Wright J, Agarwala V, Scott DA, Zhang F. Genome engineering using the CRISPR-Cas9 system. Nat Protoc. 2013;8(11):2281–308.

49. Nakano T, Kanai Y, Amano Y, Yoshimoto T, Matsubara D, Shibano T, Tamura T, Oguni S, Katashiba S, Ito T, et al. Establishment of highly metastatic KRAS mutant lung cancer cell sublines in long-term three-dimensional low attachment cultures. PLoS One. 2017;12(8):e0181342.

50. Catrysse L, Vereecke L, Beyaert R, van Loo G. A20 in inflammation and autoimmunity. Trends Immunol. 2014;35(1):22–31.

51. Zhao G, Li WY, Chen D, Henry JR, Li HY, Chen Z, Zia-Ebrahimi M, Bloem L, Zhai Y, Huss K, et al. A novel, selective inhibitor of fibroblast growth factor receptors that shows a potent broad spectrum of antitumor activity in several tumor xenograft models. Mol Cancer Ther. 2011;10(11):2200–10.

52. Gavine PR, Mooney L, Kilgour E, Thomas AP, Al-Kadhimi K, Beck S, Rooney C, Coleman T, Baker D, Mellor MJ, et al. AZD4547: an orally bioavailable, potent, and selective inhibitor of the fibroblast growth factor receptor tyrosine kinase family. Cancer Res. 2012;72(8):2045–56.

53. Busca R, Pouyssegur J, Lenormand P. ERK1 and ERK2 map kinases: specific roles or functional redundancy? Front Cell Dev Biol. 2016;4:53.

54. Welm BE, Freeman KW, Chen M, Contreras A, Spencer DM, Rosen JM. Inducible dimerization of FGFR1: development of a mouse model to analyze progressive transformation of the mammary gland. J Cell Biol. 2002;157(4):703–14.

55. Prior IA, Lewis PD, Mattos C. A comprehensive survey of Ras mutations in cancer. Cancer Res. 2012;72(10):2457–67.

56. Grabocka E, Pylayeva-Gupta Y, Jones MJ, Lubkov V, Yemanaberhan E, Taylor L, Jeng HH, Bar-Sagi D. Wild-type H- and N-Ras promote mutant K-Ras-driven tumorigenesis by modulating the DNA damage response. Cancer Cell. 2014;25(2):243–56.

9

Integrin-Rac signalling for mammary epithelial stem cell self-renewal

Safiah Olabi, Ahmet Ucar, Keith Brennan and Charles H. Streuli[*] ⓘ

Abstract

Background: Stem cells are precursors for all mammary epithelia, including ductal and alveolar epithelia, and myoepithelial cells. In vivo mammary epithelia reside in a tissue context and interact with their milieu via receptors such as integrins. Extracellular matrix receptors coordinate important cellular signalling platforms, of which integrins are the central architects. We have previously shown that integrins are required for mammary epithelial development and function, including survival, cell cycle, and polarity, as well as for the expression of mammary-specific genes. In the present study we looked at the role of integrins in mammary epithelial stem cell self-renewal.

Methods: We used an in vitro stem cell assay with primary mouse mammary epithelial cells isolated from genetically altered mice. This involved a 3D organoid assay, providing an opportunity to distinguish the stem cell- or luminal progenitor-driven organoids as structures with solid or hollow appearances, respectively.

Results: We demonstrate that integrins are essential for the maintenance and self-renewal of mammary epithelial stem cells. Moreover integrins activate the Rac1 signalling pathway in stem cells, which leads to the stimulation of a Wnt pathway, resulting in expression of β-catenin target genes such as *Axin2* and *Lef1*.

Conclusions: Integrin/Rac signalling has a role in specifying the activation of a canonical Wnt pathway that is required for mammary epithelial stem cell self-renewal.

Keywords: Mammary epithelial cells, Stem cells, β1-integrin, Rac1, Wnt

Background

The mammary gland is a highly regenerative organ that continuously undergoes tissue remodelling in female mammals during their sexually active life [29]. During each oestrous cycle, cells proliferate and form alveolar buds at the tertiary side branches and then regress in an ordered fashion [27]. A further lobuloalveolar differentiation takes place in pregnancy, with the epithelia expanding dramatically to fill the whole fat pad with milk-secreting structures [12]. Upon weaning, involution is triggered to clear up all milk-secreting cells and return the gland to a non-pregnant state [4]. These extensive tissue-remodelling processes repeat with each oestrus cycle and pregnancy.

The presence of mammary epithelial stem cells (MaSCs) is the driving force behind this high regenerative capacity [44]. Their existence and potency has been demonstrated

by serial transplantation studies. Single-cell transplant experiments have identified MaSCs as β1-integrin^{hi}CD24$^+$ cells, although α6-integrin^{hi}CD24$^+$ can also be used to identify MaSCs [33, 36]. These observations suggest that MaSCs express high levels of specific integrins, all of which are cell-extracellular matrix (ECM) receptors.

Integrins are central for the behaviour of mammary epithelial cells (MECs) [30, 37]. However, their role in MaSCs has not been elucidated. MECs can assemble several integrin heterodimers, including two collagen receptors ($\alpha_1\beta_1$ and $\alpha_2\beta_1$), three laminin receptors ($\alpha_3\beta_1$, $\alpha_6\beta_1$ and $\alpha_6\beta_4$), and three receptors that bind to RGD-containing ECM proteins such as vitronectin and fibronectin ($\alpha_5\beta_1$, $\alpha_v\beta_1$ and $\alpha_v\beta_3$) [19, 20, 31]. Because bipotent cells express high levels of β1-integrin, their signalling may play an important role. Function-perturbing antibodies that block β1-integrin, but not those that block α6-integrin, dramatically reduce the number of terminal end buds during pubertal mammary gland development [18]. Genetic deletion of β1-integrin in basal mammary cells abolishes the

* Correspondence: cstreuli@manchester.ac.uk
Wellcome Centre for Cell-Matrix Research and Manchester Breast Centre, Faculty of Biology, Medicine and Health, University of Manchester, Manchester M13 9PT, UK

regenerative potential of the epithelium and impairs ductal and lobuloalveolar development at pubertal and pregnancy stages [40]. Although these observations suggest an important role of β1-integrin in bipotent cells, direct evidence is still missing.

To directly address the functional importance of β1-integrin signalling in bipotent cells, we examined their role using a 3D organoid assay for mammary stem cells [14]. Our findings reveal that the β1-integrin/Rac1 signalling axis regulates the maintenance and self-renewal of bipotent cells through Wnt signalling. In contrast, a Rac1-independent β1-integrin signalling pathway is involved in the maintenance of the luminal progenitor pool.

Methods

Primary cell culture

Mammary glands were extracted from 8- to 12-week-old wild-type female (Institute of Cancer Research (ICR)) mice or β1-integrin, Rac1, ILK conditional knockout mice, and enzymatically digested with collagenase/trypsin mix (195 ml of H_2O + 9.8 mg F-10 medium [Sigma-Aldrich, St. Louis, MO, USA], 120 mg of $NaHCO_3$ HEPES-Na [Sigma-Aldrich], 150 mg of trypsin [840-7250; Life Technologies, Carlsbad, CA, USA], 300 mg of collagenase A [Roche Life Sciences, Indianapolis, IN, USA], 5 ml of FBS [Lonza, Walkersville, MD, USA]) for 1 h at 37 °C. Cells were spun for 1 min at 300 rpm, and the pellet was re-digested with collagenase/trypsin mix for an additional 30 min while the supernatant was spun for 3 min at 800 rpm. The pellet was kept on ice and labelled pellet 1, and the supernatant was spun at 1500 rpm for 10 min. The pellet from this wash was saved on ice and labelled pellet A. After the second digestion was completed, cells were spun at 800 rpm for 3 min. The pellet obtained was labelled pellet 2. The supernatant was spun for 10 min at 1500 rpm. The supernatant from this wash was then discarded, and the pellet was labelled pellet B. Pellets A and B were combined and washed with Ham's F-12 medium (Lonza) by spinning at 800 rpm for 3 min. This pellet was labelled pellet 3, and the supernatant was discarded. Pellets 1, 2 and 3 were pooled and washed with 15 ml of Ham's F-12 by spinning at 800 rpm for 3 min. This washing step was repeated three times. This method enriches for organoids that contain epithelial cells, whereas the washing steps removed other types of cells such as fibroblasts and haematopoietic cells. To culture cells on 2D collagen, plastic plates were coated with collagen I extracted from rat tails at a density of 100 μg/cm^2 or laminin-rich reconstituted basement membrane coating, growth factor-reduced Matrigel (EHS) (BD Biosciences, San Jose, CA, USA) at 20 μl/cm^2, conditioned for 1 h at 37 °C with 2× Ham's F-12 media, 20% FBS, 1 mg/ml fetuin (Sigma-Aldrich), 200 U/ml penicillin, 200 μg/ml streptomycin, 100 μg/ml gentamicin, 0.5 μg/ml Fungizone,

10 μg/ml insulin, 2 μg/ml hydrocortisone, and 20 ng/ml epidermal growth factor (EGF) (Sigma-Aldrich). Cells were resuspended in equal volume in Ham's F-12 media, seeded at a 2.5×10^5 cells/cm^2 on collagen or at 5×10^5 cells/cm^2 on EHS plates, fed on alternate days with Ham's F-12 media supplemented with 10% FBS, 100 U/ml penicillin, 100 μg/ml streptomycin, 50 μg/ml gentamicin, 0.25 μg/ml Fungizone, 5 μg/ml insulin, 1 μg/ml hydrocortisone, and 10 ng/ml EGF. To induce gene deletion of β1-integrin genes in cells isolated from β1-integrin$^{fx/fx}$,Cre-ER^{Tm} mice, 4-hydroxytamoxifen (4-OHT) was added at a final concentration of 100 nM. When necessary, immunoblotting was done with antibodies to β-catenin (9582; Cell Signaling Technology, Danvers, MA, USA) and Lamin-B1 (ab16048; Abcam, Cambridge, UK).

Organoid formation assay

For organoid-forming assays, cells were grown at a clonal density of 2×10^3 cells/cm^2 in 24-well ultra-low attachment plates that had been coated with 1.2% poly(2-hydroxyethyl methacrylate) to prevent adhesion and growth of the primary MECs. The cells were grown in media containing EPiCult-B media (STEMCELL Technologies, Vancouver, BC, Canada) supplemented with 5% Matrigel, 5% FBS, 10 ng/ml EGF, 20 ng/ml basic fibroblast growth factor, 4 mg/ml heparin, and 10 μM Y-27632. Cells were left for 10 days to form organoids, which were then counted. For activating Wnt signalling in organoid cultures, recombinant mouse Wnt3A (R&D Systems, Minneapolis, MN, USA) or glycogen synthase kinase 3 (GSK3) inhibitor (GSK3i, CHIR99021; Sigma-Aldrich) was added to the organoid cultures on day 0 at concentrations of 100 ng/ml or 50 nM, respectively. For gene expression analysis, RNA was collected from cells on day 2, and the RNA expression was measured using qRT-PCR. Note that addition of Rock inhibitor (Y-27632) is important for the expansion of pluripotent stem cells because it helps maintain the stem cells in their undifferentiated state, and they survive longer in culture, and note also that the Rock inhibitor increases the efficiency of colony formation.

Cell sorting and analysis using flow cytometry

To stain cells using fluorescence-activated cell sorting antibodies for analysis or sorting, cells were first dissociated into single cells. To obtain single cells from organoids, cell pellets were incubated in 2 ml of Trypsin-Versene (Lonza) for 2 min at 37 °C, mechanically dissociated with rapid pipetting, then incubated with 1 μg/ml DNase (New England BioLabs, Ipswich, MA, USA) for 5 min at 37 °C. Cells were washed with complete media and spun at 1500 rpm for 5 min, then strained through a 0.45-μm cell strainer to obtain single cells. Cells were washed with 1× PBS and resuspended in 400 μl of sorting buffer (2.5% FBS in PBS). To stain cells, 3 μl of each directly labelled antibody was added per 10 million cells and incubated on ice for 1 h, washed with sorting buffer, resuspended in sorting buffer, and sorted using a BD FACSAria cell sorter (BD Biosciences). Antibodies used for sorting experiments were as follows: epithelial cell adhesion molecule (EpCAM)-allophycocyanin (APC) (175791; eBioscience, San Diego, CA, USA), CD24-APC (170242; eBioscience), β1-integrin-eFluor 450 (48-0291; eBioscience), and α6-integrin-eFluor 450 (48-0495; eBioscience).

Lentivirus production and infection of primary cells

pLVTHM plasmid was obtained from Addgene (12247; Addgene, Cambridge, MA, USA). The lentiviral envelope plasmid CMV-VSVg (PMD2G; Addgene) and packaging plasmid psPAX2 were kindly provided by the TronoLab (Lausanne, Switzerland). All oligonucleotides for sequencing, PCR, and mutagenesis were obtained from Sigma-Aldrich. 293T cells were transfected for 6 h at a confluence of 50–70% with 6 μg of PLVTHM control vector, 3 μg of psPAX2 and 4.5 μg of PMDG.2 plasmids using 1× polyethylenimine transfection reagent. Primary MECs were transduced with virus in six-well plates under low-attachment conditions in organoid-forming media containing 1 μg/ml polybrene; media were changed the next day, another infection was performed, media were changed and the cells were left for additional 48 h before being sorted for green fluorescent protein expression. Integrin-fx mice were used for most studies where the integrin was deleted. In some experiments (e.g., Fig. 3e, f), β1-integrin was depleted using short hairpin RNA (shRNA); this approach in mammary cells is successful in reducing the integrin to barely detectable levels, as shown previously [2, 28].

RNA extraction and qPCR

Primers were designed to anneal only to complementary DNA and not to genomic DNA, at the junction between two exons. qPCR was performed using a StepOnePlus qPCR instrument (Thermo Fisher Scientific, Waltham, MA, USA): uracil DNA-glycosylase was activated (50 °C, 2 min), followed by AmpliTaq DNA polymerase (Thermo Fisher Scientific) activation (95 °C, 2 min); PCR cycles were performed by 40 repeated cycles of DNA denaturation (95 °C, 15 s), followed by DNA extension (60 °C, 1 min).

Rac1 activation assay

Lysates from primary MECs were applied to a multi-well plate containing a Rac1-GTP binding protein (GLisa Rac1 activity assay, catalogue no. BK128; Cytoskeleton, Denver, CO, USA). Active Rac1 present in the lysates was captured in the wells and detected using an anti-Rac1 antibody coupled to a colorimetric assay. Finally, absorbance was read using a PowerWave 340 plate reader (BioTek, Winooski, VT, USA) at 490 nm.

Statistical analysis

Statistical analysis was done using Excel (Microsoft, Redmond, WA, USA) or Prism (GraphPad Software, La Jolla, CA, USA) data analysis software. Statistical significance was determined by Student's t test for paired samples when comparing two groups. One-way analysis of variance was used when comparing more than two groups. Differences between samples were significantly different at $p < 0.05$. For all graphs shown, error bars represent SEM. For two groups, the means have one to four asterisks centred over the error bar to indicate the relative level of the p value: * $p < 0.05$, ** $p < 0.01$, *** $p < 0.001$, and **** $p < 0.0001$.

Results

β1-integrins are required for the maintenance and self-renewal of mammary epithelial stem cells

The initial aim of these studies was to address the functional requirement of β1-integrin for bipotent cells and luminal progenitors. Primary MECs were isolated from adult double-transgenic mice (β1-integrin$^{flox/flox}$;Rosa-CreERT2) and cultured as single cells in organoid media at a density of 5×10^5/well in ultra-low-attachment six-well plates. They were treated with 4-OHT to induce Cre-recombinase activity, thereby deleting the β1-integrin gene. Loss of β1-integrin was confirmed at both messenger RNA (mRNA) and protein levels by qRT-PCR and immunofluorescence analysis (Fig. 1a, b).

Cells were then dissociated into single cells and cultured in organoid-forming media for 10 days, and the organoids that formed were counted. Deletion of β1-integrin abolished the formation of both solid and hollow organoids (Fig. 1c, d), suggesting that β1-integrin is functionally required for both bipotent cells and luminal progenitors.

β1-integrin-null MECs analysed by flow cytometry revealed that loss of β1-integrin led to reduced populations of bipotent cell-enriched basal (CD49f^{hi}, EpCAM$^+$) and luminal (CD49f^{lo}, EpCAM$^+$, CD49b^{hi}) progenitors, but not the differentiated luminal cells (Fig. 1e, f). Treatment of wild-type MECs with 4-OHT confirmed that the observed β1-integrin-null phenotypes were due to loss of β1-integrin function rather than to 4-OHT itself (Additional file 1: Figure S1). Note that in our studies, we looked at the luminal progenitors without segregating the ER– and ER+ populations; only those expressing CD49b were able to form organoids (Additional file 2: Figure S2) [34]. These results indicate that β1-integrin is functionally required for the maintenance and self-renewal of both bipotent cells and luminal progenitor cells.

β1-integrins influence mammary stem cells via Rac1

β1-integrin can regulate cellular processes through different downstream signalling pathways via integrin-binding

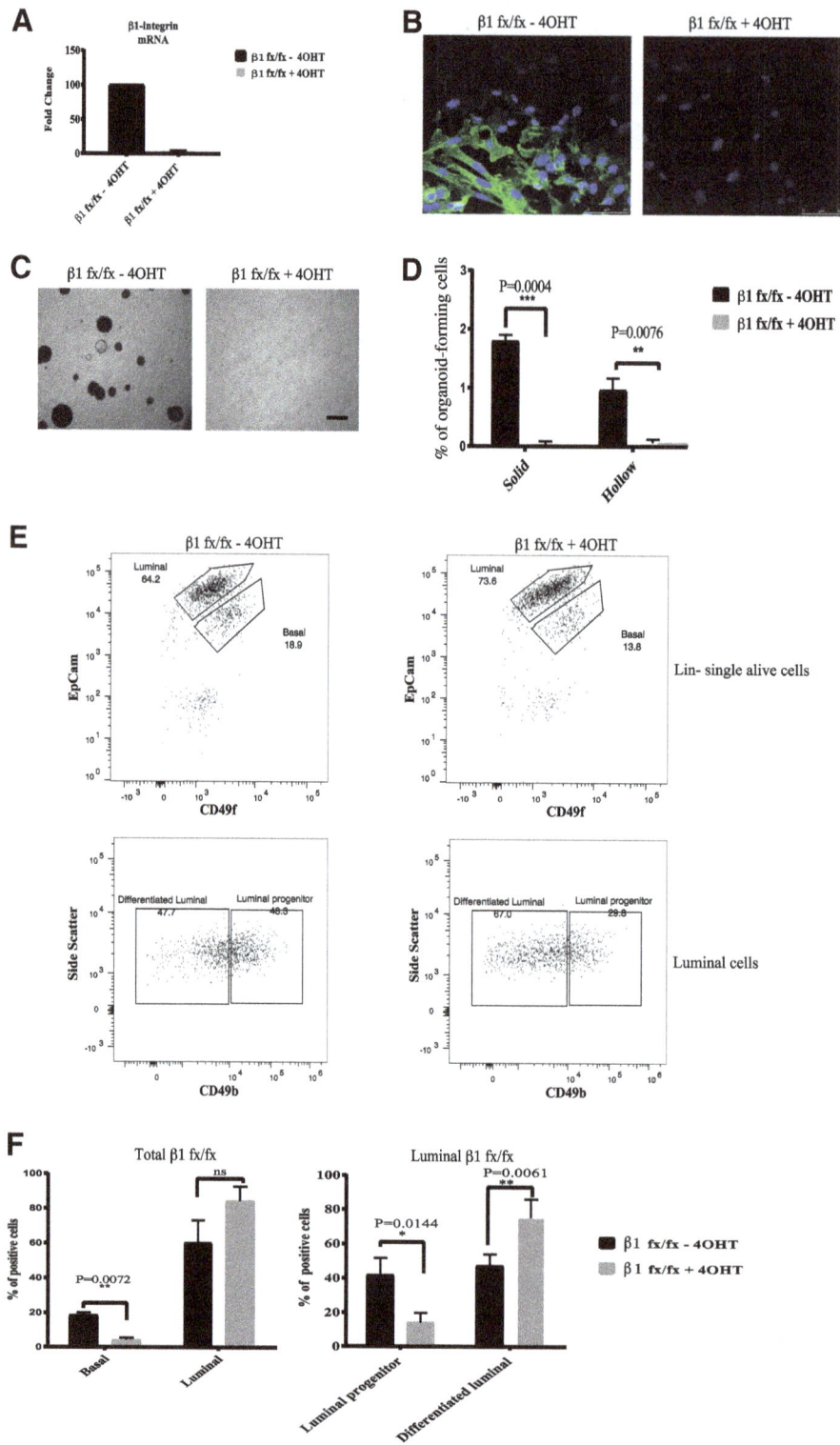

Fig. 1 (See legend on next page.)

proteins [16, 28, 32]. Loss of function of integrin-linked kinase (ILK), but not focal adhesion kinase (FAK), recapitulates, at least in part, the phenotype of β1-integrin-deficient MECs [46]. One of the major downstream effectors of β1-integrin is the small GTPase Rac1 [1, 16]. We therefore asked whether the bipotent cells and luminal progenitor phenotypes of β1-integrin-null MECs could be reiterated by either ILK or Rac1 gene deletion.

MECs were isolated from double-transgenic mice (ILK^flox/flox;Rosa-CreERT2 and Rac1^flox/flox;Rosa-CreERT2) and treated with 4-OHT to generate cells deficient in expressing ILK- or Rac1 mRNA (Fig. 2a, c) [2]. ILK gene deletion had no significant effect on the ability of MECs to form solid or hollow organoids (Fig. 2b). In contrast, Rac1 deletion decreased the formation of solid organoids, though it had no effect on hollow organoids (Fig. 2d). To confirm this result, we treated wild-type MECs with EHT1864, a specific and irreversible Rac1 inhibitor (Fig. 2e) [35]. MECs formed fewer solid organoids, but there was no effect on hollow organoids (Fig. 2f). Rac1, but not ILK, is therefore required for bipotent cell maintenance and self-renewal, though both Rac1 and ILK are dispensable for the maintenance of luminal progenitors that form hollow organoids.

To determine whether a constitutively active form of Rac1 (Rac1F28) could rescue the β1-integrin-null bipotent cell phenotype, we transduced wild-type MECs with a β1-integrin shRNA together with Rac1F28 [24]. As with β1-integrin gene deletion, β1-integrin knockdown abolished the formation of both solid and hollow organoids (Fig. 2g, h). Ectopic Rac1F28 expression in these cells rescued the formation of solid but not hollow organoids.

These results indicate that β1-integrin regulates bipotent cell maintenance and self-renewal in a Rac1-dependent manner. In contrast, the effect of β1-integrin on luminal progenitor cells is Rac1-independent.

Integrin-Rac signalling maintains mammary epithelial stem cells through a Wnt pathway

To identify downstream pathways that might link β1-integrins with bipotent cell maintenance, we examined the expression of genes previously associated with stem and progenitor identity [14]. RNA was extracted from MECs isolated from β1-integrin^flox/flox;Rosa-CreERT2 mice, which were treated with 4-OHT and cultured in organoid media for 2 days. The levels of transcription factors associated with bipotent cells such as Slug, MEF2, p63 or Twist were not altered in β1-integrin-deficient MECs (Fig. 3a). In contrast, those specifically known to mark luminal progenitors, Sox9, ELF5 and Sox10 genes, were downregulated (Fig. 3b).

Wnt is an important regulator of bipotent cell maintenance and self-renewal, so we analysed expression of known Wnt/β-catenin downstream targets. Both *Axin2* and *Lef1* transcripts were significantly downregulated in β1-integrin-deficient cells (Fig. 3c). Because β1-integrin signalling regulates bipotent cells through Rac1, we also analysed *Axin2* and *Lef1* in Rac1-deficient MECs and found that they were similarly downregulated in the absence of Rac1 (Fig. 3d). Importantly, ectopic expression of Rac1F28 rescued their levels in cells lacking β1-integrins (Fig. 3e, f). These results reveal that β1-integrin/Rac1 signalling influences canonical Wnt signalling pathway in bipotent cells.

Notch signalling is negatively regulated by Wnt [13]. Moreover it restricts bipotent cell self-renewal and promotes lineage commitment and differentiation into a luminal epithelial fate [7]. We therefore analysed expression of the Notch target genes, *Hes1*, *Hes5*, *Hey1* and *Hey2*, in β1-integrin- or Rac1-null cells. In each case, these target genes were upregulated in β1-integrin-deficient MECs (Fig. 3g). In contrast, their levels were not altered in Rac1-deficient MECs, except for a slight reduction in Hes1 transcript levels (Fig. 3h).

These results indicate that β1-integrin regulates bipotent cells through Wnt signalling in a Rac1-depenent manner. Integrins may regulate luminal progenitors via Notch signalling, but this occurs in a Rac1-independent manner.

Rac1 regulates the nuclear translocation of β-catenin in mammary epithelial stem cells

To reveal the mechanism by which β1-integrin/Rac1 signalling regulates Wnt signalling in bipotent cells, we

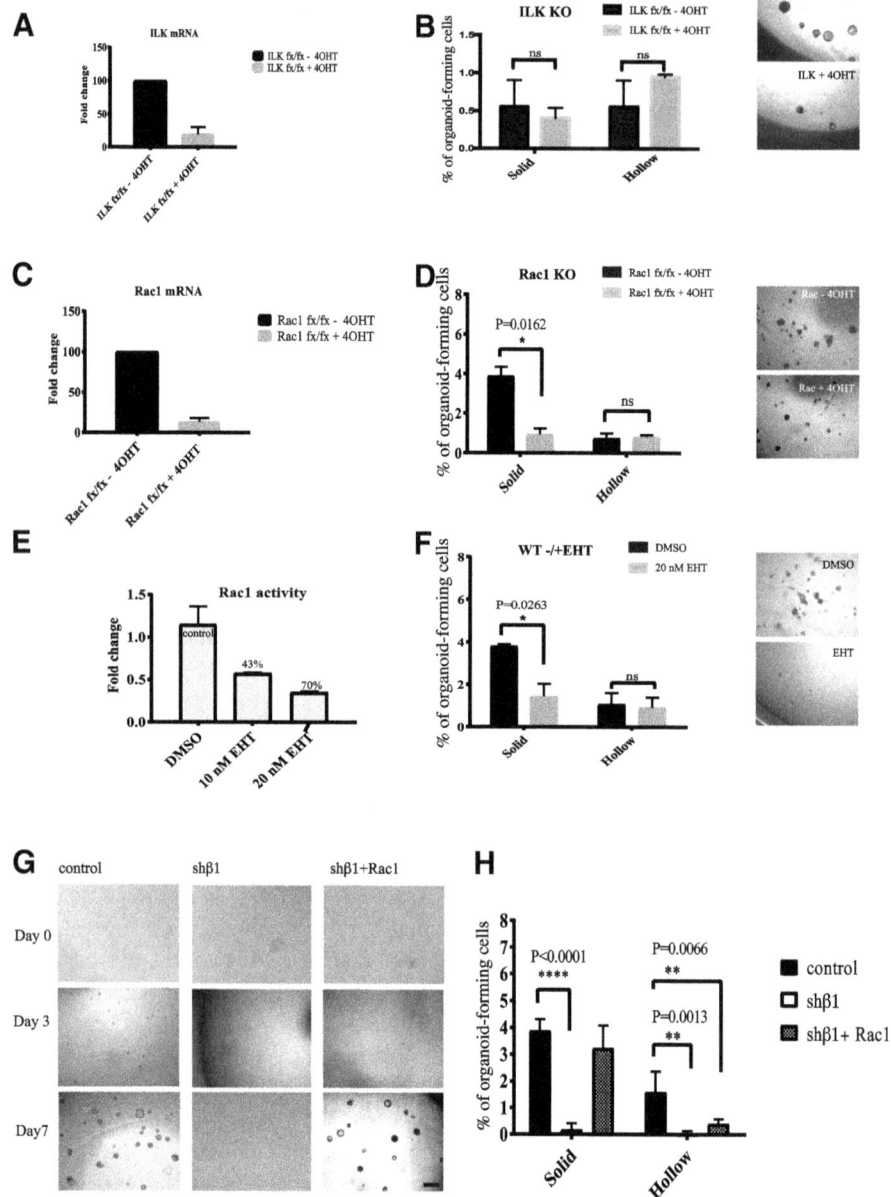

Fig. 2 Rac1, but not integrin-linked kinase (ILK), is involved in the formation of mammary organoids. **a** Primary mammary epithelial cells (MECs) were isolated from ILK^{fxfx};CreESR mice and cultured as single cells in organoid media in the absence or presence of 4-hydroxytamoxifen (4-OHT). Gene expression levels were quantified using qRT-PCR. **b** ILK gene deletion has no significant effect on solid or hollow organoid formation after 10 days of culture ($n = 2$). Error bars = SEM (Student's t test for paired samples). Representative images of organoids are shown to the right. **c** Primary MECs were isolated from Rac1^{fxfx};CreESR mice and cultured as single cells in organoid media in the absence or presence of 4-OHT. Gene expression levels were quantified using qRT-PCR. **d** Rac1 gene deletion decreases solid but not hollow organoid formation after 10 days of culture ($n = 2$). Error bars = SEM (Student's t test for paired samples). Representative images of organoids are shown to the right. **e** EHT1864 treatment reduces Rac1 activity in MECs. Primary MECs from ICR mice were cultured with 0, 10, or 20 nM EHT1864, and Rac1 activity levels were measured. **f** Inhibition of Rac1 activity using EHT1864 reduces solid organoid formation ($n = 3$). Error bars = SEM (Student's t test for paired samples). Representative images of organoids are shown to the right. **g** Rac1 rescues the impaired solid organoid formation caused by the β1-integrin knock-down, with representative images of cultures for control, sh-β1, and sh-β1 + Rac1. Scale bar = 500 μm. **h** Quantification of solid and hollow organoids demonstrates that Rac1 expression can rescue β1-integrin loss-of-function phenotype for solid but not hollow organoids ($n = 4$). Error bars = SEM (statistical significance determined by one-way analysis * = p < 0.05, ** = p < 0.01, **** = p < 0.0001 of variance)

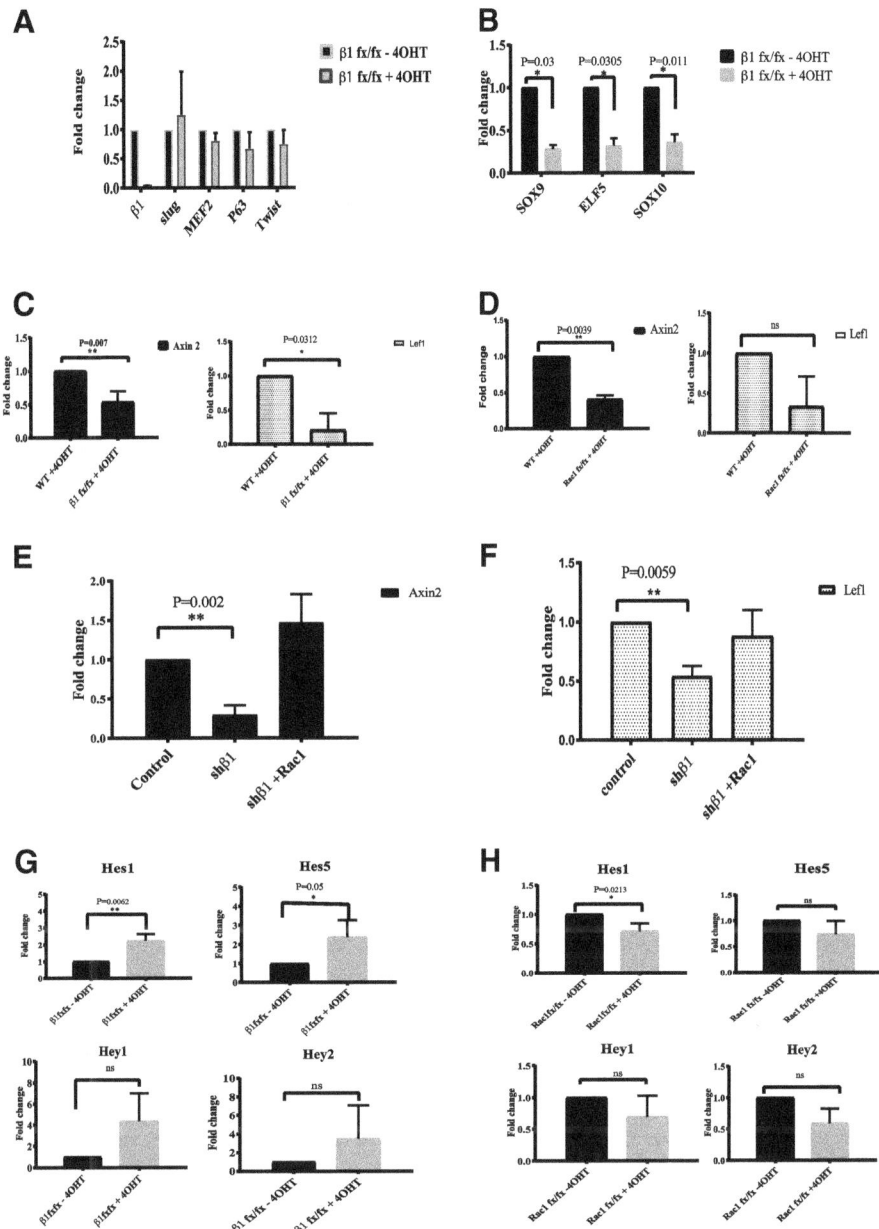

Fig. 3 β1-integrin and Rac1 are involved with Wnt and Notch signalling. **a** Expression levels of Slug, MEF2, p63 and Twist messenger RNA in control and β1-integrin knockout cells ($n = 3$). Error bars = SEM (statistical significance determined by one-way analysis of variance). **b** Expression of luminal progenitor transcription factor RNAs, SOX9, Elf5 and SOX10 in control and β1-integrin-knockout cells. **c** β1-integrin regulates the expression of Wnt target genes, *Axin2* and *Lef1*. **d** Rac1 regulates the expression of Wnt target genes, *Axin2* and *Lef1*. **e** Active Rac1 rescues downregulated Axin 2 levels in sh-β1-integrin cells. **f** Active Rac1 rescues downregulated Lef1 levels in sh-β1-integrin cells. **g** Role of β1-integrin in Notch signalling in mammary epithelial cells (MECs). RNA in primary MECs was analysed for the expression of Notch target genes, Hes1, Hes5, Hey1 and Hey2, in β1-integrin-knockout cells compared with controls (β1-integrin^{fx/fx}-4-OHT). **h** Notch target gene expression in Rac1^{fxfx} cells with or without 4-OHT. * = $p < 0.05$, ** = $p < 0.01$

performed phenotype rescue experiments. Wnt signalling was activated in β1-integrin-deficient MECs either with the soluble Wnt3A ligand or with a GSK3i.

In wild-type MECs, increased Wnt signalling via either Wnt3A or GSK3i led to an increase in solid organoids and a decrease in hollow organoids (black bars in Fig. 4a, b).

In β1-integrin-deficient MECs, GSK3i (but not Wnt3A) rescued the formation of solid organoids (Fig. 4a). In contrast, Wnt3A rescued hollow organoid formation (Fig. 4b).

Because we showed that β1-integrins influence Wnt signalling in bipotent cells, we examined whether this might occur via β-catenin localisation. β-catenin translocates

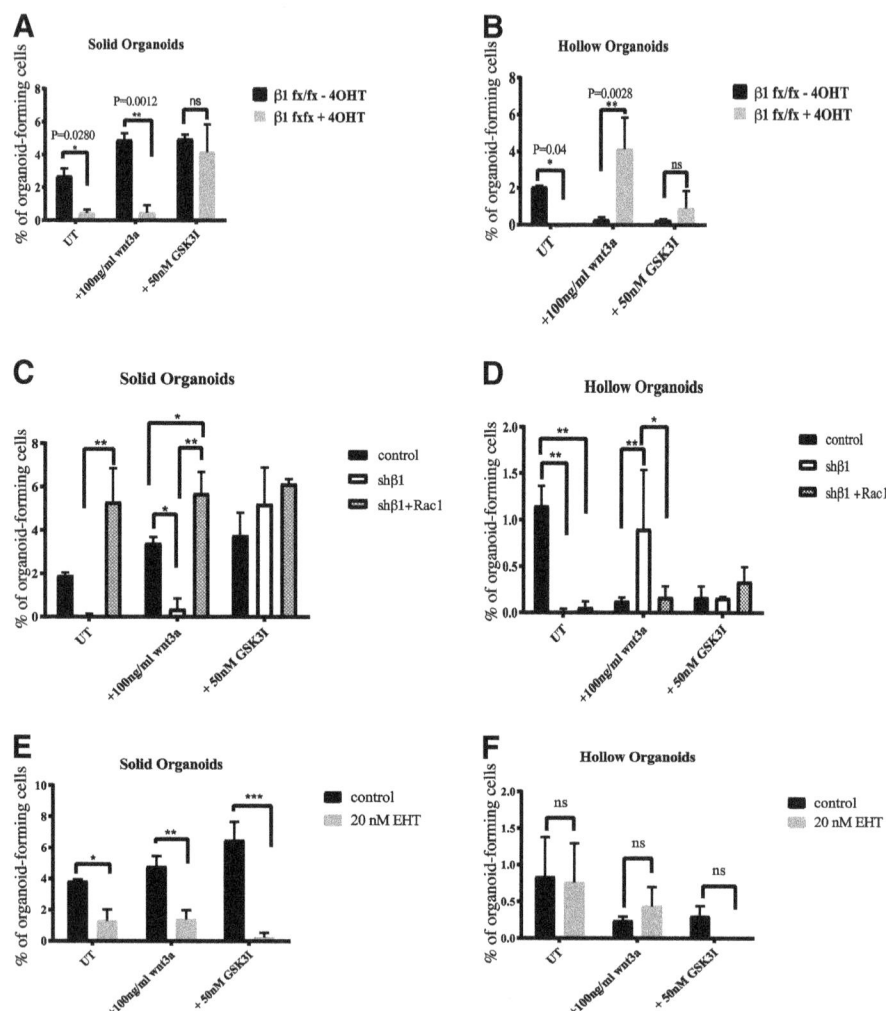

Fig. 4 Organoid formation in the presence of Wnt regulators. **a** Cells isolated from β1-integrin-flox mice treated without or with 4-OHT were incubated with either 100 ng/ml Wnt3a or 50 nM glycogen synthase kinase 3 inhibitor (GSK3i), left for 10 days in organoid media to form solid and hollow organoids, and the percentage of solid organoid-forming cells was determined. Error bars represent SEM ($n = 2$). *ns* Non-significant. **b** Quantification of the hollow organoids that formed in the experiment shown in (**a**). **c** Role of integrin-Rac signalling in the formation of solid MEC organoids, after treating control, integrin-depleted cells or those also expressing active-Rac, and treated with Wnt3a or GSK3i ($n = 3$). Error bars = SEM (statistical significance determined by one-way analysis of variance). **d** Role of integrin-Rac signalling in the formation of hollow MEC organoids. **e** Inhibiting Rac1 with EHT1864 prevents solid organoid formation. **f** Role of EHT in hollow organoid formation. * = p < 0.05, ** = p < 0.01, *** = p < 0.001

into the nucleus to interact with TCF transcription factors and thereby activate Wnt target gene expression. We examined whether GSK3i could increase nuclear β-catenin levels in β1-integrin-deleted MECs. Indeed, GSK3i-treated β1-integrin-deficient MECs showed similar levels of nuclear β-catenin as the β1-integrin-proficient MECs (not treated with 4-OHT) that were activated by either Wnt3A or GSK3i (Additional file 3: Figure S3). The Wnt3A-treated β1-integrin-deficient MECs did not show this nuclear accumulation of β-catenin. Thus, activating Wnt signalling with GSKi allows β-catenin to translocate to the nucleus, even in integrin-deleted MECs.

To determine whether Rac1 is involved with β1-integrin-dependent Wnt signalling, we examined organoid

formation after ectopic expression of RacF28. In β1-integrin-deficient MECs, Rac1F28 and GSK3i both rescued solid organoid formation (Fig. 4c).

In contrast, neither Rac1F28 nor GSK3i could rescue the impaired hollow organoid formation of β1-integrin-deficient MECs (Fig. 4b, d). Thus, crosstalk between Rac1-independent β1-integrin signalling and the non-canonical Wnt signalling pathways may regulate the luminal progenitor cell population.

Rac1 is a key node downstream of many signalling pathways. We therefore asked whether Rac1 inhibition fully recapitulated the β1-integrin-deficient Wnt phenotype. Organoid formation was assessed in EHT1846-treated cells in the absence or presence of Wnt3A or

GSK3i. This impaired solid organoid formation but had no effect on hollow organoids (Fig. 4e, f) – similar to genetic deletion of Rac1 in MECs (Fig. 2d). Neither Wnt3A nor GSK3i could rescue this phenotype, suggesting that pathways other than those involving β1-integrin signalling may also be involved in Rac1 activation in bipotent cells.

Our results indicate that integrin-Rac signalling regulates bipotent cells through Wnt in a pathway that involves nuclear translocation of β-catenin. In contrast, integrin-dependent luminal progenitors are Rac1-independent and likely involve non-canonical Wnt signalling as well as Notch signalling pathways.

Discussion

In this study, we have discovered a central role for integrins in stem cell maintenance and self-renewal within the mammary gland. Integrins are receptors for the ECM that contacts all mammary epithelia, and our genetic approach has revealed their requirement for stem cells. We found that β1-integrin maintains stem cells via a signalling pathway that involves both the small GTPase Rac1, as well as Wnt. These latter signalling proteins are known to determine the nuclear localisation of the β-catenin. We suggest that in stem cells, integrins have a new role in specifying the activation of Wnt and β-catenin.

Integrins in mammary epithelial cells

Integrins are central to the function of metazoan cells [9]. In the mammary gland, they connect cells to the ECM and activate cytoplasmic signalling pathways that control all aspects of cell function [12]. We have previously shown that integrins are essential in MECs for their survival, proliferation, and nuclear architecture; for the formation of a correctly polarised shape; and for functional differentiation into milk-producing lactating cells [2, 16, 26, 39].

In order to carry out these behaviours, integrins establish complex multi-component adhesion complexes that link ECM signals to intracellular signalling platforms and to the cytoskeleton [37]. In normal, non-transformed MECs, integrins signal directly to the cytoskeleton via talin and vinculin and to enzymatic pathways via ILK [3, 47]. Although FAK is a key integrin-binding partner, genetic studies have shown that it is not required for the development and function of normal MECs in vivo [46].

The role of integrins in bipotent cells has not been examined directly before. In this study, we have used genetic approaches to delete β1-integrin and demonstrated that both bipotent cells and luminal progenitor cells require β1-integrin function. This extends the role of integrins in mammary gland biology to include the survival and maintenance of stem cells.

Rac signalling in mammary epithelial cells

Signalling components downstream of integrins include the small GTPases. Both the Ras and Rho families of GTPases are crucial for breast cell function [50]. These proteins serve to interpret both growth factor signals as well as those within the immediate ECM microenvironment [38]. We have previously demonstrated that Rac1 is required for many aspects of MEC behaviour, including cell cycle, expression of milk proteins, and for tissue modelling during pregnancy and post-lactational involution [4].

Here we reveal a novel and central role for Rac1 in mammary epithelia, which is required for bipotent cells downstream of β1-integrin signalling. The major Rac isoform in MECs is Rac1 [28]. We found that when Rac1 is removed genetically, or if Rac is inhibited with a chemical, EHT1864, bipotent cells are deficient in their ability to form solid organoids. Moreover, the similar phenotype that occurs after β1-integrin genetic deletion is fully rescued by the expression of an active form of Rac1. Thus, integrin-Rac1 signalling is essential for MEC function, and this is now extended to the maintenance and organoid-forming ability of bipotent cells.

Wnt signalling in mammary epithelial cells

The involvement of β1-integrins in controlling key transcription factors in mammary epithelia has been studied mainly in alveolar differentiation, milk production and the cell cycle [23, 28]. It is not yet known whether β1-integrin regulates transcription factors that are required for mammary stem or progenitor cells.

Wnt signalling has a key role in stem cell activity in the mammary gland [33]. Moreover Wnt/β-catenin signalling in breast cancer is hyperactive in the basal-like and cancer stem cells that have high levels of β1-integrin [22]. In the embryo, Wnt promotes placode development and is required for initiation of mammary gland morphogenesis [6, 10, 45]. Wnt is also important in post-natal mammary branching morphogenesis, and for bud and alveolar formation during pregnancy [5, 8, 25, 41]. Lineage-tracing experiments showed that Wnt/β-catenin controls both luminal and basal lineages, depending on the developmental stage of the mammary gland [43].

However, how stem cells sense the microenvironment via adhesion receptors and then activate Wnt/β-catenin signalling to maintain their stem cell property is not understood. *Axin2* is a direct target gene of the canonical Wnt/β-catenin pathway, enabling its mRNA to be used as a readout for Wnt activity [11, 17, 21]. Moreover, Axin2-expressing cells have stem cell activity in the mammary gland [49]. Activating the canonical pathway requires the extracellular ligand for Wnt signalling to bind to receptor complexes containing Frizzled and

Lrp5/6 proteins. This recruits the Axin/APC/GSK3β destruction complex to the plasma membrane, which prevents GSK3β phosphorylating and thus marking β-catenin for degradation. Consequently, cytoplasmic β-catenin is stabilised and translocates into the nucleus, where it induces the transcription of activation of target genes such as Lef1 and Axin2 [2, 17].

Although β1-integrin and Wnt signalling are both crucial for stem cell maintenance, it has not previously been established whether these pathways interact. Rac1 may be a crucial component of Wnt signalling in lymphoid cells and fibroblasts because it controls β-catenin translocation into the nucleus. In response to activation of the Wnt pathway by Wnt3a, Rac1 activates c-Jun N-terminal kinase 2 (JNK2), which phosphorylates β-catenin and promotes its nuclear translocation [15, 48]. Rac1 may also be directly activated by Wnt3a [42, 48].

We have now established a novel link between β1-integrin-Rac and canonical Wnt signalling in the mammary gland. Notably, β1-integrin-Rac signalling affects the expression of Wnt target genes. Moreover, activating Wnt signalling by inhibiting GSK3β rescued stem cell frequency in β1-integrin-null cells.

Conclusions

The main conclusion of the present study is that integrins are essential for the maintenance of mammary epithelial progenitor cells. Our data reveal a role for β1-integrin-Rac signalling in the translocation of β-catenin into the nucleus, thereby activating the transcription of Wnt target genes and mammary stem cell pathways.

Additional files

Additional file 1: Figure S1. Tamoxifen treatment does not affect cellular distribution or organoid formation. **a** 4-OHT did not affect the frequency of basal or luminal progenitor cells. Primary MECs from WT mice were cultured at a density of 5×10^4 cells/well with or without 100 nM 4-OHT. Cells were dissociated using trypsin/EDTA at day 3, passed through a 40-μm filter and stained for CD45, CD31, EpCAM, α_6-integrin (CD49f), and α_2-integrin (CD49b) to distinguish the populations of basal/stem, total luminal, luminal progenitor, and differentiated luminal cells. **b** Quantification of the four populations with or without 4-OHT ($n = 3$). Statistical significance was determined by Student's t test for paired samples. Error bars in the graph represent SEM. *ns* Non-significant. **c** Organoid numbers in WT cells treated with 4-OHT. Primary MECs were isolated from β_1-integrin$^{fx/fx}$ mice that do not contain CreESR and cultured as single cells in organoid media at 5×10^5 cells/ml. MECs were collected at day 3, dissociated into single cells, and re-cultured at 2×10^3 cells/cm^2. Solid and hollow organoids were counted at day 10 and divided by the number of cells seeded at day 0 to calculate the percentage of organoids formed from WT cells with or without 4-OHT ($n = 3$). Statistical significance was determined by Student's t test for paired samples. Error bars in the graph represent SEM. *ns* Non-significant. (PDF 479 kb)

Additional file 2: Figure S2. Mammospheres of CD49f-, EpCAM- and CD49b-expressing cells. Before plating, the cells were selected by FACS analysis for those expressing CD49f, EpCAM and CD49b. Representative images of organoids are shown for cells with high or low levels of

CD49f, high or low levels of EpCAM, and high of low levels of CD49b. (PDF 445 kb)

Additional file 3: Figure S3. Nuclear translocation of β-catenin in response to Wnt3a and GSK3i. Immunoblotting shows nuclear fractions of control and integrin-depleted cells after cells were treated with Wnt3a or GSK3i with antibodies to β-catenin or Lamin-B1. (PDF 151 kb)

Abbreviations
ECM: Extracellular matrix; MaSC: Mammary stem cell; MEC: Mammary epithelial cell

Acknowledgements
The authors are grateful for support from Breast Cancer Now, as well as for the Wellcome Trust for funding The Wellcome Trust Centre for Cell-Matrix Research.

Funding
This work was supported by Wellcome Trust core funding for The Wellcome Trust Centre for Cell-Matrix Research, University of Manchester (grant 203128/Z/16/Z).

Authors' contributions
SO and AU conducted the experimental work. CHS, SO and KB were involved in experimental planning and study design. SO, AU and CHS wrote the manuscript. All authors read and approved the final manuscript in its submitted form.

Competing interests
The authors declare that they have no competing interests.

References
1. Akhtar N, Streuli CH. Rac1 links integrin-mediated adhesion to the control of lactational differentiation in mammary epithelia. J Cell Biol. 2006;173:781–93.
2. Akhtar N, Streuli CH. An integrin-ILK-microtubule network orients cell polarity and lumen formation in glandular epithelium. Nat Cell Biol. 2013;15:17–27.
3. Akhtar N, Marlow R, Lambert E, Schatzmann F, Lowe ET, Cheung J, Katz E, Li W, Wu C, Dedhar S, et al. Molecular dissection of integrin signalling proteins in the control of mammary epithelial development and differentiation. Development. 2009;136:1019–27.
4. Akhtar N, Li W, Mironov A, Streuli CH. Rac1 controls both the secretory function of the mammary gland and its remodeling for successive gestations. Dev Cell. 2016;38:522–35.
5. Badders NM, Goel S, Clark RJ, Klos KS, Kim S, Bafico A, Lindvall C, Williams BO, Alexander CM. The Wnt receptor, Lrp5, is expressed by mouse mammary stem cells and is required to maintain the basal lineage. PLoS One. 2009;4:e6594.
6. Boras-Granic K, Chang H, Grosschedl R, Hamel PA. Lef1 is required for the transition of Wnt signaling from mesenchymal to epithelial cells in the mouse embryonic mammary gland. Dev Biol. 2006;295:219–31.
7. Bouras T, Pal B, Vaillant F, Harburg G, Asselin-Labat ML, Oakes SR, Lindeman GJ, Visvader JE. Notch signaling regulates mammary stem cell function and luminal cell-fate commitment. Cell Stem Cell. 2008;3:429–41.
8. Brisken C, Heineman A, Chavarria T, Elenbaas B, Tan J, Dey SK, McMahon JA, McMahon AP, Weinberg RA. Essential function of Wnt-4 in mammary gland development downstream of progesterone signaling. Genes Dev. 2000;14:650–4.

9. Campbell ID, Humphries MJ. Integrin structure, activation, and interactions. Cold Spring Harb Perspect Biol. 2011;3(3):a004994.

10. Chu EY, Hens J, Andl T, Kairo A, Yamaguchi TP, Brisken C, Glick A, Wysolmerski JJ, Millar SE. Canonical WNT signaling promotes mammary placode development and is essential for initiation of mammary gland morphogenesis. Development. 2004;131:4819–29.

11. Gehrke I, Gandhirajan RK, Kreuzer KA. Targeting the WNT/β-catenin/TCF/ LEF1 axis in solid and haematological cancers: multiplicity of therapeutic options. Eur J Cancer. 2009;45:2759–67.

12. Glukhova MA, Streuli CH. How integrins control breast biology. Curr Opin Cell Biol. 2013;25:633–41.

13. Gu B, Watanabe K, Sun P, Fallahi M, Dai X. Chromatin effector Pygo2 mediates Wnt-notch crosstalk to suppress luminal/alveolar potential of mammary stem and basal cells. Cell Stem Cell. 2013;13:48–61.

14. Guo W, Keckesova Z, Donaher JL, Shibue T, Tischler V, Reinhardt F, Itzkovitz S, Noske A, Zürrer-Härdi U, Bell G, et al. Slug and Sox9 cooperatively determine the mammary stem cell state. Cell. 2012;148:1015–28.

15. Jamieson C, Lui C, Brocardo MG, Martino-Echarri E, Henderson BR. Rac1 augments Wnt signaling by stimulating β-catenin–lymphoid enhancer factor-1 complex assembly independent of β-catenin nuclear import. J Cell Sci. 2015;128:3933–46.

16. Jeanes AI, Wang P, Moreno-Layseca P, Paul N, Cheung J, Tsang R, Akhtar N, Foster FM, Brennan K, Streuli CH. Specific β-containing integrins exert differential control on proliferation and two-dimensional collective cell migration in mammary epithelial cells. J Biol Chem. 2012;287:24103–12.

17. Jho E, Zhang T, Domon C, Joo CK, Freund JN, Costantini F. Wnt/beta-catenin/Tcf signaling induces the transcription of Axin2, a negative regulator of the signaling pathway. Mol Cell Biol. 2002;22:1172–83.

18. Klinowska TC, Soriano JV, Edwards GM, Oliver JM, Valentijn AJ, Montesano R, Streuli CH. Laminin and β1 integrins are crucial for normal mammary gland development in the mouse. Dev Biol. 1999;215:13–32.

19. Klinowska TC, Alexander CM, Georges-Labouesse E, Van der Neut R, Kreidberg JA, Jones CJ, Sonnenberg A, Streuli CH. Epithelial development and differentiation in the mammary gland is not dependent on alpha 3 or alpha 6 integrin subunits. Dev Biol. 2001;233:449–67.

20. Lambert AW, Ozturk S, Thiagalingam S. Integrin signaling in mammary epithelial cells and breast cancer. ISRN Oncol. 2012;2012:493283.

21. Leung JY, Kolligs FT, Wu R, Zhai Y, Kuick R, Hanash S, Cho KR, Fearon ER. Activation of AXIN2 expression by beta-catenin-T cell factor. A feedback repressor pathway regulating Wnt signaling. J Biol Chem. 2002;277:21657–65.

22. Li Y, Welm B, Podsypanina K, Huang S, Chamorro M, Zhang X, Rowlands T, Egeblad M, Cowin P, Werb Z, et al. Evidence that transgenes encoding components of the Wnt signaling pathway preferentially induce mammary cancers from progenitor cells. Proc Natl Acad Sci U S A. 2003;100:15853–8.

23. Li N, Zhang Y, Naylor MJ, Schatzmann F, Maurer F, Wintermantel T, Schuetz G, Mueller U, Streuli CH, Hynes NE. β1 integrins regulate mammary gland proliferation and maintain the integrity of mammary alveoli. EMBO J. 2005; 24:1942–53.

24. Lin R, Cerione RA, Manor D. Specific contributions of the small GTPases rho, Rac, and Cdc42 to Dbl transformation. J Biol Chem. 1999;274:23633–41.

25. Lindvall C, Zylstra CR, Evans N, West RA, Dykema K, Furge KA, Williams BO. The Wnt co-receptor Lrp6 is required for normal mouse mammary gland development. PLoS One. 2009;4:e5813.

26. Maya-Mendoza A, Bartek J, Jackson DA, Streuli CH. Cellular microenvironment controls the nuclear architecture of breast epithelia through β1-integrin. Cell Cycle. 2016;15:345–56.

27. Metcalfe AD, Gilmore A, Klinowska T, Oliver J, Valentijn AJ, Brown R, Ross A, MacGregor G, Hickman JA, Streuli CH. Developmental regulation of Bcl-2 family protein expression in the involuting mammary gland. J Cell Sci. 1999; 112(Pt 11):1771–83.

28. Moreno-Layseca P, Ucar A, Sun H, Wood A, Olabi S, Gilmore AP, Brennan K, Streuli CH. The requirement of integrins for breast epithelial proliferation. Eur J Cell Biol. 2017;96(3):227–39.

29. Muschler J, Streuli CH. Cell–matrix interactions in mammary gland development and breast cancer. Cold Spring Harb Perspect Biol. 2010;2(10): a003202.

30. Naylor MJ, Li N, Cheung J, Lowe ET, Lambert E, Marlow R, Wang P, Schatzmann F, Wintermantel T, Schüetz G, et al. Ablation of beta1 integrin in mammary epithelium reveals a key role for integrin in glandular morphogenesis and differentiation. J Cell Biol. 2005;171:717–28.

31. Prince JM, Klinowska TCM, Marshman E, Lowe ET, Mayer U, Miner J, Aberdam D, Vestweber D, Gusterson B, Streuli CH. Cell-matrix interactions during development and apoptosis of the mouse mammary gland in vivo. Dev Dyn. 2002;223:497–516.

32. Rooney N, Wang P, Brennan K, Gilmore AP, Streuli CH. The integrin-mediated ILK-Parvin-αPix signaling axis controls differentiation in mammary epithelial cells. J Cell Physiol. 2016;231:2408–17.

33. Shackleton M, Vaillant F, Simpson KJ, Stingl J, Smyth GK, Asselin-Labat ML, Wu L, Lindeman GJ, Visvader JE. Generation of a functional mammary gland from a single stem cell. Nature. 2006;439:84–8.

34. Shehata M, Teschendorff A, Sharp G, Novcic N, Russell IA, Avril S, Prater M, Eirew P, Caldas C, Watson CJ, et al. Phenotypic and functional characterisation of the luminal cell hierarchy of the mammary gland. Breast Cancer Res. 2012;14:R134.

35. Shutes A, Onesto C, Picard V, Leblond B, Schweighoffer F, Der CJ. Specificity and mechanism of action of EHT 1864, a novel small molecule inhibitor of Rac family small GTPases. J Biol Chem. 2007;282:35666–78.

36. Stingl J. Detection and analysis of mammary gland stem cells. J Pathol. 2009;217:229–41.

37. Streuli CH. Integrins as architects of cell behavior. Mol Biol Cell. 2016;27: 2885–8.

38. Streuli CH, Akhtar N. Signal co-operation between integrins and other receptor systems. Biochem J. 2009;418:491–506.

39. Streuli CH, Bailey N, Bissell MJ. Control of mammary epithelial differentiation: basement membrane induces tissue-specific gene expression in the absence of cell-cell interaction and morphological polarity. J Cell Biol. 1991; 115:1383–95.

40. Taddei I, Deugnier MA, Faraldo MM, Petit V, Bouvard D, Medina D, Fässler R, Thiery JP, Glukhova M. Beta1 integrin deletion from the basal compartment of the mammary epithelium affects stem cells. Nat Cell Biol. 2008;10:716–22.

41. Teulière J, Faraldo MM, Deugnier MA, Shtutman M, Ben-Ze'ev A, Thiery JP, Glukhova MA. Targeted activation of β-catenin signaling in basal mammary epithelial cells affects mammary development and leads to hyperplasia. Development. 2005;132:267–77.

42. Valls G, Codina M, Miller RK, Valle-Pérez BD, Vinyoles M, Caelles C, McCrea PD, de Herreros AG, Duñach M. Upon Wnt stimulation, Rac1 activation requires Rac1 and Vav2 binding to p120-catenin. J Cell Sci. 2012;125: 5288–301.

43. van Amerongen R, Bowman AN, Nusse R. Developmental stage and time dictate the fate of Wnt/β-catenin-responsive stem cells in the mammary gland. Cell Stem Cell. 2012;11:387–400.

44. Van Keymeulen A, Rocha AS, Ousset M, Beck B, Bouvencourt G, Rock J, Sharma N, Dekoninck S, Blanpain C. Distinct stem cells contribute to mammary gland development and maintenance. Nature. 2011;479:189–93.

45. Veltmaat JM, Van Veelen W, Thiery JP, Bellusci S. Identification of the mammary line in mouse by Wnt10b expression. Dev Dyn. 2004;229:349–56.

46. Walker S, Foster F, Wood A, Owens T, Brennan K, Streuli CH, Gilmore AP. Oncogenic activation of FAK drives apoptosis suppression in a 3D-culture model of breast cancer initiation. Oncotarget. 2016;7(43):70336–52.

47. Wang P, Ballestrem C, Streuli CH. The C terminus of Talin links integrins to cell cycle progression. J Cell Biol. 2011;195:499–513.

48. Wu X, Tu X, Joeng KS, Hilton MJ, Williams DA, Long F. Rac1 activation controls nuclear localization of β-catenin during canonical Wnt signaling. Cell. 2008;133:340–53.

49. Zeng YA, Nusse R. Wnt proteins are self-renewal factors for mammary stem cells and promote their long-term expansion in culture. Cell Stem Cell. 2010;6:568–77.

50. Zuo Y, Oh W, Ulu A, Frost JA. Minireview: mouse models of rho GTPase function in mammary gland development, tumorigenesis, and metastasis. Mol Endocrinol. 2016;30:278–89.

10

The Prosigna gene expression assay and responsiveness to adjuvant cyclophosphamide-based chemotherapy in premenopausal high-risk patients with breast cancer

Maj-Britt Jensen[1]*[ID], Anne-Vibeke Lænkholm[2], Torsten O. Nielsen[3], Jens Ole Eriksen[2], Pernille Wehn[2], Tressa Hood[4], Namratha Ram[4], Wesley Buckingham[4], Sean Ferree[4] and Bent Ejlertsen[5]

Abstract

Background: The PAM50-based (Prosigna) risk of recurrence (ROR) score and intrinsic subtypes are prognostic for women with high-risk breast cancer. We investigate the predictive ability of Prosigna regarding the effectiveness of cyclophosphamide-based adjuvant chemotherapy in premenopausal patients with high-risk breast cancer.

Methods: Prosigna assays were performed on the NanoString platform in tumors from participants in Danish Breast Cancer Group (DBCG) 77B, a four-arm trial that randomized premenopausal women with high-risk early breast cancer to no systemic treatment, levamisole, oral cyclophosphamide (C) or cyclophosphamide, methotrexate and fluorouracil (CMF).

Results: In total, this retrospective analysis included 460 women (40% of the 1146 randomized patients). The continuous Prosigna ROR score was prognostic in the no systemic treatment group (unadjusted $P < 0.001$ for disease-free survival (DFS), $P = 0.001$ for overall survival (OS)). No statistically significant interaction of continuous ROR score and treatment on DFS and OS was found. A highly significant association was observed between intrinsic subtypes and C/CMF treatment for DFS ($P_{interaction} = 0.003$ unadjusted, $P = 0.001$ adjusted) and OS ($P_{interaction} = 0.04$). In the adjusted analysis treatment with C/CMF was associated with a reduced risk of DFS events in patients with basal-like (hazard ratio (HR) 0.14; 95% CI 0.06; 0.32) and luminal B (HR 0.48; 95% CI 0.27; 0.84) subtypes but not in patients with Human epidermal growth factor receptor-enriched (HR 1.05; 95% CI 0.56; 1.95) or luminal A (HR 0.61; 95% CI 0.32; 1.16) subtypes.

Conclusion: The Prosigna ROR score and intrinsic subtypes were prognostic in high-risk premenopausal patients with breast cancer, and intrinsic subtypes identify high-risk patients with or without major benefit from adjuvant C/CMF treatment.

Keywords: Breast neoplasms, Adjuvant chemotherapy, Cyclophosphamide, CMF, PAM50

* Correspondence: mj@dbcg.dk
[1]Danish Breast Cancer Cooperative Group, Rigshospitalet, Copenhagen University Hospital, DBCG Secretariat, Bldg. 2501 Rigshospitalet, Blegdamsvej 9, DK-2100 Copenhagen, Denmark
Full list of author information is available at the end of the article

Background

The early results of the first adjuvant Milan trial were published in 1976 [1], and showed a clear benefit from 4-weekly oral cyclophosphamide on days 1 to 14 combined with intravenous methotrexate and fluorouracil on days 1 and 8 (CMF). The Milan trial included patients with high-risk (node-positive) breast cancer who were randomized after mastectomy; none of whom received radiotherapy or endocrine treatment. Several cooperative groups, including the Danish Breast Cancer Group (DBCG), initiated trials to explore the results from the pivotal Milan trial. DBCG 77B included premenopausal patients with high-risk breast cancer who after mastectomy and radiotherapy and without endocrine treatment were randomized to observation, levamisole, single-agent cyclophosphamide, or CMF. Results showed a similar benefit from oral cyclophosphamide and CMF, and the survival benefit was maintained after 25 years of follow up [2]. Due to the results of these and other early clinical trials, adjuvant chemotherapy has been considered a standard in premenopausal patients with node-positive breast cancer since the National Institutes of Health Consensus Conference in 1980 [3]. Subsequent meta-analyses by the Early Breast Cancer Trialists' Collaborative Group (EBCTCG) have demonstrated that the relative benefit of CMF was largely independent of patient characteristics, nodal status and other tumor features available for analysis, and also independent of the use of concomitant tamoxifen. Furthermore, in the EBCTCG analysis an additional incremental benefit was shown from adding an anthracycline to CMF, from substituting methotrexate with doxorubicin or epirubicin, and from giving taxanes concurrently or in sequence with anthracyclines [4, 5].

Since intrinsic molecular subtypes were first described more than 15 years ago, their prognostic ability has repeatedly been demonstrated in early breast cancer [6]. However, few attempts have been made to explore the ability of these subtypes to predict benefit of chemotherapy. The prediction analysis of microarray 50 (PAM50) gene set has become a standard for identifying intrinsic subtypes from RNA expression measurements and its predictive abilities have been evaluated in the Canadian MA.5 trial comparing adjuvant cyclophosphamide, epirubicin, and fluoroucil (CEF) to CMF in patients with early breast cancer. The human epidermal growth factor receptor 2 (Her2)-enriched subtype was associated with a benefit from the anthracycline-containing chemotherapy arm while no significant differences between arms were shown for patients with basal-like, luminal A or luminal B breast cancers [7]. Additionally, a high 21-gene recurrence score (OncotypeDx) has been associated with benefit from addition of cyclophosphamide, adriamycin, and fluorouracil (CAF) to tamoxifen [8] in high-risk node-positive disease, suggesting that not all patients with high-risk early breast cancer derive a similar benefit from adjuvant chemotherapy.

The PAM50 gene signature has been developed into a clinical test, the Prosigna gene signature assay, validated to estimate the prognosis for postmenopausal patients with estrogen receptor (ER)+ early-stage breast cancer [9, 10]. In the DBCG 77B trial we randomized premenopausal patients with high-risk breast cancer to cyclophosphamide-based chemotherapy against no systemic treatment, and the two primary co-objectives of this study were to evaluate the predictive ability of the PAM50-based Prosigna risk of recurrence (ROR) score and intrinsic subtypes.

Methods

Details on DBCG 77B have been published previously [2]. In brief, this was an open-label randomized phase III trial comparing, in the adjuvant setting, radiotherapy alone (control), radiotherapy plus 2.5 mg/kg/body weight of levamisole on 2 days consecutively each week for 48 weeks, radiotherapy plus 12 cycles of single-agent cyclophosphamide (C) 130 mg/m^2 orally on days 1–14 every 4 weeks, or radiotherapy plus 12 cycles of CMF (cyclophosphamide 80 mg/m^2 orally on days 1–14, methotrexate 30 mg/m^2 intravenously on days 1 and 8, and 5-fluorouracil 500 mg/m^2 intravenously on days 1 and 8) every 4 weeks. Patients were eligible for DBCG 77B if they were without distant metastasis, were premenopausal, and had either positive lymph nodes, tumors > 5 cm, and/or invasion of the deep fascia. The DBCG prepared the original 77B trial and its biological sub-studies have previously been described in detail [2, 11]. The Biomedical Research Ethics of the Danish Capital Region approved the protocol (H-15012740).

Central assessment of Prosigna

Formalin-fixed, paraffin-embedded tumor blocks (FFPE) from primary excisional surgery specimens were collected at the Department of Pathology, Zealand University Hospital. RNA extraction and Prosigna testing were performed according to standard operating procedures [9] by investigators blinded to clinical outcome. Prosigna results were transferred to the data manager at Nanostring, who while remaining blinded to clinical data, prepared the Prosigna ROR and intrinsic subtype analysis data set. This was forwarded to the DBCG statistical office for merging with clinical data and to execute the prespecified statistical analysis plan. ROR cut offs for analysis of the combined study population (including ER +/− and Her2+/−) were prespecified in terms of the observed ROR score distribution tertiles within the study population (8–51 (low), 52–71 (intermediate), and 72–100 (high)) and were independent of nodal status.

The age of the FFPE tissue blocks resulted in decreased RNA quality compared with previous studies performed by the DBCG. In order to increase power for the exploratory analysis in the ER+/Her2- population, the Prosigna test quality control criteria for RNA quality was relaxed for this subset.

Statistical methods

A written prespecified statistical analysis plan was finalized prior to data analysis. The statistical analysis was executed by the DBCG statistical office, which was not involved in biomarker data collection. The primary endpoint for this study was disease-free survival (DFS), defined as time from randomization to any first event of invasive ipsilateral or contralateral breast cancer recurrence, local or regional invasive recurrence, distant recurrence, second (non-breast) invasive cancer, or death from any cause. The secondary endpoint was overall survival (OS), defined as time from date of randomization until death from any cause. Survival rates were estimated by the Kaplan-Meier method. Patients treated according to protocol were included. Cox proportional hazards regression models were applied to assess the unadjusted and adjusted hazard ratios (HR). The chemotherapy arms (C + CMF) were analyzed versus no chemotherapy arms (control + levamisole). The multivariate models included age at entry ($\leq$ 40, 41–45, 46–50, and 50 years), tumor size ($\leq$ 2, > 2 to $\leq$ 5, and > 5 cm), lymph node (LN) status (0–3 positive LN, 4–9, 10+ and < 10 vs 10+ retrieved), histologic type (ductal vs non-ductal), grade (ductal I, II, and III) and treatment regimen. Proportional hazards assumptions were assessed using Schoenfeld residuals and by including a time-dependent component for each covariate. The hazard rates for histologic type and grade were not proportional; therefore, stratification was used. To comply with proportional hazards assumptions about subtypes and ROR score, separate estimates were included according to time since randomization. The Wald test was used to assess heterogeneity. Associations between included and excluded patients and clinico-pathological characteristics (excluding unknowns) were analyzed using the chi-square test. P values are two-tailed, unadjusted for number of comparisons. Central review, monitoring, and statistical analyses were done by the DBCG Statistical Office using the SAS 9.4 software program package (SAS Institute, Cary, NC, USA).

Results

The DBCG 77B trial enrolled 1146 patients, among whom 1072 received treatment as allocated by randomization (Additional file 1: Figure S1). Tumor blocks were available from 649 patients, and 623 blocks contained sufficient invasive breast cancer tissue for RNA extraction. The Prosigna assay was successful in 487 patients, of which 460 were treated according to

protocol. The assessable 460 patients did differ significantly from the 612 non-assessable patients ($P < 0.05$) with regard to histologic type ($P = 0.03$) and malignancy grade ($P = 0.02$). Among the 460 patients, 231 (81%) experienced a first event within 10 years. Number of positive lymph nodes, tumor size, age, and treatment regimen were not significantly different in assessable vs non-assessable patients. The treatment effect was similar with an HR favoring chemotherapy for DFS (adjusted HR; 0.55; 95% CI, 0.38 to 0.79; $P = 0.001$) to the effect observed in the original study (HR = 0.60; 95% CI, 0.48 to 0.75). Table 1 shows the baseline characteristics according to Prosigna subtype for the 460 patients: 324 patients were included in the exploratory analysis of DFS in the ER+/Her2– patient population.

Of the 460 patients included in the primary analyses 61 (13%) were classified as having basal-like, 120 (26%) as Her2-enriched, 161 (35%) as luminal A and 116 (25%) as luminal B breast cancer, reflecting the population including patients with ER+/– and Her2+/– breast cancer.

Prognosis by Prosigna ROR score

The continuous ROR score was highly prognostic (unadjusted HR, 1.23; 95% CI, 1.09 to 1.39, $P < 0.001$ for a 10-point difference) for DFS within the group not treated systemically. For the C/CMF-treated group, the ROR continuous score had a different effect according to follow-up time (0–5 years vs 5+ years) (Fig. 1a and b). The ROR prognosis was statistically significant for the first 5 years for both the C/CMF arm and the no chemotherapy arm, and with no differential effect, whereas after 5 years no prognostic effect was apparent. There was no statistically significant differential effect according to follow-up time in the no chemotherapy arm alone. Including all patients, irrespective of hormone receptor status, the 10-year DFS rates in the untreated group were 62% (95% CI, 43 to 76), 27% (95% CI, 14 to 43) and 27% (95% CI, 15 to 41) for low, intermediate, and high ROR scores, respectively (Fig. 2a). Comparing intermediate ROR with low-risk ROR for the untreated group, unadjusted HR = 2.66; 95% CI, 1.35 to 5.24, and similarly for the high vs low-risk ROR group HR = 2.73; 95% CI, 1.43 to 5.22. Likewise, the ROR score was prognostic for OS in the untreated group (Fig. 2b) and the 10-year OS rates were 63% (95% CI, 45 to 76), 38% (95% CI, 22 to 54), and 30% (95% CI, 17 to 43) for low, intermediate, and high ROR scores, respectively.

Effect of chemotherapy according to the Prosigna ROR score

For the first co-primary objective, we examined the association between the continuous Prosigna ROR score and benefit of chemotherapy in the population including patients with ER+/– and Her2+/– breast cancer. There

Table 1 Patient and tumor characteristics by Prosigna (PAM50) subtype

Characteristics	Total study set N	%	Molecular subtype Luminal A N	%	Luminal B N	%	Basal-like N	%	Her2-E N	%
Number of patients	460	–	161	35	118	27	61	13	120	26
Age										
< 40 years	96	21	23	14	26	22	19	31	28	23
40–49 years	233	51	94	58	63	53	25	41	51	43
50–59 years	131	28	44	27	29	25	17	28	41	34
Lymph nodes excised										
None	19	4	8	5	7	6	1	2	3	3
1–3	110	24	42	26	27	23	14	23	27	23
4–9	268	58	97	60	67	57	39	64	65	54
> 9	6	14	14	9	17	14	7	11	25	21
Lymph node status										
Negative	43	9	16	10	4	3	10	16	13	11
1–3 positive	271	59	106	66	72	61	33	54	60	50
4+ positive	127	28	31	19	35	30	17	28	44	37
Unknown	19	4	8	5	7	6	1	2	3	3
Tumor size										
0–20 mm	132	29	60	37	36	31	14	23	22	18
21–50 mm	239	52	77	48	61	52	30	49	71	59
> 50 mm	85	18	24	15	21	18	13	21	27	23
Unknown	4	1	0	0	0	0	4	7	0	0
Deep fascia invasion										
Absent	346	75	127	79	93	79	45	74	81	68
Present	109	24	32	20	25	21	15	25	37	31
Unknown	5	1	2	1	0	0	1	2	2	2
Histologic type										
Ductal carcinoma	393	85	132	82	99	84	52	85	110	92
Lobular carcinoma	33	7	16	10	13	11	1	2	3	3
Other	28	6	11	7	5	4	6	10	6	5
Unknown	6	1	2	1	1	1	2	3	1	1
Malignancy grade[a]										
Grade I	65	17	46	35	15	15	1	2	3	3
Grade II	242	62	81	61	73	74	22	42	66	60
Grade III	86	22	5	4	11	11	29	56	41	37
HR status										
Positive	329	72	146	91	112	95	6	10	65	54
Negative	114	25	6	4	5	4	52	85	51	43
Unknown	17	4	9	6	1	1	3	5	4	3
Systemic treatment										
Control or levamisole	113	25	37	23	34	29	10	16	32	27
C or CMF	347	75	124	77	84	71	51	84	88	73

Table 1 Patient and tumor characteristics by Prosigna (PAM50) subtype *(Continued)*

Characteristics	Total study set		Molecular subtype							
			Luminal A		Luminal B		Basal-like		Her2-E	
	N	%	N	%	N	%	N	%	N	%
ROR score groups										
Low (0–51)	155	34	135	84	2	2	14	23	4	3
Intermediate (52–71)	148	32	26	16	50	42	40	66	32	27
High (72–100)	157	34	0	0	66	56	7	11	84	70

PAM50 prediction analysis of microarray 50, *C* cyclophosphamide, *CMF* cyclophosphamide, methotrexate and fluorouracil, *HR* hormone receptor, *Her2-E* human epidermal growth factor receptor 2-enriched, *ROR* risk of recurrence
[a]Ductal carcinomas only

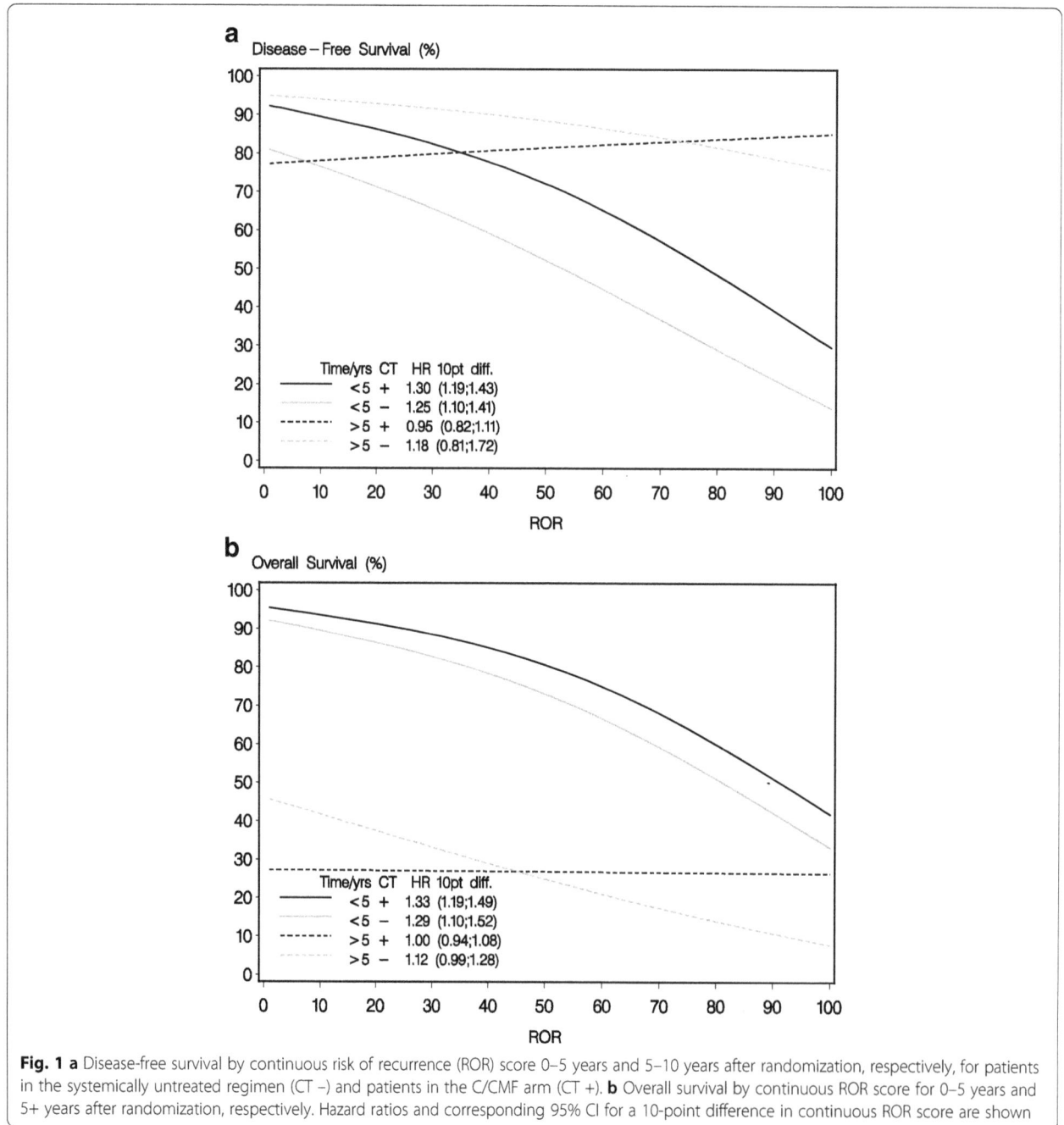

Fig. 1 a Disease-free survival by continuous risk of recurrence (ROR) score 0–5 years and 5–10 years after randomization, respectively, for patients in the systemically untreated regimen (CT –) and patients in the C/CMF arm (CT +). **b** Overall survival by continuous ROR score for 0–5 years and 5+ years after randomization, respectively. Hazard ratios and corresponding 95% CI for a 10-point difference in continuous ROR score are shown

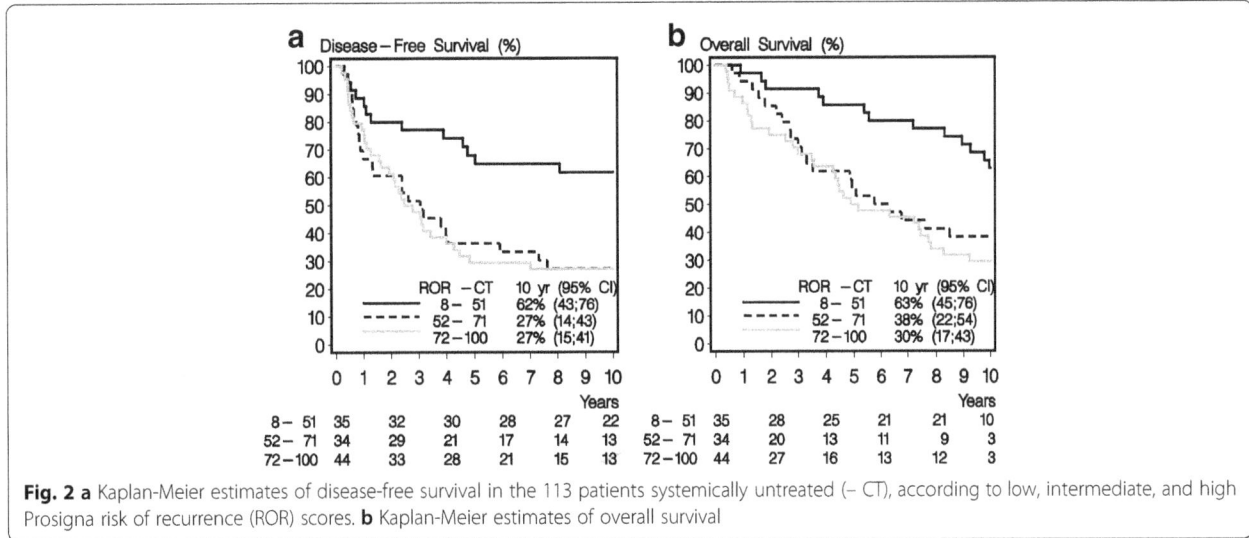

Fig. 2 a Kaplan-Meier estimates of disease-free survival in the 113 patients systemically untreated (– CT), according to low, intermediate, and high Prosigna risk of recurrence (ROR) scores. **b** Kaplan-Meier estimates of overall survival

was no significant effect of the ROR score on treatment; for the continuous ROR score $P_{interaction} = 0.66$ for DFS and $P_{interaction} = 0.32$ for OS, in unadjusted models. The benefit for DFS was significant for both intervals of intermediate (52–71) and high (72–100) Prosigna ROR scores, whereas there was a smaller, non-significant benefit for low (0–51) ROR scores, although interactions between ROR score groups and benefit of chemotherapy were not statistically significant (Table 2 for unadjusted results) ($P_{interaction} = 0.47$), also true for OS ($P_{interaction} = 0.24$). The HR for impact of the continuous ROR as the impact of the predefined intervals remained largely unchanged following adjustment for patients and tumor characteristics (Fig. 3a and b).

Prosigna has been validated and is indicated for use in ER+, Her2– disease only, therefore, an underpowered but planned exploratory analysis of DFS in the ER+, Her2- subset was also executed using the risk groups defined by the commercial cut point of low-risk ROR ≤ 40.

A benefit from chemotherapy was observed in the high-risk group (HR = 0.48, 95% CI, 0.33 to 0.69) while no benefit was demonstrated in the low-risk group (HR = 1.13, 95% CI, 0.42 to 3.07); however, no there was no statistically significant interaction between ROR risk groups and treatment effect (unadjusted $P_{interaction} = 0.11$) (Additional file 2: Figure S2) and (adjusted $P_{interaction} = 0.10$).

Effect of chemotherapy for Prosigna intrinsic subtype groups

For the second co-primary objective, we examined the association between Prosigna intrinsic subtypes and benefit of chemotherapy. A significant interaction was observed between Prosigna subtype and treatment (Table 2) for DFS ($P_{interaction} = 0.003$) and OS ($P_{interaction} = 0.04$), with the subtypes included separately. Statistically significant interactions between the Prosigna subtypes and treatment remained after multivariate adjustment both for DFS

Table 2 Unadjusted HR estimates of the treatment effect for DFS and OS according to Prosigna ROR scores and subtype

	DFS			OS		
	HR	(95% CI)	$P_{interaction}$	HR	(95% CI)	$P_{interaction}$
ROR score			0.47			0.24
Low tertile	0.79	(0.42–1.47)		1.09	(0.70–1.71)	
Intermediate tertile	0.49	(0.30–0.79)		0.75	(0.50–1.13)	
High tertile	0.64	(0.42–0.98)		0.66	(0.46–0.96)	
Subtype			0.003			0.04
Luminal A	0.64	(0.36–1.14)		0.96	(0.62–1.48)	
Luminal B	0.47	(0.28–0.77)		0.51	(0.33–0.77)	
Basal-like	0.19	(0.09–0.40)		0.52	(0.24–1.12)	
Her2-enriched	1.04	(0.62–1.75)		1.10	(0.71–1.71)	

DFS disease-free survival, *OS* overall survival, *HR* hazard ratio, *ROR* risk of recurrence, *95% CI* 95% confidence interval, *$P_{interaction}$* P derived from a Wald test for heterogeneity, *Her2* human epidermal growth factor receptor 2

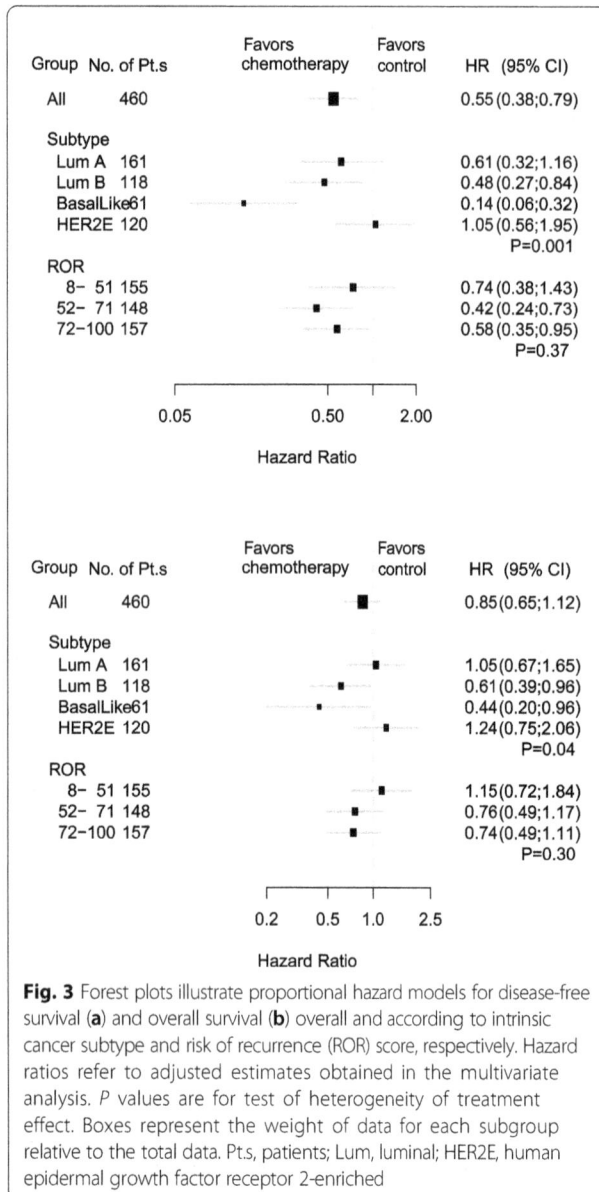

Fig. 3 Forest plots illustrate proportional hazard models for disease-free survival (**a**) and overall survival (**b**) overall and according to intrinsic cancer subtype and risk of recurrence (ROR) score, respectively. Hazard ratios refer to adjusted estimates obtained in the multivariate analysis. P values are for test of heterogeneity of treatment effect. Boxes represent the weight of data for each subgroup relative to the total data. Pt.s, patients; Lum, luminal; HER2E, human epidermal growth factor receptor 2-enriched

($P_{adjusted}$ = 0.52) or from those with non-Luminal A subtype tumors combined ($P_{adjusted}$ = 0.87). For OS the corresponding figures are $P_{adjusted}$ = 0.09 and $P_{adjusted}$ = 0.32.

Discussion

Premenopausal patients with high-risk breast cancer are generally recommended chemotherapy, but our study suggests that patients with tumors from different intrinsic molecular subtypes do not benefit equally from cyclophosphamide or CMF-based adjuvant chemotherapy. When considering a heterogeneous population of patients with ER+/– and Her2+/– disease, the continuous Prosigna ROR score was shown to be significantly associated with prognosis. The Prosigna ROR score was not significantly predictive of treatment effect in a population combining ER+/– and Her2+/– patients. However, the biology of these disease subtypes is dramatically different and it is not unexpected that a score developed to predict disease recurrence in ER+ Her2– patients does not predict benefit from chemotherapy across all ER+/– and Her2+/– patients. By focusing on the more homogenous population of ER+, Her2– patients we did observe a benefit from chemotherapy in the high-risk population and no benefit in the low-risk population though similarly, we found no statistically significant heterogeneity of treatment effect according to ROR score. This subset analysis was hindered by the limited number of patients included, especially for the group not treated with chemotherapy.

More crucially, a significantly different and clinically relevant benefit was obtained based on the major intrinsic subtypes as assigned by Prosigna. The use of cyclophosphamide-based chemotherapy in patients with basal-like breast cancer was associated with an 86% relative reduction in DFS events and a 56% relative reduction in mortality. Patients with luminal B disease also had a statistically significant benefit from chemotherapy, albeit to a lesser degree (39% reduction in DFS events and in mortality). In contrast, patients with tumors of the Her2-enriched subtype and luminal A subtype obtained no statistically measurable benefit. The gain obtained by patients with a luminal A subtype however, did not significantly differ from those with a luminal B nor from those with a non-luminal A subtype taken together.

This heterogeneity in benefit from chemotherapy according to the intrinsic subtypes explains the lack of association between the ROR score and benefit from chemotherapy in the overall population. Though the tumors with the lowest ROR are the luminal A subtype, with little sensitivity to chemotherapy, a large proportion of patients with basal-like breast cancer were assigned intermediate ROR scores and saw a large benefit from chemotherapy and most of the chemotherapy-insensitive

(Fig. 3a) and OS (Fig. 3b). Patients with a basal-like subtype of breast cancer had a pronounced benefit from cyclophosphamide-based adjuvant chemotherapy (unadjusted HR, 0.19; 95% CI, 0.09 to 0.40), and a marked benefit was also obtained by those with the luminal B subtype (unadjusted HR, 0.47; 95% CI, 0.28 to 0.77) (Fig. 4). While there was significant benefit from chemotherapy on DFS in both the subgroups with basal-like and luminal B subtype breast cancer, there was no effect in women with Her2-enriched tumors, and a less pronounced effect in those with luminal A tumors ($P_{adjusted}$ = 0.001). The benefit was not significantly different in patients with the luminal A subtype from those with the luminal B subtype

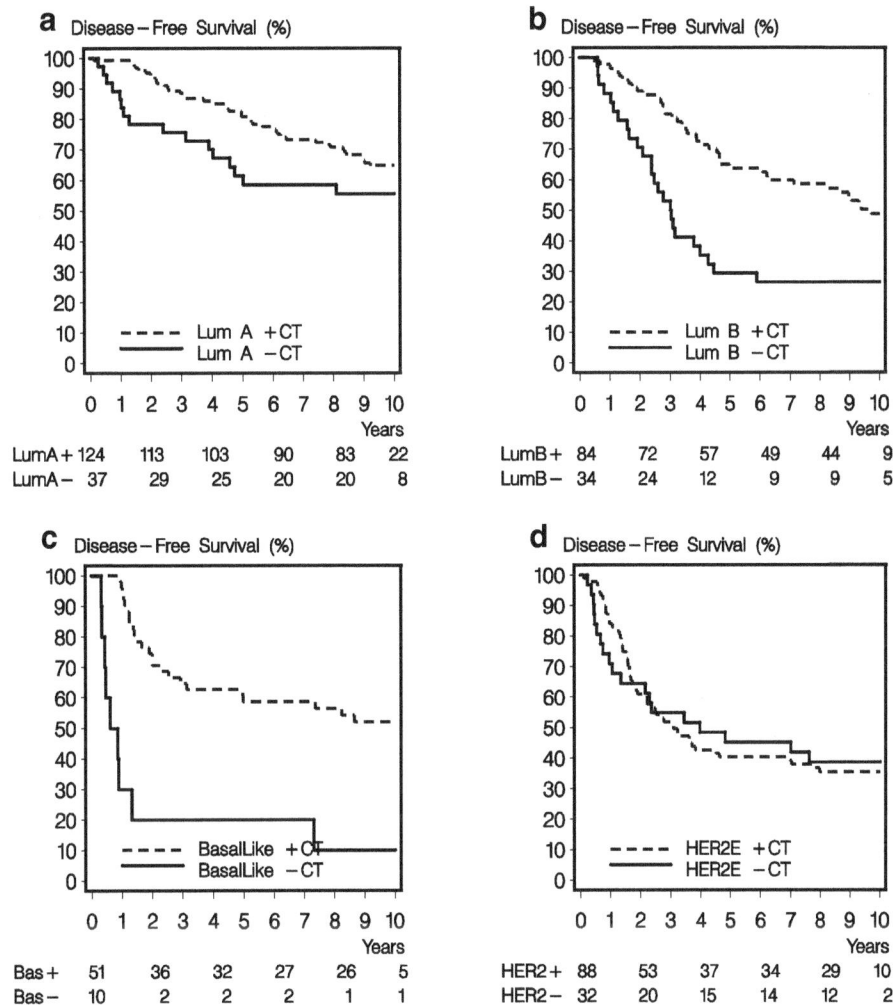

Fig. 4 Kaplan-Meier estimates of disease-free survival in patients with luminal (Lum) A (**a**), luminal B (**b**), basal-like (**c**), and human epidermal growth factor receptor 2-enriched (HER2-E) (**d**) breast cancer in the systemically untreated arm (–CT) and in the cyclophosphamide/cyclophosphamide, methotrexate and fluorouracil arm (+CT)

Her2-enriched tumors were assigned high ROR scores. Consequently, within the overall population there is not a monotonic relationship between the ROR score and benefit from chemotherapy. However, when focusing on the ER+/Her2– population, we found a more direct relationship between risk and benefit from chemotherapy, although the analysis in this subset was not powered to show an interaction.

Our results are complementary to the results from the NCIC-CTG MA.5 trial, where all patients were treated with adjuvant chemotherapy but were randomized to CMF or CEF. Cheang and colleagues showed no added benefit in basal-like breast cancer but identified a substantial benefit in Her2-enriched high-risk breast cancer from the anthracycline-containing CEF chemotherapy as compared to CMF [7]. The MA.5 and DBCG 89D trials and a pooled analysis with three

additional phase III trials showed a greater benefit of anthracyclines in patients with *TOP2A* alterations and a trend towards greater benefit in patients with Her2-amplified tumors [12–15]. More recently, the DBCG READ trial gave no evidence to support a benefit from anthracyclines in patients with early *TOP2A*-normal breast cancer while the Anthracyclines in early breast cancer (ABC) trials suggested that patients with Her2-normal breast cancer derive some benefit from anthracyclines [16, 17]. The association between the Her2-enriched subtype and alteration of *TOP2A* has not yet been clarified but may improve the clinical utility of both markers. Finally, retrospective analyses of clinical studies in the metastatic setting have shown that the intrinsic subtype may predict benefit from other specific cytotoxic agents such as gemcitabine [18] and docetaxel [19]. Together these studies emphasize that the potential benefit to patients with breast cancer from establishing an association between intrinsic subtype and type of chemotherapy could be significant.

In this subset we showed a distribution of subtypes that differs from that previously demonstrated by immunohistochemical analysis (IHC) using tissue microarrays constructed from 633 patients participating in the DBCG 77B trial [11]. The treatment effect appear less segregated between the luminal A and B subtypes using Prosigna compared to IHC, presumably due to the smaller percentage of luminal A tumors identified by the IHC definition employed in the previous study. In contrast, the effect obtained by an IHC definition of core-basal cancer was less pronounced compared to basal breast cancers as defined by Prosigna [11]. While separate studies have shown that nucleic acid-based methods surpass the analytical reproducibility of IHC, our study confirms that genomic-based tests provide also additional information on clinical benefit compared to IHC surrogates [20, 21].

Due to the very old age of the DBCG77B study, we were only able to collect tumor blocks to be used for messenger (m)RNA testing from 623 of the original 1146 patients, and samples from the no chemotherapy arms (which were closed early and recruited smaller numbers of patients) were particularly sparse (Additional file 1: Figure S1), reducing study power compared to the original [2] and even to subsequent IHC studies [11] for which more cases were available. As a consequence, the ability to conduct subgroup analysis has been limited e.g. the possible influence of chemotherapy-induced amenorrhea, which may have been particularly important in patients with luminal cancers.

Beyond power concerns, this study has other potential limitations. First, the retrospective evaluation of only a subset of patients in the biomarker analysis introduces a risk of bias and a residual risk may persist despite adjustments in the multivariate analyses. Second, the 77B study samples analyzed here had been stored for almost 40 years resulting in significant degradation in the mRNA in the samples. This degradation was evident in the higher rate of samples that were unevaluable by the assay (22%) compared to 1% in a previous study using samples banked for a median of 10 years [22]. DBCG77B only employed cyclophosphamide or classic CMF and benefit of a more pronounced effect could potentially have been obtained by more contemporary adjuvant chemotherapy. The contribution from cyclophosphamide might, however, have been inseparable from the contributions of anthracyclines, taxanes, endocrine therapy, and Her2-targeted therapy, if these treatments were combined. A possible association between molecular tumor subtype and the individual drugs may in later

studies be obtained by identifying trials with successive addition of anthracyclines and taxanes.

Strengths of this study include use of patients with high-risk breast cancer derived from a phase III randomized trial without any biomarker selection. The inclusion of a control group who were not systemically treated was crucial for our ability to isolate associations between intrinsic subtypes by Prosigna and treatment effect from cyclophosphamide based-chemotherapy. In addition, our study adhered carefully to the ReMARK guidelines [23], and used the validated and Food and Drug Association (FDA)-cleared Prosigna assay following standard operating procedures as specified by the manufacturer [24].

Conclusions

In summary, this study demonstrates that the Prosigna assay is both prognostic and predictive of benefit from cyclophosphamide-based adjuvant chemotherapy in premenopausal patients with high-risk breast cancer. These results provide further evidence that the high-risk intrinsic subtypes of breast cancer have highly differential responses to cyclophosphamide-based chemotherapy regimens, with clear benefit in the basal-like and luminal B subtypes.

Abbreviations
ABC: Anthracyclines in early breast cancer; C: Cyclophosphamide; CI: Confidence interval; CMF: Cyclophosphamide, methotrexate and fluorouracil; DBCG: Danish Breast Cancer Group; DFS: Disease-free survival; EBCTCG: Early Breast Cancer Trialists' Collaborative Group; ER: Estrogen receptor; FFPE: Formalin-fixed, paraffin-embedded blocks; Her2: Human epidermal growth factor receptor 2; Her2-E: Human epidermal growth factor receptor 2-enriched; HR: Hazard ratios; IHC: Immunohistochemistry; OS: Overall survival; PAM50: Prediction analysis of microarray 50; ROR: Risk of recurrence

Acknowledgements
We thank the Danish women who participated in this study.

Funding
The Danish Breast Cancer Cooperative Group (DBCG) prepared the original protocol (DBCG 77B) and was the sponsor of the study. Funding was not provided to the participating departments. Nanostring Technologies, Inc. kindly made the NanoString nCounter platform available, and paid expenses for the study.

Authors' contributions
Conceptualization: MBJ, AVL, TON, WB, SF, BE. Methodology: MBJ, AVL, TON, WB, SF, BE. Validation: all authors. Formal analysis: MBJ. Investigation: all authors. Resources: MBJ, AVL, JOE, PW, TH, NR, WB, SF, BE. Data curation: MBJ, AVL, JOE, PW, TH, NR, WB, SF, BE. Writing the original draft: MBJ, BE. Writing - review and editing: all authors. Visualization: MBJ, BE. Supervision: AVL, BE. Project administration: MBJ, AVL, BE. All authors read and approved the final manuscript.

Competing interests
MBJ: None. AVL: Nanostring Technologies, Inc.: grant, Roche: grant. TON:

Nanostring Technologies, Inc.: personal fees, non-financial support, other: licensing agreement, patent. JOE: none. PW: none. TH: Nanostring Technologies, Inc.: personal fees, other: employee and stock. NR: Nanostring Technologies, Inc.: personal fees: employee. WB: Nanostring Technologies, Inc.: personal fees: employee. SF: Nanostring Technologies, Inc.: other: employee and stock, patent. BE: Nanostring Technologies, Inc.:grant: institutional. Novartis: grant: institutional. Roche: Grant: institutional.

Author details

[1]Danish Breast Cancer Cooperative Group, Rigshospitalet, Copenhagen University Hospital, DBCG Secretariat, Bldg. 2501 Rigshospitalet, Blegdamsvej 9, DK-2100 Copenhagen, Denmark. [2]Department of Surgical Pathology, Zealand University Hospital, Slagelse, Denmark. [3]Department of Pathology and Laboratory Medicine, University of British Columbia, Vancouver, BC, Canada. [4]NanoString Technologies, Inc, Seattle, WA, USA. [5]Danish Breast Cancer Cooperative Group, Department of Oncology, Rigshospitalet, Copenhagen University Hospital, Copenhagen, Denmark.

References

1. Bonadonna G, Brusamolino E, Valagussa P, Rossi A, Brugnatelli L, Brambilla C, et al. Combination chemotherapy as an adjuvant treatment in operable breast cancer. N Engl J Med. 1976;294:405–10.
2. Ejlertsen B, Mouridsen HT, Jensen MB, Andersen J, Andersson M, Kamby C, et al. Cyclophosphamide, methotrexate, and fluorouracil; oral cyclophosphamide; levamisole; or no adjuvant therapy for patients with high-risk, premenopausal breast cancer. Cancer. 2010;116(9):2081–9.
3. Anonymous. Adjuvant chemotherapy of breast cancer. NIH consensus development conference, July 14–16, 1980. Cancer Treat Res. 1992;60:371–4.
4. Early Breast Cancer Trialists' Collaborative Group (EBCTCG). Effects of chemotherapy and hormonal therapy for early breast cancer on recurrence and 15-year survival: an overview of the randomised trials. Lancet. 2005;365: 1687–717.
5. Peto R, Davies C, Godwin J, Gray R, Pan HC, Clarke M, et al. Comparisons between different polychemotherapy regimens for early breast cancer: meta-analyses of long-term outcome among 100,000 women in 123 randomised trials. Lancet. 2012;379:432–44.
6. Perou CM, Sorlie T, Eisen MB, van de Rijn M, Jeffrey SS, Rees CA, et al. Molecular portraits of human breast tumours. Nature. 2000;406(6797):747–52.
7. Cheang MC, Voduc KD, Tu D, Jiang S, Leung S, Chia SK, et al. Responsiveness of intrinsic subtypes to adjuvant anthracycline substitution in the NCIC.CTG MA.5 randomized trial. Clin Cancer Res. 2012;18(8):2402–12.
8. Albain KS, Barlow WE, Shak S, Hortobagyi GN, Livingston RB, Yeh IT, et al. Prognostic and predictive value of the 21-gene recurrence score assay in postmenopausal women with node-positive, oestrogen-receptor-positive breast cancer on chemotherapy: a retrospective analysis of a randomised trial. Lancet Oncol. 2010;11(1):55–65.
9. Wallden B, Storhoff J, Nielsen T, Dowidar N, Schaper C, Ferree S, et al. Development and verification of the PAM50-based Prosigna breast cancer gene signature assay. BMC Med Genet. 2015;8:54.
10. Gnant M, Filipits M, Greil R, Stoeger H, Rudas M, Bago-Horvath Z, et al. Austrian Breast and Colorectal Cancer Study Group. Predicting distant recurrence in receptor-positive breast cancer patients with limited clinicopathological risk: using the PAM50 risk of recurrence score in 1478 postmenopausal patients of the ABCSG-8 trial treated with adjuvant endocrine therapy alone. Ann Oncol. 2014;25(2):339–45.
11. Nielsen TO, Jensen MB, Burugu S, Gao D, Joergensen CL, Balslev E, et al. High-risk premenopausal luminal a breast cancer patients derive no benefit from adjuvant cyclophosphamide-based chemotherapy: results from the DBCG77B clinical trial. Clin Cancer Res. 2017;23(4):946–53.
12. Ejlertsen B, Mouridsen HT, Jensen MB, Andersen J, Cold S, Edlund P, et al. Improved outcome from substituting methotrexate with epirubicin: results from a randomised comparison of CMF versus CEF in patients with primary breast cancer. Eur J Cancer. 2007;43:877–84.
13. Knoop AS, Knudsen H, Balslev E, Rasmussen BB, Overgaard J, Nielsen KV, et al. Retrospective analysis of topoisomerase IIa amplifications and deletions as predictive markers in primary breast cancer patients randomly assigned to cyclophosphamide, methotrexate, and fluorouracil or cyclophosphamide, epirubicin, and fluorouracil: Danish breast Cancer cooperative group. J Clin Oncol. 2005;23:7483–90.
14. O'Malley FP, Chia S, Tu D, Shepherd LE, Levine MN, Bramwell VH, et al. Topoisomerase II alpha and responsiveness of breast cancer to adjuvant chemotherapy. J Natl Cancer Inst. 2009;101(9):644–50.
15. Di Leo A, Desmedt C, Bartlett JM, Piette F, Ejlertsen B, Pritchard KI, et al. HER2/TOP2A meta-analysis study group. HER2 and TOP2A as predictive markers for anthracycline-containing chemotherapy regimens as adjuvant treatment of breast cancer: a meta-analysis of individual patient data. Lancet Oncol. 2011;12:1134–42.
16. Ejlertsen B, Tuxen MK, Jakobsen EH, Jensen MB, Knoop AS, Hoejris I, et al. Adjuvant cyclophosphamide and docetaxel with or without epirubicin for early TOP2A-normal breast cancer: DBCG 07-READ, an open-label, phase III, randomized trial. J Clin Oncol. 2017;35:2639–46.
17. Blum JL, Flynn PJ, Yothers G, Asmar L, Geyer CE Jr, Jacobs SA, et al. Anthracyclines in early breast cancer: the ABC trials–USOR 06-090, NSABP B-46-I/USOR 07132, and NSABP B-49 (NRG oncology). J Clin Oncol. 2017; 35(23):2647–55.
18. Joergensen CL, Nielsen TO, Bjerre KD, Liu S, Wallden B, Balslev E, et al. PAM50 breast cancer intrinsic subtypes and effect of gemcitabine in advanced breast cancer patients. Acta Oncol. 2014;53(6):776–87.
19. Tutt A, Ellis P, Kilburn L, Gilett C, Pinder S, Abraham J, et al. TNT: A randomized phase III trial of carboplatin compared with docetaxel for patients with metastatic or recurrent locally advanced triple negative or BRCA1/2 breast cancer. 2014 San Antonio Breast Cancer Symposium. Abstract S3-01. Presented December 11, 2014.
20. Gluz O, Liedtke C, Huober J, Peyro-Saint-Paul H, Kates RE, Kreipe HH, et al. Comparison of prognostic and predictive impact of genomic and central grade and immunohistochemical subtypes or IHC4 in HR+/HER2- early breast cancer: WSG-AGO EC-doc trial. Ann Oncol. 2016;27(6):1035–40.
21. Nielsen TO, Parker JS, Leung S, Voduc D, Ebbert M, Vickery T, et al. A comparison of PAM50 intrinsic subtyping with immunohistochemistry and clinical prognostic factors in tamoxifen-treated estrogen receptor-positive breast cancer. Clin Cancer Res. 2010;16(21):5222–32.
22. Laenkholm, AV, Jensen MB, Eriksen JO, Kiboell T, Rasmussen BB, Knoop AS, et al. Prediction of 10yr distant recurrence (DR) using the Prosigna (PAM50) assay in a Danish Breast Cancer Cooperative Group (DBCG) cohort of postmenopausal Danish women with hormone receptor-positive (HR+) early breast cancer (EBC) allocated to 5 yr of endocrine therapy (ET) alone. J Clin Oncol 2015; 33(suppl; abstr 546).
23. Altman DG, McShane LM, Sauerbrei W, Taube SE. Reporting recommendations for tumor marker prognostic studies (REMARK): explanation and elaboration. PLoS Med. 2012;9(5):e1001216.
24. Nielsen T, Wallden B, Schaper C, Ferree S, Liu S, Gao D, et al. Analytical validation of the PAM50-based Prosigna breast Cancer prognostic gene signature assay and nCounter analysis system using formalin-fixed paraffin-embedded breast tumor specimens. BMC Cancer. 2014;14:177.

11

Estrogen promotes estrogen receptor negative BRCA1-deficient tumor initiation and progression

Chuying Wang[1,2], Feng Bai[2*], Li-han Zhang[2], Alexandria Scott[2], Enxiao Li[1*] and Xin-Hai Pei[2,3*] (iD)

Abstract

Background: Estrogen promotes breast cancer development and progression mainly through estrogen receptor (ER). However, blockage of estrogen production or action prevents development of and suppresses progression of ER-negative breast cancers. How estrogen promotes ER-negative breast cancer development and progression is poorly understood. We previously discovered that deletion of cell cycle inhibitors p16^{Ink4a} (p16) or p18^{Ink4c} (p18) is required for development of *Brca1*-deficient basal-like mammary tumors, and that mice lacking *p18* develop luminal-type mammary tumors.

Methods: A genetic model system with three mouse strains, one that develops ER-positive mammary tumors (*p18* single deletion) and the others that develop ER-negative tumors (*p16;Brca1* and *p18;Brca1* compound deletion), human *BRCA1* mutant breast cancer patient-derived xenografts, and human *BRCA1*-deficient and *BRCA1*-proficient breast cancer cells were used to determine the role of estrogen in activating epithelial-mesenchymal transition (EMT), stimulating cell proliferation, and promoting ER-negative mammary tumor initiation and metastasis.

Results: Estrogen stimulated the proliferation and tumor-initiating potential of both ER-positive *Brca1*-proficient and ER-negative *Brca1*-deficient tumor cells. Estrogen activated EMT in a subset of *Brca1*-deficient mammary tumor cells that maintained epithelial features, and enhanced the number of cancer stem cells, promoting tumor progression and metastasis. Estrogen activated EMT independent of ER in *Brca1*-deficient, but not *Brca1*-proficient, tumor cells. Estrogen activated the AKT pathway in *BRCA1*-deficient tumor cells independent of ER, and pharmaceutical inhibition of AKT activity suppressed EMT and cell proliferation preventing *BRCA1* deficient tumor progression.

Conclusions: This study reveals for the first time that estrogen promotes *BRCA1*-deficient tumor initiation and progression by stimulation of cell proliferation and activation of EMT, which are dependent on AKT activation and independent of ER.

Keywords: Estrogen, Estrogen receptor, BRCA1, EMT, Cancer stem cells

Background

Estrogen plays a critical role in promoting breast cancer development and progression in addition to normal breast development [1, 2]. Although estrogen acts mainly through the estrogen receptor (ER), ovariectomy, blockage of estrogen action, or inhibition of estrogen synthesis can prevent the development of and suppress the progression of ER-negative breast cancers [3, 4]. In addition to stimulation of proliferation and induction of DNA damage in both ER-positive and ER-negative cells [1, 2], estrogen activates an epithelial-mesenchymal transition (EMT) program in ER-positive breast cancer cells to promote their stemness and invasiveness in vitro [5, 6]. Notably, it has recently been reported that estrogen promotes the number and function of ER-negative breast cancer stem cells (CSCs) through paracrine signaling produced in ER-positive cells in response to

---

* Correspondence: fbai@med.miami.edu; doclienxiao@sina.com; xhpei@med.miami.edu
[2]Molecular Oncology Program, Division of Surgical Oncology, Dewitt Daughtry Family Department of Surgery, University of Miami, Miami, FL 33136, USA
[1]Department of Medical Oncology, The First Affiliated hospital of Xi'an Jiaotong University, Xi'an, Shaanxi 710061, People's Republic of China
Full list of author information is available at the end of the article

estrogen [7, 8]. Whether and how estrogen promotes ER-negative breast cancer development and progression are poorly understood.

Breast cancer comprises, among others, three main subtypes: human epidermal growth factor receptor 2 (HER2)-positive, ER-positive luminal, and ER-negative basal-like breast cancers (BLBCs) [9]. Luminal-type tumors respond to hormone therapy. BLBCs are poorly differentiated and the most lethal, which is partly due to their enrichment of CSCs that are thought to drive clinical relapse and metastasis [10, 11]. The CSCs can be generated from luminal tumor cells by the EMT program [12, 13]. BLBCs may originate from luminal progenitors and contain a number of distinct cell types including cells that express luminal, basal, and mesenchymal biomarkers [14–19]. More than half of BLBCs are associated with functional loss of BRCA1 caused by germline or somatic mutation, or promoter methylation [9, 20, 21]. We and others have demonstrated that depletion of Brca1 in mice activates EMT and induces highly heterogeneous BLBCs [18, 22, 23]. Most importantly, only a part of the cells in both human and mouse BRCA1-deficient tumors exhibit mesenchymal features [18, 22–24], suggesting that a subset of BRCA1-deficient tumor cells have undergone EMT. Whether and how estrogen activates EMT in BRCA1-deficient, ER-negative basal-like tumor cells to promote their tumor initiation and progression remain elusive.

The phosphatidylinositol-3-kinase (PI3K)/AKT signaling pathway regulates cell proliferation, survival, metabolism, EMT, and stem cell fate [25–27], and is aberrantly activated in 77% of breast cancers [9], including BRCA1-deficient disease [28]. BRCA1 deficiency activates the PI3K/AKT pathway in immortalized fibroblasts and tumor cells by accumulating nuclear AKT [29]. Estrogen activates the PI3K/AKT pathway in both an ER-dependent and ER-independent manner [30, 31]. Estrogen also promotes the survival of Brca1-deficient tumor cells and mammary epithelial cells (MECs) [30]. Inhibition of the PI3K/AKT pathway reduces proliferation of Brca1-deficient mouse embryonic fibroblasts (MEFs) suppressing the growth of tumors generated by Brca1-deficient MEFs [28]. Whether estrogen promotes EMT and proliferation of ER-negative BRCA1-deficient tumor cells through activation of the PI3K/AKT pathway remains elusive.

The RB family of proteins (RB, p107, p130) that are phosphorylated and inactivated by CDK4 and CDK6 (CDK4/6), control the G1-to-S transition of the cell cycle. CDK4/6 are inhibited by inhibitors of CDK4/6 (INK4) including p16^{INK4A} (p16) and p18^{INK4C} (p18) [32]. Inactivation of the INK4-CDK4/6-RB pathway is a common event in breast cancers [9, 32]. p16 is inactivated in ~ 30% of and p18 expression is frequently reduced in human breast cancers [9, 32]. RB is a major target for genomic disruption in BRCA1 mutant human breast cancers, and most BRCA1-deficient BLBCs carry a dysfunctional INK4-CDK4/6-RB pathway [9, 33, 34]. All widely used BRCA1 mutant breast cancer cell lines have deletions in either RB or p16 [35, 36], reflecting the importance of inactivation of the INK4-CDK4/6-RB pathway in the proliferation of BRCA1-deficient tumor cells. We and others have reported that mice lacking p18 or Rb and p107 develop luminal-type mammary tumors [37, 38], suggesting a role of the RB pathway in controlling luminal tumorigenesis. BRCA1 deficiency in human and mouse MECs activates INK4-CDK4/6-RB pathway, inducing premature senescence [19, 39, 40]. We demonstrated that deletion of either p16 or p18 in mice rescues the premature senescence of MECs caused by Brca1 deficiency, and that p16;Brca1 and p18;Brca1 double-mutant mice develop BLBCs with EMT features [19, 23, 39]. These mutant mice provide unique mouse models to study the role of Brca1 in the suppression of EMT and basal-like mammary tumorigenesis.

In this report, we used p16;Brca1 and p18;Brca1 double-mutant mammary tumors and human BRCA1 mutant breast cancer patient-derived xenografts (PDX) to determine the function and mechanism of estrogen in promoting ER-negative BRCA1-deficient tumor initiation and progression. We demonstrate that estrogen promotes BRCA1-deficient tumor initiation and progression by stimulation of cell proliferation and activation of EMT, which are dependent on AKT activation, but independent of ER.

Methods
Mice, histopathologic analysis, and immunostaining
The generation of p18$^{-/-}$, p18$^{-/-}$;Brca1^{MGKO} (p18$^{-/-}$; Brca1$^{f/f}$;MMTV-Cre or p18$^{-/-}$;Brca1$^{f/-}$;MMTV-Cre) and p16$^{-/-}$;Brca1^{MGKO} (p16$^{-/-}$;Brca1$^{f/f}$;MMTV-Cre or p16$^{-/-}$; Brca1$^{f/-}$;MMTV-Cre) mice has been described previously [23, 37, 39]. The Institutional Animal Care and Use Committee at the University of Miami approved all animal procedures. Histopathologic analysis and immunohistochemical analysis (IHC) were performed as described previously [19, 23, 37]. The primary antibodies used were Ck14 (Thermal Scientific), ERα (Santa Cruz), p-Akt (Ser473), p-4E-bp1 (Thr37/46), vimentin (Vim), E-cadherin (E-cad), p-Fra1 (Ser265) (Cell Signaling), Ki67 and fibronectin (Fn) (Abcam). Immunocomplexes were detected using the Vectastain ABC DAB kit according to the manufacturer's instructions (Vector Laboratories) or by using Alexa Fluor 488-conjugated or Alexa Fluor 594-conjugated secondary antibodies (Biolegend). The positive results of IHC were quantified by the H score, as previously described [41].

Mammary and tumor cell preparation, fluorescence-activated cell sorting (FACS) analysis, cell sorting, and tumorsphere formation assay

Mammary glands and tumors were dissected from female mice and cell suspensions were prepared as previously described [19, 23, 37]. For surface marker analysis; mammary and tumor cells were isolated, stained, and analyzed as previously described [23, 37]. Briefly, cells were stained with anti-CD24-PE (BD Pharmingen), anti-CD29-FITC (Biolegend, San Diego, CA, USA), biotinylated and allophycocyanin (APC)-conjugated CD45, CD31 and TER119 antibodies (BD Pharmingen), and Violet dye (Dead Cell Stain, ThermoFisher Scientific). For intracellular staining of Vim, 1×10^6 cells were fixed with 4% paraformaldehyde and permeabilized with 90% methanol. Anti-Vim was added as primary antibody and Alexa Fluor 594 anti-rabbit (Invitrogen) as secondary antibody. For intracellular staining of ERα, cells were fixed and permeabilized with the Cytofix/Cytoperm fixation/permeabilization kit (BD Pharmingen). ERα staining was performed according to the manufacturer's instructions. For bromodeoxyuridine (BrdU) incorporation, tumor cells were labeled with 10 μM BrdU (Sigma) for 1.5 h, fixed with 75% ethanol, and permeabilized with 2 M HCl. The cells were then stained with fluorescein isothiocyanate (FITC)-conjugated anti-BrdU (Cell Signaling) and propidium iodide (PI) and analyzed by flow cytometry. FACS was performed using the LSR-Fortessa machine (BD Pharmingen). Data analysis was performed using Kaluza software (Beckman Coulter). To isolate tumor cells depleted of hematopoietic and endothelial cells, we stained mammary tumor cells with biotinylated and APC-conjugated CD45, CD31 and TER119 antibodies and Violet dye. Lin⁻ (CD45⁻, CD31⁻, TER119⁻) living (Violet dye negative) cells were sorted on a BD FACS SORP Aria-IIu machine. For tumorsphere formation assay, 30,000 $p18^{-/-}$; $Brca1^{MGKO}$ mammary tumor cells were plated in triplicate ultra-low attachment plates with or without addition of 17β-estradiol (E2, Sigma) in serum-free DMEM-F12 supplemented with B27, epidermal growth factor (EGF), and basic fibroblast growth factor (bFGF) as described [23, 37]. The number and size of tumorspheres formed were calculated after 7 days.

Cell culture, treatment, cell viability assay and western blot analysis

MCF7 and SUM149 cells were cultured per American Type Culture Collection (ATCC) recommendations. Primary murine mammary tumor cells were cultured in phenol-free DMEM/F12 (Gibco), with 10% charcoal-stripped FBS (Gibco), 10 μg/ml insulin, and 10 ng/ml EGF. For treatment of estrogen, AZD5363, and 4OHT, tumor cells were cultured in 10% charcoal-stripped FBS in the presence of E2, AZD5363 (ApexBio Technology), 4OHT (Sigma), or

dimethyl sulfoxide (DMSO) for the indicated times and then collected for further analysis. To determine cell viability, 50,000 cells were plated in 24-well plates and treated with DMSO or drugs at the indicated concentrations for 5 days. Viable cell numbers were determined on day 1, day 3, and day 5 by an automatic cell counter (Bio-rad) with trypan blue exclusion. For western blot, tissue and cell lysates were prepared as previously reported [19, 23, 37]. Primary antibodies used are as follows: HSP90 (Santa Cruz), Gapdh (Ambion), ERα (Santa cruz), Brca1, p-Akt (Ser473), p-4E-bp1 (Thr37/46), p-mTor (Ser2248), p-Gsk3β (Ser9), E-cad, Vim, Snail, Slug, p-Fra1 (Ser 265), p-Rb (ser780) (Cell Signaling) and Fn (Abcam).

Transplantation, analysis of metastasis, and tumor treatment

For mammary tumor cell transplantation, cells were suspended in a 50% solution of Matrigel (BD) and then inoculated into the left and/or right inguinal mammary fat pads (MFPs) of 6–8-week-old female NSG mice (Jackson Laboratory) respectively. At 6 or 7 weeks after transplantation, animals were euthanized and mammary tumors were dissected for histopathological, immunohistochemical, and biochemical analyses. For PDX tumor tissue transplantation, 4 mm × 2 mm tissue fragments prepared from BRCA1 mutant PDX tumors (TM00091, Jax lab) were transplanted into MFPs of 4-week-old female NSG mice. At 4 weeks after transplantation, or when tumor volume reached the maximal size that the Institutional Animal Care and Use Committee (IACUC) allowed, animals were euthanized and tumors were analyzed. For estrogen treatment in vivo, 0.72 mg E2 (SE-121, IRA, Sarasota, FL, USA) or placebo beeswax pellet was implanted subcutaneously in mice receiving tumor cell or tissue transplants. To analyze the estrogen-induced metastasis from mammary tumors, metastatic $p18^{-/-}$;$Brca1^{MGKO}$ tumor cells were inoculated into the MFPs of 4-week-old female NSG mice in which either E2 or placebo beeswax pellet was implanted subcutaneously. When newly generated tumors reached the maximum size (1.3 cm³) allowed by the IACUC in 3–6 weeks, or the mice became moribund, the lungs and other major organs were examined for detection of metastasis. For quantification of the number of metastatic nodules in the lungs, fixed lung tissues of all five lobes were sagittally sectioned at 200-μm intervals. At least three sections for each lobe were prepared and stained with H.E. The metastatic nodules in each lobe of lung tissue were confirmed by H.E. staining, counted under a microscope, and averaged. The number of nodules in all lobes was then calculated. For AZD5363 treatment of pre-existing mammary tumors, $p18^{-/-}$;$Brca1^{MGKO}$ tumor cells were transplanted into MFPs of NSG mice and allowed to reach ~ 250 mm³ in size. Mice were then treated with AZD5363 ((150 mg/kg solubilized in a 10% DMSO 25% w/v (2-Hydroxypropyl)-β-cyclodextrin buffer (Sigma)) or vehicle by oral gavage once a day. The tumor size was measured daily with a caliper. Tumor volumes were calculated as:

$$V = a \times b^2/2$$

where "a" is the largest diameter and "b" is the smallest. Statistical significance was evaluated using the two-tailed t test.

Statistical analysis

All data are presented as the mean ± SD for at least three repeated individual experiments for each group. Quantitative results were analyzed by the two tailed Fisher exact test or two-tailed Student's t test. $P < 0.05$ was considered statistically significant.

Results

Deletion of Brca1 in p16 and p18 null epithelia results in ER-negative mammary tumors

We previously discovered that the expression of p16 and p18 along with senescence markers was increased in MECs of $Brca1^{+/-}$ (heterozygous germline deletion of $Brca1$) and $Brca1^{MGKO}$ (specific deletion of $Brca1$ in epithelia) mice [19, 23, 39]. $p18^{-/-}$ mice in the Balb/c background developed ER-positive luminal-type mammary tumors [37] whereas $p18^{-/-};Brca1^{+/-}$ double mutant mice formed ER-negative basal-like mammary tumors [19]. We generated $p16^{-/-};Brca1^{MGKO}$ and $p18^{-/-};Brca1^{MGKO}$ double-mutant mice in the Balb/c-B6 mixed background. We found that 47% of $p18^{-/-}$, 73% of $p18^{-/-};Brca1^{MGKO}$, 60% of $p16^{-/-};Brca1^{MGKO}$, and 8% of $Brca1^{MGKO}$ mice in the Balb/c-B6 mixed background developed mammary tumors, yet no $p16^{-/-}$ mice developed mammary tumors at similar ages (Table 1 and Additional file 1: Figure S1). Though the mammary tumor incidence of $p18^{-/-}$ mice in the Balb/c-B6 mixed background was lower than those in the Balb/c background (47% vs. 83%) (Table 1 and Reference [19, 37]), $p18^{-/-}$ tumors in the Balb/c-B6 mixed

background were also predominantly ERα-positive, Ck5/CK14 negative tumors (Table 1 and Additional file 1: Figure S1). These results indicate that loss of p18 induces ER-positive mammary tumors independent of mouse genetic background. Further analysis revealed that only 18% ($n = 11$) of $p18^{-/-};Brca1^{MGKO}$ and none ($n = 6$) of $p16^{-/-};Brca1^{MGKO}$ tumors were positive for ERα. These rates were significantly lower than that of $p18^{-/-}$ tumors (71%, $n = 7$). Consistent with these results, 82% of $p18^{-/-};Brca1^{MGKO}$ and all of $p16^{-/-};Brca1^{MGKO}$ tumors were positive for Ck5 or Ck14, whereas only 29% of $p18^{-/-}$ tumors were positive for Ck5 or Ck14 (Table 1 and Additional file 1: Figure S1). These data confirm the role of Brca1 in the suppression of ER-negative, basal-like tumorigenesis in an epithelium autonomous manner.

Deletion of Brca1 stimulates the tumor-initiating potential of the tumor cells

We transplanted 10^6 primary tumor cells from three individual $p16^{-/-};Brca1^{MGKO}$ and four $p18^{-/-};Brca1^{MGKO}$ tumors into MFPs of NSG mice respectively and found that all of these cells efficiently generated tumors in 6–7 weeks. Furthermore, we found that as few as 4000 $p16^{-/-};Brca1^{MGKO}$ or $p18^{-/-};Brca1^{MGKO}$ tumor cells efficiently generated tumors in the same period (Table 2 and data not shown). In contrast, as many as 10^7 tumor cells from three individual $p18^{-/-}$ tumors did not generate tumors in 6–7 weeks when transplanted (experiment 1 in Table 2 and data not shown). Since $p16^{-/-}$ mice did not develop mammary tumors, we were unable to determine the tumor initiating potential of $p16^{-/-}$ mammary tumor cells by transplantation assay. These results suggest that the deletion of $Brca1$ enhances the tumor-initiating potential of tumor cells, which is consistent with our previous finding that loss of $Brca1$ activates EMT and induces ER-negative basal-like mammary tumors with enriched CSCs [23].

Table 1 Deletion of *Brca1* in *p18* and *p16* null epithelia induces estrogen receptor (ER)-negative mammary tumors

Genotype[a]	Mammary tumor number	ERα + tumor number	% ERα + cells/tumor	Ck5/Ck14+ tumor number	% Ck5/Ck14+ cells/tumor
Wild-type	0/9				
$p18^{-/-}$	7/15 (47%)	5/7 (71%)	2% - 50%	2/7 (29%)	2%, 5%
$Brca1^{MGKO}$ [b]	1/13 (8%)	0/1		1/1(100%)[c]	20%
$p18^{-/-};Brca1^{MGKO}$	11/15 (73%)	2/11 (18%)[d]	2%, 5%	10/11 (82%)[d]	2–80%
$p16^{-/-}$	0/20				
$p16^{-/-};Brca1^{MGKO}$	6/10 (60%)	0/6[e]		6/6(100%)[e]	2%-80%

[a]All mice were in the Balb/c-B6 mixed background and were at the age of 12–26 months
[b]$Brca1^{MGKO}$, $Brca1^{f/f}$;MMTV-Cre or $Brca1^{f/-}$;MMTV-Cre
[c]A mouse with tumor harboring p53 mutation was 24 months of age
[d]Significance for $p18^{-/-};Brca1^{MGKO}$ and $p18^{-/-}$ tumors analyzed by the two-tailed Fisher's exact test
[e]Significance for $p16^{-/-};Brca1^{MGKO}$ and $p18^{-/-}$ tumors analyzed by the two-tailed Fisher's exact test

Table 2 Brca1 deficiency promotes mammary tumor initiation

Genotype	p18^(-/-)-Donor A		p18^(-/-);Brca1^(MGKO)- Donor A
Number of tumor cell transplanted [a]	1×10^7/mouse		1×10^6/mouse
Experiment number	1	2	1
Tumor incidence [b] (7 weeks)	0/6	3/6 (50%) [c]	4/4 (100%)
Genotype	p18^(-/-)-Donor B		p16^(-/-);Brca1^(MGKO)- Donor A
Number of tumor cell transplanted [a]	3×10^6/mouse		1×10^6/mouse
Experiment number	1	2	1
Tumor incidence (6 weeks)	0/6	1/4 (25%) [c]	4/4 (100%)

[a]Unsorted primary tumor cells were used
[b]Tumors generated larger than 12mm^3 in size were counted
[c]Tumor cells were transplanted into MFPs of NSG mice with E2 supplement. A statistical significance from E2-treated and non-E2 treated groups combining both p18^(-/-)-Donor A and -B transplants by two tailed Fisher Exact test

Generation of transplantable ER-negative Brca1-deficient mammary tumor models

In mammary and tumor cells ERα expression is restricted to the CD24$^+$CD29^{low} luminal population while the CD24$^+$CD29^{high} population is ERα negative while also enriched with basal and stem cells [42, 43]. Consistently, we previously reported that 40–60% of the cells in most of the ER-positive p18$^{-/-}$ tumors and less than 10% of the cells in most of the ER-negative p18$^{-/-}$;Brca1^{MGKO} tumors were CD24$^+$CD29^{low} [23, 37]. We detected a predominant CD24$^+$CD29^{high} population containing 60–81% of the cells in most of the p18$^{-/-}$;Brca1^{MGKO} and p16$^{-/-}$;Brca1^{MGKO} tumors (Additional file 2: Figure S2A) [23]. We chose and further characterized two individual p18$^{-/-}$;Brca1^{MGKO} tumors in addition to two individual p16$^{-/-}$;Brca1^{MGKO} tumors in which ERα was undetectable by western blot and IHC (Table 1, Additional file 1: Figure S1, and Fig. 3c); there were more than 75% CD24$^+$CD29^{high} cells and less than 2% CD24$^+$CD29^{low} cells (Additional file 2: Figure S2A and data not shown). Taking advantage of the tumors predominantly composed of CD24$^+$CD29^{high} cells, we transplanted 6×10^4 FACS-sorted Lin$^-$ cells (depleted of hematopoietic and endothelial cells) from a p18$^{-/-}$;Brca1^{MGKO} tumor and a p16$^{-/-}$;Brca1^{MGKO} tumor into eight MFPs of NSG mice (four for each cell type). After 1–2 months all recipient mice produced mammary tumors that were ERα negative (placebo group in Table 3, Additional file 2: Figure S2B, C, and data not shown). We cultured these tumor cells and found that most (> 90%) of the cells maintained their CD24$^+$CD29^{high} feature and less than 2% of the cells were CD24$^+$CD29^{low}, whereas, as a control, about half of the p18$^{-/-}$ tumor cells were CD24$^+$CD29^{low} (Additional file 2: Figure S2D). We determined expression of ERα by FACS and found that all cells derived from four individual p18$^{-/-}$;Brca1^{MGKO} and p16$^{-/-}$;Brca1^{MGKO} tumors were ERα negative whereas, as controls, 59% of

MCF7 and 43% of p18$^{-/-}$ tumor cells were ERα positive, respectively (Additional file 2: Figure S2E). We transplanted 1×10^6 cultured cells from each of the two individual p18$^{-/-}$;Brca1^{MGKO} and p16$^{-/-}$;Brca1^{MGKO} tumors into MFPs of NSG mice. We found all recipient mice also generated ERα-negative mammary tumors, which were indistinguishable from tumors generated by Lin$^-$ primary tumor cells in respect to ERα negativity (placebo group in Table 3, Additional file 2: Figure S2F, G, and data not shown). In summary these results demonstrate that transplantation of representative p18$^{-/-}$;Brca1^{MGKO} and p16$^{-/-}$;Brca1^{MGKO} tumor cells into MFPs of NSG mice generate reproducible ER-negative tumors, which build a model system to study BRCA1-deficient mammary tumor development and progression.

Table 3 Estrogen promotes Brca1-deficient mammary tumor initiation and progression

Genotype	p18^(-/-);Brca1^(MGKO)- Donor A	
number of tumor cell transplanted [a]	1×10^6/mouse	
Treatment	Placebo	E2
Tumor incidence (7 weeks)	4/4 (100%)	4/4 (100%)
Tumor size (mm^3)	426 ± 98	1294 ± 265 [c]
Tumor number with metastasis	0/4	1/4 [d]
Genotype	p16^(-/-);Brca1^(MGKO)- Donor B	
number of tumor cell transplanted [b]	6×10^4/mouse	
Treatment	Placebo	E2
Tumor incidence (6 weeks)	4/4 (100%)	4/4 (100%)
Tumor size (mm^3)	50 ± 22	785 ± 452 [c]

[a]Cultured tumor cells were used
[b]FACS-sorted Lin- tumor cells were used
[c]A statistical significance from E2-and Placebo-treated groups by two tailed t test
[d]A tumor metastasized to the lung and liver. No statistical significance was detected in tumor metastasis between E2- and placebo-treated groups by two tailed Fisher Exact test

Estrogen promotes Brca1-deficient mammary tumor initiation and metastasis

To determine the role of estrogen in *Brca1*-deficient mammary tumorigenesis, we transplanted *Brca1*-proficient and *Brca1*-deficient mammary tumor cells into MFPs of NSG mice with or without estrogen (17β-estradiol, E2) supplement. We found with E2 supplement, a half (3 out of 6) and a quarter (1 out of 4) of the mice that received two individual $p18^{-/-}$ tumor cell transplants yielded small tumors, respectively (experiment 2 in Table 2 and Additional file 3: Figure S3). Importantly, all $p18^{-/-};Brca1^{MGKO}$ and $p16^{-/-};Brca1^{MGKO}$ tumor cells yielded significantly larger tumors in NSG mice when transplanted with E2 supplement compared with those with placebo treatment (Table 3). IHC and western blot analysis confirmed the expression of Brca1 and ERα in regenerated mammary tumors by $p18^{-/-}$ tumor cells and lack of Brca1 and ERα in regenerated tumors by $p18^{-/-};Brca1^{MGKO}$ cells with E2 supplement (Additional file 3: Figure S3 and Additional file 4: Figure S4B, C). Pathologic analysis revealed that relative to placebo-treated tumors, E2-treated $p18^{-/-};Brca1^{MGKO}$ and $p16^{-/-};Brca1^{MGKO}$ tumors were poorly differentiated, more aggressive (increased necrosis, squamous metaplasia, spindle cells, nuclear-cytoplasm ratio, and mitotic indices) and contained highly heterogeneous cell types, whereas, E2-treated $p18^{-/-}$ tumors retained well-differentiated glandular structures (Fig. 1a and Additional file 3: Figure S3). Notably, one out of four $p18^{-/-};Brca1^{MGKO}$ tumors that were treated with E2 metastasized to the lungs and liver (Table 3 and Fig. 1a). We found that 51% (25/49) of DMSO-treated tumorspheres were smaller than 50 μm whereas 63% (47/74) of E2-treated tumorspheres were larger than 50 μm. The number of E2-treated tumorspheres that were larger than 100 μm or that were 50–100 μm was significantly more than that of DMSO-treated tumorspheres. Notably, the increased number of $p18^{-/-};Brca1^{MGKO}$ tumorspheres was not inhibited by 4OHT, an ER antagonist (Fig. 1b). These data suggest that E2 stimulates *Brca1*-deficient CSCs independent of ER. Together, these results demonstrate that in addition to the increased tumor-initiating potential of ER-positive *Brca1*-proficient tumor cells, estrogen enhances the number of *Brca1*-deficient CSCs and promotes ER-negative basal-like tumor initiation and progression.

Consistent with the findings derived from E2-treated $p18^{-/-};Brca1^{MGKO}$ and $p16^{-/-};Brca1^{MGKO}$ tumors, we also found that *BRCA1* mutant PDX tumor development was significantly enhanced by E2 treatment relative to that by placebo (Fig. 1c). E2-treated *BRCA1* mutant PDX tumors were also less differentiated, but more heterogeneous and invasive than placebo-treated tumors (Fig. 1d). These data further support the finding that estrogen promotes human *BRCA1*-deficient tumor initiation and progression.

To further investigate the role of estrogen in *Brca1*-deficient mammary tumor progression, we isolated a highly metastatic $p18^{-/-};Brca1^{MGKO}$ tumor cell line from a mammary tumor (tumor B) that was metastasized to lung. We then transplanted metastatic $p18^{-/-};Brca1^{MGKO}$ tumor cells into the MFPs of NSG mice with the supplement of either E2 or placebo pellet. We found that all newly generated mammary tumors metastasized to lung in 3–6 weeks. Notably, E2-treated mice with mammary tumors developed significantly more metastatic nodules in their lungs when compared with placebo-treated animals (115 ± 62 vs 241 ± 75, $p < 0.05$) (Fig. 2a-c, and Additional file 5: Figure S5). IHC analysis revealed that metastasized tumors in lung were negative for ER (Fig. 2d). These results confirm that estrogen promotes ER-negative *Brca1*-deficient mammary tumor metastasis.

Estrogen activates EMT in a subset of Brca1-deficient tumor cells

Estrogen has been found to activate EMT and stimulate the function of ER-negative breast CSCs through paracrine signaling produced in ER-positive cells in response to estrogen [7, 8]. However, clinically hormone therapy prevents development and suppresses the progression of *BRCA1*-deficient, ER-negative breast cancers [3, 4]. Inspired by the finding that a fraction of *BRCA1*-deficient human and mouse tumor cells harbor EMT features [16–19, 22–24, 39, 44], and the finding that E2 enhanced the heterogeneity of $p18^{-/-};Brca1^{MGKO}$ and $p16^{-/-};Brca1^{MGKO}$ tumors with elevated squamous metaplasia and spindle-shaped cells (typical morphological characteristics of mesenchymal cells), we hypothesized that estrogen promotes EMT and stimulates *BRCA1*-deficient, ER-negative tumorigenesis independent of ER. We found by western blot analysis that E2-treated $p18^{-/-};Brca1^{MGKO}$ tumors expressed a higher level of EMT marker (Vim) and EMT-inducing transcription factors (EMT-TFs) including p-Fra1 and Snail, than placebo-treated tumors. Importantly, we noticed by IHC that the number of cells that are positive for EMT markers and EMT-TFs was drastically enhanced in E2-treated $p18^{-/-};Brca1^{MGKO}$ tumors than in placebo-treated counterparts (Fig. 3a and Additional file 4: Figure S4A). We confirmed, as expected, that metastasized mammary tumors in lung were positive for Vim and p-Fra1 (Fig. 2d). These data suggest that estrogen activates EMT in a subset of ER-negative *Brca1*-deficient epithelial tumor (carcinoma) cells that have not undergone EMT, leading to an increase in the fraction of mesenchymal-like cells in *Brca1*-deficient tumors.

We examined *BRCA1* mutant PDX tumors and discovered that more than 80% of tumor cells expressed a

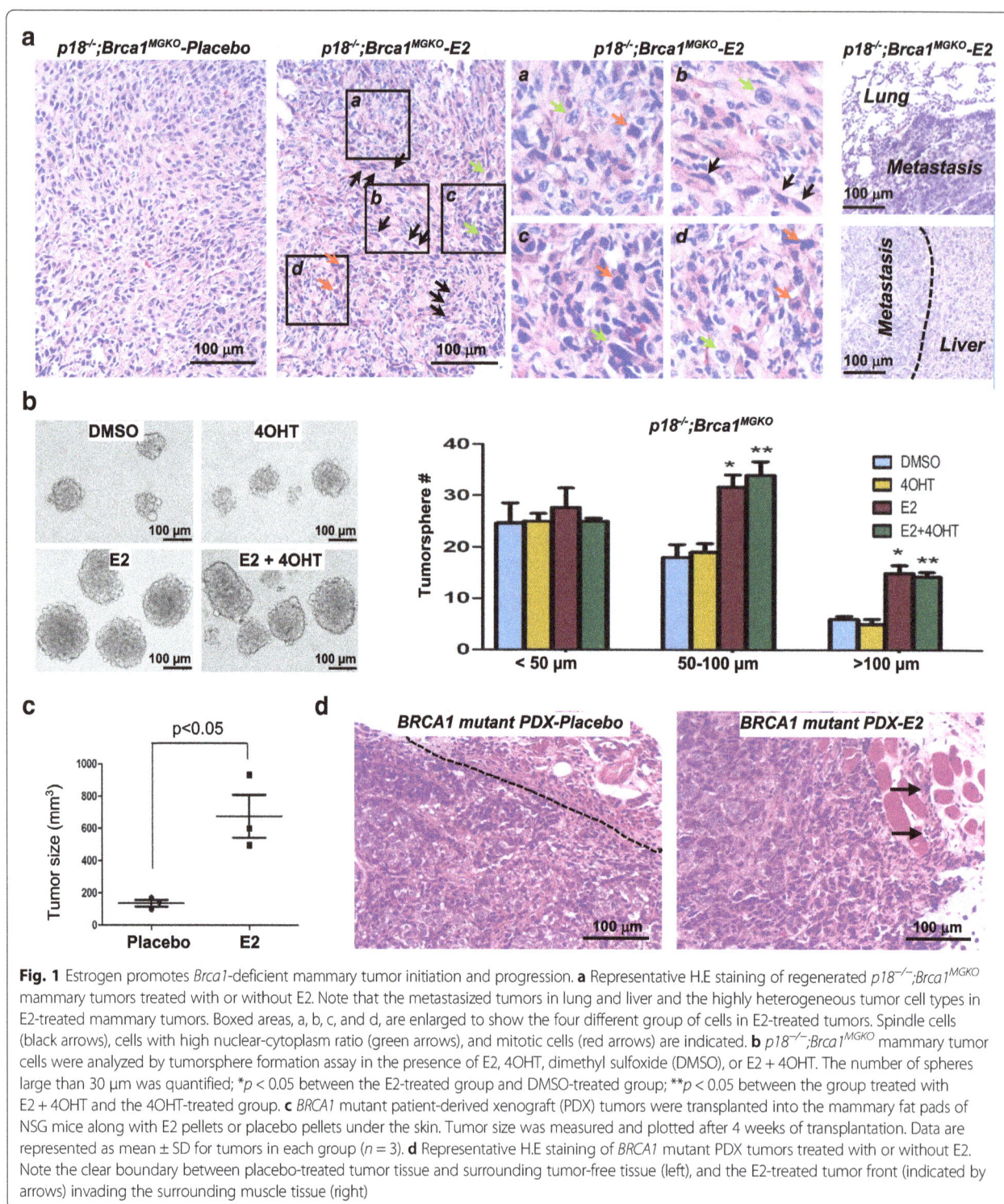

Fig. 1 Estrogen promotes *Brca1*-deficient mammary tumor initiation and progression. **a** Representative H.E staining of regenerated *p18⁻/⁻;Brca1^MGKO^* mammary tumors treated with or without E2. Note that the metastasized tumors in lung and liver and the highly heterogeneous tumor cell types in E2-treated mammary tumors. Boxed areas, a, b, c, and d, are enlarged to show the four different group of cells in E2-treated tumors. Spindle cells (black arrows), cells with high nuclear-cytoplasm ratio (green arrows), and mitotic cells (red arrows) are indicated. **b** *p18⁻/⁻;Brca1^MGKO^* mammary tumor cells were analyzed by tumorsphere formation assay in the presence of E2, 4OHT, dimethyl sulfoxide (DMSO), or E2 + 4OHT. The number of spheres large than 30 μm was quantified; *$p < 0.05$ between the E2-treated group and DMSO-treated group; **$p < 0.05$ between the group treated with E2 + 4OHT and the 4OHT-treated group. **c** *BRCA1* mutant patient-derived xenograft (PDX) tumors were transplanted into the mammary fat pads of NSG mice along with E2 pellets or placebo pellets under the skin. Tumor size was measured and plotted after 4 weeks of transplantation. Data are represented as mean ± SD for tumors in each group ($n = 3$). **d** Representative H.E staining of *BRCA1* mutant PDX tumors treated with or without E2. Note the clear boundary between placebo-treated tumor tissue and surrounding tumor-free tissue (left), and the E2-treated tumor front (indicated by arrows) invading the surrounding muscle tissue (right)

high level of VIM without treatment (Fig. 3b). These data are supported by the findings in both mouse [23] and human mammary tumors [24, 44] that most *BRCA1* mutant tumors are VIM positive and some of them are predominantly composed of VIM-positive cells. Though we failed to detect a further increase in the number of VIM-positive cells by E2-treatment in *BRCA1* mutant PDX tumors (Fig. 3b), the number of tumor cells that are positive for fibronectin, another key marker of mesenchymal cells, and for SNAIL and SLUG was drastically enhanced by E2 relative to the placebo (Fig. 3b). These results indicate that estrogen also

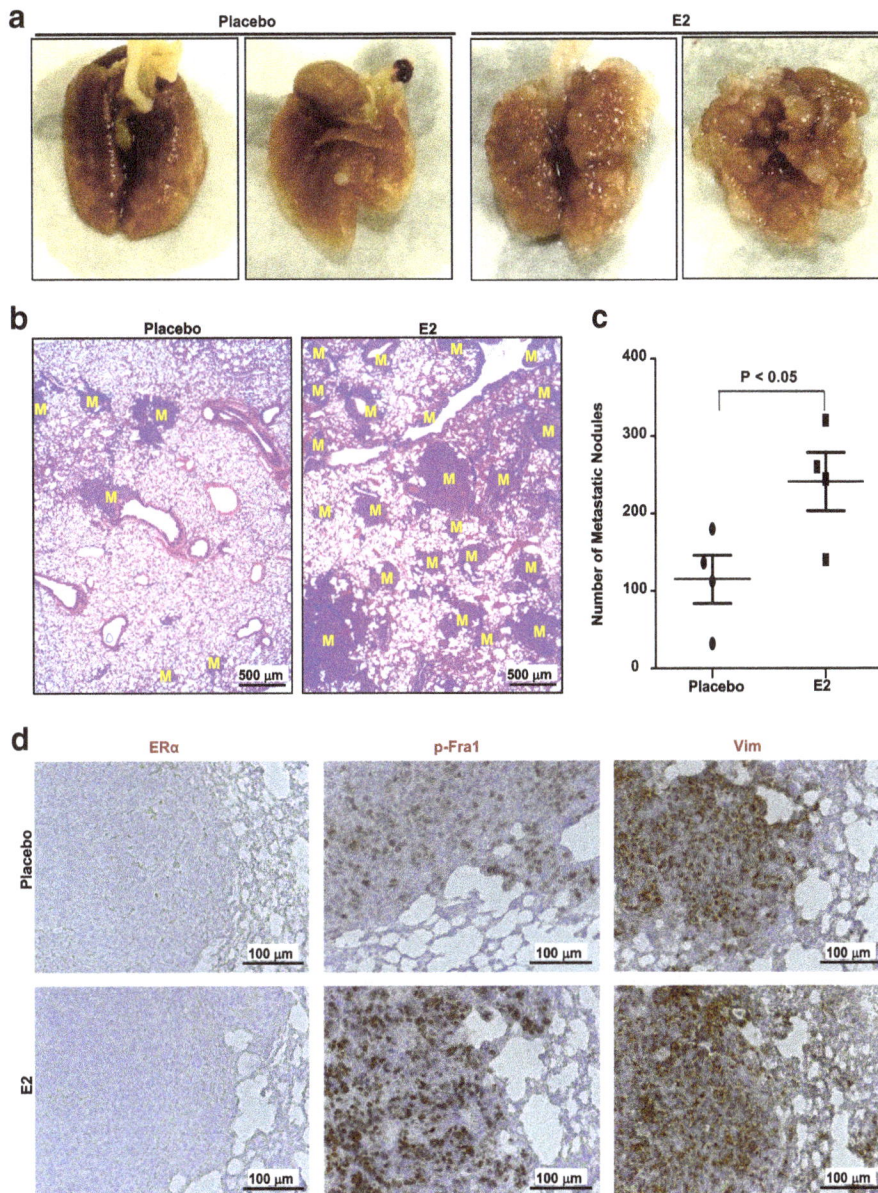

Fig. 2 Estrogen promotes *Brca1*-deficient mammary tumor metastasis. **a-d** We inoculated 1×10^6 metastatic $p18^{-/-}$;*Brca1*^{MGKO} tumor (donor B) cells into the mammary fat pads of 4-week-old female NSG mice in which either E2 or placebo Beeswax pellet was implanted subcutaneously. When newly generated tumors reached maximum size (1.3 cm^3) allowed by the IACUC in 3–6 weeks, or the mice became moribund, lungs were examined for gross appearance (**a**), H.E. staining (**b**), and quantification of the number of metastatic nodules (**c**). M, metastatic nodules. Data in (**c**) are mean ± SD for the numbers of metastatic nodules detected in all lobes of the lungs in each group (*n* = 4). **d** Representative immunohistochemical analysis of lung metastasis with antibodies against estrogen receptor (ER)α, p-fos-related antigen 1 (Fra1), and vimentin (Vim)

activates EMT in a subset of human BRCA1 mutant tumor cells.

As no tumor formed after the transplantation of $p18^{-/-}$ tumor cells without an E2 supplement (Table 2), we determined EMT markers in E2-treated tumors and primary tumors. We found no significant change in the expression of E-cad, p-Fra1, and Snail in E2-treated $p18^{-/-}$ tumors compared to $p18^{-/-}$ primary tumors (Fig. 3c, Additional file 4: Figure S4C,

and data not shown). Notably, except for a slight increase in Slug in a longer treatment, the expression of E-cad, Vim, Snail, and p-Fra1 in $p18^{-/-}$ tumor cells in culture was not affected by E2 either, whereas, the expression of Vim, Snail, and Slug in $p18^{-/-}$;*Brca1*^{MGKO} tumor cells was clearly enhanced by E2 under the same culture conditions (Fig. 3e, g and Additional file 6: Figure S6A-D). Together, these results indicate that estrogen promotes EMT in

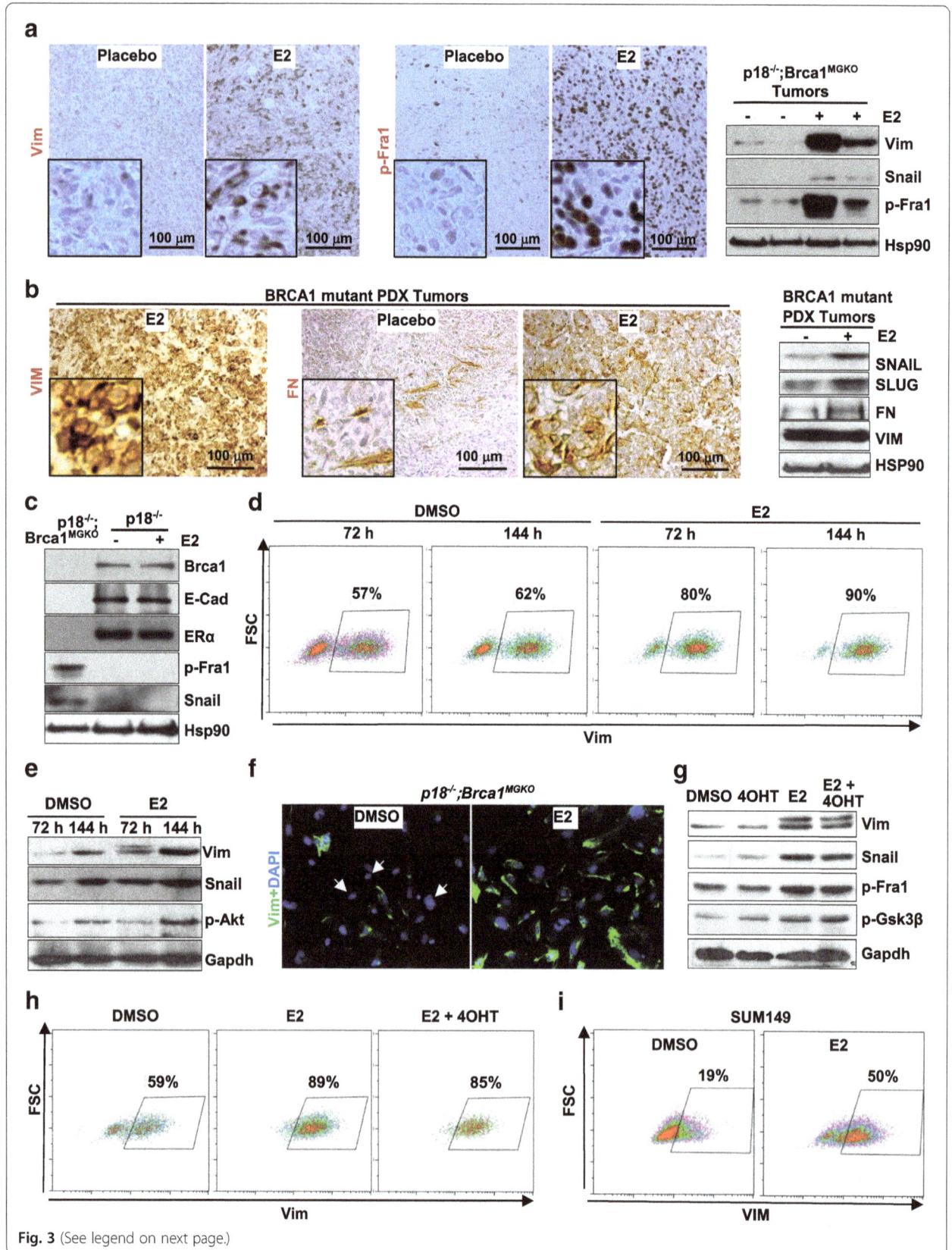

Fig. 3 (See legend on next page.)

Fig. 3 Estrogen activates epithelial-mesenchymal transition in *Brca1*-deficient and estrogen receptor (ER)-negative tumor cells. **a, b** $p18^{-/-}$;*Brca1*^{MGKO} (**a**) and *BRCA1* mutant patient-derived xenograft (PDX) (**b**) tumors treated with E2 or placebo were analyzed by immunohistochemical staining and western blot. Samples in (**a**) were derived from four different tumors developed in four individual mice. **c** The expression of genes indicated in the regenerated $p18^{-/-}$ tumors treated with E2 and primary $p18^{-/-}$ tumors was determined by western blot; $p18^{-/-}$;*Brca1*^{MGKO} tumor was used as a control. **d, e** $p18^{-/-}$;*Brca1*^{MGKO} tumor cells were treated with 50 nM E2 and dimethyl sulfoxide (DMSO) for 72 h and 144 h, respectively, and analyzed by fluorescence-activated cell sorting (FACS) (**d**) and western blot (**e**). The percentages of vimentin (Vim)-positive cells in (**d**) are indicated. **f** $p18^{-/-}$; *Brca1*^{MGKO} tumor cells were treated with 50 nM E2 or DMSO for 120 h and stained with anti-Vim. **g, h** $p18^{-/-}$;*Brca1*^{MGKO} tumor cells were treated with DMSO or 50 nM E2 in the presence or absence of 5 μM 4OHT for 72 h and analyzed by western blot (**g**) and FACS (**h**). **i** SUM149 breast cancer cells were treated with DMSO or 50 nM for 72 h and analyzed by FACS. The percentages of VIM-positive cells are indicated

Brca1-deficient, but not in *Brca1*-proficient, tumor cells.

Because the number of cells with mesenchymal features varies in different *BRCA1*-deficient tumors, we screened a panel of primary $p18^{-/-}$;*Brca1*^{MGKO} tumor cells by FACS for expression of Vim and identified at least two types of $p18^{-/-}$;*Brca1*^{MGKO} tumor cells, and in one of these, Vim-positive cells constituted 30–65% of the total tumor cells (type 1) and in the other, Vim-positive cells constituted > 90% of the total cells (type 2) (Fig. 3d-h and Additional file 6: Figure S6C). Due to the enrichment of EMT-promoting factors including transforming growth factors (TGFs) in serum, culture immortalized MECs in serum in vitro activates EMT [45]. Therefore, we cultured tumor cells in charcoal-stripped FBS with minimal hormones and cytokines (http://www.thermofisher.com) and performed all of our in vitro experiments using either primary or early passaged (before passage 3) tumor cells.

We treated $p18^{-/-}$;*Brca1*^{MGKO} tumor cells with E2 in multiple time periods and observed by western blot that E2 stimulated expression of Vim and EMT-TFs including p-Fra1 and/or Snail/Slug in both type of cells (Fig. 3d-h, Additional file 6: Figure S6), indicating E2 promotes EMT in *Brca1*-deficient tumor cells in vitro. As the majority of *BRCA1*-deficient tumors contain a fraction of cells that are positive for VIM and/or other mesenchymal markers, and only a small number of human *BRCA1*-deficient tumors, i.e. metaplastic breast cancers, are predominantly composed of mesenchymal/VIM-positive cells [16–19, 24, 39, 44, 46], we therefore focused on type 1 $p18^{-/-}$;*Brca1*^{MGKO} tumor cells. When type 1 $p18^{-/-}$;*Brca1*^{MGKO} tumor cells were examined by immunofluorescent staining and FACS, we found that E2 treatment enhanced the number of Vim-positive cells - converting Vim-positive cells from 57-62% to 80–90% after 72 h (Fig. 3d, f, h). Furthermore, the increase in Vim expression and conversion of cells from Vim-negative to positive by E2 in $p18^{-/-}$;*Brca1*^{MGKO} tumor cells was not blocked by 4OHT (Fig. 3g, h), whereas, 4OHT effectively blocked E2-enhanced cell proliferation and RB phosphorylation in ER-positive MCF7 cells, as expected (Additional file 7: Figure S7). These results demonstrated that estrogen activates EMT

in a subset of *Brca1*-deficient tumor cells that have not undergone EMT, and further indicated that estrogen promotes EMT in ER-negative *Brca1*-deficient tumor cells independent of ER.

We then selected a *BRCA1* mutant, ER-negative human breast cancer cell line, SUM149, in which p16 is deleted and VIM is expressed in 10–30% of total cells [35, 47–49]. This cell line shares many genetic (*p16/p18* and *Brca1* loss-of-function mutation) and phenotypical (ER negative with a subset of cells exhibiting EMT features) similarities with *p16;Brca1* and *p18;Brca1* mutant murine mammary tumor cells. We found that E2 treatment also drastically enhanced the number of Vim-positive cells - from 19% to 50% after 72 h (Fig. 3i). Notably, it has been reported that in the SUM149 cell line, VIM-positive, stem/basal cells are able to efficiently generate both basal and luminal cells, whereas, VIM-negative, luminal cells rarely generate VIM-positive, stem/basal cells under serum-containing culture condition [47]. In addition, we also detected by western blot the increase in VIM, p-FRA1, and SNAIL in SUM149 cells in response to E2 treatment (Additional file 6: Figure S6E), indicating the activation of EMT by estrogen.

In summary, these in vitro results confirmed that estrogen activates EMT in a subset of *Brca1*-deficient tumor cells with epithelial features, which is independent of ER.

Estrogen stimulates Brca1-deficient tumor cell proliferation

We performed IHC of mammary tumors generated by primary tumor cells derived from three individual $p16^{-/-}$; *Brca1*^{MGKO} and four $p18^{-/-}$;*Brca1*^{MGKO} tumors. We found that all newly generated tumors contained Ck5 or Ck14 (Ck5/Ck14)-positive cells. We observed that the more Ck5/Ck14-positive cells in primary tumors, the more Ck5/Ck14-positive cells will be detected in the regenerated tumors, though the percentages of Ck5-positive or Ck14-positive cells varied among tumors (Figs. 4, 6 and data not shown) [19, 23, 39]. These results suggest that newly generated $p16^{-/-}$;*Brca1*^{MGKO} and $p18^{-/-}$; *Brca1*^{MGKO} mammary tumors maintain their basal-like tumor phenotype. We investigated cell proliferation in tumors by Ki67 staining and found that there were more Ki67-positive cells in E2-treated tumors than in

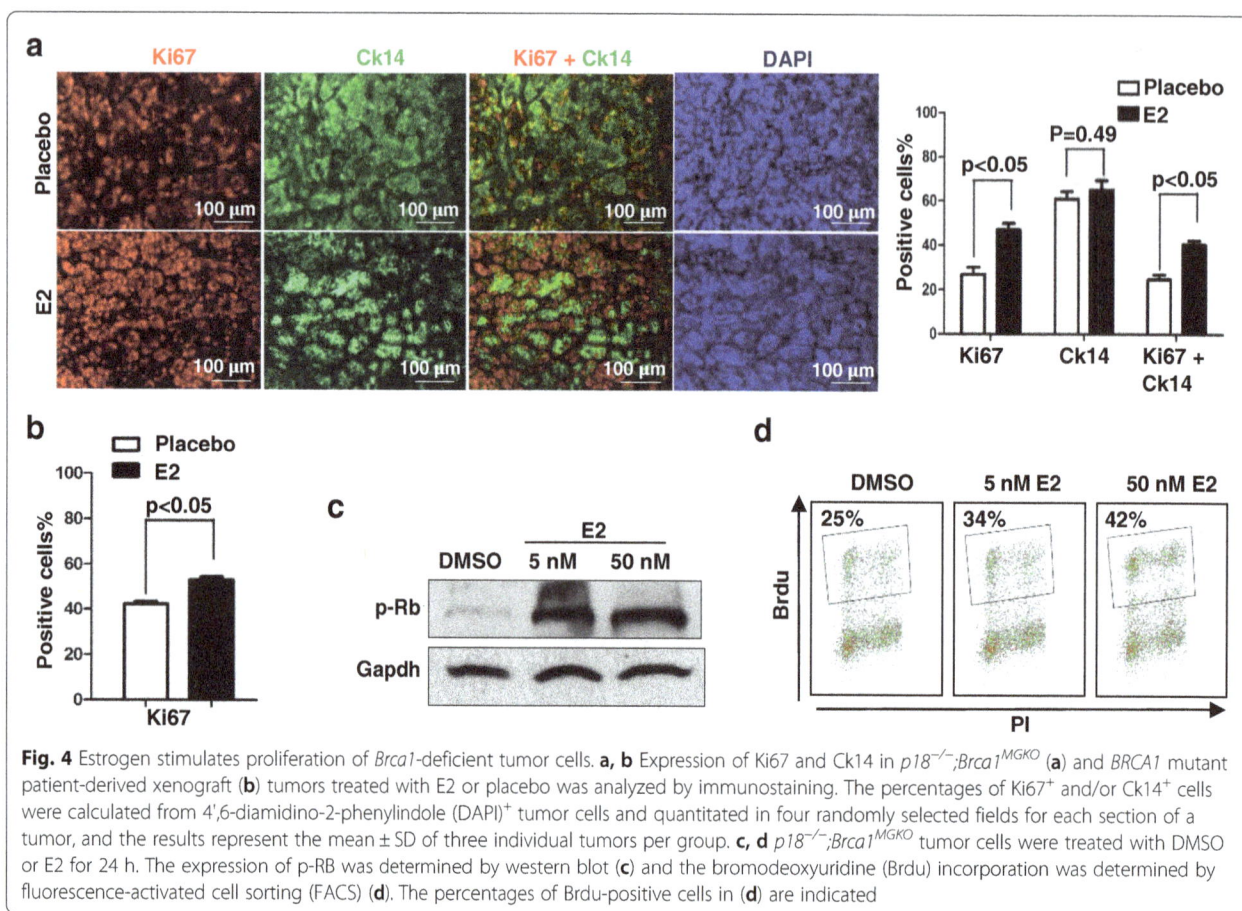

Fig. 4 Estrogen stimulates proliferation of *Brca1*-deficient tumor cells. **a, b** Expression of Ki67 and Ck14 in *p18⁻/⁻;Brca1^MGKO* (**a**) and *BRCA1* mutant patient-derived xenograft (**b**) tumors treated with E2 or placebo was analyzed by immunostaining. The percentages of Ki67⁺ and/or Ck14⁺ cells were calculated from 4',6-diamidino-2-phenylindole (DAPI)⁺ tumor cells and quantitated in four randomly selected fields for each section of a tumor, and the results represent the mean ± SD of three individual tumors per group. **c, d** *p18⁻/⁻;Brca1^MGKO* tumor cells were treated with DMSO or E2 for 24 h. The expression of p-RB was determined by western blot (**c**) and the bromodeoxyuridine (Brdu) incorporation was determined by fluorescence-activated cell sorting (FACS) (**d**). The percentages of Brdu-positive cells in (**d**) are indicated

placebo-treated tumors. Furthermore, the majority of Ki67 positive cells in E2-treated tumors were also positive for CK14 (Fig. 4a). We then performed similar analysis for *BRCA1* mutant PDX tumors and found that E2 treatment also enhanced the number of Ki67-positive cells in tumors, most of which are also CK14 positive (Fig. 4b, and data not shown). These results indicate that estrogen stimulates proliferation of *Brca1*-deficient basal-like tumor cells in vivo.

We cultured cells derived from three individual *p18⁻/⁻;Brca1^MGKO* tumors and found that E2 treatment in both type 1 and type 2 tumor cells enhanced the number of cells (Fig. 6b, Additional file 8: Figure S8C), promoted phosphorylation of RB (Fig. 4c), and stimulated incorporation of BrdU in cells (Fig. 4d). These data confirm the role of estrogen in stimulation of proliferation of *Brca1*-deficient tumor cells.

Estrogen activates the AKT pathway in BRCA1-deficient mammary tumors

During the course of analysis of the role of estrogen in activating EMT, we observed that E2 stimulated expression of p-Akt, p-Gsk3β, and p-4Ebp1, downstream targets of Akt, in *p18⁻/⁻;Brca1^MGKO* tumor cells, which was not blocked by 4OHT (Fig. 3e, g). We examined tumors

by IHC and western blot analysis, and found that the expression of p-Akt and its targets, p-4Ebp1, p-mTor, and p-Gsk3β, was significantly enhanced in E2-treated tumors when compared with placebo-treated tumors. (Fig. 5a, b). We treated *p18⁻/⁻;Brca1^MGKO* and SUM149 tumor cells with or without E2 and found that E2 stimulated expression of p-Akt, p-4Ebp1, p-mTor, and p-Gsk3β in all time points tested from 2 to 144 h (Fig. 3e, g, Fig. 5c, Fig. 6a and Additional file 6: Figure S6A, B, E). Consistent with the data derived from *p18⁻/⁻;Brca1^MGKO* tumors, E2 treatment also significantly enhanced the expression of p-AKT, p-4EBP1, p-mTOR, and p-GSK3β in *BRCA1* mutant PDX tumors relative to placebo treatment (Fig. 5d, e and Additional file 8: Figure S8A, B). These results indicate that estrogen activates the AKT pathway in *BRCA1*-deficient mammary tumor cells independent of ER.

Inhibition of AKT suppresses EMT and cell proliferation preventing Brca1-deficient tumor progression

Along with activation of the Akt pathway, estrogen promoted EMT and proliferation in *Brca1*-deficient mammary tumor cells, which prompted us to test whether pharmaceutical inhibition of Akt activity has any effect

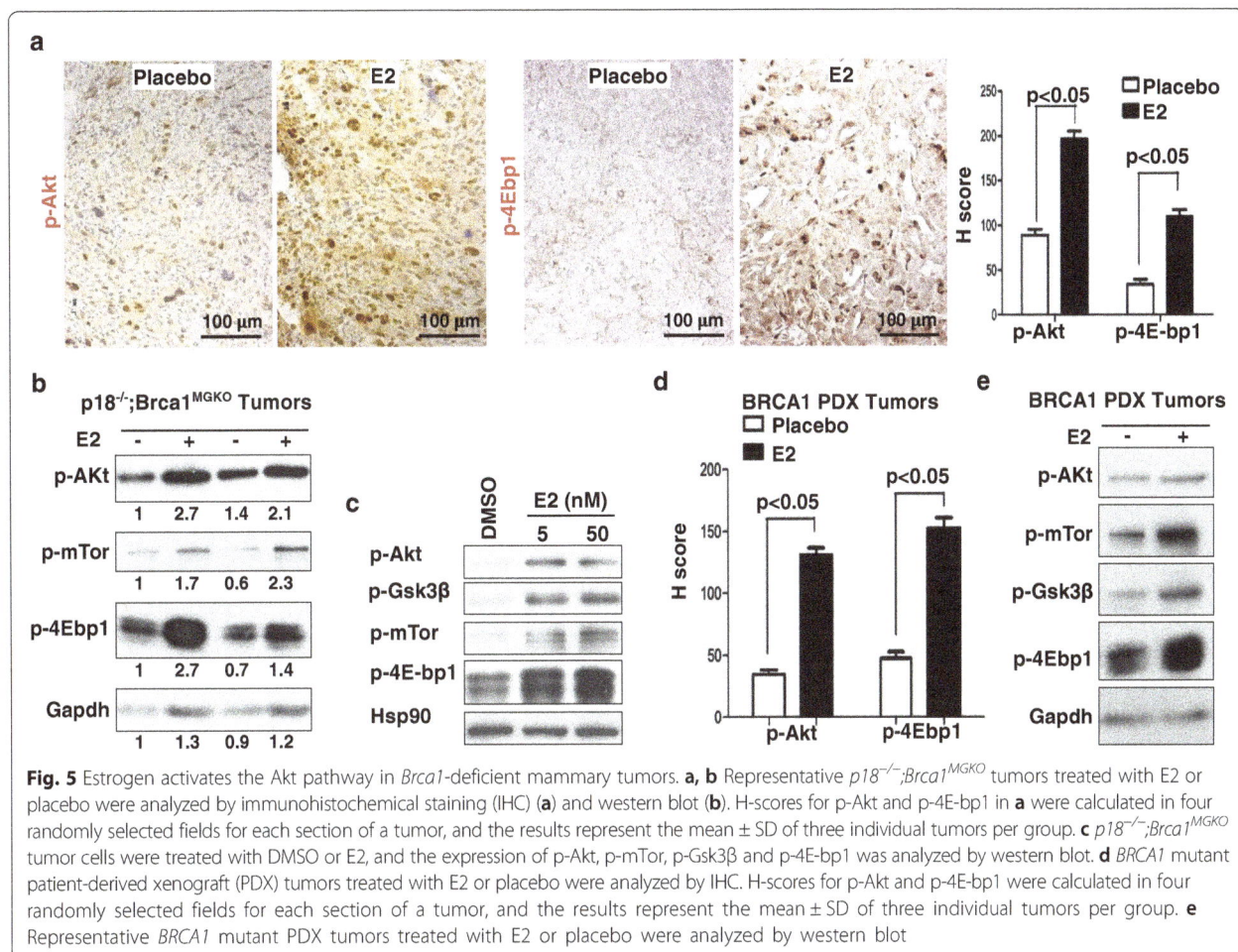

Fig. 5 Estrogen activates the Akt pathway in *Brca1*-deficient mammary tumors. **a, b** Representative *p18^{−/−};Brca1^{MGKO}* tumors treated with E2 or placebo were analyzed by immunohistochemical staining (IHC) (**a**) and western blot (**b**). H-scores for p-Akt and p-4E-bp1 in **a** were calculated in four randomly selected fields for each section of a tumor, and the results represent the mean ± SD of three individual tumors per group. **c** *p18^{−/−};Brca1^{MGKO}* tumor cells were treated with DMSO or E2, and the expression of p-Akt, p-mTor, p-Gsk3β and p-4E-bp1 was analyzed by western blot. **d** *BRCA1* mutant patient-derived xenograft (PDX) tumors treated with E2 or placebo were analyzed by IHC. H-scores for p-Akt and p-4E-bp1 were calculated in four randomly selected fields for each section of a tumor, and the results represent the mean ± SD of three individual tumors per group. **e** Representative *BRCA1* mutant PDX tumors treated with E2 or placebo were analyzed by western blot

on *Brca1*-deficient cell proliferation and tumor progression. We treated *p18^{−/−};Brca1^{MGKO}* tumor cells with E2 in the presence or absence of AZD5363, a well-studied preclinical Akt inhibitor [50]. We found that AZD5363 drastically inhibited E2-enhanced expression of p-4Ebp1, p-mTor, and p-Gsk3β, and that of Vim and p-Fra1 (Fig. 6a), suggesting that AZD5363 efficiently suppresses estrogen-enhanced Akt pathway and EMT program in Brca1 deficient tumor cells. Treatment of *p18^{−/−};Brca1^{MGKO}* tumor cells including both type 1 and type 2 cells with AZD5363 significantly reduced the E2-enhanced number of cells and incorporation of BrdU (Fig. 6b, c and Additional file 8: Figure S8C), indicating that AZD5363 inhibits estrogen-enhanced proliferation of *Brca1*-deficient tumor cells.

We then determined if pharmaceutical inhibition of Akt activity suppresses the progression of pre-existing *Brca1*-deficient tumors. Transplanted *p18^{−/−};Brca1^{MGKO}* tumors with E2 supplement were allowed to reach ~ 250 mm³ in size and then mice were treated with vehicle or AZD5363 daily. Three days after treatment, tumors from AZD5363-treated mice began to show a significant size reduction in comparison with the tumors

from vehicle-treated animals. After 7-day treatment, tumors from vehicle-treated mice reached ~ 1475 mm³ in size, whereas those from AZD5363 -treated mice only reached ~ 188 mm³, which was comparable with that of the tumor size at the start of treatment (~ 224 mm³) (*p* = 0.59) (Fig. 6d), indicating that treatment with AZD5363 prevents estrogen-enhanced *Brca1*-deficient tumor progression.

Further analysis of tumors by IHC and western blot revealed that in tumors from mice with E2 supplement the expression of p-4Ebp1, p-mTor, and p-Gsk3β was clearly reduced by AZD5363 treatment relative to vehicle treatment (Fig. 6e and Additional file 8: Figure S8D), confirming the role of AZD5363 in inhibition of the estrogen-induced Akt pathway in *Brca1*-deficient tumor progression. Notably, the expression of Vim, Fn and Slug in tumors with E2 was drastically reduced and that of E-cad was enhanced in AZD5363-treated mice relative to control (Fig. 6e, f). These data demonstrate that AZD5363 efficiently suppresses estrogen-activated EMT in *Brca1*-deficient tumors in vivo. Consistent with the findings derived from *p18^{−/−};Brca1^{MGKO}* tumor cells in vitro (Fig. 6b),

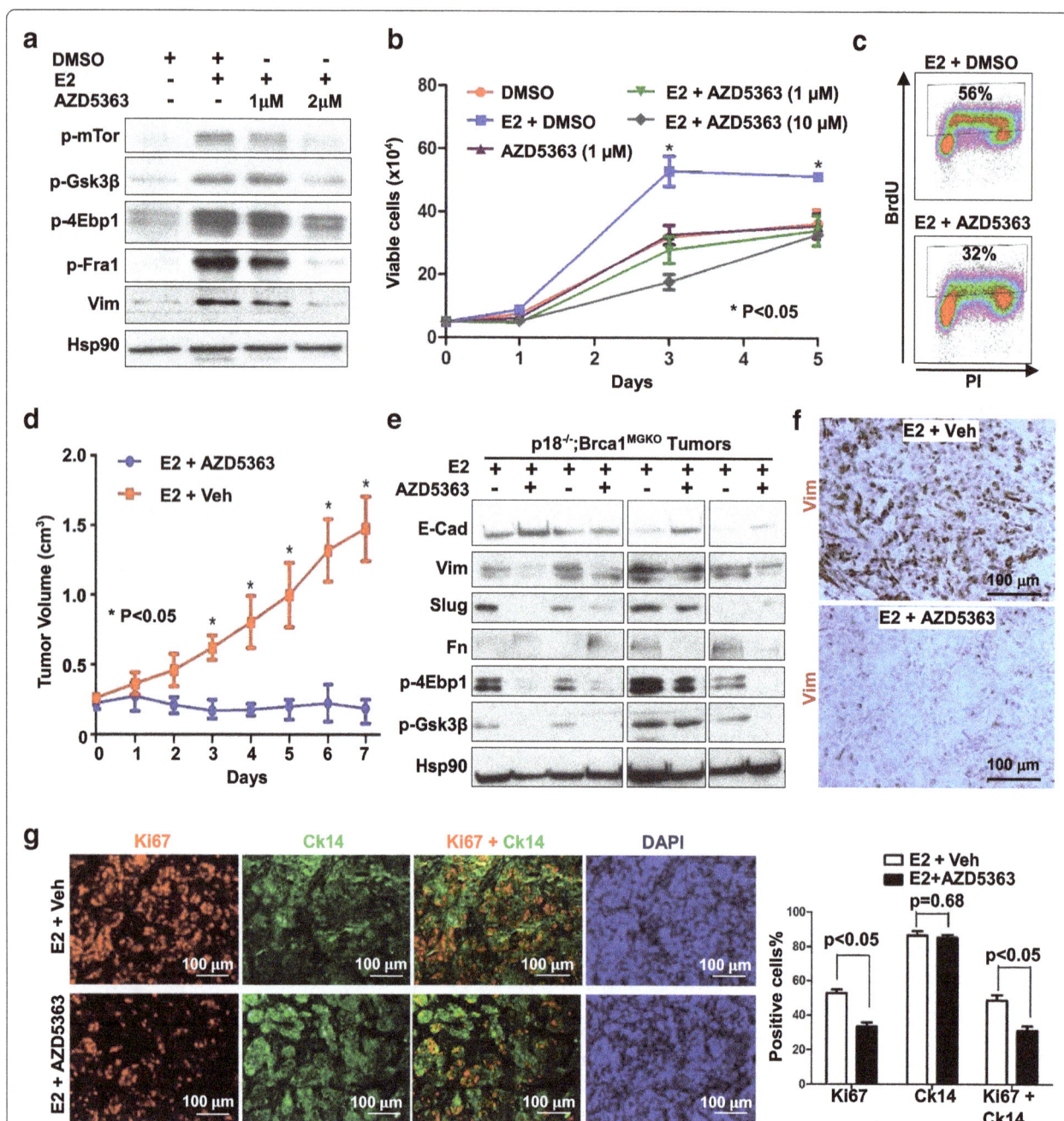

Fig. 6 Pharmaceutical inhibition of Akt suppresses epithelial-mesenchymal transition and cell proliferation preventing *Brca1*-deficient tumor progression. **a** *p18⁻/⁻;Brca1^MGKO* tumor cells were treated with dimethyl sulfoxide (DMSO) or 5 nM E2 in the presence or absence of different dosage of AZD5363 for 2 h, the expression of p-mTor, p-4E-bp1, p-Gsk3β, p-Fra1 and vimentin (Vim) were analyzed by western blot. **b** *p18⁻/⁻; Brca1^MGKO* tumor cells were treated with DMSO or 5 nM E2 in the presence or absence of different dosage of AZD5363, and the numbers of viable cells were determined on day 1, day 3, and day 5. *$p < 0.05$ between E2-treated and E2 + AZD5363-treated groups at the time points (Student *t* test). Data are represented as mean ± SD (n = 4). **c** *p18⁻/⁻;Brca1^MGKO* tumor cells were treated with 5 nM E2 with or without 1 μM AZD5363 for 24 h, and bromodeoxyuridine (Brdu) incorporation was then determined by fluorescence-activated cell sorting (FACS). **d-g** We transplanted 1 × 10⁶ *p18⁻/⁻; Brca1^MGKO* tumor cells into the mammary fat pads of NSG mice along with E2 pellet under the skin, and tumors were allowed to reach ~ 250 mm³ in size. Mice were then treated with AZD5363 at 150 mg/kg body weight or vehicle daily by oral gavage. The tumor size was determined and plotted (**d**). Data in **d** are represented as mean ± SD of four tumors in each group. *$p < 0.05$ between two groups at each time point (Student *t* test). *p18⁻/⁻; Brca1^MGKO* tumors treated with AZD5363 or vehicle for 7 days (**d**) were analyzed by western blot (**e**), immunohistochemical staining (**f**), and immunofluorescent staining (**g**). Samples in **e** were derived from eight different tumors developed in eight individual mice. The percentages of Ki67⁺ and/or Ck14⁺ cells (**g**) were quantitated in four randomly selected fields for each section of a tumor, and the results represent the mean ± SD of three individual tumors per group

we also detected that AZD5363 significantly reduced the number of Ki67 and Ck14 double-positive cells stimulated by E2 in $p18^{-/-};Brca1^{MGKO}$ tumors (Fig. 6g). Together, these results indicate that estrogen promotes EMT and proliferation of $Brca1$-deficinet tumor cells leading to tumor progression, which is dependent on the activation of the Akt pathway.

Discussion

In this study, we found that deletion of $Brca1$ enhances the tumor-initiating potential of tumor cells, and that estrogen stimulates proliferation and the tumor-initiating potential of both $Brca1$-proficient ER-positive and $Brca1$-deficient ER-negative tumor cells. We discovered that estrogen activates EMT in a subset of $Brca1$-deficient tumor cells that maintain epithelial features, and enhances the number of CSCs, promoting ER-negative basal-like tumor progression and metastasis. We found that estrogen activates EMT independent of ER in $Brca1$-deficient but not $Brca1$-proficient tumor cells. We further discovered that estrogen activates the Akt pathway in $Brca1$-deficient mammary tumor cells independent of ER, and that pharmaceutical inhibition of Akt activity suppresses EMT and cell proliferation preventing $Brca1$-deficient tumor progression. To the best of our knowledge, this study reveals for the first time that estrogen promotes $BRCA1$-deficient tumor initiation and progression by stimulation of cell proliferation and activation of EMT, which are dependent on AKT activation and independent of ER.

It has long been known that estrogen is required for normal mammary development and that it promotes mammary tumorigenesis and progression [1, 2]. Not until recently has the role of estrogen in stimulation of normal and cancerous mammary stem cells been investigated. Though mammary stem cells lack the ER [43], they are highly responsive to estrogen [51]. Estrogen expands the number and promotes the function of mammary stem cells, likely mediated through paracrine signaling from RANK ligand produced in ER-positive luminal epithelial cells [51]. More recently, it has been reported that estrogen promotes mammary stem cells by paracrine signaling from IGF and WNT provided in stromal cells, in which Gli2 induces expression of ER and coordinates the induction of stem cell support factors including insulin-like growth factor (IGF) and WNT [52]. Interestingly, estrogen has been found to promote ER-negative breast CSCs derived from ER-positive cell lines through paracrine FGF-Tbx3, EGFR, and Notch signaling provided in ER-positive cells [5, 7, 8]. Notably, paracrine factors produced in response to estrogen in ER-positive cancer cells also expands CSCs derived from ER-negative breast cancer cell lines [7]. However, all of these findings on the role of estrogen in promoting breast CSCs were obtained from cell lines

in vitro, and were dependent on the paracrine stem cell supporting and promoting factors that were provided by ER-positive cells. It remains elusive whether estrogen directly regulates breast CSCs in ER-negative breast cancers. We have previously reported that heterozygous germline deletion or mammary epithelial specific deletion of $Brca1$ in mice promotes CSCs and induces development of ER-negative mammary tumors [19, 23, 39]. We report in this paper that estrogen enhances the number of breast CSCs in $Brca1$-deficient, ER-negative mammary tumors independent of ER. Our results indicate that $BRCA1$ deficiency caused by somatic mutation or promoter methylation of $BRCA1$ in sporadic ER-negative breast cancers sensitizes tumor cells to endogenous estrogen activating EMT, promoting CSCs and, therefore, inducing tumor progression. Our finding supports the development of strategies to inhibit estrogen synthesis for treatment of $BRCA1$-deficient BLBCs.

EMT plays a critical role in generating CSCs in tumor development and progression [12, 13]. The role of estrogen in regulation of EMT in breast cancer is controversial. On one hand, it is extensively studied and reported that estrogen activates ERα signaling, maintaining epithelial phenotype and suppressing EMT (as reviewed [53]), but on the other hand, estrogen has been found to activate EMT in ER-positive breast and ovarian cancer cells, promoting their stemness and invasiveness [5–7, 54]. Again, all the findings on promotion of EMT by estrogen were obtained from cancer cell lines and are dependent on activation of ER signaling. However, it remains obscure whether estrogen regulates EMT in ER-negative cancer cells and alters their properties in tumor initiation and progression. We showed that estrogen does not activate EMT in ER-positive and $Brca1$-proficient tumor cells in vitro and tumorigenesis in vivo. These data warrant further investigation of the role of estrogen/ER signaling in regulation of EMT in tumorigenesis. Importantly, we demonstrated that estrogen activates EMT in a subset of ER-negative and $Brca1$-deficient mammary tumor cells, promoting their properties in tumor initiation and progression. These results provide the first genetic evidence demonstrating that estrogen activates EMT in ER-negative breast cancer cells independent of paracrine factors produced by ER-positive cells.

The PI3K/AKT pathway stimulates tumor development and progression through multiple mechanisms including promotion of cell proliferation, survival, and EMT [25, 26]. Estrogen activates the PI3K/AKT pathway in ER-negative breast cancer cells, and promotes survival of $Brca1$-deficient tumor cells, which stimulate tumor growth [30]. Estrogen also stimulates proliferation of $Brca1$-mutant cells through activation of remaining ERα, which is gradually diminished during tumor progression in $Brca1^{\Delta11/\Delta11}p53^{+/-}$

mice [55]. Depletion or inhibition of the PI3K/Akt pathway reduces proliferation of *BRCA1*-deficient MEFs suppressing growth of tumors generated by transplantation of *BRCA1*-deficient MEFs [28]. However, it remains elusive whether estrogen stimulates proliferation of ER-negative *BRCA1*-deficient tumor cells in vivo through activation of the Akt pathway. Further, due to the lack of a proper model system, i.e. ER-negative *BRCA1*-deficient tumor cells that can be induced by estrogen to EMT in vitro and in vivo, it is unknown if estrogen-activated EMT in ER negative *BRCA1*-deficient tumor cells is dependent on AKT activation. In the present study, we demonstrated that estrogen activates the Akt pathway not only stimulating proliferation but also promoting EMT in ER-negative, *BRCA1*-deficient tumor cells, which further enhances tumor progression.

In this study, we investigated the effect of estrogen on ER-negative *BRCA1*-deficient tumor progression by transplantation of tumor cells into the MFPs of NSG mice that did not receive ovariectomy. Host estrogen in recipient mice may play a role in ER-negative *BRCA1*-deficient tumor growth and progression. Transplantation of ER-positive $p18^{-/-}$ tumor cells into NSG mice did not produce tumors, whereas, with exogenous E2 supplement, $p18^{-/-}$ tumor cells generated ER-positive tumors in NSG mice, suggesting that host estrogen is not sufficient to induce $p18$ deficient, *Brca1*-proficient tumor initiation. Notably, transplantation of either $p18^{-/-}$; $Brca1^{MGKO}$ or $p16^{-/-}$;$Brca1^{MGKO}$ tumor cells into NSG mice generated tumors efficiently, which were further promoted by exogenous E2 administration. Taking into consideration our finding that estrogen promotes EMT, proliferation, sphere-forming potential, and Akt activation in *Brca1*-deficient tumor cells in vitro, these results suggest that host estrogen likely promotes *Brca1*-deficient tumor initiation, which support our conclusion. Importantly, it has been demonstrated that the E2 pellet (0.72 mg pellet) we used produces between 18 and 40 times higher concentrations of serum E2 than the physiological range in intact mice [56], suggesting that the effect of host estrogen on tumor growth in recipient mice is minor on supplementation with the E2 pellet. Furthermore, as estrogen is produced in the ovaries, adrenal glands, and fat tissues, an ovariectomy reduces only about 1/3 of the serum E2 concentration in female mice when compared with the serum E2 concentration in mice with intact ovaries [57]. Whether the reduced host estrogen due to ovariectomy in recipient mice impacts *Brca1*-deficient tumorigenesis remains elusive.

Conclusions

Our finding, for the first time, demonstrates that estrogen promotes *BRCA1*-deficient tumor initiation and progression by stimulation of cell proliferation and activation of EMT, which are dependent on AKT activation and

independent of ER. This study not only reveals the molecular mechanisms underlying the role of estrogen in promoting development and progression of ER-negative basal-like breast cancers but also identifies a druggable AKT pathway that is activated by estrogen in *BRCA1*-deficient breast cancers. This investigation will support to develop strategies to inhibit estrogen synthesis and to target AKT for treatment of *BRCA1*-deficient basal-like breast cancers.

Additional file

Additional file 1: Figure S1. Characterization of mammary tumors developed in mutant mice in Balb/cB6 mixed background. Representative mammary tumors spontaneously developed in $p18^{-/-}$;$Brca1^{MGKO}$, $p16^{-/-}$;$Brca1^{MGKO}$ and $p18^{-/-}$ mice were immunostained with the antibodies indicated. The representative cells are enlarged in the insets.

Additional file 2: Figure S2. $p18^{-/-}$;$Brca1^{MGKO}$ and $p16^{-/-}$;$Brca1^{MGKO}$ tumor cells generate reproducible ER-negative *Brca1*-deficient mammary tumors. (A) A primary mammary tumor (donor tumor A) developed in a 15-month-old $p16^{-/-}$;$Brca1^{MGKO}$ mouse was analyzed by FACS. As a control, tumor-free mammary glands from age-matched $p16^{-/-}$ mice were analyzed. Note a predominant CD24$^+$?$^+$CD29^{high} population in the tumor. (B, C) We transplanted 6?×?10^4 FACS-sorted Lin- cells from a $p16^{-/-}$;$Brca1^{MGKO}$ tumor (donor tumor B) into MFPs of four NSG mice. Representative tumors generated were analyzed by IHC (B) and western blot (C). (D, E) Representative $p18^{-/-}$ and $p18^{-/-}$;$Brca1^{MGKO}$ tumor cells were cultured and analyzed. MCF7 cells were used as a positive control of ERa expression. (F, G) We transplanted 1?×?10^6 cultured $p18^{-/-}$;$Brca1^{MGKO}$ tumor (donor tumor A) cells into MFPs of four NSG mice. Representative tumors generated were analyzed by IHC (F) and western blot (G). $p18^{-/-}$ tumors were used as control in (C) and (G).

Additional file 3: Figure S3. Estrogen promotes *Brca1*-proficient and deficient mammary tumor initiation (A) Western blot analysis of mammary tumors regenerated by $p18^{-/-}$ or $p18^{-/-}$;$Brca1^{MGKO}$ tumor cells with E2 supplement. (B) Representative gross pictures of $p18^{-/-}$ and $p16^{-/-}$;$Brca1^{MGKO}$ tumors generated by transplantation. We transplanted 1 × 10^7 $p18^{-/-}$ or 6 × 10^4 $p16^{-/-}$;$Brca1^{MGKO}$ tumor cells into MFPs of NSG mice with or without E2 supplement. Gross pictures were taken 6-7 weeks post-transplantation. (C) Representative H.E. staining of primary $p18^{-/-}$ tumors and tumors generated by $p18^{-/-}$ tumor cells with E2 supplement. Note the well-differentiated cells with glandular structure in both primary and regenerated tumors. (D) Representative H.E. staining of $p16^{-/-}$;$Brca1^{MGKO}$ tumors generated in the presence or absence of E2 supplement. Note the poorly differentiated cells with increased fibroblast-like cells in the tumors with E2 treatment. Spindle cells (black arrows), cells with high nuclear-cytoplasm ratio (green arrows), mitotic cells (red arrows), and necrosis (yellow arrows) are indicated.

Additional file 4: Figure S4. Estrogen promotes lung metastasis of *Brca1*-deficient mammary tumors. (A, B) Metastatic $p18^{-/-}$;$Brca1^{MGKO}$ tumor cells were inoculated into the MFPs of NSG mice with either E2 or placebo supplement. When newly generated tumors reached maximum size allowed by the IACUC in 3–6 weeks, or the mice became moribund, lungs were dissected for analysis. Representative gross pictures (A) and H.E. staining (B) of lungs are shown.

Additional file 5: Figure S5. IHC analysis of ERa and EMT markers for tumors with or without E2 treatment. (A-C) Representative $p18^{-/-}$;$Brca1^{MGKO}$ and $p18^{-/-}$ mammary tumors treated with E2 or placebo were immunostained with the antibodies indicated. Note the negative ERa staining in E2-treated $p18^{-/-}$;$Brca1^{MGKO}$ tumors (B) and positive ERa staining in E2-treated $p18^{-/-}$ tumors (C).

Additional file 6: Figure S6. Estrogen promotes EMT in *Brca1*-deficient tumor cells (A, B) $p18^{-/-}$;$Brca1^{MGKO}$ type 1 (A) and $p18^{-/-}$ tumor cells (B) were treated with DMSO or E2 for the indicated time and analyzed by western blot. (C, D) $p18^{-/-}$;$Brca1^{MGKO}$ type 2 tumor cells were treated with

DMSO or 50 nM E2 for 2 h or 72 h, and then analyzed by FACS (C) and western blot (D). (E) SUM149 cells were treated with DMSO or 50 nM E2 for 72 h and analyzed by western blot.

Additional file 7: Figure S7. Estrogen stimulates ER-positive cell proliferation that is blocked by 4OHT. MCF-7 cells were treated with DMSO and 5 nM E2 with or without 5 μM 4OHT. The number of viable cells was determined on day 1, day 3, and day 5 (A). Cells treated for 72 h were collected and analyzed by western blot (B); *p?<?0.05 between E2-treated and E2?+?4OHT-treated groups at the time points (Student t test). Data are represented as mean?±?SD (n?=?4).

Additional file 8: Figure S8. E2 activates the AKT pathway in *BRCA1* mutant PDX tumors, and inhibition of Akt suppresses proliferation of *Brca1*-deficient tumor cells. (A, B) Representative *BRCA1* mutant PDX tumors treated with E2 or placebo were immunostained with the antibodies indicated. (C) *p18$^{-/-}$; Brca1^{MGKO}* type 2 tumor cells were treated with DMSO or 5 nM E2 in the presence of different dosage of AZD5363. The number of viable cells were determined on day 1, day 3, and day 5; *p?<?0.05 between E2-treated and E2?+?AZD5363-treated groups at the time points (Student t test). Data are represented as mean?±?SD (n?=?4). (D) Representative *p18$^{-/-}$; Brca1^{MGKO}* tumors treated with AZD5363 or vehicle for 7 days were analyzed by IHC. (PDF 3678 kb)

Abbreviations

BLBCs: Basal-like breast cancers; *Brca1^{MGKO}*: *Brca1$^{f/f}$;MMTV-Cre* or *Brca1$^{f/-}$;MMTV-Cre*); BrdU: Bromodeoxyuridine; CSCs: Cancer stem cells; DMEM: Dulbecco's modified Eagle's medium; DMSO: Dimethyl sulfoxide; E2: 17β-estradiol; E-cad: E-cadherin; EMT: Epithelial-mesenchymal transition; EMT-TFs: Epithelial-mesenchymal transition-inducing transcription factors; ER: Estrogen receptor; FACS: Fluorescence-activated cell sorting; FBS: Fetal bovine serum; Fn: Fibronectin; H.E.: Hematoxylin and eosin; IACUC: Institutional Animal Care and Use Committee; IHC: Immunohistochemical analysis; INK4: Inhibitors of CDK4/6; MECs: Mammary epithelial cells; MEFs: Mouse embryonic fibroblasts; MFPs: Mammary fat pads; p16: p16^{Ink4a}; p18: p18^{Ink4c}; PDX: Patient-derived xenografts; PI3K: Phosphatidylinositol-3-kinase; Vim: Vimentin

Acknowledgements

We thank Drs. Beverly Koller, Chuxia Deng, Norman Sharpless, and Lothar Hennighausen for *Brca1* mutant, p16 null, and MMTV-cre mice; Yue Xiong for discussion; Emely Pimentel for technical support; Jun-Zhu (Jenny) Pei for proofreading; the FACS core facility at University of Miami for cell sorting; and the DVR core facility for animal husbandry. Chuying Wang thanks Xi'an Jiaotong University for financial support.

Funding

This study was supported by DOD Idea Expansion Award (W81XWH-13-1-0282), the Woman's Cancer Association Grant, the Bankhead-Coley Cancer Research grant (TBC07), and research funds from the University of Miami Department of Surgery and Sylvester Comprehensive Cancer Center to Xin-Hai Pei.

Authors' contributions

CW, FB, and XHP designed the research; CW, FB, and LZ performed the research; AS generated and characterized *p16;Brca1* mice; CW, FB, and XHP analyzed the data; EL provided administrative, technical, and material support; CW, FB, and XHP wrote the paper; XHP provided financial support and supervised the project. All authors read and approved the final manuscript.

Competing interests

The authors declare that they have no competing interests.

Author details

[1]Department of Medical Oncology, The First Affiliated hospital of Xi'an Jiaotong University, Xi'an, Shaanxi 710061, People's Republic of China. [2]Molecular Oncology Program, Division of Surgical Oncology, Dewitt Daughtry Family Department of Surgery, University of Miami, Miami, FL 33136, USA. [3]Sylvester Comprehensive Cancer Center, Miller School of Medicine, University of Miami, Miami, FL 33136, USA.

References

1. Yue W, Yager JD, Wang JP, Jupe ER, Santen RJ. Estrogen receptor-dependent and independent mechanisms of breast cancer carcinogenesis. Steroids. 2013;78:161–70.
2. Dall GV, Britt KL. Estrogen effects on the mammary gland in early and late life and breast cancer risk. Front Oncol. 2017;7:110.
3. Swain SM. Tamoxifen for patients with estrogen receptor-negative breast cancer. J Clin Oncol. 2001;19:93S–7S.
4. Rebbeck TR, Kauff ND, Domchek SM. Meta-analysis of risk reduction estimates associated with risk-reducing salpingo-oophorectomy in BRCA1 or BRCA2 mutation carriers. J Natl Cancer Inst. 2009;101:80–7.
5. Sun Y, Wang Y, Fan C, Gao P, Wang X, Wei G, Wei J. Estrogen promotes stemness and invasiveness of ER-positive breast cancer cells through Gli1 activation. Mol Cancer. 2014;13:137.
6. Planas-Silva MD, Waltz PK. Estrogen promotes reversible epithelial-to-mesenchymal-like transition and collective motility in MCF-7 breast cancer cells. J Steroid Biochem Mol Biol. 2007;104:11–21.
7. Fillmore CM, Gupta PB, Rudnick JA, Caballero S, Keller PJ, Lander ES, Kuperwasser C. Estrogen expands breast cancer stem-like cells through paracrine FGF/Tbx3 signaling. Proc Natl Acad Sci U S A. 2010;107:21737–42.
8. Harrison H, Simoes BM, Rogerson L, Howell SJ, Landberg G, Clarke RB. Oestrogen increases the activity of oestrogen receptor negative breast cancer stem cells through paracrine EGFR and notch signalling. Breast Cancer Res. 2013;15:R21.
9. Koboldt DC, Fulton RS, McLellan MD, Schmidt H, Kalicki-Veizer J, McMichael JF, Fulton LL, Dooling DJ, Ding L, Mardis ER, et al. Comprehensive molecular portraits of human breast tumours. Nature. 2012;487:330–7.
10. Fedele M, Cerchia L, Chiappetta G. The epithelial-to-mesenchymal transition in breast cancer: focus on basal-like carcinomas. Cancers (Basel). 2017;9(10):134.
11. Wicha MS. Cancer stem cell heterogeneity in hereditary breast cancer. Breast Cancer Res. 2008;10:105.
12. Ye X, Weinberg RA. Epithelial-mesenchymal plasticity: a central regulator of cancer progression. Trends Cell Biol. 2015;25:675–86.
13. Mani SA, Guo W, Liao MJ, Eaton EN, Ayyanan A, Zhou AY, Brooks M, Reinhard F, Zhang CC, Shipitsin M, et al. The epithelial-mesenchymal transition generates cells with properties of stem cells. Cell. 2008;133:704–15.
14. Kim MJ, Ro JY, Ahn SH, Kim HH, Kim SB, Gong G. Clinicopathologic significance of the basal-like subtype of breast cancer: a comparison with hormone receptor and Her2/neu-overexpressing phenotypes. Hum Pathol. 2006;37:1217–26.
15. Livasy CA, Karaca G, Nanda R, Tretiakova MS, Olopade OI, Moore DT, Perou CM. Phenotypic evaluation of the basal-like subtype of invasive breast carcinoma. Mod Pathol. 2006;19:264–71.
16. Lim E, Vaillant F, Wu D, Forrest NC, Pal B, Hart AH, Asselin-Labat ML, Gyorki DE, Ward T, Partanen A, et al. Aberrant luminal progenitors as the candidate target population for basal tumor development in BRCA1 mutation carriers. Nat Med. 2009;15:907–13.
17. Proia TA, Keller PJ, Gupta PB, Klebba I, Jones AD, Sedic M, Gilmore H, Tung N, Naber SP, Schnitt S, et al. Genetic predisposition directs breast cancer phenotype by dictating progenitor cell fate. Cell Stem Cell. 2011;8:149–63.
18. Molyneux G, Geyer FC, Magnay FA, McCarthy A, Kendrick H, Natrajan R, Mackay A, Grigoriadis A, Tutt A, Ashworth A, et al. BRCA1 basal-like breast cancers originate from luminal epithelial progenitors and not from basal stem cells. Cell Stem Cell. 2010;7:403–17.
19. Bai F, Smith MD, Chan HL, Pei XH. Germline mutation of Brca1 alters the fate of mammary luminal cells and causes luminal-to-basal mammary tumor transformation. Oncogene. 2013;32:2715–25.
20. De Summa S, Pinto R, Sambiasi D, Petriella D, Paradiso V, Paradiso A, Tommasi S. BRCAness: a deeper insight into basal-like breast tumors. Ann Oncol. 2013;24(Suppl 8):viii13–21.

21. Zhu X, Shan L, Wang F, Wang J, Wang F, Shen G, Liu X, Wang B, Yuan Y, Ying J, Yang H. Hypermethylation of BRCA1 gene: implication for prognostic biomarker and therapeutic target in sporadic primary triple-negative breast cancer. Breast Cancer Res Treat. 2015;150:479–86.

22. Liu X, Holstege H, van der Gulden H, Treur-Mulder M, Zevenhoven J, Velds A, Kerkhoven RM, van Vliet MH, Wessels LF, Peterse JL, et al. Somatic loss of BRCA1 and p53 in mice induces mammary tumors with features of human BRCA1-mutated basal-like breast cancer. Proc Natl Acad Sci U S A. 2007;104: 12111–6.

23. Bai F, Chan HL, Scott A, Smith MD, Fan C, Herschkowitz JI, Perou CM, Livingstone AS, Robbins DJ, Capobianco AJ, Pei XH. BRCA1 suppresses epithelial-to-mesenchymal transition and stem cell dedifferentiation during mammary and tumor development. Cancer Res. 2014;74:6161–72.

24. Rodriguez-Pinilla SM, Sarrio D, Honrado E, Moreno-Bueno G, Hardisson D, Calero F, Benitez J, Palacios J. Vimentin and laminin expression is associated with basal-like phenotype in both sporadic and BRCA1-associated breast carcinomas. J Clin Pathol. 2007;60:1006–12.

25. Xu W, Yang Z, Lu N. A new role for the PI3K/Akt signaling pathway in the epithelial-mesenchymal transition. Cell Adhes Migr. 2015;9:317–24.

26. Yang SX, Polley E, Lipkowitz S. New insights on PI3K/AKT pathway alterations and clinical outcomes in breast cancer. Cancer Treat Rev. 2016; 45:87–96.

27. Yu JS, Cui W. Proliferation, survival and metabolism: the role of PI3K/AKT/mTOR signalling in pluripotency and cell fate determination. Development. 2016;143:3050–60.

28. Xiang T, Jia Y, Sherris D, Li S, Wang H, Lu D, Yang Q. Targeting the Akt/mTOR pathway in Brca1-deficient cancers. Oncogene. 2011;30:2443–50.

29. Xiang T, Ohashi A, Huang Y, Pandita TK, Ludwig T, Powell SN, Yang Q. Negative regulation of AKT activation by BRCA1. Cancer Res. 2008;68:10040–4.

30. Gorrini C, Gang BP, Bassi C, Wakeham A, Baniasadi SP, Hao Z, Li WY, Cescon DW, Li YT, Molyneux S, et al. Estrogen controls the survival of BRCA1-deficient cells via a PI3K-NRF2-regulated pathway. Proc Natl Acad Sci U S A. 2014;111:4472–7.

31. Renoir JM, Marsaud V, Lazennec G. Estrogen receptor signaling as a target for novel breast cancer therapeutics. Biochem Pharmacol. 2013;85:449–65.

32. Pei XH, Xiong Y. Biochemical and cellular mechanisms of mammalian CDK inhibitors: a few unresolved issues. Oncogene. 2005;24:2787–95.

33. Jonsson G, Staaf J, Vallon-Christersson J, Ringner M, Gruvberger-Saal SK, Saal LH, Holm K, Hegardt C, Arason A, Fagerholm R, et al. The retinoblastoma gene undergoes rearrangements in BRCA1-deficient basal-like breast cancer. Cancer Res. 2012;72:4028–36.

34. Stefansson OA, Jonasson JG, Olafsdottir K, Hilmarsdottir H, Olafsdottir G, Esteller M, Johannsson OT, Eyfjord JE. CpG island hypermethylation of BRCA1 and loss of pRb as co-occurring events in basal/triple-negative breast cancer. Epigenetics. 2011;6:638–49.

35. Hollestelle A, Nagel JH, Smid M, Lam S, Elstrodt F, Wasielewski M, Ng SS, French PJ, Peeters JK, Rozendaal MJ, et al. Distinct gene mutation profiles among luminal-type and basal-type breast cancer cell lines. Breast Cancer Res Treat. 2010;121:53–64.

36. Stephens PJ, McBride DJ, Lin ML, Varela I, Pleasance ED, Simpson JT, Stebbings LA, Leroy C, Edkins S, Mudie LJ, et al. Complex landscapes of somatic rearrangement in human breast cancer genomes. Nature. 2009;462:1005–10.

37. Pei XH, Bai F, Smith MD, Usary J, Fan C, Pai SY, Ho IC, Perou CM, Xiong Y. CDK inhibitor p18(INK4c) is a downstream target of GATA3 and restrains mammary luminal progenitor cell proliferation and tumorigenesis. Cancer Cell. 2009;15:389–401.

38. Jiang Z, Deng T, Jones R, Li H, Herschkowitz JI, Liu JC, Weigman VJ, Tsao MS, Lane TF, Perou CM, Zacksenhaus E. Rb deletion in mouse mammary progenitors induces luminal-B or basal-like/EMT tumor subtypes depending on p53 status. J Clin Invest. 2010;120:3296–309.

39. Scott A, Bai F, Chan HL, Liu S, Ma J, Slingerland JM, Robbins DJ, Capobianco AJ, Pei XH. p16INK4a suppresses BRCA1-deficient mammary tumorigenesis. Oncotarget. 2016;7:84496–507.

40. Sedic M, Skibinski A, Brown N, Gallardo M, Mulligan P, Martinez P, Keller PJ, Glover E, Richardson AL, Cowan J, et al. Haploinsufficiency for BRCA1 leads to cell-type-specific genomic instability and premature senescence. Nat Commun. 2015;6:7505.

41. Goulding H, Pinder S, Cannon P, Pearson D, Nicholson R, Snead D, Bell J, Elston CW, Robertson JF, Blamey RW, et al. A new immunohistochemical antibody for the assessment of estrogen receptor status on routine formalin-fixed tissue samples. Hum Pathol. 1995;26:291–4.

42. Visvader JE, Stingl J. Mammary stem cells and the differentiation hierarchy: current status and perspectives. Genes Dev. 2014;28:1143–58.

43. Asselin-Labat ML, Shackleton M, Stingl J, Vaillant F, Forrest NC, Eaves CJ, Visvader JE, Lindeman GJ. Steroid hormone receptor status of mouse mammary stem cells. J Natl Cancer Inst. 2006;98:1011–4.

44. Hassanein M, Huiart L, Bourdon V, Rabayrol L, Geneix J, Nogues C, Peyrat JP, Gesta P, Meynard P, Dreyfus H, et al. Prediction of BRCA1 germ-line mutation status in patients with breast cancer using histoprognosis grade, MS110, Lys27H3, vimentin, and KI67. Pathobiology. 2013;80:219–27.

45. Dumont N, Wilson MB, Crawford YG, Reynolds PA, Sigaroudinia M, Tlsty TD. Sustained induction of epithelial to mesenchymal transition activates DNA methylation of genes silenced in basal-like breast cancers. Proc Natl Acad Sci U S A. 2008;105:14867–72.

46. Turner NC, Reis-Filho JS, Russell AM, Springall RJ, Ryder K, Steele D, Savage K, Gillett CE, Schmitt FC, Ashworth A, Tutt AN. BRCA1 dysfunction in sporadic basal-like breast cancer. Oncogene. 2007;26:2126–32.

47. Gupta PB, Fillmore CM, Jiang G, Shapira SD, Tao K, Kuperwasser C, Lander ES. Stochastic state transitions give rise to phenotypic equilibrium in populations of cancer cells. Cell. 2011;146:633–44.

48. Prat A, Parker JS, Karginova O, Fan C, Livasy C, Herschkowitz JI, He X, Perou CM. Phenotypic and molecular characterization of the claudin-low intrinsic subtype of breast cancer. Breast Cancer Res. 2010;12:R68.

49. Jordan NV, Prat A, Abell AN, Zawistowski JS, Sciaky N, Karginova OA, Zhou B, Golitz BT, Perou CM, Johnson GL. SWI/SNF chromatin-remodeling factor Smarcd3/Baf60c controls epithelial-mesenchymal transition by inducing Wnt5a signaling. Mol Cell Biol. 2013;33:3011–25.

50. Hyman DM, Smyth LM, Donoghue MTA, Westin SN, Bedard PL, Dean EJ, Bando H, El-Khoueiry AB, Perez-Fidalgo JA, Mita A, et al. AKT inhibition in solid tumors with AKT1 mutations. J Clin Oncol. 2017;35:2251–9.

51. Asselin-Labat ML, Vaillant F, Sheridan JM, Pal B, Wu D, Simpson ER, Yasuda H, Smyth GK, Martin TJ, Lindeman GJ, Visvader JE. Control of mammary stem cell function by steroid hormone signalling. Nature. 2010;465:798–802.

52. Zhao C, Cai S, Shin K, Lim A, Kalisky T, Lu WJ, Clarke MF, Beachy PA. Stromal Gli2 activity coordinates a niche signaling program for mammary epithelial stem cells. Science. 2017;356:eaal3485.

53. Guttilla IK, Adams BD, White BA. ERalpha, microRNAs, and the epithelial-mesenchymal transition in breast cancer. Trends Endocrinol Metab. 2012;23: 73–82.

54. Park SH, Cheung LW, Wong AS, Leung PC. Estrogen regulates snail and Slug in the down-regulation of E-cadherin and induces metastatic potential of ovarian cancer cells through estrogen receptor alpha. Mol Endocrinol. 2008; 22:2085–98.

55. Li W, Xiao C, Vonderhaar BK, Deng CX. A role of estrogen/ERalpha signaling in BRCA1-associated tissue-specific tumor formation. Oncogene. 2007;26: 7204–12.

56. Ingberg E, Theodorsson A, Theodorsson E, Strom JO. Methods for long-term 17beta-estradiol administration to mice. Gen Comp Endocrinol. 2012;175: 188–93.

57. Haisenleder DJ, Schoenfelder AH, Marcinko ES, Geddis LM, Marshall JC. Estimation of estradiol in mouse serum samples: evaluation of commercial estradiol immunoassays. Endocrinology. 2011;152:4443–7.

12

Tumor-derived granulocyte colony-stimulating factor diminishes efficacy of breast tumor cell vaccines

Sruthi Ravindranathan[1], Khue G. Nguyen[2,3], Samantha L. Kurtz[1], Haven N. Frazier[4], Sean G. Smith[1,5], Bhanu prasanth Koppolu[1,5], Narasimhan Rajaram[1] and David A. Zaharoff[1,2,3,4,5]* (iD)

Abstract

Background: Although metastasis is ultimately responsible for about 90% of breast cancer mortality, the vast majority of breast-cancer-related deaths are due to progressive recurrences from non-metastatic disease. Current adjuvant therapies are unable to prevent progressive recurrences for a significant fraction of patients with breast cancer. Autologous tumor cell vaccines (ATCVs) are a safe and potentially useful strategy to prevent breast cancer recurrence, in a personalized and patient-specific manner, following standard-of-care tumor resection. Given the high intra-patient and inter-patient heterogeneity in breast cancer, it is important to understand which factors influence the immunogenicity of breast tumor cells in order to maximize ATCV effectiveness.

Methods: The relative immunogenicity of two murine breast carcinomas, 4T1 and EMT6, were compared in a prophylactic vaccination-tumor challenge model. Differences in cell surface expression of antigen-presentation-related and costimulatory molecules were compared along with immunosuppressive cytokine production. CRISPR/Cas9 technology was used to modulate tumor-derived cytokine secretion. The impacts of cytokine deletion on splenomegaly, myeloid-derived suppressor cell (MDSC) accumulation and ATCV immunogenicity were assessed.

Results: Mice vaccinated with an EMT6 vaccine exhibited significantly greater protective immunity than mice vaccinated with a 4T1 vaccine. Hybrid vaccination studies revealed that the 4T1 vaccination induced both local and systemic immune impairments. Although there were significant differences between EMT6 and 4T1 in the expression of costimulatory molecules, major disparities in the secretion of immunosuppressive cytokines likely accounts for differences in immunogenicity between the cell lines. Ablation of one cytokine in particular, granulocyte-colony stimulating factor (G-CSF), reversed MDSC accumulation and splenomegaly in the 4T1 model. Furthermore, G-CSF inhibition enhanced the immunogenicity of a 4T1-based vaccine to the extent that all vaccinated mice developed complete protective immunity.

Conclusions: Breast cancer cells that express high levels of G-CSF have the potential to diminish or abrogate the efficacy of breast cancer ATCVs. Fortunately, this study demonstrates that genetic ablation of immunosuppressive cytokines, such as G-CSF, can enhance the immunogenicity of breast cancer cell-based vaccines. Strategies that combine inhibition of immunosuppressive factors with immune stimulatory co-formulations already under development may help ATCVs reach their full potential.

Keywords: Breast cancer vaccine, Autologous tumor cell vaccine, MDSCs, Breast cancer immunogenicity

* Correspondence: dazaharo@ncsu.edu
[1]Department of Biomedical Engineering, University of Arkansas, Fayetteville, AR, USA
[2]Cell and Molecular Biology Program, University of Arkansas, Fayetteville, AR, USA
Full list of author information is available at the end of the article

Background

In 2018, approximately 41,400 breast-cancer-related deaths will occur in the USA [1]. About 90% of these deaths will be due to metastases. Since only about 4% of the 265,000+ new patients with breast cancer are typically diagnosed with stage IV metastatic cancer, the vast majority of breast-cancer-related deaths are due to the recurrence and progression of breast cancers initially diagnosed at stages I–III. In an attempt to prevent tumor recurrence, approximately four out of every five patients with breast cancer receive adjuvant therapies such as chemotherapy, hormone therapy, and/or radiotherapy following tumor resection [2]. Even with state-of-the-art adjuvant treatments, the 5-year recurrence rates for stage I, II, and III breast cancer are 7%, 11%, and 13%, respectively [3]. After 10 years, the overall breast cancer recurrence rate increases to 20% [3]. Furthermore, side effects associated with current adjuvant therapies can be life-altering and even life-threatening [4]. Thus, strategies capable of more effectively and more safely preventing progressive breast cancer recurrences, particularly after standard-of-care tumor resection, are urgently needed.

Adjuvant breast cancer vaccines are of interest due to their potential to educate a patient's immune system to recognize and eliminate occult tumor cells before a recurrence can develop. In particular, autologous tumor cell vaccines (ATCVs) comprise a promising class of vaccines capable of inducing personalized, polyclonal anti-tumor immune responses [5–14]. Patient/tumor-specific polyclonal immune responses are especially relevant for breast cancer with high intra-patient and inter-patient molecular heterogeneity that facilitates resistance to targeted therapies [15–19]. Because ATCVs are generated from a patient's own malignant cells, they present a complete and personalized library of tumor-associated antigens (TAAs). In contrast, peptide-based vaccines deliver one or a couple different peptides and are prone to tumor escape through downregulation of the targeted epitope(s). Furthermore, since ATCVs are "antigen agnostic," they could be used in the management of any subtype of breast cancer including triple-negative breast cancers (TNBCs), which lack hormone and human epidermal growth factor receptor 2 (HER2) receptors, the usual targets for breast cancer therapies.

While ATCVs have been shown to be safe and active in numerous clinical studies, a major barrier to their widespread clinical use is inconsistent, if not limited, immunogenicity. Patient-derived cancer cells, which form the basis of the vaccine, have undergone extensive immunoediting to avoid elimination by the host's immune system [20]. Common mechanisms that cancer cells use during immune escape include (1) downregulation of major histocompatibility complex (MHC I/II) molecules and development of defects in antigen presentation; (2) downregulation of costimulatory molecules, such as B7–1 and B7–2; (3) upregulation of immunoinhibitory molecules, such as programmed death-ligand 1 (PD-L1); (4) loss or modification of tumor-associated antigen(s); and (5) increased production of immunosuppressive factors such as indoleamine 2,3-dioxygenase (IDO), IL-10 and tumor growth factor (TGF)β [21]. As a result, nearly all ATCVs currently under development utilize strategies to boost tumor cell immunogenicity through one or more of the following: transfection of autologous tumor cells with costimulatory molecules [22–26], conjugation of immunostimulatory moieties to autologous tumor cells [10, 27]; co-formulation with immunostimulatory molecules [6, 8, 27–30]; or engineering autologous tumor cells to secrete adjuvant cytokines [9, 31–41]. Employing these strategies has demonstrated significant increases in antitumor immunity against various malignancies in clinical studies [8–10, 26, 27, 33, 36, 37, 39, 41–43].

For breast cancer, ATCV clinical studies have been limited to three completed [44–46] and two active trials [47, 48]. All three completed studies show promise in generating antitumor responses [49]. Despite the relatively small number of clinical studies, breast cancer remains an ideal indication for ATCV deployment as (1) 62% of breast cancer cases are diagnosed at stage I, where the tumor is still localized in the breast with minimal impact on the patient's immune status [50]; (2) nearly all patients with breast cancer undergo tumor resection, thus ensuring a source of tumor cells for ATCV production; and (3) the vast majority of patients with breast cancer have minimal, if any, detectable disease after resection so the tumor burden is low.

Because of the aforementioned heterogeneity in breast cancer, it is expected that breast ATCVs will display varying degrees of immunogenicity. Thus, the goal of this study was to begin to define the primary determinants of ATCV immunogenicity by comparing two murine models of breast adenocarcinoma, 4T1 and EMT6: 4T1 is a poorly immunogenic murine breast cancer cell line that shares many features with human stage IV breast cancer [51–53]. EMT6 on the other hand, is a highly aggressive, yet immunogenic cell line [54–56]. By understanding the key drivers of breast cancer immunogenicity, we may be able to directly and more efficiently enhance ATCVs during ex vivo modifications. At the very least, data gathered could be used to identify which patients are better candidates for adjuvant ATCV therapy. During the study, we observed that myeloid-derived suppressor cells (MDSCs) played a dominant role in influencing breast ATCV immunogenicity. The immunosuppressive role of MDSCs in breast cancer progression and metastasis is well-documented [57–60]. In particular, the levels of circulating MDSCs were found to correlate with clinical stage and metastatic tumor burden [61]. However, to the best of our knowledge, the influence of MDSCs on ATCV efficacy has not been explored. Thus, the focus of the latter stages of this study shifted towards identifying and blocking the origin of breast-cancer-related MDSCs as a strategy to enhance ATCV immunogenicity.

Methods

Cell culture

Murine breast adenocarcinoma cells 4T1 and EMT6 were purchased from American Type Culture Collection (Manassas, VA, USA). The rest of the breast cancer cells, namely 4T07, 67NR, 66Cl4, 168FARN were a generous gift from Dr Fred Miller (Karmanos Cancer Institute, Detroit, MI, USA). All cell lines except EMT6 cells were maintained in Dulbecco's modified eagle medium (DMEM), supplemented with 10% fetal bovine serum (FBS) and 1% penicillin/streptomycin (P/S). EMT6 cells were maintained in Roswell Park Memorial Institute-1640 (RPMI-1640) medium, supplemented with 15% FBS and 1% P/S. All cells were cultured at 37 °C in a humidified incubator with 5% CO_2.

Mice

All experimental procedures were approved by the Institutional Animal Care and Use Committee at University of Arkansas. Female Balb/cByJ mice were purchased from The Jackson Laboratory (Bar Harbor, ME, USA) and were housed in microisolator cages. Mice were utilized for experiments at 8–12 weeks of age and animal care followed *The Guide for Care and Use of Laboratory Animals* (National Research Council).

In vitro proliferation assay

The 4T1 and EMT6 cells were irradiated at 0, 20, 40, 60, 80, or 100 Gy using a Gammacell 1000 cesium irradiator. Cells were then plated in triplicate on a 96-well plate and incubated at 37 °C for 24, 48, 72, or 96 h. After incubation, 20 µl of CellTiter 96 Aqueous One Solution Reagent from Promega (Madison, WI, USA) was added to each well and incubated for another hour. Using a Biotek Synergy 2 plate reader from Biotek Instruments Inc. (Winooski, VT, USA), absorbance was measured at 490 nm and compared to the absorbance of similarly treated known numbers of irradiated 4T1/EMT6 cells to determine the number of viable cells in the sample wells.

Expression of MHC and costimulatory molecules

Irradiated (100 Gy) and non-irradiated 4T1 and EMT6 cells (5×10^5) were stained with fluorochrome-conjugated anti-CD80 (clone 16-10A1), anti-CD86 (clone GL1), anti-H-$2K^b$ (MHC I) (clone AF6–88.5), anti-I-A^d/I-E^d (MHC II) (clone M5/114.15.2), anti-CD54 (ICAM-1) (clone 3E2), and anti-CD95 (FasR) (clone Jo2) (BD Biosciences). Cells were analyzed on a FACSCantoII and differences in median fluorescence intensities (ΔMFI) between unstained and stained cells were determined using FlowJo software (Tree Star, San Carlos, CA, USA).

In vitro cytokine analysis

The cells (5×10^5 4T1 or EMT6 cells, untouched or irradiated, and 5×10^5 untouched 4T07, 67NR, 168FARN or 66Cl4 cells) were seeded in separate T25 flasks and cultured for 48 h. Cell culture supernatants were collected and centrifuged to remove any non-adherent cells and stored at −80 °C until analysis. From the untouched and irradiated 4T1 or EMT6 cells, levels of monocyte-colony stimulating factor (M-CSF), vascular endothelial growth factor (VEGF), transforming growth factor-β (TGF-β), interleukin-6 (IL-6), monocyte chemotactic protein (MCP-1), GM-CSF and G-CSF in cell culture supernatants were quantified. On the other hand, the cell culture supernatants from untouched 4T07, 67NR, 168FARN and 66Cl4 were only evaluated for G-CSF. Levels of M-CSF, VEGF and TGF-β were analyzed using ELISA kits from R&D systems Inc. (Minneapolis, MN, USA) and Biolegend (San Diego, CA, USA). Levels of IL-6, MCP-1, GM-CSF, and G-CSF were analyzed using a cytometric bead array (CBA) on a FACSCantoII from BD Biosciences.

CRISPR/Cas9 genomic deletion of G-CSF

Using the CRISPR design tool provided by the Zhang laboraoty at Massachussetts Institute of Technology (MIT) (http://crispr.mit.edu/), a 20-bp guide sequence targeting the *G-CSF* gene in 4T1 cells was identified. Guide sequences were cloned into separate pCas-Guide-EF1a-green fluorescent protein (GFP) plasmid via Origene's cloning service. Plasmids were amplified in *Escherichia coli* and isolated via QIAGEN Plasmid Maxi Kit. For transfection, plasmid encoding guide RNA (gRNA) (10 µg) was mixed with Lipofectamine™ 3000 reagent (ThermoFisher) and added to 1×10^6 4T1 cells pre-seeded in a 6-well plate. After 48 h, cells expressing GFP were sorted using a FACSAriaIII system (BD Biosciences). Sorted cells were subsequently cloned by limiting dilution. G-CSF expression was quantified by enzyme-linked immunosorbent assay (ELISA) from R&D systems Inc. (Minneapolis, MN, USA). A mixture of clones producing lower than detectable levels of G-CSF were identified and denoted as 4T1.G-CSF⁻.

Prophylactic vaccination studies

Tumor cell vaccines were generated by irradiating 4T1 or EMT6 cells at 100 Gy using a Gammacell 1000 cesium irradiator. Mice were subcutaneously vaccinated with a primary and booster vaccine 10 days apart, which comprised 1×10^6 irradiated 4T1 cells (4T1 vaccine) or 5×10^5 irradiated EMT6 cells (EMT6 vaccine). For mice in the ipsilateral and contralateral hybrid vaccine groups, 1×10^6 irradiated 4T1 cells and 5×10^5 irradiated EMT6 cells were subcutaneously injected on the same and opposite flanks, respectively. In some instances, where the effect of G-CSF on overall survival was investigated, mice received 4T1.G-CSF⁻ cells in place of 4T1 cells.

Further, all vaccinated mice were challenged with 1×10^6 live 4T1, 5×10^5 live EMT6 cells or 1×10^6 live 4T1.G-CSF⁻ cells, 10 days after the booster vaccine. Tumor volumes were recorded 2–3 times per week using the formula:

$$V = (w \times w \times l)/2,$$

where V is tumor volume, w is tumor width and l is tumor length.

G-CSF in serum from mice

When tumor volumes in mice bearing 4T1, 4T1.GCSF⁻, 4T07, 67NR, 168FARN and 66Cl4 reached about 500 mm³, about 400–500 µl of blood was collected in microcentrifuge tubes by submandibular bleeding. After allowing the blood to clot for 30 min at room temperature, samples were centrifuged at 2000 × g for 10 min at 4 °C. The serum was carefully collected from each sample and the levels of G-CSF were determined by ELISA (R&D systems Inc.; Minneapolis, MN, USA).

Tissue collection and analysis of immune cell subsets

Spleens and draining lymph nodes (DLNs) from 4T1 and 4T1.GCSF⁻ tumor-bearing mice were isolated when tumors reached 500–700 mm³. Single cell suspensions were prepared by mechanically dissociating spleen and DLNs with a syringe plunger and passing samples through a 40-µm nylon mesh cell strainer. Splenocytes were additionally treated with ammonium-chloride-potassium buffer (Lonza, Allendale, NJ, USA) for 10 min to lyse red blood cells. Single cell suspensions were then blocked with purified rat anti-mouse CD16/CD32 monoclonal antibody (BD Biosciences) and stained with fluorochrome-conjugated anti-CD11b (clone M1/70), anti-CD19 (clone 1D3), anti-Ly6G and Ly6C (clone RB6-8C5), anti-CD25 (clone PC61), anti-CD4 (clone GK1.5), and anti-CD3ε (clone 145-2C11) (BD Biosciences).

Cells were then rinsed, fixed and permeabilized with 1× Perm/Wash buffer from BD Biosciences. The permeabilized cells were further stained with fluorochrome-conjugated anti-FoxP3 and read on a BD FACSCanto II flow cytometer. Frequencies of MDSCs, T cells, B cells, and regulatory T cells (T_{regs}) in the single cell suspensions were determined using FlowJo software (Tree Star, San Carlos, CA, USA). For mice bearing 4T07, 67NR, 66Cl4 and 168FARN tumors, only the spleens were isolated and stained for MDSCs.

Statistical analysis

All data were analyzed using GraphPad Prism software, version 7 (GraphPad Software, Inc., San Diego, CA, USA). For all in vivo vaccine studies, Kaplan-Meier tumor-free survival curves were plotted and statistical comparisons made using the log rank test. For all other studies, data are represented as mean ± standard deviation. For the experiments that compare cytokine release and expression of MHC and costimulatory molecules by 4T1 and EMT6 before and after irradiation, statistical comparisons were made using two-way analysis of variance (ANOVA) followed by Tukey's multiple comparison post-hoc test. For experiments where different immune cell subsets in spleen and DLN of mice bearing 4T1 or 4T1.G-CSF⁻ tumors are compared to subsets in naïve mice, statistical comparisons were made using the Kruskal-Wallis test followed by Dunn's post-hoc test. For all other experiments, statistical comparisons were made using one-way ANOVA followed by Tukey's post-hoc analysis.

Results

Effect of irradiation on proliferation of breast cancer cells

Prior to using irradiated 4T1 or EMT6 cells as tumor cell vaccines, an appropriate dose of irradiation that effectively prevents tumor cell proliferation was determined using an in-vitro proliferation assay. In the absence of irradiation, both 4T1 and EMT6 cells effectively proliferated over the time observed in this study (24–96 h). However, in the presence of varying doses of irradiation (20–100 Gy), there was no significant difference in viable cell numbers during the study period (Fig. 1).

Immunogenicity of murine breast carcinoma lines

A standard prophylactic vaccine model was used to evaluate the immunogenicities of 4T1 and EMT6 cells. Mice were vaccinated twice with either irradiated 4T1 or EMT6 cells and challenged with live 4T1 or EMT6 cells, respectively. While all mice in both 4T1 and EMT6 control groups developed tumors, upon vaccination, some of the mice in the EMT6 vaccinated group did not develop any tumor. Moreover, the mice that developed tumors in the EMT6 vaccinated group, showed a delayed tumor incidence when compared to the EMT6 control (Fig. 2a). In both groups, vaccinated mice exhibited some level of protective immunity as demonstrated by extended survival compared to mice in unvaccinated control groups (Fig. 2b). However, EMT6 vaccinated mice exhibited higher overall survival with a p value < 0.01 when compared to EMT6 control. On the other hand, 4T1 vaccinated mice had a p value < 0.05 when compared to 4T1 control. Additionally, while all mice in the 4T1 vaccinated group developed and succumbed to tumors within 50 days of tumor inoculation, 75% of the mice in the EMT6 vaccinated group are tumor free survivors.

Costimulatory molecule and MHC expression on breast cancer cell lines

The elaboration of robust adaptive immunity requires antigen presentation in MHC I or MHC II complexes (signal 1) and simultaneous engagement of costimulatory molecules (signal 2), such as B7-1, B7-2, ICAM-1 and FasR, on APCs, with their cognate receptors, i.e. T cell

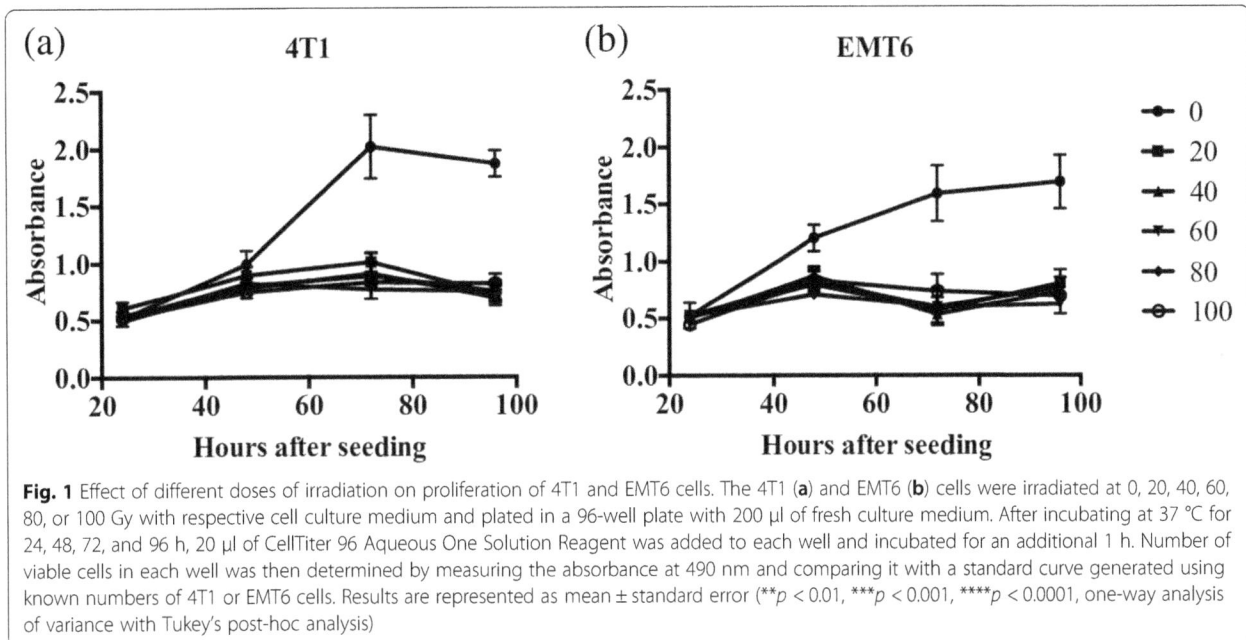

Fig. 1 Effect of different doses of irradiation on proliferation of 4T1 and EMT6 cells. The 4T1 (**a**) and EMT6 (**b**) cells were irradiated at 0, 20, 40, 60, 80, or 100 Gy with respective cell culture medium and plated in a 96-well plate with 200 μl of fresh culture medium. After incubating at 37 °C for 24, 48, 72, and 96 h, 20 μl of CellTiter 96 Aqueous One Solution Reagent was added to each well and incubated for an additional 1 h. Number of viable cells in each well was then determined by measuring the absorbance at 490 nm and comparing it with a standard curve generated using known numbers of 4T1 or EMT6 cells. Results are represented as mean ± standard error (**p < 0.01, ***p < 0.001, ****p < 0.0001, one-way analysis of variance with Tukey's post-hoc analysis)

receptor (TCR), CD28, lymphocyte function-associated antigen 1 (LFA-1) and Fas ligand (Fas-L), on lymphocytes. Thus, MHC and costimulatory molecules on 4T1 and EMT6 cells were evaluated to determine if differences in expression levels could explain the observed differences in immunogenicity. Since irradiated cells displayed higher levels of autofluorescence [62] differences in mean fluorescence intensity values, ΔMFI, between unstained and stained irradiated cells and between unstained and stained non-irradiated cells were analyzed.

Prior to irradiation, 4T1 cells expressed slightly higher levels MHC I when compared to EMT6 cells (4T1: 25.2 ± 3.4; EMT6: 16.6 ± 2.3). However, upon irradiation, EMT6 cells expressed significantly higher level of MHC I which was 49.9 ± 3.3 when compared to 4T1 cells which was only 25.3 ± 3.6. On the other hand, EMT6 cells expressed higher levels of MHC II both before and after irradiation (Table 1).

B7-1 and B7-2 are costimulatory molecules that bind to CD28 on T cells. This binding provides a second signal that is required for generation of an adaptive immune response. Prior to irradiation, though the level of B7-1 expressed by EMT6 cells was higher than 4T1 cells, the difference was not significant. (Table 1). However, upon irradiation, the ΔMFI value of EMT6 cells (263.6 ± 45.1) was significantly higher than 4T1 cells (14.8 ± 2.8). On the other hand, the ΔMFI value of B7-2 for EMT6 cells were significantly higher than 4T1 cells, before and after irradiation.

ICAM-1 is a ligand for LFA-1, which is expressed on a number of cell types, including T cells, APCs and some cancer cells. In general, the high levels of expression of ICAM-1 by cancer cells could promote an increased

level of transcellular migration of leukocytes to the tumor site. Additionally, ICAM-1 expression also acts as a costimulatory signal for CTL activation [63]. Our analysis found no significant difference in the ΔMFI values of ICAM-1 between 4T1 and EMT6 before and after irradiation (Table 1).

FasR is a death receptor, which when bound to Fas-L on CTLs, can cause apoptosis of the cell expressing FasR. The ΔMFI value of FasR for EMT6 cells was significantly higher than that of 4T1 cells, both before and after irradiation. Specifically, ΔMFI of FasR for 4T1 cells were only 405.3 ± 20.4 and 1073.0 ± 71.6, compared to 2396.0 ± 159.0 and 4688.2 ± 99.9 for EMT6 cells, before and after irradiation, respectively (Table 1).

Differences in cytokine release

Another factor that could influence the immunogenicity of a tumor cell vaccine is its spontaneous release of cytokines and growth factors. To this end, IL-6, VEGF, TGF-β, MCP-1 and colony stimulating factors G-CSF, M-CSF and GM-CSF secreted by 4T1 and EMT6, before and after irradiation were compared (Fig. 3).

Colony stimulating factors, G-CSF, GM-CSF and M-CSF, at physiological levels, stimulate the proliferation, differentiation and survival of immune-supporting myeloid cells. However, at higher levels, these growth factors are associated with aberrant myeloid differentiation and accumulation of immunosuppressive MDSCs [64]. All three colony stimulating factors were produced at significantly higher levels by irradiated 4T1 cells compared to irradiated EMT6 cells (Fig. 3a, b, c). Most strikingly, the levels of G-CSF released by 4T1 cells before irradiation (5765 ± 80.9 pg/10^5 cells) and after irradiation

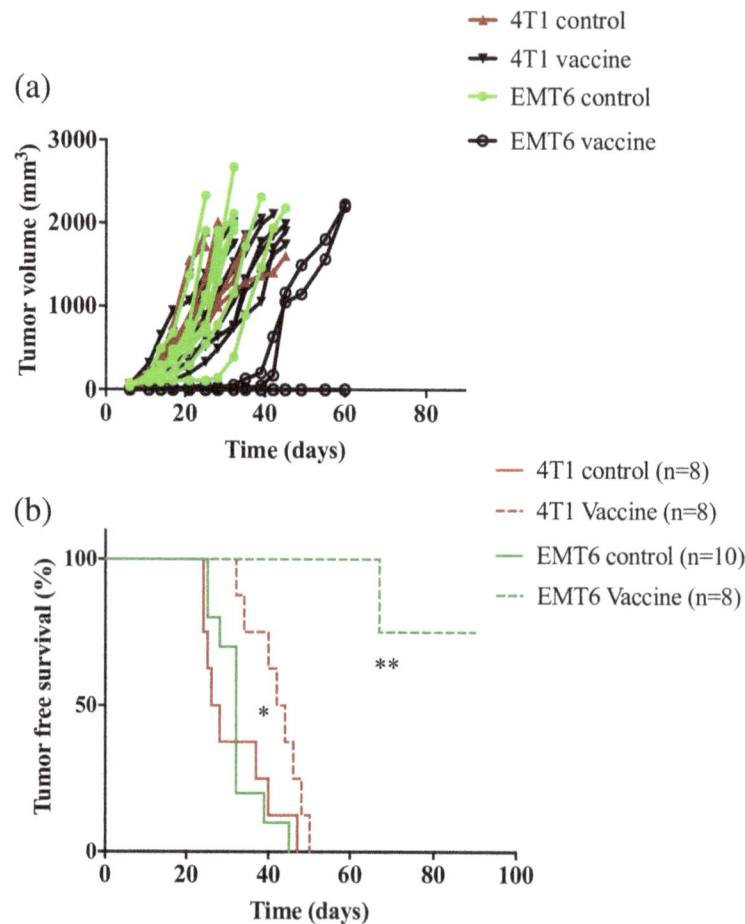

Fig. 2 Differences in protective immunity induced by irradiated breast cancer cell lines. Balb/cByJ mice ($n = 8$ per group) received 1×10^6 irradiated 4T1 cells (4T1 vaccine) or 5×10^5 irradiated EMT6 cells (EMT6 vaccine) twice, 10 days apart. Ten days after the booster vaccination, mice were challenged with live 5×10^5 4T1 or EMT6 cells, respectively. Additionally, naive mice that received only 5×10^5 live EMT6 cells (EMT6 control) or live 4T1 cells (4T1 control) served as controls for each group. Tumor volumes (**a**) and tumor-free survival (**b**) were recorded. (*$p < 0.05$ vs. naïve/4T1 challenge group, **$p < 0.01$ vs. naïve/EMT6 challenge group, log rank test)

Table 1 Differences in expression of MHC and costimulatory molecules in non-irradiated and irradiated breast cancer cells

	B7–1	B7–2	ICAM-1	MHCI	MHCII	FasR
4T1						
Non-irradiated	6.7 ± 1.3^a	28.6 ± 6.6	20.6 ± 2.2^a	25.2 ± 3.4^a	43.4 ± 1.8	405.3 ± 20.4
Irradiated	14.8 ± 2.8^{ab}	50.2 ± 1.4	35.7 ± 4.0^c	25.3 ± 3.6^a	133.3 ± 4.2	1073.0 ± 71.6
% change	150 ± 47.1	57.1 ± 19.7	79.3 ± 3.5	11.7 ± 15.4	209.6 ± 31.4	171.8 ± 6
			EMT6			
Non-irradiated	61.3 ± 7.2^{ab}	75 ± 5.7	22.0 ± 3.0^{ab}	16.6 ± 2.3	94.3 ± 3.6	2396.0 ± 159.0
Irradiated	263.6 ± 45.1	93.1 ± 5.3	30.5 ± 4.0^{bc}	49.9 ± 3.3	164.1 ± 12.5	4688.2 ± 99.9
% change	356.6 ± 7	19.1 ± 13.5	22.5 ± 8.5	203 ± 36.1	76.8 ± 2.8	102.7 ± 7.5

The 4T1 and EMT6 cells were exposed to 0 Gy (non-irradiated) or 100 Gy. At 24 h after irradiation, cells were harvested and stained with fluorochrome conjugated anti-CD80 (B7–1), anti-CD86 (B7–2), anti-H2-K^b (MHC I), anti-I-A^d/I-E^d (MHC II), anti-CD54 (ICAM-1), and anti-CD95 (FasR). The samples were analyzed on a multiparameter flow cytometer (FACSCantoII). The differences in mean fluorescence intensities, ΔMFI, between unstained and stained non-irradiated cells, and unstained and stained irradiated cells were tabulated. The experiment was repeated twice and one representative experiment with triplicates is shown. The results are represented as ΔMFI ± standard deviation. Means with the same letter are not statistically significant from each other ($p > 0.05$, two-way analysis of variance followed by Tukey's multiple comparison)

$(5334 \pm 114.2$ pg/10^5 cells) were exceptionally high even when compared to the levels released by EMT6 cells before $(1100 \pm 98.84$ pg/10^5 cells) and after irradiation $(1760 \pm 145.1$ pg/10^5 cells) (Fig. 3a).

IL-6 has been shown to exhibit both pro- and anti-tumor activities. Among its suppressive activities, IL-6 directly promotes cancer cell proliferation, survival and metastasis while indirectly supporting angiogenesis in the tumor microenvironment [65]. Here, IL-6 was released at modest levels with no major changes before irradiation (4T1: 62.6 ± 8.4 pg/10^5 cells; EMT6: 25.6 ± 3.7 pg/10^5 cells) or after irradiation (4T1: 21.3 ± 1.8 pg/10^5 cells; EMT6: 44.3 ± 6.6 pg/10^5 cells) (Fig. 3d).

Tumor-derived MCP-1 promotes infiltration of monocytes and macrophages. MCP-1 as well as VEGF are associated with promoting angiogenesis [66, 67]. Additionally, tumor secretion of VEGF blocks normal myeloid differentiation, resulting in MDSC accumulation [68, 69]. 4T1 cells produced higher levels of MCP-1 only after irradiation (4T1: 1596 ± 123.6 pg/10^5 cells; EMT6: 744.7 ± 58.91 pg/10^5 cells) (Fig. 3e). On the contrary, EMT6 cells produced higher levels of VEGF before $(833 \pm 41.19$ pg/10^5 cells) and after $(371.3 \pm 8.09$ pg/10^5 cells) irradiation, when compared to 4T1 cells before $(10 \pm 1.1$ pg/10^5 cells) and after $(8.6 \pm 0.6$ pg/10^5 cells) (Fig. 3f).

TGF-β, an immunosuppressive cytokine that plays a role in the induction of T_{regs}, was produced at higher levels by EMT6 cells before irradiation (4T1: 108 ± 7.6 pg/10^5 cells; EMT6: 832 ± 49 pg/10^5 cells) (Fig. 3g). However, upon irradiation, the difference between cell lines was not statistically significant (4T1: 355 ± 22.1 pg/10^5 cells; EMT6: 274 ± 17 pg/10^5 cells) (Fig. 3g).

Local and systemic effects of 4T1 mediated immunosuppression

Based on differences in cytokine release (Fig. 3), we explored if immunosuppressive cytokines released by 4T1 cells would abrogate the protective immunity established by the irradiated EMT6 vaccine. To explore the potential for localized immune suppression, mice were immunized with a heterogeneous mixture of irradiated 4T1 and EMT6 cells (ipsilateral hybrid vaccine). To explore possible systemic immune suppression mediated by 4T1 cells, mice were vaccinated with irradiated 4T1 cells and irradiated EMT6 cells on opposite flanks (contralateral hybrid vaccine). The efficacy of these vaccines was compared using mice immunized with irradiated EMT6 cells alone (EMT6 vaccine). The study design is shown in Fig. 4a.

When all groups of mice were challenged with live EMT6 cells, unlike the EMT6 vaccine group, both ipsilateral and contralateral hybrid vaccine group did not exhibit a delayed tumor incidence (Fig. 4b). Additionally, the presence of irradiated 4T1 cells in the hybrid vaccines diminished the protective immunity induced by irradiated EMT6 cells, as the percentage of tumor free survival in the ipsilateral and contralateral vaccine groups were only about 34% and 27%, respectively (Fig. 4c). The long term, tumor-free survival for mice receiving the EMT6 vaccine alone was significantly higher at 71%.

The immunosuppressive role of G-CSF

Due to the exceptionally high levels of G-CSF produced by 4T1 cells with and without irradiation, we hypothesized that it played a key role in inhibiting the efficacy of ipsilateral and contralateral vaccines. To test this hypothesis, we functionally deleted the G-CSF gene via CRISPR/Cas9 genomic editing.

4T1 cells before G-CSF deletion released 4550 ± 604 pg G-CSF per 10^5 cells, whereas after G-CSF deletion, cells only released 386 ± 31 pg G-CSF/10^5 cells. Clonal selection led to the propagation of a 4T1 colony, called 4T1.G-CSF$^-$, that released lower than detectable levels of G-CSF in vitro (Fig. 5a). The G-CSF deletion did not affect tumor establishment or growth in vivo (Fig. 5b). To further verify G-CSF ablation, G-CSF serum concentrations were assessed in mice bearing 4T1.G-CSF$^-$ tumors when tumor volumes reached 500–700 mm^3. 4T1.G-CSF$^-$ tumor bearing mice contained only 10 ± 2.9 pg/ml of G-CSF in their sera, which was comparable to G-CSF in the sera of naïve mice $(59 \pm 34$ pg/ml). On the other hand, mice with similarly sized, unmodified 4T1 tumors contained $13,096 \pm 1947$ pg/ml G-CSF in their sera (Fig. 5c).

Additionally, spleens and DLNs from 4T1 and 4T1.G-CSF$^-$ tumor bearing mice were harvested to determine the frequency of T cells, B cells, MDSCs and T_{regs} in each lymphoid tissue. MDSCs were of particular interest as immature myeloid cells have often been associated with high levels of colony stimulating factors [70, 71]. Prior to immunophenotyping we noted remarkable differences in the sizes and weights of spleens removed from mice bearing 4T1 tumors, 4T1.GCSF$^-$ tumors or no tumors (Fig. 6a, b). G-CSF appeared to be driving the extreme splenomegaly observed in 4T1-bearing mice. In addition, spleens from 4T1 tumor bearing mice contained significantly higher levels of MDSCs $(213 \pm 21 \times 10^6$ MDSCs) when compared to naive $(1.7 \pm 0.3 \times 10^6$ MDSCs) spleens. On the other hand, there was no significant difference between the levels of MDSCs in naïve and 4T1.G-CSF$^-$ tumor bearing mice $(26 \pm 10 \times 10^6$ MDSCs)(Fig. 6c). The same trends held when analyzing the percentages of MDSCs in the spleens of mice from the three groups (see Additional file 1).

Though there was no significant difference in the number of T cells in the spleens of mice among the different groups, there was a significant difference in the number of B cells and T_{regs} between 4T1 tumor bearing and naïve mice (4T1: $37 \pm 8 \times 10^6$ B cells and $4.2 \pm 0.5 \times 10^6$ T_{regs}; naïve: $2.3 \pm 0.4 \times 10^6$ B cells and $0.08 \pm 0.01 \times 10^6$ T_{regs}) (Fig. 6d, e, f).

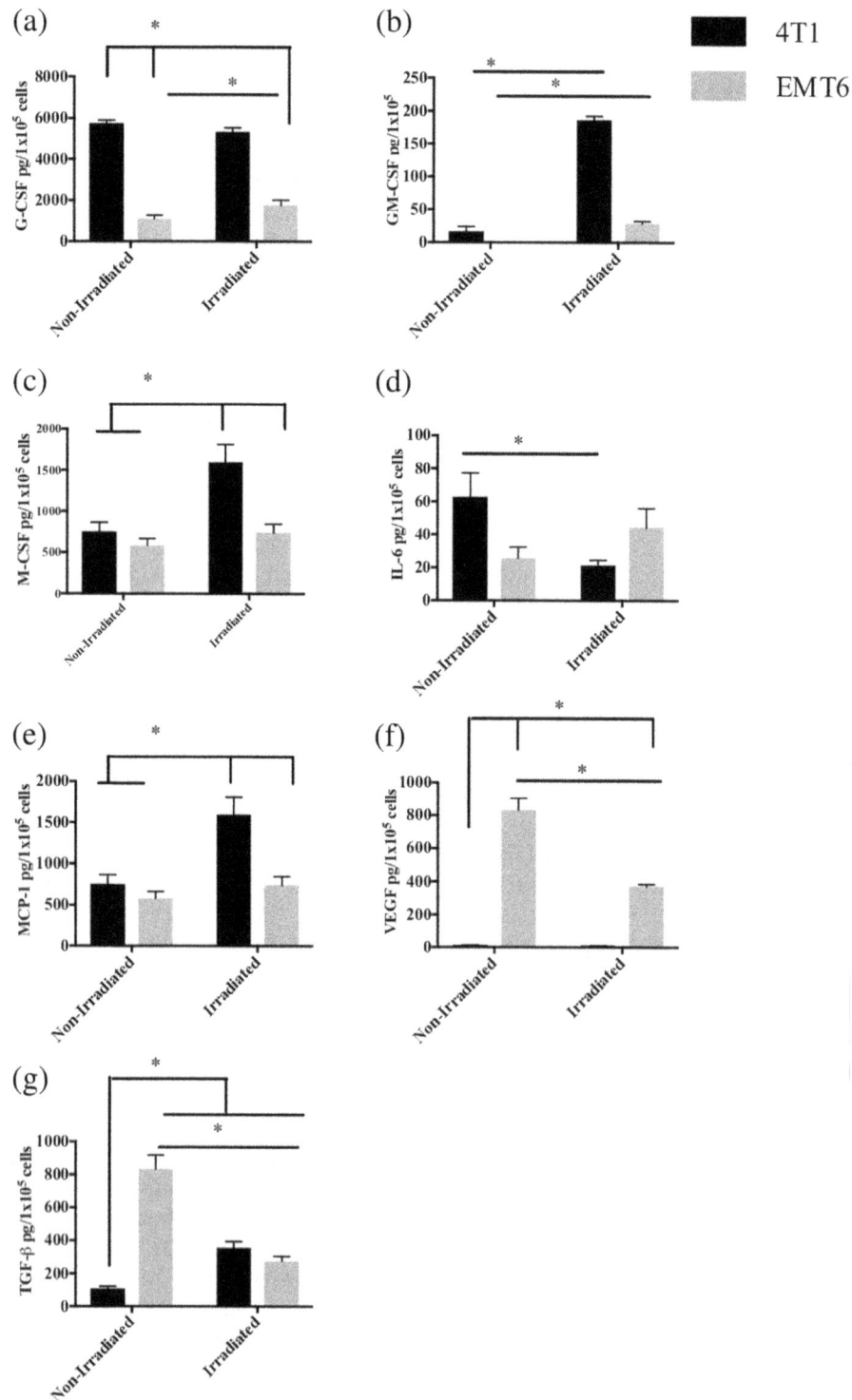

Fig. 3 Cytokine release profile of 4T1 and EMT6 cells before and after irradiation. The 4T1 or EMT6 cells were exposed to 0 Gy (non-irradiated) or 100 Gy. The cells (5 × 10⁵ non-irradiated (4T1 and EMT6) and irradiated (4T1 Irr and EMT6 Irr) cells) were seeded on separate T25 flasks and cultured for 48 h. Cell culture supernatants were collected from each flask and centrifuged to remove debris. Levels of IL-6 (**a**), granulocyte-macrophage colony-stimulating factor (GM-CSF) (**b**), monocyte chemotactic protein-1 (MCP-1) (**c**), and granulocyte colony-stimulating factor (G-CSF) (**d**) in cell-free supernatants were quantified using cytometric bead array. Levels of macrophage colony-stimulating factor (M-CSF) (**e**), vascular endothelial growth factor (VEGF) (**f**), and tumor growth factor-beta (TGF-β) (**g**) were quantified by ELISA. The experiment was repeated thrice and the results represent the mean ± standard error from one representative experiment (*$p < 0.05$, two-way analysis of variance with Tukey's multiple comparisons post-hoc analysis)

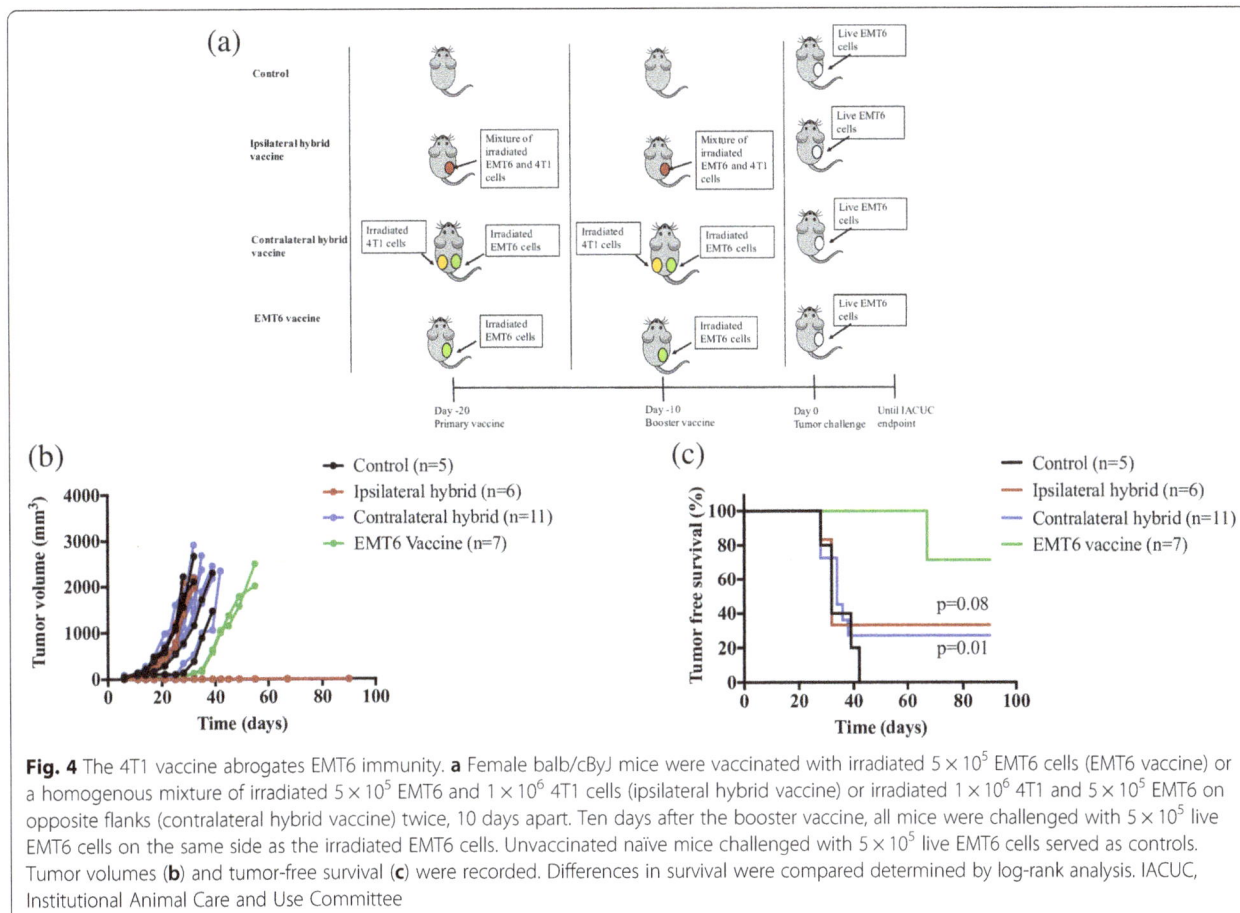

Fig. 4 The 4T1 vaccine abrogates EMT6 immunity. **a** Female balb/cByJ mice were vaccinated with irradiated 5×10^5 EMT6 cells (EMT6 vaccine) or a homogenous mixture of irradiated 5×10^5 EMT6 and 1×10^6 4T1 cells (ipsilateral hybrid vaccine) or irradiated 1×10^6 4T1 and 5×10^5 EMT6 on opposite flanks (contralateral hybrid vaccine) twice, 10 days apart. Ten days after the booster vaccine, all mice were challenged with 5×10^5 live EMT6 cells on the same side as the irradiated EMT6 cells. Unvaccinated naïve mice challenged with 5×10^5 live EMT6 cells served as controls. Tumor volumes (**b**) and tumor-free survival (**c**) were recorded. Differences in survival were compared determined by log-rank analysis. IACUC, Institutional Animal Care and Use Committee

Immune subset populations from 4T1.G-CSF$^-$ tumor bearing mice were comparable with those found in naïve mice. Percentages of splenic T cells, B cells and T$_{regs}$ were not statistically different among the cohorts (see Additional file 1).

In DLNs, numbers of MDSCs in 4T1 tumor bearing mice ($35 \pm 0.5 \times 10^4$ MDSCs) was significantly higher than the levels in naïve mice ($1.2 \pm 0.3 \times 10^4$ MDSCs) but not 4T1.G-CSF$^-$ tumor bearing mice (Fig. 7a). Similarly, DLNs contained significant differences in the numbers of T cells between 4T1 bearing and naïve mice, whereas the T cell levels were similar between 4T1.G-CSF$^-$ and naïve mice (4T1: $335 \pm 81 \times 10^4$ T cells; 4T1.G-CSF$^-$: $194 \pm 42 \times 10^4$ T cells; naïve: $45 \pm 5 \times 10^4$ T cells) (Fig. 7b). No significant differences in the numbers of B cells and T$_{regs}$ between the three groups was observed (Fig. 7c, d). In terms of percentages, both 4T1 and 4T1.G-CSF$^-$ tumor bearing mice had higher percentages of MDSCs in their DLNs than naïve mice, while there were no differences in T cell or B cell percentages (see Additional file 2).

G-CSF secretion versus MDSC accumulation in different breast cancers

To further establish the correlation between tumor secreted G-CSF levels and MDSC accumulation, we used four different 4T1sister cell lines, namely 4 T07, 67NR, 66Cl4 and 168 FARN, that share a common origin, a single, spontaneously arising breast tumor, but differ in their metastatic ability [72]. 4T1 metastasizes to lung, liver, brain and bone; 66Cl4 metastasizes to lungs and liver; 168 FARN metastasizes to regional lymph nodes; whereas 67NR and 4T07 do not form visible metastases although 4T07 cells can be found in blood and lungs [73]. In vitro studies revealed that 4T1 and 4 T07 cells secreted high levels of G-CSF (4T1: 5182 ± 814 pg/10^5 cells, 4T07: 3032 ± 476 pg/10^5 cells), while 66Cl4 secreted only about 68.5 ± 10.6 pg/10^5 cells. On the other hand, G-CSF secretion by 67NR and 168FARN cells was undetectable (Fig. 8a). Similarly, we found that serum G-CSF levels in mice bearing 4T1 and 4T07 tumors were much higher (4T1: $19,100 \pm 2274$ pg/ml, 4T07: $17,600 \pm 10,220$ pg/ml) than the other tumor models (Fig. 8b). mice bearing 67NR, 66Cl4, and 168FARN had only 165 ± 53 pg/ml, 117 ± 16 pg/ml and 46 ± 6 pg/ml, of serum G-CSF respectively. These levels were not significantly different from serum G-CSF in naïve mice (59 ± 34 pg/ml) (Fig. 8b). To determine the relationship between serum G-CSF levels and accumulation of MDSCs, cohorts of mice were implanted with each of the tumor

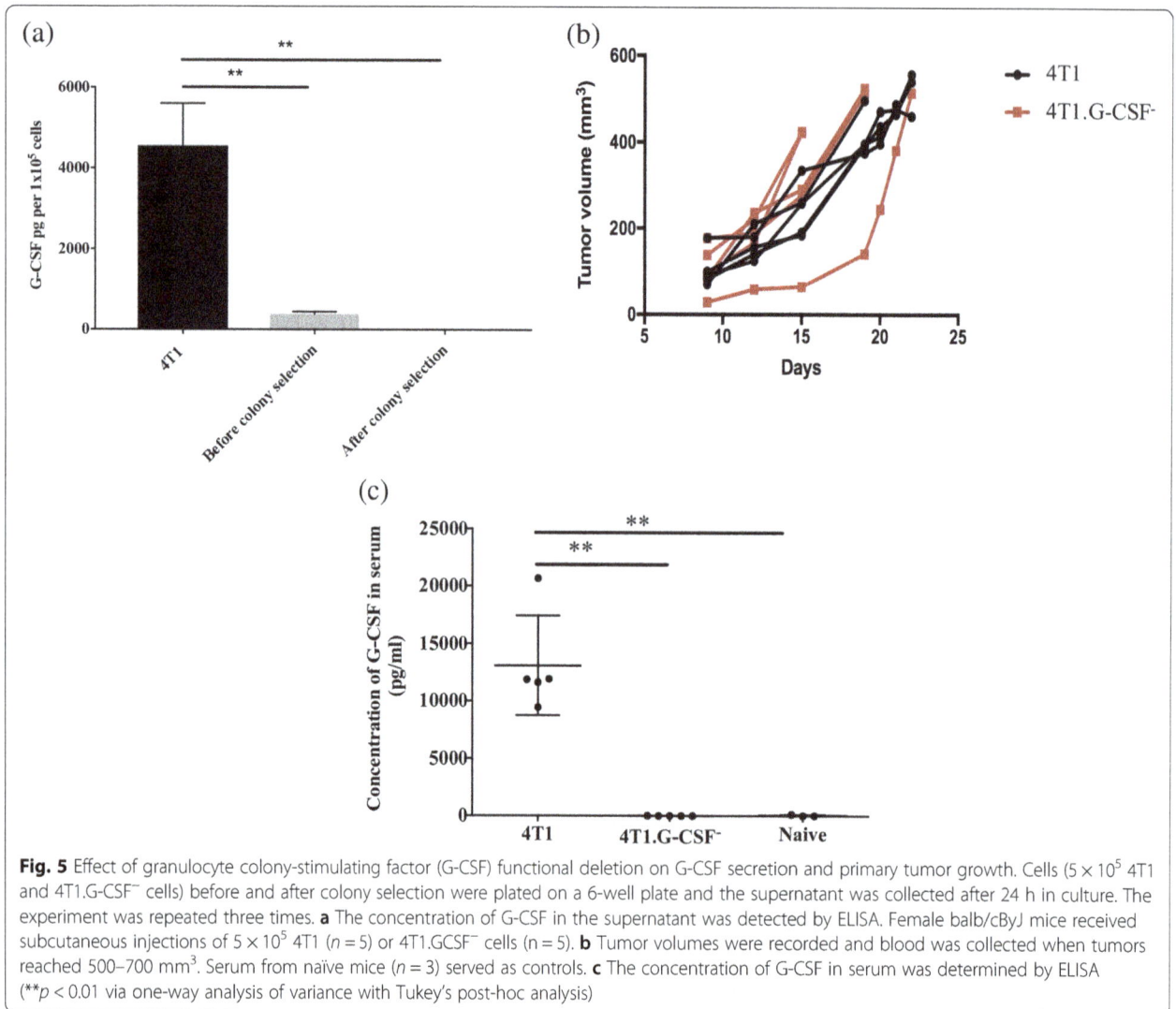

Fig. 5 Effect of granulocyte colony-stimulating factor (G-CSF) functional deletion on G-CSF secretion and primary tumor growth. Cells (5×10^5 4T1 and 4T1.G-CSF⁻ cells) before and after colony selection were plated on a 6-well plate and the supernatant was collected after 24 h in culture. The experiment was repeated three times. **a** The concentration of G-CSF in the supernatant was detected by ELISA. Female balb/cByJ mice received subcutaneous injections of 5×10^5 4T1 ($n = 5$) or 4T1.GCSF⁻ cells (n = 5). **b** Tumor volumes were recorded and blood was collected when tumors reached 500–700 mm³. Serum from naïve mice ($n = 3$) served as controls. **c** The concentration of G-CSF in serum was determined by ELISA (**$p < 0.01$ via one-way analysis of variance with Tukey's post-hoc analysis)

cell lines and spleens harvested for enumeration of MDSCs. Spleens from 4T1 and 4T07 tumor-bearing mice contained $1.27 \pm 0.1 \times 10^8$ and $1.9 \pm 0.3 \times 10^8$ MDSCs, respectively. This was significantly higher MDSC accumulation compared to the remaining breast tumor models (67NR: $4 \pm 0.4 \times 10^6$; 66Cl4: $3 \pm 0.2 \times 10^6$; 168FARN: $5 \pm 0.7 \times 10^6$ MDSCs) (Fig. 8c).

Effect of G-CSF on protective immunity

From the aforementioned studies, it appeared that MDSCs arising from high levels of G-CSF released by 4T1 vaccine were directly responsible for the impaired response to the EMT6 vaccine. To test this hypothesis, we repeated the contralateral hybrid vaccine study (Fig. 4) with irradiated 4T1.GCSF⁻ plus EMT6 cells followed by a live EMT6 challenge. We found that only 30% of mice receiving a hybrid vaccine containing 4T1.G-CSF⁻ cells developed and succumbed to tumors (Fig. 9a). This was significantly different from a hybrid vaccine containing parental 4T1 cells,

where 70% of the mice developed tumors (Fig. 9a). Additionally, we recorded survival in mice that were vaccinated and challenged with 4T1 or 4T1.G-CSF⁻ cells alone, i.e. without including EMT6 cells. We found that in the 4T1 group, all mice developed tumors similar to unvaccinated controls (Fig. 9b). On the other hand, none of the mice in the 4T1.G-CSF⁻ vaccine group developed tumors (Fig. 9b). Thus, deleting G-CSF in 4T1 cells appears to render them more immunogenic than EMT6 cells (Figs. 2 and 4).

Discussion

A major barrier to the widespread development of ATCVs as an adjuvant to breast tumor resection is the sporadic, often poor, immunogenicity of resected breast cancer cells. Thus, in this study, we set out to determine the key factors influencing the immunogenicity of breast cancer ATCVs by comparing two murine breast cancer cells, 4T1 and EMT6. This study was not meant to

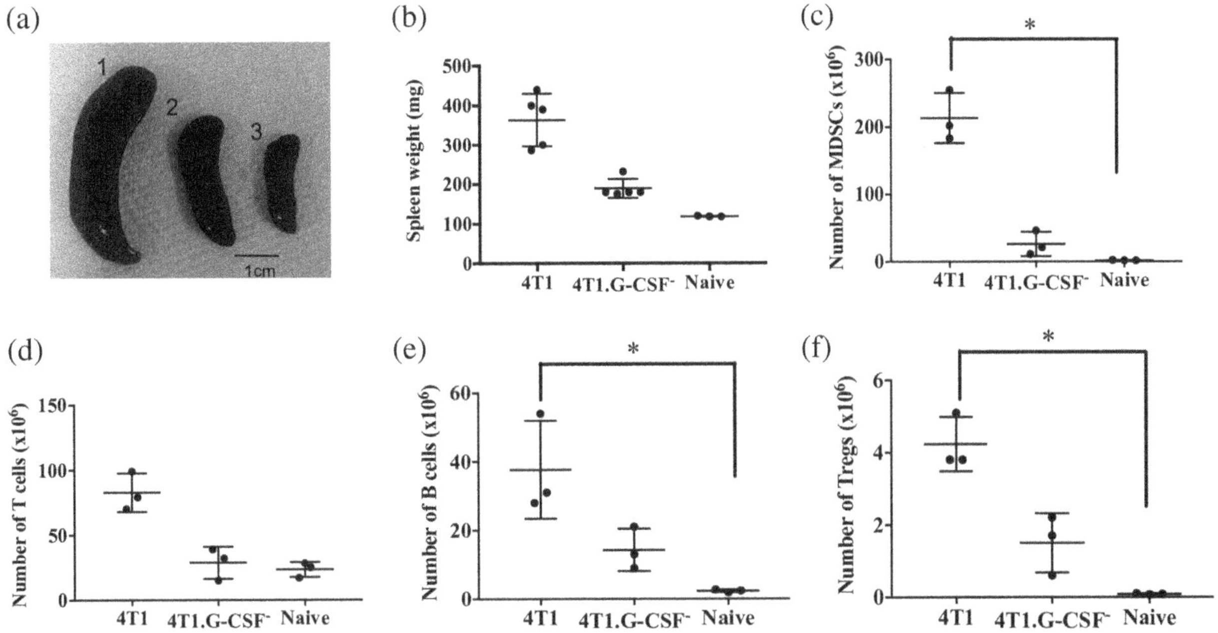

Fig. 6 Comparison of spleen size, spleen weight and immune cell subsets in spleen of 4T1 and 4T1.G-CSF$^-$ tumor-bearing mice and naïve mice. Female balb/cByJ mice received subcutaneous injections of 1×10^6 4T1 or 4T1.G-CSF$^-$ cells. Spleens were harvested when tumor volumes reached 500–700 mm^3. **a** Spleens from representative mice bearing (1) 4T1, (2) 4T1.G-CSF$^-$ tumors and from (3) a naïve mouse. **b** Spleen weight at the time of harvest. The spleens were processed and flow cytometric analysis was performed to determine the percentage of myeloid derived suppressor cells (MDSCs) (CD11b$^+$Ly6G$^+$Ly6C$^+$), B cells (CD19$^+$), T cells (CD3$^+$) and regulatory T cells (T$_{regs}$) (CD4$^+$CD25$^+$FoxP3$^+$). Absolute numbers of MDSCs (**c**), T cells (**d**), B cells (**e**), and T$_{regs}$ (**f**) were quantified and results are presented as mean ± standard error (*$p < 0.05$, Kruskal-Wallis test with Dunn's post-hoc test)

provide a comprehensive account of immunogenic and immunosuppressive elements in breast cancer, but rather a springboard for further exploration of key factors in other tumor models and clinical samples.

Though the use of irradiated tumor cells to develop autologous tumor cell vaccines is reported extensively in the literature, we first wanted to demonstrate that we could effectively inactivate 4T1 and EMT6 cells using this approach. We tested for the effect of different doses of irradiation (20, 40, 60, 80, and 100 Gy) on tumor cell proliferation using a proliferation assay as described in "Methods". We confirmed that at all five doses, both 4T1 and EMT6 cells failed to proliferate over the observed period of 4 days (Fig. 1). Thus, for experiments throughout this study, we chose 100 Gy, the highest dose tested, as a standard to develop our tumor cell vaccines.

The 4T1 cell line is often referred to as poorly immunogenic, while EMT6 is considered as a highly immunogenic cell line. Since the immunogenicity of these two cell lines has never been directly compared in any study, we first confirmed the differences in their immunogenicity in the ATCV setting. We vaccinated mice with irradiated 4T1 or EMT6 cells and subsequently challenged with live 4T1 or EMT6 cells. We found that mice immunized with EMT6 cells developed partial-to-complete protective immunity against live

EMT6 challenge. On the other hand, 4T1 vaccine failed to provide any measurable protective immunity (Fig. 2). These data were consistent with previous publications [54, 74].

To explore potential causes of immunogenic differences, we first looked at the expression of the immunologically relevant surface molecules MHC I, MHC II, B7–1, B7–2, ICAM-1, and FasR. We found that irradiated EMT6 cells express significantly higher levels of MHC I, B7–1, B7–2, and FasR, which could be responsible for the enhanced immune response to EMT6 vaccine (Table 1). We next analyzed cytokines released by each cell line and found that irradiated 4T1 cells released very high levels of GM-CSF, M-CSF, and in particular G-CSF (Fig. 3). Each of these cytokines can be immune-activating or immune-suppressive depending on their concentrations and context [75–78].

The hybrid vaccine studies (Fig. 4) were designed to help tease out the relative contributions of cell surface markers versus cytokines on ATCV responses. The 4T1 vaccine was unlikely to improve the activity of the EMT6 vaccine as the former was found to be non-immunogenic. However, if the 4T1 vaccine had no effect on the EMT6 vaccine, or if the 4T1 vaccine reduced the efficacy of the EMT6 vaccine only locally, i.e. in the ipsilateral setting, then decreased costimulation (signal 2) on the part of the 4T1 vaccine could

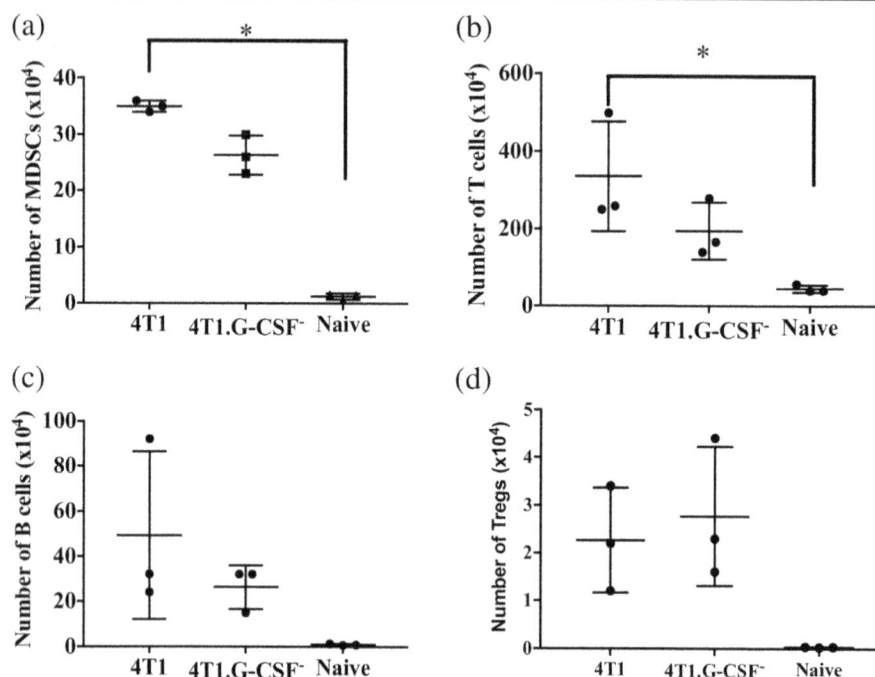

Fig. 7 Comparison of immune cell subsets in draining lymph nodes (DLNs) from mice bearing 4T1 and 4T1.G-CSF⁻ and naïve mice. Female balb/cByJ mice (n = 3) received subcutaneous injections of 1 × 10⁶ 4T1 or 4T1.G-CSF⁻ cells. Once tumors reached 500–700 mm³, DLNs were harvested and single cell suspensions obtained. Leukocytes isolated from naïve mice served as control (n = 3). Flow cytometric analysis was performed to determine the percentage of myeloid derived suppressor cells (MDSCs) (CD11b⁺Ly6G⁺Ly6C⁺), B cells (CD19⁺), T cells (CD3⁺) and regulatory T cells (T_regs) (CD4⁺CD25⁺FoxP3⁺). Absolute numbers of MDSCs (**a**), T cells (**b**), B cells (**c**), and T_regs (**d**) were quantified and results are represented as mean ± standard error (*$p < 0.05$, Kruskal-Wallis test with Dunn's post-hoc test)

have induced a localized tolerogenic effect. One also could have argued that local immunosuppressive cytokines may have inhibited the EMT6 vaccine as well. Conversely, if the 4T1 vaccine inhibited the EMT6 vaccine both locally and systemically, as was observed, then a soluble factor secreted at high levels by 4T1 cells must be responsible for the inhibited EMT6 vaccine response.

Of the different cytokines released by 4T1 cells, G-CSF was produced at exceptional levels (Fig. 3). At such high levels, G-CSF and other colony stimulating factors have been associated with MDSC expansion and immune impairment [71, 79–82]. Not surprisingly, we found that MDSC levels more or less correlated with G-CSF concentrations produced by five sister breast cancer cell lines: 4T1, 4T07, 67NR, 66Cl4 and 168FARN (Fig. 8). Although they did not measure cytokine production, Talmadge et al., also found significant differences in MDSC frequency among different breast tumor models, with 4T1 inducing the highest levels [83]. It should also be noted that, although other publications have suggested a link between G-CSF and/or MDSCs and tumor metastasis [64, 80, 84, 85], mice bearing 4T07 tumors, which do not induce visible metastatic lesions [73], produced high levels of G-CSF and more

splenic MDSCs than mice bearing any other tumor including highly metastatic 4T1 or 66CL4 tumors. These data suggest that other factors, such as IL-6 [86], may be involved in breast cancer metastasis. At the very least, the relationship between G-CSF/MDSCs and metastasis may be model-dependent.

The correlation between G-CSF and MDSC accumulation was further solidified by functional deletion of G-CSF. Mice with 4T1 tumors, when compared to mice with 4T1.G-CSF⁻ tumors, had increased amounts of MDSCs in both spleens and DLNs (Figs. 6, 7). It should be noted that relatively high levels of CD11b⁺Ly6-G⁺Ly6C⁺ cells were found in the DLNs of mice bearing 4T1.G-CSF tumors (Fig. 7). We did not evaluate the immunosuppressive activity of these cells, but it is unlikely that they were highly suppressive, if at all, given that mice vaccinated with 4T1.G-CSF⁻ cells were protected from a 4T1.G-CSF⁻ tumor challenge. This is a reminder that MDSCs are a diverse family of cells and that not all CD11b⁺Ly6G⁺Ly6C⁺ can be classified as MDSC [87]. While there were other differences in immune subset populations between 4T1 and 4T1.G-CSF⁻ tumor-bearing mice (Figs. 6, 7), similar to differences in costimulatory molecules, these were overshadowed by the enormous differences in the MDSC populations. To

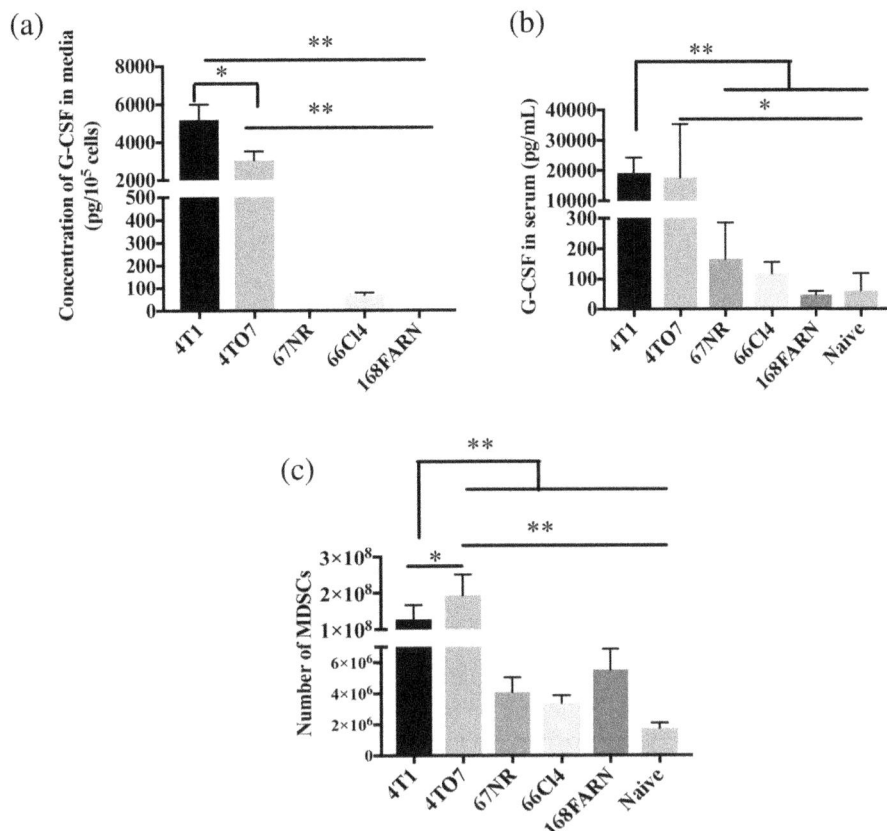

Fig. 8 Concentration of granulocyte colony-stimulating factor (G-CSF) in culture (in vitro) and in serum (in vivo) in mice bearing different breast cancer cell lines compared to the number of myeloid derived suppressor cells (MDSCs) in spleen. **a** The 4T1, 4T07, 67NR, 66Cl4 and 168FARN were seeded on separate T25 flasks and cultured for 48 h. G-CSF concentrations from culture supernatants were determined by ELISA. **b** Balb/cByJ mice were subcutaneously injected with 1×10^6 4T1 cells ($n = 5$), 5×10^6 4T07 cells ($n = 3$), 1×10^6 168FARN ($n = 3$), 1×10^6 67NR ($n = 5$) and 3×10^6 66Cl4 ($n = 5$). When tumor volumes reached 500 mm³, blood and spleens were harvested. Serum G-CSF concentrations were determined by ELISA. **c** Absolute numbers of MDSCs (CD11b⁺Ly6G⁺Ly6C⁺) among splenocytes from the same tumor-bearing mice were determined by flow cytometry. Results are representative of two independent experiments. Data are presented as mean ± standard error (*$p < 0.05$, **$p < 30.01$ via one-way analysis of variance with Tukey's post-hoc analysis)

verify that tumor-derived G-CSF was responsible for abrogating vaccine efficacy, we repeated the hybrid vaccine study utilizing 4T1.G-CSF⁻ cells in the contralateral vaccine group. We found that the hybrid vaccine containing 4T1.G-CSF⁻ cells was far less immunosuppressive than the hybrid vaccine containing parental 4T1 cells (Fig. 9). Overall, the findings from this study establish a causal link between tumor-derived G-CSF and a loss of responsiveness to breast ATCVs.

As mentioned previously, the finding that 4T1-derived G-CSF leads to MDSC accumulation and immune suppression is not novel. However, that this immune impairment can be eliminated by knocking out a single, non-essential protein, G-CSF, despite an otherwise aggressive phenotype was somewhat surprising. In fact, it should be noted that after G-CSF deletion, the 4T1.G-CSF⁻ vaccine was more immunogenic and more protective than the EMT6 vaccine (Fig. 9b versus Figs. 2, 4). These data imply that tumor

cell surface phenotype is not as important as tumor-derived secreted factors when establishing breast ATCV immunogenicity.

Although this study has provided useful insight into the effect of tumor-derived factors on ATCV efficacy, we acknowledge that it has a few limitations and opportunities for additional exploration. First, through the entirety of the study, tumor cell vaccines were only used in a prophylactic setting. To truly recapitulate the effect of the tumor-derived factors, future studies ought to focus on vaccinating the mice post tumor resection. Second, this study only used the 4T1 cell line to establish the causal link between G-CSF secretion and ATCV efficacy. Future studies that involve either knocking in or knocking out G-CSF in the other cancer cell lines that intrinsically secrete low or high levels of G-CSF will further strengthen the findings of this study. Third, there is no question that G-CSF-induced MDSCs are responsible for vaccine impairment in our models.

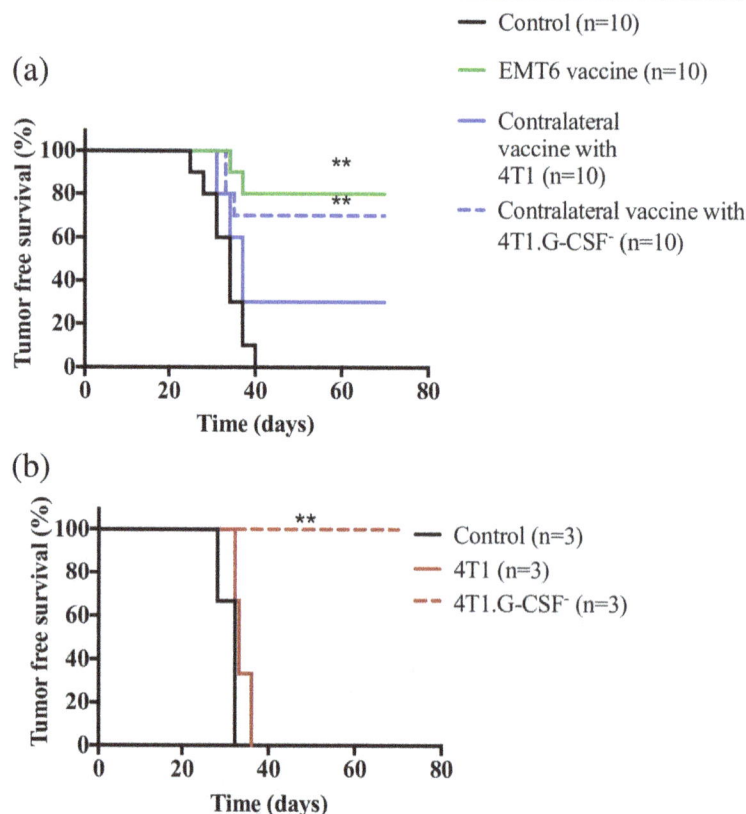

Fig. 9 Prophylactic vaccination with 4T1.G-CSF⁻ cells. **a** Balb/cByJ mice received 5 × 10⁵ irradiated EMT6 cells or 5 × 10⁵ irradiated EMT6 cells and 1 × 10⁶ irradiated 4T1 cells on opposite sides (contralateral 4T1 vaccine) or 5 × 10⁵ irradiated EMT6 cells and 1 × 10⁶ irradiated 4T1.G-CSF⁻ cells on opposite sides (contralateral 4T1.G-CSF⁻ vaccine) twice, 10 days apart. Ten days after the booster vaccination, all mice were challenged with 5 × 10⁵ live EMT6 cells. Additionally, naive mice that received only 5 × 10⁵ live EMT6 cells served as controls. Tumor-free survival was recorded. **b** Balb/cByJ mice were vaccinated with 1 × 10⁶ 4T1 cells or 1 × 10⁶ 4T1.G-CSF⁻ cells, twice 10 days apart. Ten days after the booster vaccination, mice were challenged with live 5 × 10⁵ 4T1 cells or 5 × 10⁵ 4T1.G-CSF⁻ cells, respectively. Naive mice that received only 5 × 10⁵ live 4T1 cells, served as controls. Tumor-free survival was recorded (**p < 0.01, log-rank analysis)

However, G-CSF could also be causing immune suppression through additional pathways. In a recent clinical study, G-CSF was highly expressed in tumors in patients with breast cancer with more aggressive disease and was correlated with poorer overall survival [88]. As this study illustrates, tumor-associated macrophages (TAMs) are another key immunosuppressive subset that is strongly influenced by G-CSF. Assessing differences in TAM number and function between 4T1 and 4T1.G-CSF⁻ tumors is the subject of ongoing research. Likewise, while G-CSF is clearly an important target in breast cancer, it is important to note that our findings do not eliminate the possibility of other mechanisms that could be involved in MDSC expansion. For instance, knocking out other colony stimulating factors such as GM-CSF may have a similar effect on vaccine efficacy. Last, given that G-CSF and GM-CSF are routinely administered to prevent neutropenia in patients with breast cancer undergoing chemotherapy, a closer look at the immunosuppressive impacts of these cytokines, particularly in a setting of minimal residual disease, is warranted.

Conclusion

ATCVs represent a safe and potentially effective weapon to prevent breast cancer recurrence in a patient-specific manner. A better understanding of factors that influence the effectiveness of breast cancer ATCVs will facilitate continued development and eventual clinical application. Here, our study began with an initial comparison of surface marker expression between a non-immunogenic and an immunogenic breast cancer cell line. While some differences were noted, the most obvious being the increase in B7–1 on the surfaces of EMT6 cells, these differences were far less striking when compared to differences in cytokine expression levels. The exceptionally high levels of G-CSF released by 4T1 cells were found to be responsible for MDSC accumulation, splenomegaly, and the associated abrogation of EMT6 vaccine responses. After knocking out G-CSF expression, 4T1 cells became as immunogenic as EMT6 cells in a prophylactic vaccination-tumor challenge experiment.

These results imply that similar inhibition of immuno-suppressive signals may help enhance, if not standardize, the immunogenicity of breast ATCVs.

Abbreviations

ANOVA: Analysis of variance; APC: Antigen presenting cell; ATCV: Autologous tumor cell vaccine; CBA: Cytokine bead array; CRISPR: Clustered regularly interspaced short palindromic repeats; DLN: Draining lymph node; ELISA: Enzyme-linked immunosorbent assay; FasR: Fas receptor; G-CSF: Granulocyte colony-stimulating factor; GM-CSF: Granulocyte-macrophage colony-stimulating factor; ICAM-1: Intracellular adhesion molecule-1; IDO: Indoleamine-pyrrole 2,3-dioxygenase; IL-10: Interleukin-10; IL-6: Interleukin-6; LFA-1: Lymphocyte function-associated antigen-1; MCP-1: Monocyte chemotactic protein-1; M-CSF: Macrophage colony-stimulating factor; MDSC: Myeloid-derived suppressor cell; MFI: Median fluorescence intensity; MHC: Major histocompatibility complex; PD-1: Programmed cell death protein 1; PD-L1: Programmed death-ligand 1; TAM: Tumor associated macrophage; TCR: T cell receptor; TGF-b: Tumor growth factor-beta; TNBC: Triple-negative breast cancer; T_{reg}: Regulatory T cell; VEGF: Vascular endothelial growth factor

Funding
This work was supported by grants from the National Institutes of Health, National Cancer Institute (R01CA172631, R15CA176648), and the Arkansas Breast Cancer Research Programs.

Authors' contributions
SR and DAZ designed the research. SR, KGN, SLK, HNF, SGS, and BK performed the research. SR, KGN, SGS, BK, NR, and DAZ analyzed and interpreted the data. SR and DAZ wrote and edited the manuscript. All authors read and approved the final manuscript.

Competing interests
The authors declare that they have no competing interests.

Author details
[1]Department of Biomedical Engineering, University of Arkansas, Fayetteville, AR, USA. [2]Cell and Molecular Biology Program, University of Arkansas, Fayetteville, AR, USA. [3]Department of Microbiology and Immunology, University of North Carolina, Chapel Hill, NC, USA. [4]Honors College, University of Arkansas, Fayetteville, AR, USA. [5]Joint Department of Biomedical Engineering, University of North Carolina, Chapel Hill, NC and North Carolina State University, Raleigh, NC, USA.

References
1. Siegel RL, Miller KD, Jemal A. Cancer statistics, 2018. Ca-Cancer J Clin. 2018; 68(1):7–30.
2. Weigelt B, Peterse JL, van 't Veer LJ. Breast cancer metastasis: markers and models. Nat Rev Cancer. 2005;5(8):591–602.
3. Brewster AM, Hortobagyi GN, Broglio KR, Kau SW, Santa-Maria CA, Arun B, Buzdar AU, Booser DJ, Valero V, Bondy M, et al. Residual risk of breast cancer recurrence 5 years after adjuvant therapy. J Natl Cancer Inst. 2008; 100(16):1179–83.
4. Baum M. Harms from breast cancer screening outweigh benefits if death caused by treatment is included. BMJ. 2013;346:f385.
5. Baskar S, Kobrin CB, Kwak LW. Autologous lymphoma vaccines induce human T cell responses against multiple, unique epitopes. J Clin Invest. 2004;113(10):1498–510.
6. Curry WT Jr, Gorrepati R, Piesche M, Sasada T, Agarwalla P, Jones PS, Gerstner ER, Golby AJ, Batchelor TT, Wen PY, et al. Vaccination with irradiated autologous tumor cells mixed with irradiated GM-K562 cells stimulates antitumor immunity and T lymphocyte activation in patients with recurrent malignant glioma. Clin Cancer Res. 2016;22(12):2885–96.
7. de Gruijl TD, van den Eertwegh AJ, Pinedo HM, Scheper RJ. Whole-cell cancer vaccination: from autologous to allogeneic tumor- and dendritic cell-based vaccines. Cancer Immunol Immunother. 2008;57(10):1569–77.
8. Hanna MG Jr, Hoover HC Jr, Vermorken JB, Harris JE, Pinedo HM. Adjuvant active specific immunotherapy of stage II and stage III colon cancer with an autologous tumor cell vaccine: first randomized phase III trials show promise. Vaccine. 2001;19(17–19):2576–82.
9. Luiten RM, Kueter EWM, Mooi W, Gallee MPW, Rankin EM, Gerritsen WR, Clift SM, Nooijen WJ, Weder P, van de Kasteele WF, et al. Immunogenicity, including vitiligo, and feasibility of vaccination with autologous GM-CSF-transduced tumor cells in metastatic melanoma patients. J Clin Oncol. 2005; 23(35):8978–91.
10. Manne J, Mastrangelo MJ, Sato T, Berd D. TCR rearrangement in lymphocytes infiltrating melanoma metastases after administration of autologous dinitrophenyl-modified vaccine. J Immunol. 2002;169(6):3407–12.
11. Ophir E, Bobisse S, Coukos G, Harari A, Kandalaft LE. Personalized approaches to active immunotherapy in cancer. Biochim Biophys Acta. 2016;1865(1):72–82.
12. Parmiani G, Pilla L, Maccalli C, Russo V. Autologous versus allogeneic cell-based vaccines? Cancer J. 2011;17(5):331–6.
13. Thompson PL, Dessureault S. Tumor cell vaccines. Adv Exp Med Biol. 2007; 601:345–55.
14. Wittke S, Baxmann S, Fahlenkamp D, Kiessig ST. Tumor heterogeneity as a rationale for a multi-epitope approach in an autologous renal cell cancer tumor vaccine. Oncotargets Ther. 2016;9:523–37.
15. Ellsworth RE, Blackburn HL, Shriver CD, Soon-Shiong P, Ellsworth DL. Molecular heterogeneity in breast cancer: state of the science and implications for patient care. Semin Cell Dev Biol. 2017;64:65–72.
16. Lehmann BD, Pietenpol JA. Clinical implications of molecular heterogeneity in triple negative breast cancer. Breast. 2015;24:S36–40.
17. Ma D, Jiang YZ, Liu XY, Liu YR, Shao ZM. Clinical and molecular relevance of mutant-allele tumor heterogeneity in breast cancer. Breast Cancer Res Treat. 2017;162(1):39–48.
18. Braga S. Resistance to targeted therapies in breast cancer. Methods Mol Biol. 2016;1395:105–36.
19. Zuo WJ, Jiang YZ, Yu KD, Shao ZM. Activating HER2 mutations promote oncogenesis and resistance to HER2-targeted therapies in breast cancer. Cancer Res. 2015;75.
20. Schreiber RD, Old LJ, Smyth MJ. Cancer immunoediting: integrating immunity's roles in cancer suppression and promotion. Science. 2011; 331(6024):1565–70.
21. Beatty GL, Gladney WL. Immune escape mechanisms as a guide for cancer immunotherapy. Clin Cancer Res. 2015;21(4):687–92.
22. Litzinger MT, Foon KA, Tsang KY, Schlom J, Palena C. Comparative analysis of MVA-CD40L and MVA-TRICOM vectors for enhancing the immunogenicity of chronic lymphocytic leukemia (CLL) cells. Leukemia Res. 2010;34(10):1351–7.
23. Sharma RK, Yolcu ES, Elpek KG, Shirwan H. Tumor cells engineered to codisplay on their surface 4-1BBL and LIGHT costimulatory proteins as a novel vaccine approach for cancer immunotherapy. Cancer Gene Ther. 2010;17(10):730–41.
24. Mazzocco M, Martini M, Rosato A, Stefani E, Matucci A, Dalla Santa S, De Sanctis F, Ugel S, Sandri S, Ferrarini G, et al. Autologous cellular vaccine overcomes cancer immunoediting in a mouse model of myeloma. Immunology. 2015;146(1):33–49.
25. Sule-Suso J, Arienti F, Melani C, Colombo MP, Parmiani G. A B7-1-transfected human melanoma line stimulates proliferation and cytotoxicity of autologous and allogeneic lymphocytes. Eur J Immunol. 1995;25(10):2737–42.
26. Fishman M, Hunter TB, Soliman H, Thompson P, Dunn M, Smilee R, Farmelo MJ, Noyes DR, Mahany JJ, Lee JH, et al. Phase II trial of B7-1 (CD-86) transduced, cultured autologous tumor cell vaccine plus subcutaneous interleukin-2 for treatment of stage IV renal cell carcinoma. J Immunother. 2008;31(1):72–80.
27. Lotem M, Merims S, Frank S, Hamburger T, Nissan A, Kadouri L, Cohen J, Straussman R, Eisenberg G, Frankenburg S, et al. Adjuvant autologous melanoma vaccine for macroscopic stage III disease: survival, biomarkers, and improved response to CTLA-4 blockade. J Immunol Res. 2016;2016:8121985.

28. Berd D, Maguire HC Jr, McCue P, Mastrangelo MJ. Treatment of metastatic melanoma with an autologous tumor-cell vaccine: clinical and immunologic results in 64 patients. J Clin Oncol. 1990;8(11):1858–67.

29. Pyo KH, Lee YW, Lim SM, Shin EH. Immune adjuvant effect of a Toxoplasma gondii profilin-like protein in autologous whole-tumor-cell vaccination in mice. Oncotarget. 2016;7(45):74107–19.

30. Yannelli JR, Wouda R, Masterson TJ, Avdiushko MG, Cohen DA. Development of an autologous canine cancer vaccine system for resectable malignant tumors in dogs. Vet Immunol Immunop. 2016;182:95–100.

31. Olivares J, Kumar P, Yu Y, Maples PB, Senzer N, Bedell C, Barve M, Tong A, Pappen BO, Kuhn J, et al. Phase I trial of TGF-beta 2 antisense GM-CSF gene-modified autologous tumor cell (TAG) vaccine. Clin Cancer Res. 2011;17(1):183–92.

32. Cicchelero L, de Rooster H, Sanders NN. Various ways to improve whole cancer cell vaccines. Expert Rev Vaccines. 2014;13(6):721–35.

33. Soiffer R, Hodi FS, Haluska F, Jung K, Gillessen S, Singer S, Tanabe K, Duda R, Mentzer S, Jaklitsch M, et al. Vaccination with irradiated, autologous melanoma cells engineered to secrete granulocyte-macrophage colony-stimulating factor by adenoviral-mediated gene transfer augments antitumor immunity in patients with metastatic melanoma. J Clin Oncol. 2003;21(17):3343–50.

34. Goldberg JM, Fisher DE, Demetri GD, Neuberg D, Allsop SA, Fonseca C, Nakazaki Y, Nemer D, Raut CP, George S, et al. Biologic activity of autologous, granulocyte-macrophage colony-stimulating factor secreting alveolar soft-part sarcoma and clear cell sarcoma vaccines. Clin Cancer Res. 2015;21(14):3178–86.

35. Chen X, Ni J, Meng H, Li D, Wei Y, Luo Y, Wu Y. Interleukin15: a potent adjuvant enhancing the efficacy of an autologous wholecell tumor vaccine against Lewis lung carcinoma. Mol Med Rep. 2014;10(4):1828–34.

36. Salgia R, Lynch T, Skarin A, Lucca J, Lynch C, Jung K, Hodi FS, Jaklitsch M, Mentzer S, Swanson S, et al. Vaccination with irradiated autologous tumor cells engineered to secrete granulocyte-macrophage colony-stimulating factor augments antitumor immunity in some patients with metastatic non-small-cell lung carcinoma. J Clin Oncol. 2003;21(4):624–30.

37. Simons JW, Mikhak B, Chang JF, DeMarzo AM, Carducci MA, Lim M, Weber CE, Baccala AA, Goemann MA, Clift SM, et al. Induction of immunity to prostate cancer antigens: results of a clinical trial of vaccination with irradiated autologous prostate tumor cells engineered to secrete granulocyte-macrophage colony-stimulating factor using ex vivo gene transfer. Cancer Res. 1999;59(20):5160–8.

38. Alkayyal AA, Tai LH, Kennedy MA, de Souza CT, Zhang JQ, Lefebvre C, Sahi S, Ananth AA, Mahmoud AB, Makrigiannis AP, et al. NK-cell recruitment is necessary for eradication of peritoneal carcinomatosis with an IL12-expressing Maraba virus cellular vaccine. Cancer Immunol Res. 2017;5(3):211–21.

39. Ghisoli M, Barve M, Mennel R, Lenarsky C, Horvath S, Wallraven G, Pappen BO, Whiting S, Rao D, Senzer N, et al. Three-year follow up of GMCSF/bi-shRNA(furin) DNA-transfected autologous tumor immunotherapy (Vigil) in metastatic advanced Ewing's sarcoma. Mol Ther. 2016;24(8):1478–83.

40. Zhao L, Mei Y, Sun Q, Guo L, Wu Y, Yu X, Hu B, Liu X, Liu H. Autologous tumor vaccine modified with recombinant new castle disease virus expressing IL-7 promotes antitumor immune response. J Immunol. 2014;193(2):735–45.

41. Russell HV, Strother D, Mei Z, Rill D, Popek E, Biagi E, Yvon E, Brenner M, Rousseau R. A phase 1/2 study of autologous neuroblastoma tumor cells genetically modified to secrete IL-2 in patients with high-risk neuroblastoma. J Immunother. 2008;31(9):812–9.

42. May M, Brookman-May S, Hoschke B, Gilfrich C, Kendel F, Baxmann S, Wittke S, Kiessig ST, Miller K, Johannsen M. Ten-year survival analysis for renal carcinoma patients treated with an autologous tumour lysate vaccine in an adjuvant setting. Cancer Immunol Immun. 2010;59(5):687–95.

43. Nemunaitis J, Sterman D, Jablons D, Smith JW 2nd, Fox B, Maples P, Hamilton S, Borellini F, Lin A, Morali S, et al. Granulocyte-macrophage colony-stimulating factor gene-modified autologous tumor vaccines in non-small-cell lung cancer. J Natl Cancer Inst. 2004;96(4):326–31.

44. Ahlert T, Sauerbrei W, Bastert G, Ruhland S, Bartik B, Simiantonaki N, Schumacher J, Hacker B, Schumacher M, Schirrmacher V. Tumor-cell number and viability as quality and efficacy parameters of autologous virus-modified cancer vaccines in patients with breast or ovarian cancer. J Clin Oncol. 1997; 15(4):1354–66.

45. Jiang XP, Yang DC, Elliott RL, Head JF. Vaccination with a mixed vaccine of autogenous and allogeneic breast cancer cells and tumor associated antigens CA15-3, CEA and CA125 - Results in immune and clinical responses in breast cancer patients. Cancer Biother Radio. 2000;15(5):495–505.

46. Elliott RL, Head JF. Adjuvant breast cancer vaccine improves disease specific survival of breast cancer patients with depressed lymphocyte immunity. Surg Oncol. 2013;22(3):172–7.

47. Vaccination with autologous breast cancer cells engineered to secrete granulocyte-macrophage colony-stimulating factor (GM-CSF) in metastatic breast cancer patients (NCT00317603). Available at: clinicaltrials.gov. Accessed 2 Aug 2017.

48. Autologous vaccination with lethally irradiated, autologous breast cancer cells engineered to secrete GM-CSF in women with operable breast cancer (NCT00880464). Available at: clinicaltrials.gov. Accessed 2 Aug 2017.

49. Kurtz SL, Ravindranathan S, Zaharoff DA. Current status of autologous breast tumor cell-based vaccines. Expert Rev Vaccines. 2014;13(12):1439–45.

50. Berg W, Hendrick E, Kopans D, Smith R. Frequently asked questions about mammography and the USPSTF recommendations: a guide for practitioners. Reston: Society of Breast Imaging; 2009.

51. Brockstedt DG, Diagana M, Zhang Y, Tran K, Belmar N, Meier M, Yang A, Boissiere F, Lin A, Chiang Y. Development of anti-tumor immunity against a non-immunogenic mammary carcinoma through in vivo somatic GM-CSF, IL-2, and HSVtk combination gene therapy. Mol Ther. 2002;6(5):627–36.

52. Majumdar AS, Zolotorev A, Samuel S, Tran K, Vertin B, Hall-Meier M, Antoni B-A, Adeline E, Philip M, Philip R. Efficacy of herpes simplex virus thymidine kinase in combination with cytokine gene therapy in an experimental metastatic breast cancer model. Cancer Gene Ther. 2000;7(7):1086.

53. Tsai SJ, Gransbacher B, Tait L, Miller FR, Heppner GH. Induction of antitumor immunity by interleukin-2 gene-transduced mouse mammary tumor cells versus transduced mammary stromal fibroblasts. JNCI. 1993;85(7):546–53.

54. Gorczynski RM, Chen Z, Erin N, Khatri I, Podnos A. Comparison of immunity in mice cured of primary/metastatic growth of EMT6 or 4THM breast cancer by chemotherapy or immunotherapy. PLoS One. 2014;9(11):e113597.

55. Rockwell SC, Kallman RF, Fajardo LF. Characteristics of a serially transplanted mouse mammary tumor and its tissue-culture-adapted derivative. J Natl Cancer Inst. 1972;49(3):735–49.

56. Korbelik M, Dougherty GJ. Photodynamic therapy-mediated immune response against subcutaneous mouse tumors. Cancer Res. 1999;59(8):1941–6.

57. Shou D, Wen L, Song Z, Yin J, Sun Q, Gong W. Suppressive role of myeloid-derived suppressor cells (MDSCs) in the microenvironment of breast cancer and targeted immunotherapies. Oncotarget. 2016;7(39):64505.

58. Gonda K, Shibata M, Ohtake T, Matsumoto Y, Tachibana K, Abe N, Ohto H, Sakurai K, Takenoshita S. Myeloid-derived suppressor cells are increased and correlated with type 2 immune responses, malnutrition, inflammation, and poor prognosis in patients with breast cancer. Oncol Lett. 2017;14(2):1766–74.

59. Toor SM, Khaja ASS, El Salhat H, Faour I, Kanbar J, Quadri AA, Albashir M, Elkord E. Myeloid cells in circulation and tumor microenvironment of breast cancer patients. Cancer Immunol Immunother. 2017;66(6):753–64.

60. Markowitz J, Wesolowski R, Papenfuss T, Brooks TR, Carson WE. Myeloid-derived suppressor cells in breast cancer. Breast Cancer Res Treat. 2013;140(1):13–21.

61. Diaz-Montero CM, Salem ML, Nishimura MI, Garrett-Mayer E, Cole DJ, Montero AJ. Increased circulating myeloid-derived suppressor cells correlate with clinical cancer stage, metastatic tumor burden, and doxorubicin-cyclophosphamide chemotherapy. Cancer Immunol Immunother. 2009; 58(1):49–59.

62. Schaue D, Ratikan JA, Iwamoto KS. Cellular autofluorescence following ionizing radiation. PLoS One. 2012;7(2):e32062.

63. Deeths MJ, Mescher MF. ICAM-1 and B7-1 provide similar but distinct costimulation for CD8+ T cells, while CD4+ T cells are poorly costimulated by ICAM-1. Eur J Immunol. 1999;29(1):45–53.

64. Talmadge JE, Gabrilovich DI. History of myeloid-derived suppressor cells. Nat Rev Cancer. 2013;13(10):739–52.

65. Fisher DT, Appenheimer MM, Evans SS. The two faces of IL-6 in the tumor microenvironment. Semin Immunol. 2014;26(1):38–47.

66. Hoeben A, Landuyt B, Highley MS, Wildiers H, Van Oosterom AT, De Bruijn EA. Vascular endothelial growth factor and angiogenesis. Pharmacol Rev. 2004;56(4):549–80.

67. Niu J, Azfer A, Zhelyabovska O, Fatma S, Kolattukudy PE. Monocyte chemotactic protein (MCP)-1 promotes angiogenesis via a novel transcription factor, MCP-1-induced protein (MCPIP). J Biol Chem. 2008; 283(21):14542–51.

68. Bronte V, Serafini P, Apolloni E, Zanovello P. Tumor-induced immune dysfunctions caused by myeloid suppressor cells. J Immunother. 2001;24(6):431–46.

69. Almand B, Clark JI, Nikitina E, van Beynen J, English NR, Knight SC, Carbone DP, Gabrilovich DI. Increased production of immature myeloid cells in

cancer patients: a mechanism of immunosuppression in cancer. J Immunol. 2001;166(1):678–89.

70. Gabrilovich DI, Ostrand-Rosenberg S, Bronte V. Coordinated regulation of myeloid cells by tumours. Nat Rev Immunol. 2012;12(4):253–68.

71. Waight JD, Hu Q, Miller A, Liu S, Abrams SI. Tumor-derived G-CSF facilitates neoplastic growth through a granulocytic myeloid-derived suppressor cell-dependent mechanism. PLoS One. 2011;6(11):e27690.

72. Aslakson CJ, Miller FR. Selective events in the metastatic process defined by analysis of the sequential dissemination of subpopulations of a mouse mammary tumor. Cancer Res. 1992;52(6):1399–405.

73. Heppner GH, Miller FR, Shekhar PM. Nontransgenic models of breast cancer. Breast Cancer Res. 2000;2(5):331–4.

74. Pulaski BA, Ostrand-Rosenberg S. Reduction of established spontaneous mammary carcinoma metastases following immunotherapy with major histocompatibility complex class II and B7.1 cell-based tumor vaccines. Cancer Res. 1998;58(7):1486–93.

75. Parmiani G, Castelli C, Pilla L, Santinami M, Colombo MP, Rivoltini L. Opposite immune functions of GM-CSF administered as vaccine adjuvant in cancer patients. Ann Oncol. 2007;18(2):226–32.

76. Sivakumar R, Atkinson MA, Mathews CE, Morel M. G-CSF: a friend or foe. Immunome Res. 2015;S2:007.

77. Martins A, Han J, Kim SO. The multifaceted effects of granulocyte colony-stimulating factor in immunomodulation and potential roles in intestinal immune homeostasis. IUBMB Life. 2010;62(8):611–7.

78. Eubank TD, Galloway M, Montague CM, Waldman WJ, Marsh CB. M-CSF induces vascular endothelial growth factor production and angiogenic activity from human monocytes. J Immunol. 2003;171(5):2637–43.

79. Serafini P, Carbley R, Noonan KA, Tan G, Bronte V, Borrello I. High-dose granulocyte-macrophage colony-stimulating factor-producing vaccines impair the immune response through the recruitment of myeloid suppressor cells. Cancer Res. 2004;64(17):6337–43.

80. Kowanetz M, Wu X, Lee J, Tan M, Hagenbeek T, Qu X, Yu L, Ross J, Korsisaari N, Cao T, et al. Granulocyte-colony stimulating factor promotes lung metastasis through mobilization of Ly6G+Ly6C+ granulocytes. Proc Natl Acad Sci U S A. 2010;107(50):21248–55.

81. Waight JD, Netherby C, Hensen ML, Miller A, Hu Q, Liu S, Bogner PN, Farren MR, Lee KP, Liu KB, et al. Myeloid-derived suppressor cell development is regulated by a STAT/IRF-8 axis. J Clin Investig. 2013;123(10):4464–78.

82. Rutella S, Zavala F, Danese S, Kared H, Leone G. Granulocyte colony-stimulating factor: a novel mediator of T cell tolerance. J Immunol. 2005; 175(11):7085–91.

83. Donkor MK, Lahue E, Hoke TA, Shafer LR, Coskun U, Solheim JC, Gulen D, Bishay J, Talmadge JE. Mammary tumor heterogeneity in the expansion of myeloid-derived suppressor cells. Int Immunopharmacol. 2009;9(7–8):937–48.

84. Agarwal S, Lakoma A, Chen Z, Hicks J, Metelitsa LS, Kim ES, Shohet JM. G-CSF promotes neuroblastoma tumorigenicity and metastasis via STAT3-dependent cancer stem cell activation. Cancer Res. 2015;75(12):2566–79.

85. Anderson RL, Swierczak A, Cao Y, Hamilton JA. G-CSF promotes metastasis in preclinical models of breast cancer. Asia-Pac J Clin Onco. 2014;10:89–90.

86. Oh K, Lee OY, Shon SY, Nam O, Ryu PM, Seo MW, Lee DS. A mutual activation loop between breast cancer cells and myeloid-derived suppressor cells facilitates spontaneous metastasis through IL-6 trans-signaling in a murine model. Breast Cancer Res. 2013;15(5):R79.

87. Ostrand-Rosenberg S, Sinha P. Myeloid-derived suppressor cells: linking inflammation and cancer. J Immunol. 2009;182(8):4499–506.

88. Hollmen M, Karaman S, Schwager S, Lisibach A, Christiansen AJ, Maksimow M, Varga Z, Jalkanen S, Detmar M. G-CSF regulates macrophage phenotype and associates with poor overall survival in human triple-negative breast cancer. Oncoimmunology. 2016;5(3):e1115177.

13

The added value of mammography in different age-groups of women with and without *BRCA* mutation screened with breast MRI

Suzan Vreemann[1]*(iD), Jan C. M. van Zelst[1], Margrethe Schlooz-Vries[2], Peter Bult[3], Nicoline Hoogerbrugge[4], Nico Karssemeijer[1], Albert Gubern-Mérida[1] and Ritse M. Mann[1]

Abstract

Background: Breast magnetic resonance imaging (MRI) is the most sensitive imaging method for breast cancer detection and is therefore offered as a screening technique to women at increased risk of developing breast cancer. However, mammography is currently added from the age of 30 without proven benefits. The purpose of this study is to investigate the added cancer detection of mammography when breast MRI is available, focusing on the value in women with and without *BRCA* mutation, and in the age groups above and below 50 years.

Methods: This retrospective single-center study evaluated 6553 screening rounds in 2026 women at increased risk of breast cancer (1 January 2003 to 1 January 2014). Risk category (*BRCA* mutation versus others at increased risk of breast cancer), age at examination, recall, biopsy, and histopathological diagnosis were recorded. Cancer yield, false positive recall rate (FPR), and false positive biopsy rate (FPB) were calculated using generalized estimating equations for separate age categories (< 40, 40–50, 50–60, ≥ 60 years). Numbers of screens needed to detect an additional breast cancer with mammography (NSN) were calculated for the subgroups.

Results: Of a total of 125 screen-detected breast cancers, 112 were detected by MRI and 66 by mammography: 13 cancers were solely detected by mammography, including 8 cases of ductal carcinoma in situ. In *BRCA* mutation carriers, 3 of 61 cancers were detected only on mammography, while in other women 10 of 64 cases were detected with mammography alone. While 77% of mammography-detected-only cancers were detected in women ≥ 50 years of age, mammography also added more to the FPR in these women. Below 50 years the number of mammographic examinations needed to find an MRI-occult cancer was 1427.

Conclusions: Mammography is of limited added value in terms of cancer detection when breast MRI is available for women of all ages who are at increased risk. While the benefit appears slightly larger in women over 50 years of age without *BRCA* mutation, there is also a substantial increase in false positive findings in these women.

Keywords: Mammography, Breast MRI, High-risk screening, Age-categories, Screen-detected breast cancer, False positives

* Correspondence: Suzan.Vreemann@radboudumc.nl
[1]Department of Radiology and Nuclear Medicine, Radboud University Medical Center, Geert Grooteplein 10, 6525 GA Nijmegen, the Netherlands
Full list of author information is available at the end of the article

Background

Mammography-based screening for breast cancer reduces breast cancer-related mortality in the general female population [1]. However, in women at increased risk (e.g. those with a germline mutation in the BRCA1 or BRCA2 genes) biennial mammographic screening is insufficient due to low sensitivity and high rates of interval cancers [2–5]. Consequently, these women who have a higher-than-average lifetime risk of breast cancer (approximately ≥ 20–25% life time risk (LTR)) are invited to intensified screening programs [6, 7], consisting of dynamic contrast-enhanced magnetic resonance imaging (DCE-MRI) and mammography. The sensitivity and specificity of these screening programs have been reported to be as high as 97% and 98%, respectively [4, 8–12].

Recent studies question the added cancer detection of mammography in this population, especially in BRCA mutation carriers [13]. In the study of Kuhl et al. [10], MRI proved to be the most important contributor to stage reduction. Although these results show the superiority of breast MRI compared to mammography for the detection of cancers, routine mammography is currently recommended for all women, even at a relatively young age. Various authors have proposed to cancel mammographic screening in young women also screened with breast MRI, especially in BRCA1 mutation carriers. In these BRCA1 mutation carriers, the mammographic sensitivity is exceedingly low, reported as low as 35% [14]. This is believed to be caused not only by the on-average dense breasts of these women, but also by the mammographic benign-like features of BRCA1-associated cancers [15, 16]. Berrington de Gonzalez et al. reported that there is little to no benefit of mammographic screening under the age of 35 [17]. Additionally, concerns are raised about the risk of radiation-induced cancers in these women, as BRCA mutation carriers have increased susceptibility to radiation [17, 18].

Although guidelines may vary per country, mammographic screening in BRCA mutation carriers is advised from the age of 30 years [6, 7]. However, the actual benefits in terms of tumor detection of the addition of mammography at such a young age are still unclear. Furthermore, additional findings on the mammogram might lead to an increase in false positive recalls in the screening program.

Hence, there is a clinical need to find an optimal regimen for intensified screening programs to prevent unnecessary recalls, biopsies, and radiation exposure. The purpose of this study is to evaluate the added cancer detection and false positive rates with mammography when breast MRI is available in a population of women at increased risk of developing breast cancer. Differences in the complementary value of mammography in women below and above 50 years of age, and in BRCA mutation carriers versus others at increased risk of breast cancer were assessed.

Methods

This retrospective study was approved by our local institutional review board and the requirement for informed consent was waived.

Screening program

The increased risk screening program was evaluated for the period 1 January 2003 until 1 January 2014. The program starts at age 25 years for BRCA mutation carriers, who undergo yearly MRI. At the age of 30 years a yearly mammography is added. Women with an LTR of ≥ 20–25% are screened from the start with mammography and MRI; starting ages differ by the reason for screening [19]. Furthermore, women may have been enrolled in the program at a later point in time after detection of a specific factor that increases their personal risk. We previously reported on the overall screening performance in this cohort [20].

Case selection

The local database was searched to identify all screening MRI and mammography examinations. Women were included when an MRI examination was considered a screening examination (inquiry at the radiology department was for screening purposes in asymptomatic women). Women were excluded when no mammography was performed within 6 months of the screening MRI. Risk category, age, screening tests performed, eventual recall for workup of screen-detected abnormalities and histopathological diagnosis were recorded when available.

Image acquisition

MRI acquisition and protocols varied over time and have previously been reported in detail [21]. In short: examinations were performed on either a 1.5 or 3.0 Tesla Siemens scanner (Magnetom Avanto, Magnetom Sonata, Magnetom symphony or Magnetom Trio) using a dedicated bilateral breast coil. Patients were imaged in the prone position. A transverse or coronal three-dimensional T1-weighted gradient-echo dynamic sequence was performed before contrast agent administration followed by four or five post-contrast sequences. Various gadolinium chelates were used as a contrast agent, administered at a dose of 0.1 mmol/kg or 0.2 mmol/kg body weight using a power injector (Medrad, Warrendale, PA, USA) at a flow rate of 2.5 mL/s, followed by a saline flush. Premenopausal women were scheduled in the 6th to 12th day of their menstrual cycle.

Mammograms were obtained in two directions (medio-lateral oblique and cranio-caudal) with a full-field digital mammography machine (GE Senograph 2000 or GE Senograph DS, GE, Fairfield, CT, USA). Additional views and spot compression views were performed at request of the evaluating radiologist.

Image interpretation

The Breast Imaging Reporting and Data system (BI-R-ADS) [22, 23] was used for evaluation. All examinations were evaluated by one of eight breast radiologists with experience ranging from 0.5 to 23 years after certification. Images were reported using a dedicated breast MRI workstation (versions of DynaCAD, Invivo, Philips, Best, the Netherlands). Mammograms were evaluated together with MRI examinations when these examinations were acquired the same day. In general, biopsies were performed for lesions classified as BI-RADS 4 and 5, and a subset of lesions classified as BI-RADS 3. The remainder of BI-RADS 3 lesions underwent short-term follow up.

Ground truth

For BI-RADS 3 lesions with a short-term follow-up recommendation, at least 1 year of clinical follow up was required to confirm benignity. A cross-computer search of our pathology records was performed to identify all biopsies performed. We subsequently analyzed if the biopsy was triggered by screening results or whether the woman presented with symptoms. To ensure detection of all cancers, the database was also linked to the nationwide population-based Netherlands Cancer Registry (NCR).

Data analysis

Pathology results were grouped into malignant (in situ, invasive, and metastatic cancer) and benign lesions (all other findings). Only screen-detected cancers were investigated, which were defined as cancers diagnosed after diagnostic workup initiated by screening results. We separated screen-detected cancers by mammography, MRI, or both based on radiological reports of the respective modalities (or report sections when mammograms and MRI were reported simultaneously).

Cancer yield, false positive recall rate (FPR) and false positive biopsy rate (FPB) for mammography, MRI, and the combination were calculated. Cancer yield was defined as the number of screen-detected cancers per 1000 screening rounds. An FPR or FPB was defined as a woman who was recalled/biopsied and was considered disease-free after workup and/or after at least 1 year of clinical follow up. The FPR/FPB were defined as the number of FPRs/FPBs per 1000 screening rounds.

Two risk categories were evaluated (*BRCA* mutation carriers and all others). The *BRCA* mutation carriers group also included first-degree untested relatives. Examinations were grouped into four age categories to investigate the influence of age ($<$ 40, 40–50, 50–60, $\geq$ 60 years).

Statistical analysis

Descriptive statistics were extracted. The chi-square (χ^2) test was applied to compare differences between groups in demographics, in proportion of breast cancer, invasive cancer, ductal carcinoma in situ (DCIS), tumor grade, and false positives. Chi-square trend-tests were performed to investigate the distribution of parameters across age categories. Repeated screening results were summarized to form binomial counts for each woman to estimate cancer yield, FPR, and FPB. For each woman, the number of true-positive and true-negative screens per modality, and the number of screening visits with or without breast cancer detected were counted. In this way, binomial counts per modality were calculated and analyzed. As the dependent variable was assumed to follow a binomial distribution, generalized estimating equations (GEE) were applied. The binomial proportions were modeled and conducted separately for cancer yield, FPR, and FPB, using a compound symmetry correlation structure. The analysis was conducted separately for each age category, modality, and risk category. After applying the Bonferroni correction, a two-sided p value of 0.013 was considered statistically significant. The number of mammography screens needed (NSN) to detect one breast cancer that was missed by MRI was calculated by dividing the number of mammography screens performed by the number of breast cancers detected by mammography alone. All statistics were performed using SPSS (version 22, SPSS Inc., Chicago, IL, USA).

Results
Study population

Final analysis included 2026 women with 6553 screening rounds (Table 1 and Table 2): 125 screen-detected cancers were identified of which 13 and 59 were only detected by mammography or MRI, respectively ($p < 0.001$). In total, 112 cancers were seen on MRI and 66 on mammography. Overall, no significant difference was found between tumor grade of cancers detected by mammography or MRI ($p = 0.193$). Mammography detected a significantly larger proportion of pure DCIS (16/66 (24%) and 15/112 (13%) for mammography or MRI, respectively, $p < 0.001$). We did not observe a difference in the grade of DCIS detected with mammography or MRI ($p = 0.436$).

Mammography-detected breast cancers

The majority of cancers detected only with mammography consisted of pure DCIS (pTis) (8/13, 62%, Table 3). Most women who were diagnosed with pure DCIS were $\geq$ 50 years of age (6/8, 75%, Table 3). The remaining five women with an invasive cancer detected only at

Table 1 Demographic data and risk profile

	All women	BRCA mutation carriers[a]	Others at increased risk[b]
Number	2026	744	1282
Age			
Mean	44.7	40.4	47.2
SD	11.7	11.0	11.3
Median	44	39	47
Range	21–91	23–75	21–91
Number of cancers	125	61	64
Number of false positive recalls	502	165	337
Number of false positive biopsies	331	117	214

[a]BRCA mutation carriers include 454 BRCA1 mutation carriers and 290 BRCA2 mutation carriers
[b]Others at increased risk include 561 women with a family history of breast cancer, 515 women with a personal history of breast cancer, and 206 others

mammography were aged 35, 53, 54, 55, and 56 years, respectively. Overall, cancer detection with mammography only was higher in women ≥ 50 years old, than in those below 50, though this was not significant (3/58 vs. 10/67, $p = 0.07$). All pure mammography-detected breast cancers were detected in follow-up rounds. The NSN for the overall population and the defined subgroups are presented in Table 4. There was no cancer that was not reported by MRI in the first rounds of screening, making an estimate of NSN not applicable. Our results show that the NSN was highest in the lowest age categories. Whether there is a difference in age groups between women with a proven BRCA mutation and women without is difficult to determine, since we did not observe only mammographically detected breast cancers in BRCA mutation carriers under 50 years of age, but overall the added cancer detection in BRCA mutation carriers was slightly lower than in other women at increased risk (3/61 vs. 10/64, $p = 0.05$).

Cancer yield
Cancer yield increased over time, with a peak at the 50–60 years age category (Fig. 1). The difference between cancers detected by MRI and the combination (mammography + MRI) seemed to increase with age (< 40 years, 0.47; 40–50 years, 0.93; 50–60 years, 4.26; ≥ 60 years, 2.93 per 1000 examinations), pointing to a possible increased added value of mammography in higher age categories (Fig. 2), which was the strongest in the 50–60 years categories both in the BRCA mutation carriers and others. The increase in breast cancer yield by the addition of mammography was not significant in any risk category ($p ≥ 0.303$). Table 5 summarizes cancer yield, FPR, and FPB.

False positives
For FPRs, mammography added 103 FPRs on top of 112 FPRs based on both mammography and MRI, and 287 FPRs based on MRI alone. Overall, mammography significantly added to the FPRs ($p = 0.001$), especially in the

group of women without a BRCA mutation ($p = 0.001$). The relative increase in the FPR due to mammography was greater in the higher age groups (< 40 years, 14%; 40–50 years, 27%; 50–60 years, 44%; ≥ 60 years, 61%, Fig. 2). This was significant in women without a BRCA mutation ($p < 0.001$). In total 35 FPBs were performed based on mammography alone. This did not lead to a significant increase in the overall FPBs ($p = 0.013$), or in any of the subcategories ($p ≥ 0.323$). Completely omitting mammography from the screening regimen would have led to a reduction of 21% (103/502) in FPRs and 11% (35/331) in FPBs.

Discussion
This study evaluated the added value of mammography on top of MRI in a multimodal imaging screening program for women who are at intermediate or high risk of developing breast cancer in a single academic institute. The addition of mammography translated mostly to the detection of a small number of DCIS cases that were occult on MRI. However, five additional invasive carcinomas were also detected. The number of mammography screening examinations needed to detect an MRI occult cancer depended on age, and was very high in women under 40 years old. In addition, adding mammography led to a slight increase in false-positive recalls and biopsies.

Screening, with the aim of early detection of (pre-) malignant breast lesions to decrease breast cancer-related mortality, is a well-accepted risk-reducing strategy for most women at increased risk of developing breast cancer [24]. MRI is considered the most accurate imaging modality [10, 12, 25, 26]. Mammography is currently added to most screening regimens that include MRI to detect calcified breast lesions that may be visualized with mammography but not with MRI [27, 28]. In our study, 8 out of 13 cancers (62%) were MRI-occult DCIS that were detected based on microcalcifications on the mammogram. The five invasive cancers that were detected only with mammography, were also found because of microcalcifications.

Table 2 Population and breast cancer characteristics in the cohort

	Age < 40 years	Age 40–50 years	Age 50–60 years	Age ≥ 60 years	Overall	p value[a]
Women (N)						
BRCA	388	258	182	75	903	<0.001
Others	329	504	482	273	1588	0.014
Overall	717	762	664	348	2491	<0.001
Exams (N)						
BRCA	1113	737	568	190	2608	<0.001
Others	716	1313	1265	651	3945	0.046
Overall	1829	2050	1833	841	6553	<0.001
BC (N)						
Mammography	13	13	25	15	66	0.253
Mammography only	1	2	8	2	13	0.202
MRI	25	30	37	20	112	0.697
MRI only	13	19	20	7	59	0.254
Overall	26	32	45	22	125	0.963
Invasive tumor (N)						
Mammography	13	9	16	12	50	0.771
Mammography only	1	0	4	0	5	0.822
MRI	24	25	30	18	97	0.496
MRI only	12	16	18	6	52	0.253
Overall	25	25	34	18	102	0.540
DCIS (N)						
Mammography	0	4	9	3	16	0.073
Mammography only	0	2	5	1	8	0.281
MRI	1	5	7	2	15	0.036
MRI only	1	3	2	1	7	0.848
Overall	1	7	11	4	23	0.164
Tumor grade of all cancers (invasive and in situ) (N)						
Grade 1						
Mammography	1	1	4	1	7	0.536
Mammography only	0	0	1	0	1	0.655
MRI	3	4	5	5	17	0.384
MRI only	2	3	2	4	11	0.442
Grade 2						
Mammography	1	5	7	4	17	0.171
Mammography only	0	1	2	1	4	0.317
MRI	3	10	17	6	36	0.170
MRI only	2	6	12	3	23	0.335
Grade 3						
Mammography	11	7	11	6	35	0.339
Mammography only	1	1	2	1	5	0.822
MRI	17	15	15	5	52	0.010
MRI only	7	9	6	0	22	0.009
Missing	2	1	3	4	10	0.197
FPR (N)						

Table 2 Population and breast cancer characteristics in the cohort *(Continued)*

	Age < 40 years	Age 40–50 years	Age 50–60 years	Age ≥ 60 years	Overall	p value[a]
Mammography	63	75	55	22	215	<0.001
Mammography only	22	38	28	15	103	0.115
MRI	159	143	72	25	399	<0.001
MRI only	118	106	45	18	287	<0.001
Overall	181	181	100	40	502	<0.001
FPB (*N*)						
Mammography	35	46	32	9	122	<0.001
Mammography only	6	15	11	3	35	0.258
MRI	114	113	51	18	296	<0.001
MRI only	85	82	30	12	209	<0.001
Overall	120	128	62	21	331	<0.001

BC breast cancer (invasive cancer and ductal carcinoma in situ (DCIS)), *MRI* magnetic resonance imaging, *FPR* false positive recall, *FPB* false positive biopsy
[a]Chi-square test for trend was performed for the fraction of the overall population

By mammography alone, only one invasive cancer (grade 3) was detected in a *BRCA* mutation carrier, at the age of 56 years. Our results are in line with the meta-analysis of Heijnsdijk et al. [29], who reported only one invasive cancer detected by mammography alone in *BRCA1* mutation carriers across four breast cancer screening trials of women at high risk of developing breast cancer. Obdeijn et al. [13] also reported little benefit of mammography screening in younger women with a *BRCA1* mutation. In their study, omitting mammography from the screening regimen would have led to two missed DCIS cases in women aged 50 and 67 years. Obdeijn et al. suggested to

increase the starting age for mammography screening in women with *BRCA1* mutations to 40 years. Interestingly, in our study all cancers detected by mammography alone were detected in follow-up rounds, which might point to some increased value in higher age groups. It may also be partly explained by the fact that *BRCA* mutation carriers start with MRI alone, and only from the age of 30 years is mammography added. Our results suggest that the detection of MRI-occult breast cancers is very rare in all women younger than 40 years. Of 13 MRI-occult cancers (both DCIS and invasive cancers and both high and low grade), 10 were observed in women ≥ 50 years old in our

Table 3 Breast cancers detected solely by mammography

Number	Risk category	Ipsi/ contra[b]	Age	Tumor type	Tumor size[a]	Tumor grade	ER-status	PR- status	H2N-status	Nodal status	1st round versus FU
1	*BRCA1*	N/A	50	DCIS	6	2	–	–	–	0	FU
2	Family	N/A	43	DCIS	7	2	–	–	–	0	FU
3	Family	N/A	48	DCIS	–	3	–	–	–	0	FU
4	Personal	Ipsi	55	DCIS	23	–	–	–	–	0	FU
5	Personal	Contra	58	DCIS	–	–	–	–	–	0	FU
6	Personal	Contra	69	DCIS	6	2	–	–	–	0	FU
7	Other	N/A	61	DCIS	21	3	–	–	–	–	FU
8	Personal	Contra	55	DCIS	–	3	–	–	–	0	FU
9	*BRCA2*	N/A	57	DCIS[1]	6	–	Positive	Positive	Negative	0	FU
10	*BRCA1*	N/A	56	IDC	8	3	Positive	Positive	Negative	0	FU
11	Family	N/A	35	IDC	4	3	Positive	Positive	–	0	FU
12	Family	N/A	53	Tubular	3	1	Positive	Positive	Negative	0	FU
13	Other	N/A	54	ILC	23	2	Positive	Positive	Negative	1mi	FU

The symbol "–" indicates not available
N/A not applicable, *ipsi* ipsilateral, *contra* contralateral, *ER* estrogen receptor, *PR* progesterone receptor, *DCIS* ductal carcinoma in situ, *IDC* invasive ductal carcinoma, *ILC* invasive lobular carcinoma, *FU* follow up
[a]Pathological tumor size (in mm), in case of multi-centric tumors (case 13) the diameter of the largest tumor is mentioned
[b]Breast cancer in the ipsilateral or contralateral breast in patients with a personal history of breast cancer
[1]DCIS with micro-invasive growth

Table 4 Number of screens needed (NSN) for one additional mammography-only detected cancer

	Age group (years)	Number of breast cancers	Number of screens	Breast cancers detected by mammography only	NSN for mammography to detect breast cancer missed by MRI
Overall	< 40 years	26	1829	1	1829
	40–50 years	32	2050	2	1025
	50–60 years	45	1833	8	229
	≥ 60 years	22	841	2	421
BRCA	< 40 years	17	1113	0	N/A
	40–50 years	14	737	0	N/A
	50–60 years	26	568	3	189
	≥ 60 years	4	190	0	N/A
No BRCA	< 40 years	9	716	1	716
	40–50 years	18	1313	2	657
	50–60 years	19	1265	5	253
	≥ 60 years	18	651	2	326
Follow up	< 40 years	17	1112	1	1112
	40–50 years	20	1447	2	724
	50–60 years	28	1342	8	168
	≥ 60 years	11	626	2	313
BRCA	< 40 years	12	725	0	N/A
	40–50 years	9	554	0	N/A
	50–60 years	18	433	3	144
	≥ 60 years	0	152	0	N/A
No BRCA	< 40 years	5	387	1	387
	40–50 years	11	893	2	447
	50–60 years	10	909	5	182
	≥ 60 years	11	474	2	237

MRI magnetic resonance imaging, N/A not applicable, the first round was not shown in the table as no mammography-only cancers were detected in the first round

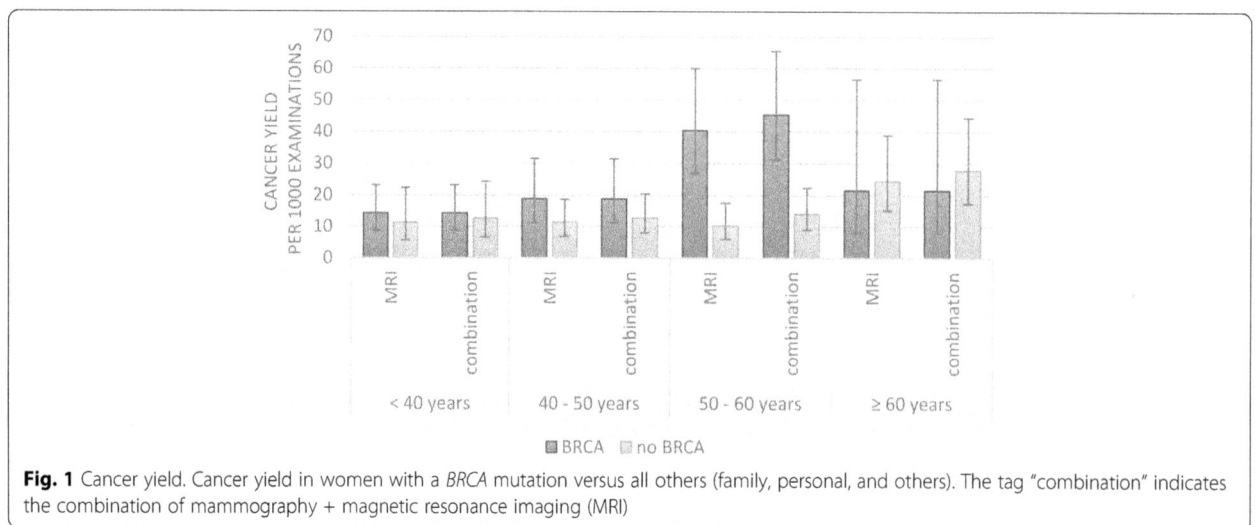

Fig. 1 Cancer yield. Cancer yield in women with a BRCA mutation versus all others (family, personal, and others). The tag "combination" indicates the combination of mammography + magnetic resonance imaging (MRI)

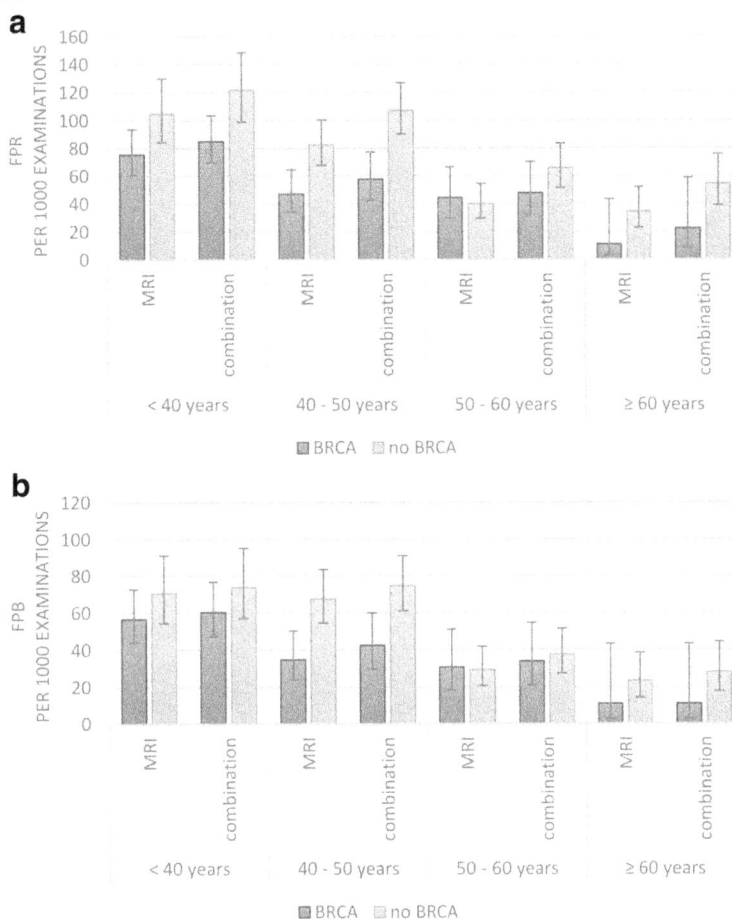

Fig. 2 False positive rates. False positive rates for recall (FPR) (**a**) and for biopsy (FPB) (**b**) for women with a *BRCA* mutation versus all others (family, personal, and others). The tag "combination" indicates the combination of mammography + magnetic resonance imaging (MRI)

population, which is in line with the results reported by Narayan et al. [30]. It should be noted that according to Vreemann et al. [31] 3 of the 13 MRI-occult cancers in this study were in retrospect visible on MRI, including 2 invasive ductal carcinoma (IDC) and 1 DCIS. In our study, raising the starting age of mammography to 40 years would have led to missing one invasive ductal cancer (high grade) in a woman with a positive family history of breast cancer but without a known *BRCA* mutation, and no DCIS would have been missed. In retrospect, this invasive cancer was one of the visible lesions on the MRI and was therefore not truly occult [31, 32]. Additionally, while in older women the additional detection of breast cancer increases with the addition of mammography, this is counterbalanced by an increase in false positive findings. These results are supported by the data of Phi and coworkers [33].

Other imaging modalities may be used to detect additional cancers on top of MRI. Unfortunately, handheld ultrasound or even automated breast ultrasound has been shown to be of limited value in a screening setting where MRI is available [10–12, 25, 34]. Digital breast

tomosynthesis (DBT) has also been shown to increase the cancer detection rate and decrease the number of FPRs when compared to mammography alone in women at average risk [35, 36]. However, there is no consensus on the added value of DBT when breast MRI is available [37]. Therefore, current guidelines only include mammography. The gain in sensitivity with mammography seems to come mostly from the detection of lesions presenting with calcifications. DBT appears to be of relatively equal value to mammography for this purpose, but at a higher dose [38, 39]. Since younger women at high risk and in particular *BRCA* mutation carriers have been shown to be more susceptible to developing radiation-induced cancers [17, 18], replacing mammography with DBT might not be beneficial for women screened with MRI. Berrington de Gonzalez et al. [17] reported no net benefit of mammography surveillance before the age of 35 years in women with a *BRCA* mutation and recommended to limit the radiation dose by raising the age for undergoing mammography. Our results indicate that raising the age

Table 5 Cancer yield, FPR and FPB results for mammography (A), MRI (B), and the combination (C)

Age category	Risk category	Cancer yield[a] (95% CI)	FPR[a] (95% CI)	FPB[a] (95% CI)
A. Mammography				
< 40 years	Overall	6.54 (3.73–11.46)	36.06 (27.57–47.03)	19.48 (13.73–27.58)
	BRCA	7.17 (3.61–14.18)	26.96 (18.07–40.03)	15.52 (9.03–26.57)
	No BRCA	5.61 (2.10–14.89)	49.62 (34.62–70.64)	24.94 (15.94–38.83)
40–50 years	Overall	6.35 (3.71–10.83)	40.44 (31.53–51.72)	24.23 (17.66–33.16)
	BRCA	6.78 (2.85–16.02)	18.90 (11.26–31.56)	12.21 (6.37–23.30)
	No BRCA	6.11 (3.08–12.06)	52.66 (39.80–69.38)	30.56 (21.36–43.55)
50–60 years	Overall	13.57 (9.21–19.94)	33.28 (24.94–44.29)	18.38 (12.60–26.75)
	BRCA	26.10 (15.93–42.47)	10.56 (4.75–23.31)	8.85 (3.67–21.15)
	No BRCA	7.89 (4.26–14.58)	43.06 (31.68–58.27)	22.16 (14.61–33.47)
≥ 60 years	Overall	17.72 (10.81–28.93)	25.82 (16.76–39.58)	10.88 (5.64–20.90)
	BRCA	21.48 (7.99–56.49)	10.69 (2.64–42.22)	0.00 (N/A)
	No BRCA	16.90 (9.54–29.77)	30.38 (19.27–47.57)	14.14 (7.31–27.15)
Overall	Overall	9.95 (7.80–12.69)	36.42 (31.42–42.19)	20.05 (16.49–24.37)
	BRCA	12.44 (8.75–17.65)	20.65 (15.32–27.77)	12.56 (8.50–18.51)
	No BRCA	8.33 (5.95–11.65)	47.08 (39.74–55.71)	24.95 (19.91–31.24)
B. MRI				
< 40 years	Overall	13.09 (8.80–19.44)	87.25 (74.68–101.71)	62.30 (51.89–74.63)
	BRCA	14.31 (8.81–23.16)	75.49 (60.59–93.70)	56.72 (44.03–72.79)
	No BRCA	11.22 (5.61–22.31)	104.96 (84.38–129.84)	70.70 (54.44–91.35)
40–50 years	Overall	14.06 (9.83–20.07)	70.45 (59.44–83.31)	55.95 (46.39–67.33)
	BRCA	18.86 (11.26–31.42)	47.03 (34.06–64.61)	34.73 (23.93–50.15)
	No BRCA	11.37 (6.91–18.66)	82.49 (67.63–100.27)	67.55 (54.44–83.53)
50–60 years	Overall	19.56 (14.16–26.96)	41.64 (32.53–53.16)	29.88 (22.29–39.94)
	BRCA	40.37 (27.00–59.96)	44.36 (29.42–66.36)	30.66 (18.27–51.02)
	No BRCA	10.25 (5.97–17.55)	40.08 (29.42–54.38)	29.41 (20.59–41.84)
≥ 60 years	Overall	23.56 (15.39–35.93)	29.04 (19.45–43.15)	20.49 (12.72–32.85)
	BRCA	21.48 (7.99–56.49)	10.85 (2.66–43.12)	10.85 (2.66–43.12)
	No BRCA	24.40 (15.23–38.87)	34.37 (22.63–51.89)	23.31 (14.04–38.45)
Overall	Overall	16.64 (13.81–20.04)	62.52 (56.37–69.29)	46.27 (41.11–52.06)
	BRCA	22.08 (17.03–28.60)	56.98 (48.07–67.42)	41.81 (34.35–50.80)
	No BRCA	13.10 (10.02–17.10)	66.13 (58.03–75.27)	49.21 (42.42–57.03)
C. Combination				
< 40 years	Overall	13.56 (9.24–20.10)	99.78 (86.35–115.04)	65.68 (54.96–78.31)
	BRCA	14.31 (8.81–23.16)	85.01 (69.45–103.66)	60.34 (47.29–76.70)
	No BRCA	12.65 (6.58–24.21)	121.64 (99.00–148.59)	73.85 (56.96–95.26)
40–50 years	Overall	15.02 (10.64–21.17)	89.74 (77.29–103.98)	63.26 (53.13–75.18)
	BRCA	18.86 (11.26–31.42)	57.42 (42.61–76.97)	42.39 (29.86–59.85)
	No BRCA	12.89 (8.10–20.48)	107.19 (90.27–126.84)	74.68 (61.11–90.97)
50–60 years	Overall	23.82 (17.82–31.76)	60.11 (48.79–73.85)	36.58 (28.05–47.59)
	BRCA	45.29 (31.14–65.43)	47.62 (32.20–69.90)	33.91 (20.91–54.54)
	No BRCA	14.16 (8.97–22.29)	65.53 (51.26–83.42)	37.51 (27.28–51.37)
≥ 60 years	Overall	26.49 (17.31–40.36)	46.86 (34.05–64.17)	24.16 (15.57–37.33)
	BRCA	21.48 (7.99–56.49)	22.05 (8.12–58.46)	10.85 (2.66–43.12)

Table 5 Cancer yield, FPR and FPB results for mammography (A), MRI (B), and the combination (C) *(Continued)*

Age category	Risk category	Cancer yield[a] (95% CI)	FPR[a] (95% CI)	FPB[a] (95% CI)
	No *BRCA*	27.87 (17.39–44.38)	54.21 (38.71–75.43)	28.06 (17.67–44.30)
Overall	Overall	18.68 (15.65–22.27)	79.65 (72.70–87.21)	51.73 (46.28–57.78)
	BRCA	23.17 (18.00–29.79)	65.59 (56.09–76.55)	46.14 (38.31–55.47)
	No *BRCA*	15.74 (12.28–20.15)	89.14 (79.65–99.64)	55.39 (48.20–63.57)

[a]General estimating equations were used to calculate performance measures, correcting for multiple screening rounds within the same patient. All measurements are per 1000 examinations

MRI magnetic resonance imaging, *N/A* no cancers, recalls, or biopsies were found in this category and no 95% CI of this measure could be calculated, *95% CI* Wald 95% confidence intervals

limit of supplemental mammography screening to the age of 40 years should be considered, not only for *BRCA* germline mutation carriers, but for all women at increased risk of developing breast cancer.

A further reason for this recommendation is that population-based mammography screening programs have been criticized because of overdiagnosis and overtreatment of non-fatal breast disease detected during screening [40]. Overdiagnosis, defined as the detection of a breast cancer at screening that would have never been identified clinically in the lifetime of the woman, has been reported as between 1 and 10% [41]. Our results suggest that adding mammography screening to breast MRI may contribute to overdiagnosis because of the preferential detection of relatively indolent (pre-) malignant subtypes such as low-grade calcified ductal in situ carcinoma as described in a previous study [20]. These cancers might be biologically irrelevant compared to invasive and in situ cancers detected with MRI that tend to be of higher grade and are usually detected at an earlier stage [10, 37]. However, this is not evident from our data.

Our study has some limitations. It is a single-center study in a tertiary referral center with a large, high-risk screening program that might not be fully generalizable to the whole breast imaging community. In addition, due to the retrospective nature of the study, some of the MRI and mammography examinations were evaluated simultaneously, which might affect the screening outcomes either positively or negatively. Breast density and background parenchymal enhancement were often not reported and therefore not used in this analysis. While the study describes a long time-span, the absolute number of cancers detected is still small, which might lead to underpowered results. Therefore, more studies are required to confirm our findings.

Conclusions

In conclusion, mammography does not appear to significantly add to cancer yield, albeit our results must be interpreted with the relatively small number of cancers in our study. In *BRCA* mutation carriers the added cancer detection with mammography is even less than for women without *BRCA* mutation. Especially in younger women, the number of mammography screens needed to detect one additional cancer is very high, and increasing the starting age for mammography (if at all) seems safe to maximize the benefits of MRI screening. In higher age groups mammography does add to the detection rates, but also leads to an increase in FPR and FPB.

Acknowledgements
The authors thank the registration team of the Netherlands Comprehensive Cancer Organization (IKNL) for the collection of data for the Netherlands Cancer Registry, and the IKNL staff for scientific advice.

Funding
This work received funding from the European Union's Seventh Framework Programme for research, technological development and demonstration (grant agreement number 601040) and The Netherlands Organization for Health Research and Development (grant agreement number 9051 4524).

Authors' contributions
Study concepts/study design or data acquisition or data analysis/interpretation - all authors; manuscript drafting or manuscript revision for important intellectual content - all authors; approval of the final version of the submitted manuscript - all authors; agree to ensure any questions related to the work are appropriately resolved - all authors; literature research - SV, JCMvZ, AGM, and RMM; clinical studies - SV, JCMvZ, and RMM; experimental studies - SV and JCMvZ; statistical analysis - SV and JCMvZ; manuscript editing - all authors.

Competing interests
The authors declare that they have no competing interests.

Author details
[1]Department of Radiology and Nuclear Medicine, Radboud University Medical Center, Geert Grooteplein 10, 6525 GA Nijmegen, the Netherlands. [2]Department of Surgery, Radboud University Medical Center, Nijmegen, the Netherlands. [3]Department of Pathology, Radboud University Medical Center, Nijmegen, the Netherlands. [4]Department of Human Genetics, Radboud University Medical Center, Nijmegen, the Netherlands.

References
1. Nystrom L, Bjurstam N, Jonsson H, Zackrisson S, Frisell J. Reduced breast cancer mortality after 20+ years of follow-up in the Swedish randomized

controlled mammography trials in Malmo, Stockholm, and Goteborg. J Med Screen. 2017;24(1):34-42.

2. Ford D, Easton DF, Stratton M, Narod S, Goldgar D, Devilee P, Bishop DT, Weber B, Lenoir G, Chang-Claude J, et al. Genetic heterogeneity and penetrance analysis of the BRCA1 and BRCA2 genes in breast cancer families. The Breast Cancer Linkage Consortium. Am J Hum Genet. 1998; 62(3):676–89.

3. Tilanus-Linthorst MM, Obdeijn IM, Bartels KC, de Koning HJ, Oudkerk M. First experiences in screening women at high risk for breast cancer with MR imaging. Breast Cancer Res Treat. 2000;63(1):53–60.

4. Kriege M, Brekelmans CT, Boetes C, Besnard PE, Zonderland HM, Obdeijn IM, Manoliu RA, Kok T, Peterse H, Tilanus-Linthorst MM, et al. Efficacy of MRI and mammography for breast-cancer screening in women with a familial or genetic predisposition. N Engl J Med. 2004;351(5):427–37.

5. Komenaka IK, Ditkoff BA, Joseph KA, Russo D, Gorroochurn P, Ward M, Horowitz E, El-Tamer MB, Schnabel FR. The development of interval breast malignancies in patients with BRCA mutations. Cancer. 2004;100(10):2079–83.

6. Mann RM, Kuhl CK, Kinkel K, Boetes C, Breast MRI. Guidelines from the European Society of Breast Imaging. Eur Radiol. 2008;18(7):1307–18.

7. Saslow D, Boetes C, Burke W, Harms S, Leach MO, Lehman CD, Morris E, Pisano E, Schnall M, Sener S, et al. American Cancer Society guidelines for breast screening with MRI as an adjunct to mammography. CA Cancer J Clin. 2007;57(2):75–89.

8. Leach MO, Boggis CR, Dixon AK, Easton DF, Eeles RA, Evans DG, Gilbert FJ, Griebsch I, Hoff RJ, Kessar P, et al. Screening with magnetic resonance imaging and mammography of a UK population at high familial risk of breast cancer: a prospective multicentre cohort study (MARIBS). Lancet. 2005;365(9473):1769–78.

9. Rijnsburger AJ, Obdeijn IM, Kaas R, Tilanus-Linthorst MM, Boetes C, Loo CE, Wasser MN, Bergers E, Kok T, Muller SH, et al. BRCA1-associated breast cancers present differently from BRCA2-associated and familial cases: long-term follow-up of the Dutch MRISC Screening Study. J Clin Oncol. 2010; 28(36):5265–73.

10. Kuhl C, Weigel S, Schrading S, Arand B, Bieling H, Konig R, Tombach B, Leutner C, Rieber-Brambs A, Nordhoff D, et al. Prospective multicenter cohort study to refine management recommendations for women at elevated familial risk of breast cancer: the EVA trial. J Clin Oncol. 2010;28(9): 1450–7.

11. Warner E, Plewes DB, Hill KA, Causer PA, Zubovits JT, Jong RA, Cutrara MR, DeBoer G, Yaffe MJ, Messner SJ, et al. Surveillance of BRCA1 and BRCA2 mutation carriers with magnetic resonance imaging, ultrasound, mammography, and clinical breast examination. JAMA. 2004;292(11):1317–25.

12. Riedl CC, Luft N, Bernhart C, Weber M, Bernathova M, Tea MK, Rudas M, Singer CF, Helbich TH. Triple-modality screening trial for familial breast cancer underlines the importance of magnetic resonance imaging and questions the role of mammography and ultrasound regardless of patient mutation status, age, and breast density. J Clin Oncol. 2015;33(10):1128–35.

13. Obdeijn IM, Winter-Warnars GA, Mann RM, Hooning MJ, Hunink MG, Tilanus-Linthorst MM. Should we screen BRCA1 mutation carriers only with MRI? A multicenter study. Breast Cancer Res Treat. 2014;144(3):577–82.

14. Plevritis SK, Kurian AW, Sigal BM, Daniel BL, Ikeda DM, Stockdale FE, Garber AM. Cost-effectiveness of screening BRCA1/2 mutation carriers with breast magnetic resonance imaging. JAMA. 2006;295(20):2374–84.

15. Schrading S, Kuhl CK. Mammographic, US, and MR imaging phenotypes of familial breast cancer. Radiology. 2008;246(1):58–70.

16. Tilanus-Linthorst M, Verhoog L, Obdeijn IM, Bartels K, Menke-Pluymers M, Eggermont A, Klijn J, Meijers-Heijboer H, van der Kwast T, Brekelmans C. A BRCA1/2 mutation, high breast density and prominent pushing margins of a tumor independently contribute to a frequent false-negative mammography. Int J Cancer. 2002;102(1):91–5.

17. Berrington de Gonzalez A, Berg CD, Visvanathan K, Robson M. Estimated risk of radiation-induced breast cancer from mammographic screening for young BRCA mutation carriers. J Natl Cancer Inst. 2009;101(3):205–9.

18. Andrieu N, Easton DF, Chang-Claude J, Rookus MA, Brohet R, Cardis E, Antoniou AC, Wagner T, Simard J, Evans G, et al. Effect of chest X-rays on the risk of breast cancer among BRCA1/2 mutation carriers in the international BRCA1/2 carrier cohort study: a report from the EMBRACE, GENEPSO, GEO-HEBON, and IBCCS Collaborators' Group. J Clin Oncol. 2006;24(21):3361–6.

19. NABON: Breast Cancer Guideline. 2012.

20. Vreemann S, Gubern-Merida A, Schlooz-Vries MS, Bult P, van Gils CH, Hoogerbrugge N, Karssemeijer N, Mann RM. Influence of risk category and screening round on the performance of an MR imaging and mammography screening program in carriers of the BRCA mutation and other women at increased risk. Radiology. 2018;286(2):443-51.

21. Dalmis MU, Litjens G, Holland K, Setio A, Mann R, Karssemeijer N, Gubern-Merida A. Using deep learning to Segment breast and fibroglanduar tissue in MRI volumes. Med Phys. 2017;44(2):533-46.

22. Edwards SD, Lipson JA, Ikeda DM, Lee JM. Updates and revisions to the BI-RADS magnetic resonance imaging lexicon. Magn Reson Imaging Clin N Am. 2013;21(3):483–93.

23. Molleran V, Mahoney MC. The BI-RADS breast magnetic resonance imaging lexicon. Magn Reson Imaging Clin N Am. 2010;18(2):171–85. vii

24. Metcalfe KA, Lubinski J, Ghadirian P, Lynch H, Kim-Sing C, Friedman E, Foulkes WD, Domchek S, Ainsworth P, Isaacs C, et al. Predictors of contralateral prophylactic mastectomy in women with a BRCA1 or BRCA2 mutation: the Hereditary Breast Cancer Clinical Study Group. J Clin Oncol. 2008;26(7):1093–7.

25. van Zelst JCM, Mus RDM, Woldringh G, Rutten M, Bult P, Vreemann S, de Jong M, Karssemeijer N, Hoogerbrugge N, Mann RM. Surveillance of women with the BRCA1 or BRCA2 mutation by using biannual automated breast US, MR imaging, and mammography. Radiology. 2017;285(2):376-88.

26. Sardanelli F, Podo F, Santoro F, Manoukian S, Bergonzi S, Trecate G, Vergnaghi D, Federico M, Cortesi L, Corcione S, et al. Multicenter surveillance of women at high genetic breast cancer risk using mammography, ultrasonography, and contrast-enhanced magnetic resonance imaging (the high breast cancer risk Italian 1 study): final results. Investig Radiol. 2011;46(2):94–105.

27. Sung JS, Stamler S, Brooks J, Kaplan J, Huang T, Dershaw DD, Lee CH, Morris EA, Comstock CE. Breast cancers detected at screening MR imaging and mammography in patients at high risk: method of detection reflects tumor histopathologic results. Radiology. 2016;280(3):716–22.

28. Lord SJ, Lei W, Craft P, Cawson JN, Morris I, Walleser S, Griffiths A, Parker S, Houssami N. A systematic review of the effectiveness of magnetic resonance imaging (MRI) as an addition to mammography and ultrasound in screening young women at high risk of breast cancer. Eur J Cancer. 2007; 43(13):1905–17.

29. Heijnsdijk EA, Warner E, Gilbert FJ, Tilanus-Linthorst MM, Evans G, Causer PA, Eeles RA, Kaas R, Draisma G, Ramsay EA, et al. Differences in natural history between breast cancers in BRCA1 and BRCA2 mutation carriers and effects of MRI screening-MRISC, MARIBS, and Canadian studies combined. Cancer Epidemiol Biomark Prev. 2012;21(9):1458–68.

30. Narayan AK, Visvanathan K, Harvey SC. Comparative effectiveness of breast MRI and mammography in screening young women with elevated risk of developing breast cancer: a retrospective cohort study. Breast Cancer Res Treat. 2016;158(3):583–9.

31. Vreemann S, Gubern-Merida A, Lardenoije S, Bult P, Karssemeijer N, Pinker K, Mann RM. The frequency of missed breast cancers in women participating in a high-risk MRI screening program. Breast Cancer Res Treat. 2018;169(2):323-31.

32. Gubern-Merida A, Vreemann S, Marti R, Melendez J, Lardenoije S, Mann RM, Karssemeijer N, Platel B. Automated detection of breast cancer in false-negative screening MRI studies from women at increased risk. Eur J Radiol. 2016;85(2):472–9.

33. Phi XA, Saadatmand S, De Bock GH, Warner E, Sardanelli F, Leach MO, Riedl CC, Trop I, Hooning MJ, Mandel R, et al. Contribution of mammography to MRI screening in BRCA mutation carriers by BRCA status and age: individual patient data meta-analysis. Br J Cancer. 2016;114(6):631–7.

34. Berg WA, Zhang Z, Lehrer D, Jong RA, Pisano ED, Barr RG, Bohm-Velez M, Mahoney MC, Evans WP 3rd, Larsen LH, et al. Detection of breast cancer with addition of annual screening ultrasound or a single screening MRI to mammography in women with elevated breast cancer risk. JAMA. 2012; 307(13):1394–404.

35. Lang K, Andersson I, Rosso A, Tingberg A, Timberg P, Zackrisson S. Performance of one-view breast tomosynthesis as a stand-alone breast cancer screening modality: results from the Malmo Breast Tomosynthesis Screening Trial, a population-based study. Eur Radiol. 2016;26(1):184–90.

36. Lang K, Andersson I, Zackrisson S. Breast cancer detection in digital breast tomosynthesis and digital mammography-a side-by-side review of discrepant cases. Br J Radiol. 2014;87(1040):20140080.

37. Kuhl CK. Abbreviated breast MRI for screening women with dense breast: the EA1141 trial. Br J Radiol. 2017:20170441. [Epub ahead of print].

38. Svahn TM, Houssami N, Sechopoulos I, Mattsson S. Review of radiation dose estimates in digital breast tomosynthesis relative to those in two-view full-field digital mammography. Breast. 2015;24(2):93–9.

39. Clauser P, Nagl G, Helbich TH, Pinker-Domenig K, Weber M, Kapetas P, Bernathova M, Baltzer PAT. Diagnostic performance of digital breast tomosynthesis with a wide scan angle compared to full-field digital mammography for the detection and characterization of microcalcifications. Eur J Radiol. 2016;85(12):2161–8.

40. Bleyer A, Welch HG. Effect of three decades of screening mammography on breast-cancer incidence. N Engl J Med. 2012;367(21):1998–2005.

41. Puliti D, Duffy SW, Miccinesi G, de Koning H, Lynge E, Zappa M, Paci E. Overdiagnosis in mammographic screening for breast cancer in Europe: a literature review. J Med Screen. 2012;19(Suppl 1):42–56.

14

Pyruvate carboxylase supports the pulmonary tropism of metastatic breast cancer

Aparna Shinde[1,2], Tomasz Wilmanski[1,3], Hao Chen[1,2], Dorothy Teegarden[1,3] and Michael K. Wendt[1,2*]

Abstract

Background: Overcoming systemic dormancy and initiating secondary tumor grow under unique microenvironmental conditions is a major rate-limiting step in metastatic progression. Disseminated tumor cells encounter major changes in nutrient supplies and oxidative stresses compared to the primary tumor and must demonstrate significant metabolic plasticity to adapt to specific metastatic sites. Recent studies suggest that differential utilization of pyruvate sits as a critical node in determining the organotropism of metastatic breast cancer. Pyruvate carboxylase (PC) is key enzyme that converts pyruvate into oxaloacetate for utilization in gluconeogenesis and replenishment of the TCA cycle.

Methods: Patient survival was analyzed with respect to gene copy number alterations and differential mRNA expression levels of PC. Expression of PC was analyzed in the MCF-10A, D2-HAN and the 4 T1 breast cancer progression series under in vitro and in vivo growth conditions. PC expression was depleted via shRNAs and the impact on in vitro cell growth, mammary fat pad tumor growth, and pulmonary and non-pulmonary metastasis was assessed by bioluminescent imaging. Changes in glycolytic capacity, oxygen consumption, and response to oxidative stress were quantified upon PC depletion.

Results: Genomic copy number increases in *PC* were observed in 16–30% of metastatic breast cancer patients. High expression of PC mRNA was associated with decreased patient survival in the MCTI and METABRIC patient datasets. Enhanced expression of PC was not recapitulated in breast cancer progression models when analyzed under glucose-rich in vitro culture conditions. In contrast, PC expression was dramatically enhanced upon glucose deprivation and in vivo in pulmonary metastases. Depletion of PC led to a dramatic decrease in 4 T1 pulmonary metastasis, but did not affect orthotopic primary tumor growth. Tail vein inoculations confirmed the role of PC in facilitating pulmonary, but not extrapulmonary tumor initiation. PC-depleted cells demonstrated a decrease in glycolytic capacity and oxygen consumption rates and an enhanced sensitivity to oxidative stress.

Conclusions: Our studies indicate that PC is specifically required for the growth of breast cancer that has disseminated to the lungs. Overall, these findings point to the potential of targeting PC for the treatment of pulmonary metastatic breast cancer.

Keywords: Breast cancer, Metastasis, Pyruvate carboxylase, Metabolism, Glycolysis, Hypoxia, Oxidative stress

* Correspondence: mwendt@purdue.edu
[1]Purdue University Center for Cancer Research, Purdue University, West Lafayette, IN 47907, USA
[2]Department of Medicinal Chemistry and Molecular Pharmacology, Purdue University, West Lafayette, IN 47907, USA
Full list of author information is available at the end of the article

Background

Metastasis of primary mammary tumors to vital secondary organs is the primary cause of breast cancer-associated death, with no effective treatment [1]. Metastasis is a highly selective process that requires cancer cells to overcome multiple barriers to escape the primary tumor, survive in circulation, and eventually colonize distant secondary organs. The major sites of breast cancer metastasis include bone, liver, brain, and lungs [2]. Understanding the unique drivers of organ-specific metastases could hold the key to more personalized and more effective therapies for stage 4 patients. Previous studies have sought to characterize stable genetic and gene expression changes that drive metastatic tropism of individual cancer cells [3, 4]. However, the plasticity of metastatic breast cancer cells in response to specific growth environments makes identification of in vivo tropic factors difficult.

Metabolic reprogramming is a hallmark of cancer, and is implicated in cell proliferation, survival, and metastatic progression [5]. Considerable progress has been made in understanding the unique metabolic changes cancer cells must undergo to adapt to the hypoxic and acidic microenvironment of the primary tumor [6]. Furthermore, the Warburg effect dictates that tumor cells will continue to utilize glycolysis for energy production even in the presence of abundant oxygen. However, recent studies suggest that metastatic cells have an increased ability to alternate between usage of glycolysis or oxidative phosphorylation (OXPHOS) for energy production in response to particular environmental stresses [7]. Furthermore, expression of the master transcriptional regulator of mitochondrial biogenesis, peroxisome proliferator-activated receptor gamma coactivator 1-alpha (PGC-1α), has recently been linked to the pulmonary metastasis of breast cancer [8]. Overall, these and other studies support the notion that breast cancers capable of reversing the Warburg effect and reactivating mitochondrial OXPHOS are at a selective advantage during initiation of metastatic tumor growth, particularly within the oxygen-rich pulmonary microenvironment.

The axis of pyruvate utilization is emerging as a key regulatory point in cancer cell metabolism, and may be critical to organotropism of metastatic breast cancer [9–11]. The majority of pyruvate in primary tumors is converted into lactate to sustain high rates of glycolysis. Indeed, depletion of lactate dehydrogenase (LDH), the enzyme responsible for lactate production inhibited primary tumor growth and subsequently metastasis [12]. Alternatively, pyruvate may enter the TCA cycle via its metabolism by pyruvate dehydrogenase (PDH) or pyruvate carboxylase (PC). Dupuy et al. demonstrated that a key negative regulator of PDH, pyruvate dehydrogenase kinase (PDK1), is essential for liver metastasis [13]. These data suggest that modulation of mitochondrial pyruvate metabolism may determine successful colonization of specific organs by metastatic cancer cells. PC is a mitochondrial enzyme which sustains anaplerosis through its carboxylation of pyruvate into oxaloacetate. PC has recently been shown to be upregulated in lung metastases [8]. Given these data and the critical role of pyruvate metabolism in metastasis, we sought to address the hypothesis that PC is specifically required for the initiation of metastatic outgrowth within the pulmonary microenvironment.

The current study characterizes PC expression and genomic amplification in relation to breast cancer patient survival. Furthermore, we utilize several models of breast cancer to delineate the pulmonary tropism that is dictated by PC. Overall, our data clearly indicate that PC is specifically required for initiation of pulmonary metastatic breast cancer, but it is not required for extrapulmonary tumor growth. These findings suggest inhibition of PC may serve as an effective therapeutic target for the treatment of pulmonary metastasis.

Methods

Cell lines and reagents

The five different TRC lentiviral mouse *Pcx*-targeting short hairpin RNAs (shRNAs) (lentiviral pLKO.1 TRC cloning vector) were purchased from GE Dharmacon, Lafayette, CO USA. The shRNA lentiviral plasmids were cotransfected with psPAX2 and pMD2.G into HEK293T cells using polyethylenimine to obtain lentiviral particles. The 4 T1, 4 T07, and D2.A1 cells were transduced with lentiviral particles for 48 h and stably transduced cells were selected over a span of 14 days in puromycin (5μg/ml). In all cases, separate cells were transduced with scrambled non-silencing shRNAs as a control. The target shRNA sequences were 5′- AAAGGACAAATAGC TGAAGGG-3′(shPC 25) and 5′ –TTGACCTCGATGAA GTAGTGC-3′ (shPC28). The scrambled sequence was 5′-TTCTCCGAACGTGTCACGT-3′. All cells were culture in DMEM containing, 10% fetal bovine serum (FBS), penicillin/streptomycin, 25 mM glucose, 1 mM sodium pyruvate and 4 mM glutamine. Where indicated glucose concentrations were decreased to 5.6 mM.

Immunological assays

For immunoblot analyses cells were lysed using a modified RIPA lysis buffer containing 50 mM Tris, 150 mM NaCl, 0.25% sodium deoxycholate, 1.0% NP40, 0.1% SDS, protease inhibitor cocktail, 10 mM activated sodium orthovanadate, 40 mM β-glycerolphosphate, and 20 mM sodium fluoride. These lysates were separated by reducing SDS PAGE and probed for PC (Santa Cruz Biotechnology, Dallas, TX, USA), actin (Santa Cruz Biotechnology, Dallas, TX, USA), or β-tubulin (DSHB, Iowa City, IA, USA). Immunohistochemical analyses of formalin-fixed paraffin-embedded tissue sections from 4 T1 primary and metastatic tumors were conducted by deparfinization of in xylene, rehydration, and antigen retrieval using 10 mM sodium citrate (pH 6.0) under pressurized boiling. After inactivation of endogenous peroxidases in 3% H_2O_2, primary antibodies specific for PC (Sigma-Aldrich, St. Louis, MO, USA) or hypoxia inducible factor (HIF)1-α (Novus, Littleton, CO, USA) were added and incubated overnight. Protein-specific staining was detected through the use of appropriate biotinylated secondary antibodies in conjunction with ABC reagent (Vector, Burlingame, CA, USA). These sections were counterstained with hematoxylin, dehydrated, and mounted.

Three-dimensional (3D) culture

Bioluminescent 4 T1 scram, shPC 25 and shPC 28 cells were grown under 3D culture conditions. Cell growth was quantified via addition of luciferin (GoldBio, St. Louis, MO< USA). Briefly, 1000 cells were plated in each well of a white-walled 96-well dish on top of a solidified 50 μl bed of Cultrex basement membrane extract (BME) from (Trevigen, Gaithersburg, MD, USA). These cells were suspended in growth media containing DMEM (low or high glucose), 10% FBS, and 5% of the BME.

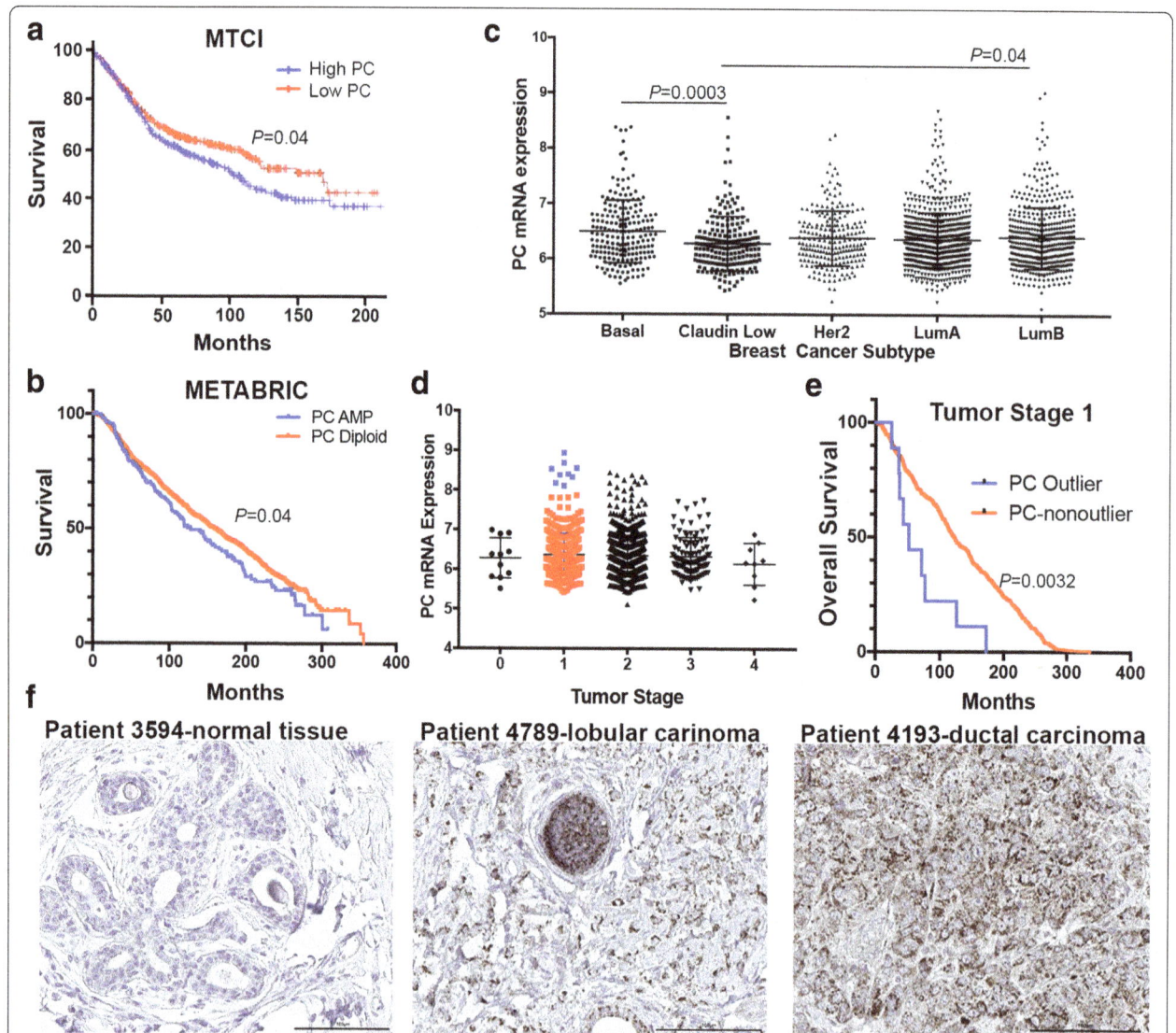

Fig. 1 PC expression is increased in more aggressive breast cancers. **a** Patients with lymph node-positive breast cancer from the MTCI dataset were split into two groups split based on mean expression of PC and the resultant differences in patient survival are shown. **b** Patients within the METABRIC dataset were separated into two groups based on increased genomic copy numbers of *PC*. Differences in patient survival are shown. **c** Expression levels of PC are plotted across the different breast cancer subtypes within the METABRIC dataset. Subtypes were defined by the PAM50 expression analysis. Differences in PC expression levels were analyzed by a Kruskal-Wallis test resulting in the indicated *P* values. **d** PC expression levels within the METABRIC data set are plotted based on tumor stage. Significant outliers in the stage 1 group as determined by a ROUT analysis are shown in *blue*. **e** The stage 1 patients shown in panel **d** were separated based on PC outlier status and differences in overall survival are shown. Data in panels **a**, **b** and **e** were analyzed by a log-rank test resulting in the indicated *P* values. **f** IHC analyses for PC expression within normal mammary tissue, lobular breast carcinoma, and ductal breast carcinoma. Data in panel F are representative of three normal samples and ten primary breast tumors

Table 1 Gene copy numbers of *PC* are increased in metastatic breast cancer patients. Copy number alterations in the *PC* gene (chromosome 11q13.2) were analyzed in the indicated datasets. The percentage of patient tumors demonstrating increases in *PC* gene copy number was calculated for each dataset

Dataset	Deep deletion	Shallow deletion	Diploid	Gain	Amplification	% samples with gain in PC
METABRIC	0	145	1575	232	98	16.09
MBC Project	0	5	75	16	7	22.30
TCGA, Nature 2012	0	64	558	121	35	20.00
Mutational profiles of metastatic breast cancer	1	31	117	49	15	30.04

METABRIC Molecular Taxonomy of Breast Cancer International Consortium, *MBC Project* Metastatic Breast Cancer Project, *TCGA* The Cancer Genome Atlas

Invasion and migration assays

Control and PC depleted 4 T1 cells were plated at equal cell density in serum-free medium containing either 1 or 4 mM pyruvate into 8µm fluoroBlok 24-well transwell inserts (Corning, Corning, NY, USA). The bottom well was filled with 10% FBS medium containing either 1 mM or 4 mM pyruvate. Serum-free medium in the bottom well was used as a negative control. Cell migration was quantified after 12 h of incubation using 5 µg/mL of Calcein AM in phosphate-buffered saline (PBS) and a Synergy H1 Multi-mode reader (bottom read: ex./em. 495/530). For wound closure assays control and PC-depleted 4 T1 cells were plated onto six-well plates and grown till 90–95%

confluence. Once nearly confluent, each well was scratched using a 200 ul pipette tip and cell media was replaced to 0.5% serum. Wound images were taken at time 0,15 and 24 h. The open wound area was quantified using TScratch software [14] and percent wound closure was calculated using the following formula: [(open area at time 0 - open area at time x)/open area at time 0] *100.

Metabolic and oxidative stress analysis

Rate of glycolysis and oxygen consumption were analyzed using the Seahorse XFe24 Analyzer (Agilent, Santa Clara, CA, USA). 4 T1 shScram and shPC25 cells were plated at a concentration of 20,000 cells/well on a

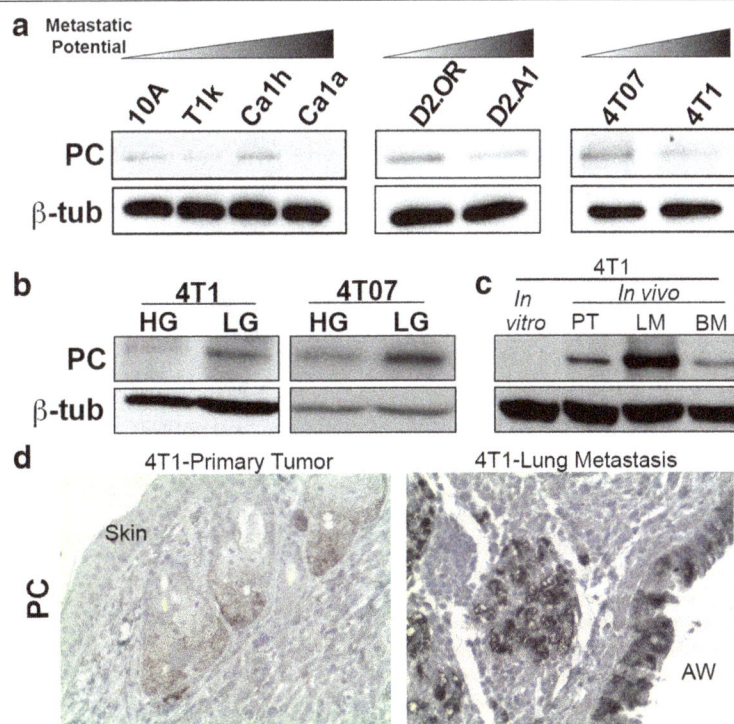

Fig. 2 PC expression is enhanced in the pulmonary microenvironment. **a** Expression of PC protein was assessed by immunoblot across the indicated cell lines of varying metastatic potential. **b** 4 T07 and 4 T1 cells were cultured in the absence of exogenous glucose for 4 days and PC expression was assessed by immunoblot. **c** Expression of PC proteins was analyzed in 4 T1 lysates harvested from in vitro culture, mammary fat pad primary tumors (PT), and their resultant metastases growing within the lung (LM) and bone marrow (BM). **d** IHC analyses for PC expression within 4 T1 primary tumors pushing directly against the skin and the resulting pulmonary metastases growing near an airway (AW) in the lungs. Data are representative of at least three tumors from each location. For panel A-C expression of β-tubulin (β-tub) served as a loading control

Seahorse bioanalyzer plate 24 h before analysis. 4 T07 shScram and shPC25 cells were plated at a concentration of 40,000 cells/well on the same Seahorse bioanalyzer plate to achieve comparable viable cell number at the time of experiment. The glycolytic stress test was conducted according to the manufacturer's instructions with 10 mM glucose concentration in the media while oxygen consumption rate (OCR) was measured in the presence of 10 mM glucose, 2 mM glutamine, and 1 mM pyruvate. After the assay was completed, cells within each well were lysed into 25 ul of 1× RIPA buffer and protein content was measured using a BCA Assay. Where indicated 4 T1 cells were plated overnight and treated with hydrogen peroxide (H_2O_2) at multiple concentrations on day 2. The cells were washed with PBS twice on day 7, and stained with crystal violet, lysed, and absorbance was read at 600 nm.

In vivo studies

Control or PC-depleted 4 T1 cells previously engineered to express firefly luciferase stably were resuspended in sterile PBS (50 μl) and injected orthotopically into the mammary fat pad (2.5×10^4 cells/mouse) of 6-week-old female Balb/c mice. Primary tumor growth and metastasis development was assessed by using digital calipers and by weekly bioluminescent imaging on an advanced molecular imager (AMI, Spectral Instruments; Tucson, AZ, USA). For tail vein assays, control or PC-depleted 4 T07 or D2.A1 cells previously engineered to express

firefly luciferase were resuspended in sterile PBS (200 μl) and injected into lateral tail vein (5×10^5 cells/injection) of 6-week-old female Balb/c mice. Mice were assessed for tumor development by weekly bioluminescent imaging on an AMI in vivo imager. All animal studies were performed in accordance with the animal protocol procedures approved by the Purdue Animal Care and Use Committee of Purdue University.

Statistical analyses

One way ANOVA or two-sided t tests were used where the data met the assumptions of these tests and the variance was similar between the two groups being compared. Expression values for PC across breast cancer subtypes were analyzed using a Kruskal-Wallis test, together with a Dunn's multiple comparisons test. P values of less than 0.05 were considered significant. No exclusion criteria were utilized in these studies.

Results

PC expression is increased in more aggressive breast cancers

To evaluate the importance of PC in breast cancer progression we initially utilized the BreastMark Kaplan-Meier analysis program to analyze the Molecular Therapeutics for Cancer, Ireland (MTCI) dataset [15]. There was a significant decrease in survival of patients whose tumors express high versus low levels of PC based on the mean value of

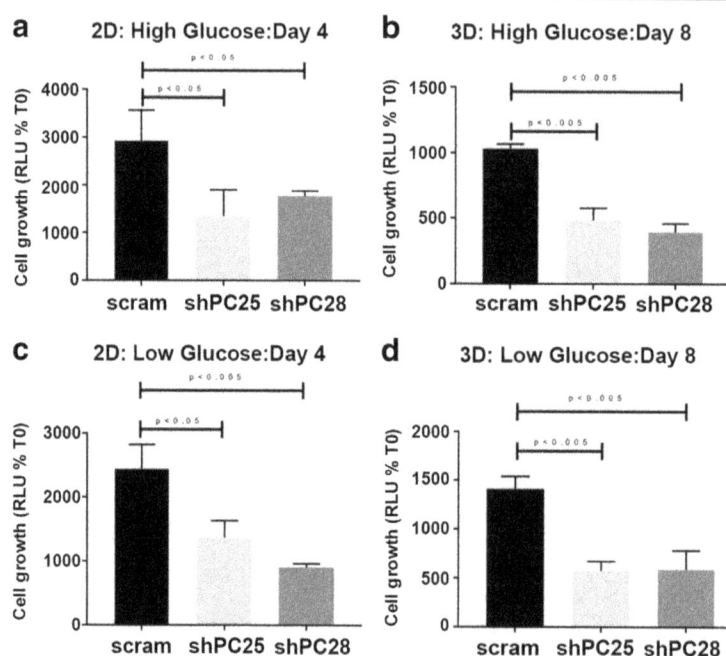

Fig. 3 Depletion of the PC inhibits in vitro cell growth. Two different shRNA sequences targeting PC (shPC25 and shPC28) were stably expressed in the 4 T1 cells and cellular viability was assessed under two-dimensional (**a** and **c**) and three-dimensional (**b** and **d**) culture conditions containing high (4.5 mg/ml; **a** and **b**) or low (1 mg/ml; **c** and **d**) amounts of glucose. Data are the mean ± SE of the three separate experiments completed in triplicate resulting in the indicated P values

the entire cohort (Fig. 1a). We also analyzed the Molecular Taxonomy of Breast Cancer International Consortium (METABRIC) dataset consisting of 2509 patient samples annotated for several pieces of the patient-specific data including breast cancer subtype and tumor stage [16]. Analysis of PC gene copy number in the METABRIC and other invasive and metastatic breast cancer datasets indicated that 16–30% of patients demonstrate copy number gains in PC (Table 1). All patient datasets analyzed and the cell line encyclopedia indicated increased PC gene copy number directly correlates with increased PC mRNA expression levels (not shown). Importantly, patients with PC gene amplification in the METABRIC data set displayed significantly reduced survival times as compared to the rest of the cohort (Fig. 1b). Significant differences in PC mRNA expression were observed between subtypes, with the aggressive basal subtype showing the highest mean level of PC expression (Fig. 1c). Changes in PC mRNA expression were also analyzed across tumor stage. No significant correlation in PC expression was observed in regard to tumor stage or tumor size (Fig. 1d, Additional file 1: Figure S1). However, significant outliers were determined by a ROUT analysis in both stage 1 and stage 2 patients (Fig. 1d). The high-level PC outlier patients in the stage 1 group demonstrated a

significant decrease in survival as compared to the rest of the stage 1 patients (Fig. 1e). These data suggest that high-level PC expression does not contribute to primary tumor growth, but may be involved in the later stages of breast cancer progression, contributing to decreased patient survival. Further supporting these genomic and mRNA analyses, immunohistochemical (IHC) analysis of lobular and ductal breast carcinoma tissues ($n = 10$) demonstrated the detection of PC-expressing tumor cells, something that was not observed in normal mammary epithelium ($n = 3$) (Fig. 1f and Additional file 2: Figure S2). Overall, these data clearly demonstrate genomic amplification and increased expression of PC in more aggressive breast cancers. Furthermore, lack of PC correlation with primary tumor stage/ size suggests a functional role for this protein in driving the later stages of breast cancer progression.

PC expression is increased in the pulmonary microenvironment

To examine the functional role of PC in breast cancer metastasis, we first assessed PC expression levels across several breast cancer progression series. In contrast to the patient data shown in Fig. 1, PC expression failed to correlate with increasing metastatic capacity of the MCF10A series, the

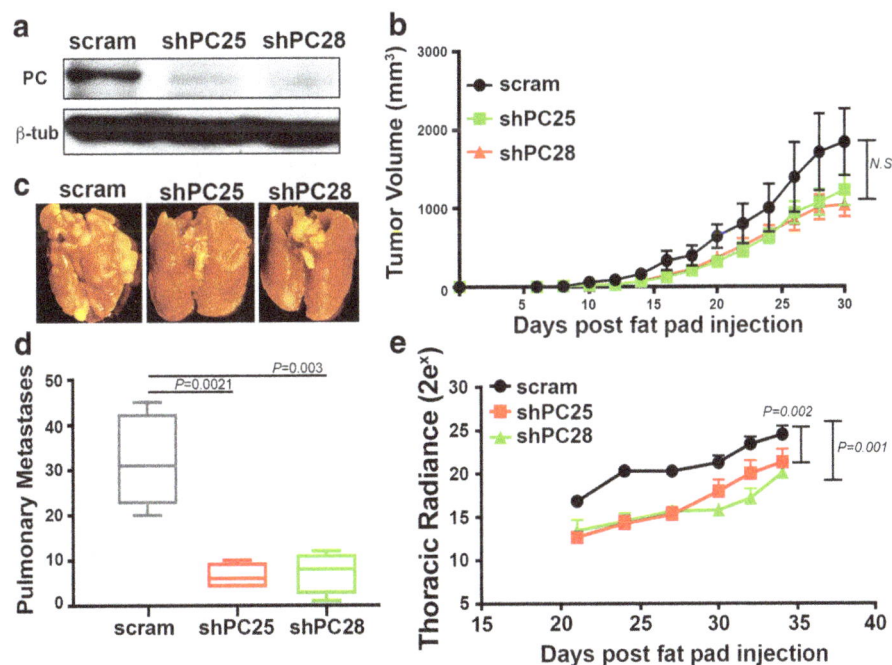

Fig. 4 PC is required for 4 T1 metastasis but not primary tumor growth. **a** Immunoblot analysis for PC in 4 T1 cells expressing control (*scram*) or PC-targeted (*shPC25* and *shPC28*) shRNAs. Analysis of β-tubulin (*β-tub*) served as a loading control. **b** 4 T1 cells (2.5×10^4/mouse) were engrafted onto the mammary fat pad via an intraductal inoculation and primary tumor growth was measured by digital caliper measurements at the indicated time points. Any differences between groups were found to be not significant (NS). **c** Necropsy pictures showing lungs of mice bearing the indicated 4 T1 primary tumors. **d** The numbers of metastatic pulmonary nodules resulting in mice bearing control (*scram*) and PC-depleted (*shPC25* and *shPC28*) 4 T1 primary tumors. Data are the mean ± SE of five mice per group resulting in the indicated P values. **e** Bioluminescent intensity (Radiance) measurements of thoracic metastases of control (scram) or PC-depleted (shPC25 and shPC28) 4 T1 tumor-bearing mice. Data are the mean radiance measurements ±SE of five mice per group resulting the in the indicated P values

D2-hyperplastic alveolar nodule (HAN) series, and the 4 T1 series (Fig. 2a) [17–19]. Previous studies suggest that PC expression can be increased during epithelial-mesenchymal transition (EMT) through the transcription factor Snail [9, 20]. While stimulation of the 4 T1 cells with transforming growth factor (TGF)-β1 induced a robust morphological change consistent with EMT, we did not observe any change in PC expression (Additional file 3: Figure S3A and S3B). Furthermore, expression of Snail in the MCF-10-T1 k cells did not robustly increase PC expression (Additional file 3: Figure S3C). The presence of glucose can enhance expression of PC through activation of one of two distinct promoters [21]. In contrast, PC is also required for gluconeogenesis, and therefore its expression can be selectively enhanced under glucose-deprived conditions [22]. We observed that depletion of exogenous glucose from sodium pyruvate-containing growth media of 4 T1 and 4 T07 cells led to increased expression of PC (Fig. 2b). We also observed an increase in PC expression in orthotopic 4 T1 primary tumors (Fig. 2c). However, upon IHC analysis we found that PC was highly expressed in the murine sebaceous glands within these tumors, but was still not detectable in 4 T1 tumor cells (Fig. 2c and d). Expression of PC was further enhanced in 4 T1 lung metastases and IHC

analyses clearly indicated that PC was expressed in both bronchial epithelial cells and tumor cells (Fig. 2c and d; [11]). Taken together these data suggest that in contrast to the primary tumor, growth within the pulmonary microenvironment demands high levels of PC.

Depletion of PC inhibits spontaneous metastasis

We next depleted PC expression in the highly metastatic 4 T1 cells using two independent shRNAs [19]. Depletion of PC did not affect cellular migration as assessed by both a transwell and a wound healing assay (Additional file 4: Figure S4). However, depletion of PC did result in inhibition of cell growth irrespective of glucose concentration or whether cells were grown on two-dimensional (2D) plastic or within 3D hydrogel cultures (Fig. 3). In contrast to in vitro culture, there were no significant differences in the growth of PC-depleted primary tumors as compared to control (Fig. 4a and b). However, resultant pulmonary metastases observed in these mice were drastically inhibited upon depletion of PC (Fig. 4c-e).

PC expression is required for pulmonary tumor growth

Inhibition of pulmonary metastasis was quite dramatic in the 4 T1 model, but overall inhibition of thoracic

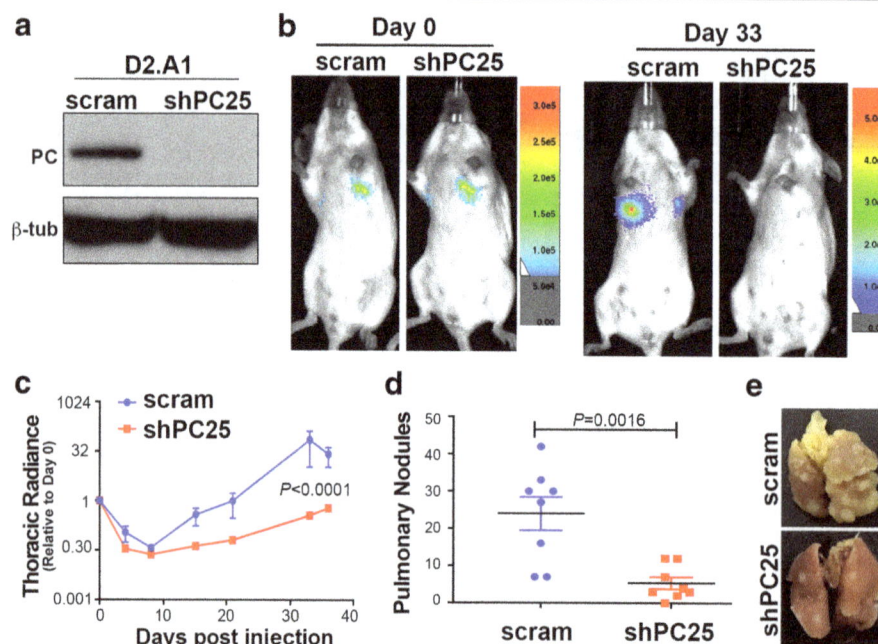

Fig. 5 PC expression is required for pulmonary outgrowth of D2.A1 cells. **a** Immunoblot analysis for PC in D2.A1 cells expressing control (scram) or PC-targeted (shPC25) shRNAs. Analysis of β-tubulin (β-tub) served as a loading control. **b** D2.A1 cells (5.0 × 10⁵/ mouse) were injected into the lateral tail vein of female Balb/c mice. Pulmonary tumor cell delivery (Day 0) and pulmonary tumor growth (Day 33) were visualized by bioluminescent imaging. **c** Bioluminescent intensity (Radiance) values were normalized to the injected values for each group and used to quantify pulmonary tumor seeding and outgrowth at the indicated time points. Growth curves were analyzed two-way ANOVA differences resulting in the indicated P value (n = 4 mice per group). **d** The number of pulmonary tumor nodules per lobe resulting in mice injected with control (scram) and PC-depleted (shPC25) D2.A1 cells. Data are the mean ± SE of four mice per group resulting in the indicated P values. **e** Necropsy pictures showing representative lungs of mice 35 days after tail vein injections of control (scram) and PC depleted (shPC25) D2.A1 cells. PC pyruvate carboxylase

metastasis, which includes pulmonary metastases, cells within the pleural space, and bone metastases throughout the spine and rib cage, was not as robust (Fig. 4d and e). These data, together with the lack of change in primary tumor growth (Fig. 4b), and enhanced expression of PC in lung metastases (Fig. 2d) led us to hypothesize that PC may be specifically required for tumor growth within the pulmonary microenvironment. To examine the role of PC in pulmonary tumors, we utilized a tail vein injection approach with the D2.A1 cells. These cells grow very well when delivered into the lungs via the tail vein, but do not demonstrate extrapulmonary metastasis beyond this site [23, 24]. Similar to the 4 T1 cells, PC could be readily depleted from these cells using stable expression of shRNAs (Fig. 5a). Equal pulmonary delivery of control and PC-depleted cells was verified by bioluminescent imaging (Fig. 5b). Furthermore, early bioluminescence readings taken 3 and 8 days after tumor cell injection indicated that initial seeding within in the lungs was not affected by PC depletion (Fig. 5c). However, pulmonary outgrowth was drastically decreased in D2.A1 cells lacking PC (Fig. 5c-e). These findings

strongly suggest that PC is required for initiation of tumor growth within the pulmonary microenvironment.

PC is not required for growth of extrapulmonary metastases

We have previously established that unlike the D2.A1 cells, the 4 T07 cell model will not only grow in the lungs following tail vein inoculation, but will also form extrapulmonary metastases primarily in the upper thoracic region of the animal [25]. Therefore, we depleted PC in 4 T07 cells to evaluate the role of PC in pulmonary versus extrapulmonary tumor growth following injection into the lateral tail vein (Fig. 6a and b). Bioluminescent imaging verified equal pulmonary delivery, but a decrease in ultimate thoracic luminescence generated by PC-depleted 4 T07 cells 21 days after tumor cell injection (Fig. 6b and c). Upon necropsy, a dramatic difference in macroscopic pulmonary tumor nodules once again confirmed the requirement of PC for robust tumor growth within the lungs (Fig. 6d and e). In contrast, luminescent imaging of carcasses in which tumor-bearing lungs had been removed demonstrated a significant increase in extrapulmonary metastases generated

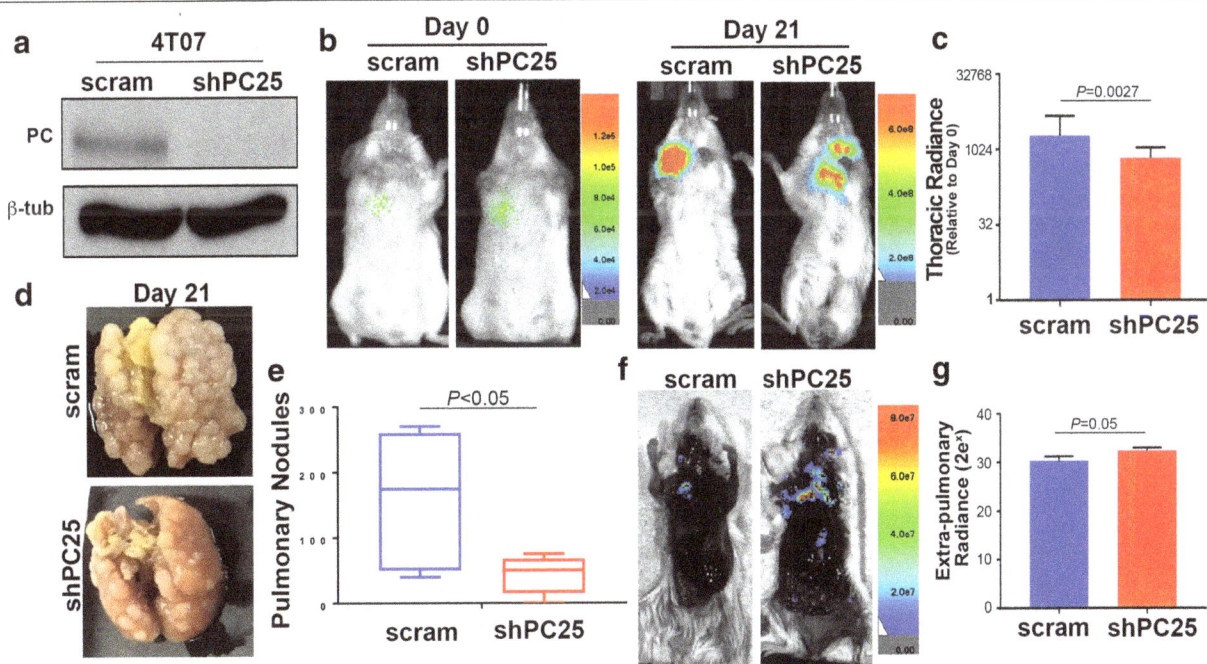

Fig. 6 PC is not required for the growth of extrapulmonary metastases. **a** Immunoblot analysis for PC in 4 T07 cells expressing control (*scram*) or PC-targeted (*shPC25*) shRNAs. Analysis of β-tubulin (*β-tub*) served as a loading control. **b** 4 T07 cells (5.0×10^5/mouse) were injected into the lateral tail vein of female Balb/c mice. Pulmonary tumor cell delivery (Day 0) and tumor formation (Day 21) were visualized by bioluminescent imaging. **c** Bioluminescent intensity (Radiance) values were normalized to the injected values for each group and used to quantify thoracic tumor growth in intact mice 21 days after tumor cell injections. Data are the mean normalized values ±SE of five mice per group resulting in the indicated *P* value. **d** Necropsy pictures showing representative lungs of mice 21 days after tail vein injections of control (scram) and PC depleted (shPC25) 4 T07 cells. **e** The numbers of pulmonary tumor nodules per lobe was quantified in mice injected with control (scram) and PC-depleted (shPC25) 4 T07 cells. Data are the mean ± SE of five mice per group resulting in the indicated *P* value. **f** The lungs of mice injected with control (scram) and PC-depleted (shPC25) 4 T07 cells were removed upon necropsy and the carcasses were immediately imaged. Shown are representative images from each group. **g** Whole animal bioluminescent intensity measurements were taken for dissected carcasses described in panel F. Data are the mean radiance values ±SE of five mice per group resulting in the indicated *P* value. *PC* pyruvate carboxylase

by PC-depleted cells as compared to control cells (Fig. 6f and g). These data strongly suggest that while PC is required for growth in the lungs its expression is not required, or maybe inhibitory to the growth of extrapulmonary metastases.

PC is required for the metabolic plasticity of metastatic breast cancer

To investigate the importance of PC in the metabolic plasticity of metastatic breast cancer cells, rates of glycolysis and oxygen consumption were measured using the XFe24 Seahorse bioanalyzer. Both glycolysis, as measured by the extracellular acidification rate (ECAR), and oxygen consumption rate (OCR) were significantly higher in 4 T1 versus 4 T07 cells (Fig. 7; [7]). Along these lines, PC depletion resulted in a

significant decrease in both glycolysis and OCR in 4 T1 cells, but not 4 T07 cells (Fig. 7a and c). Glycolytic capacity was further measured by injecting oligomycin (Fig. 7b), an ATP synthase inhibitor that shifts cell dependence on ATP generation towards glycolysis. Consistent with previous reports, 4 T1 cells demonstrated significantly higher glycolytic capacity than the 4 T07 cells, and again this was dependent upon expression of PC (Fig. 7a; [26]).

The hypoxic environment of the primary tumor induces the stabilization of HIF-1α and shutdown of the TCA cycle, but newly developing pulmonary metastases lose HIF-1α expression (Additional file 5: Figure S5; [27]). Thus, metabolic adaptation upon loss of HIF-1α is a major hurdle that must be overcome during initiation of pulmonary metastatic outgrowth. HIF-1α levels are

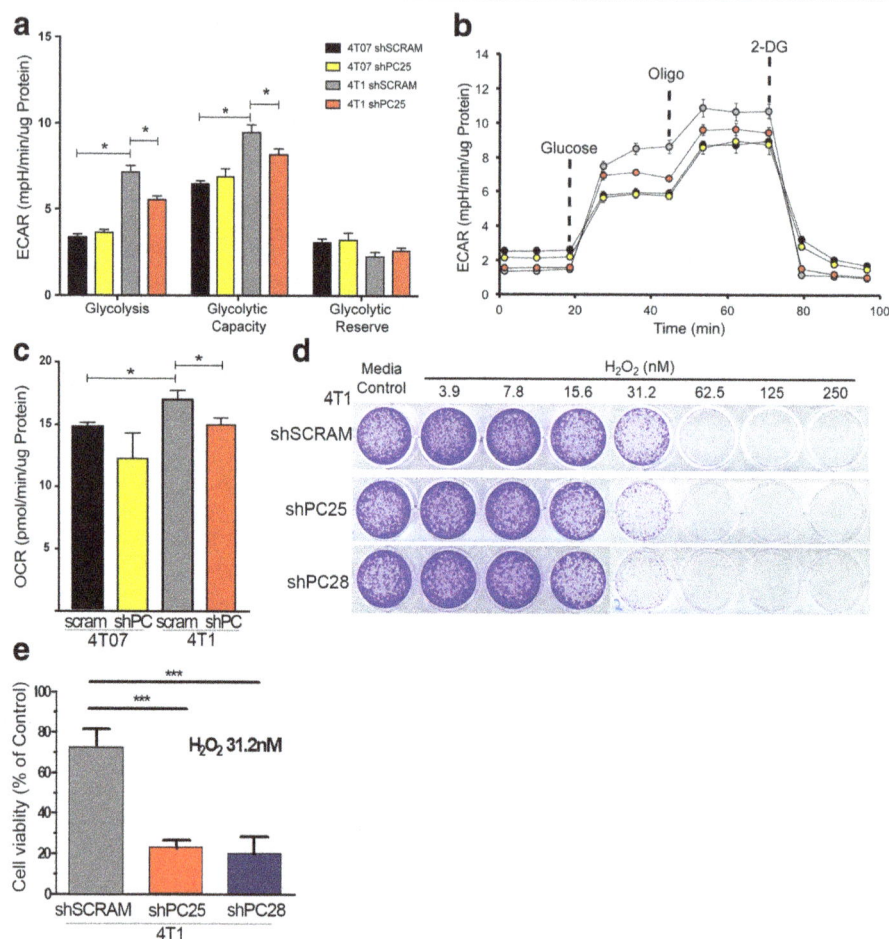

Fig. 7 PC supports metabolic flexibility and oxidative stress defense. **a** Glycolytic stress test analysis of 4 T07 and 4 T1 control (*shscram*) and PC-depleted (*shPC25*) cells. **b** ECAR measurements obtained upon injections of glucose (10 mM), oligomycin (Oligo) and 2-deoxglucose (2-DG) used to calculate glycolysis and glycolytic capacity in each cell line. **c** OCR measurements for 4 T07 and 4 T1 control (shscram) and PC depleted (shPC25) cells in the presence of 10 mM glucose, 2 mM glutamine and 1 mM pyruvate. Data are the mean ± SE of measurements per μg protein. **d** Control (shscram) and PC-depleted (shPC25 and *shPC28*) 4 T1 cells were treated with the indicated concentrations of H_2O_2 and viable cells were visualized with crystal violet. **e** Stained cells from panel D were solubilized and quantified via absorbance at 600 nm. Data are the mean ± SD of three independent experiments. Asterisks indicates statistical significance (*$P < 0.05$, ***$P < 0.01$). *ECAR* extracellular acidification rate, *OCR* oxygen consumption rate

constitutively low in in vitro culture, consistent with the requirement of PC for in vitro cell growth (Fig. 3). Therefore, to further recapitulate the enhanced oxidative stress within the pulmonary microenvironment, we treated cells with increasing concentrations of hydrogen peroxide (H_2O_2). Consistent with our recent studies we observed an enhanced sensitivity to H_2O_2 upon depletion of PC (Fig. 7d and e; [28]).

Discussion

Herein, we utilized several syngeneic models of breast cancer to demonstrate that initiation of pulmonary metastatic outgrowth is strongly dependent on PC. We also demonstrate that PC is not required for primary mammary tumor growth or extrapulmonary metastasis. Our findings are nicely supported by previous studies in lung cancer that similarly demonstrate the requirement of PC for in vivo tumor growth [10, 29]. The specific aspects of the pulmonary microenvironment that demand PC expression remain to be determined definitively. However, enhanced oxygen content and increased oxidative stress are very unique aspects of the pulmonary microenvironment with respect to pyruvate utilization. Under hypoxic conditions of primary tumors, extrapulmonary metastases, and macroscopic pulmonary tumors, pyruvate utilization mainly occurs through anaerobic glycolysis that is driven by HIF-1α-induced expression of hexokinase, LDH, and pyruvate kinase M2 [27]. HIF-1α also inhibits pyruvate dehydrogenase via upregulation of PDK1, further blocking aerobic glycolysis and increasing lactate production [30]. Depletion of HIF-1α or HIF-1α target genes such as LDH or carbonic anhydrase IX (CAIX) in 4 T1 cells inhibits primary tumor growth, therefore decreasing subsequent macrometastasis [12, 13, 31]. In contrast, we propose a model that in the oxygen- and pyruvate-rich microenvironment of the lungs HIF-1α is directed to proteosomal degradation and metastatic cells must transiently shift to PC-mediated aerobic utilization of pyruvate to initiate metastatic outgrowth. Only once macroscopic metastases are formed and hypoxia is reestablished are tumors able to reengage HIF-1α and return to anaerobic glycolysis.

Our analysis of the METABRIC dataset demonstrates decreased survival of stage 1 breast cancer patients with genomic amplification of PC. These findings are completely consistent with our mouse studies in that high-level PC expression does not contribute to primary tumor growth, but these cells have an enhanced antioxidant defense system and are more metabolically fit for aerobic initiation of pulmonary metastatic outgrowth following systemic dissemination. Indeed, recent studies clearly indicate that systemic dissemination of primary tumor cells is an early step in metastasis whereas overcoming dormancy within secondary organs is the rate-limiting process leading to patient lethality [32]. Therefore, our findings suggest

assessment of PC genomic amplification or mRNA expression could serve as an effective prognostic biomarker to predict for metastatic relapse in patients diagnosed with early-stage primary tumors. Additionally, PC could also serve as therapeutic biomarker in conjunction with application of direct pharmacological inhibitors of PC or more general inhibitors of oxidative phosphorylation such as IACS-010759, which is currently in clinical trials (NCT03291938).

Conclusions

Overall, the data herein present a comprehensive analysis of patient data and syngeneic mouse models that uniformly support a specific role for PC in facilitating initiation of pulmonary metastatic tumor growth. Moreover, we present findings that demonstrate a role for PC in facilitating metabolic plasticity of disseminated breast cancer cells. Our findings clearly point to the potential of genomic amplification of PC as prognostic biomarker and as a therapeutic target for the treatment of pulmonary metastatic breast cancer.

Additional files

Additional file 1: Figure S1. PC expression is not correlated with primary tumor size. Patient samples within the METABRIC dataset were analyzed for PC expression in relation to primary tumor size. Data are analyzed by a nonparametric Spearman correlation resulting in the indicated r and P values. The linear regression for these data is also shown. (PDF 235 kb)

Additional file 2: Figure S2. PC expression in primary breast tumors. PC expression within tumor cells was rated as high, medium, low, or negative (n = 10). Representative sections from each group are shown. Data was obtained from the protein atlas dataset (www. proteinatlas.org) [33]. (PDF 2805 kb)

Additional file 3: Figure S3. Transient induction of EMT does not induce expression of PC. (A) Photomicrographs showing EMT-like changes in cellular morphology of the control (scram) and PC-depleted (shPC25 and shPC28) 4 T1 cells upon treatment with exogenous TGF-β1 (5 ng/ml) for 4 days. (B) Immunoblot analyses for PC in cells shown in Panel A. β-tubulin served as a loading control. (C) The RAS transformed MCF-10A-T1 k cells were constructed to express a doxycycline-inducible vector encoding the EMT transcription factor Snail. Expression of PC was analyzed upon addition of doxycycline (Dox) at the indicated concentrations. Expression of Snail and β-tubulin (β-Tub) served as loading controls. (PDF 1401 kb)

Additional file 4: Figure S4. PC is not required for cell migration. (A) Control (shScram) and PC depleted (shPC28) cells were plated into 8 μm transwell inserts in serum-free media containing 1 or 4 mM pyruvate. Cell migration was quantified 12 h after plating using calcein AM. SFM represents wells where the bottom chamber was filled with serum-free media as negative control. Values are presented as mean relative fluorescence units, ±SEM. (B) Control (shScram) and PC-depleted (shPC28) 4 T1 monolayers were wounded and closure was measured 15 and 24 h later. Values are presented as mean percent would closure, ±SEM. (PDF 372 kb)

Additional file 5: Figure S5. HIF-1α expression that characterizes primary tumors is lost in pulmonary metastases. 4 T1 cells were engrafted onto the mammary fat pad via an intraductal injection and grown as primary tumors. These tumors gave rise to spontaneous pulmonary metastases. Upon necropsy both primary and metastatic tumors were analyzed by immunohistochemistry for the expression of HIF-1α. Nuclear expression of HIF-1α is very high in viable primary tumor tissue. In contrast, nuclear HIF-1α is drastically reduced in pulmonary metastases. Data are representative of three separate mice bearing primary tumors and metastases. (PDF 1389 kb)

Abbreviations
ECAR: Extracellular acidification rate; EMT: Epithelial-mesenchymal transition; HAN: Hyperplastic alveolar nodule; HIF1-α: Hypoxia inducible factor; IMH: Immunohistochemical; LDH: Lactate dehydrogenase; METABRIC: Molecular Taxonomy of Breast Cancer International Consortium; MTCI: Molecular Therapeutics of Cancer, Ireland; OCR: Oxygen consumption rate; OXPHOS: Oxidative phosphorylation; PC: Pyruvate carboxylase; PDH: Pyruvate dehydrogenase; PDK1: Pyruvate dehydrogenase kinase; PGC-1α: Peroxisome proliferator-activated receptor gamma coactivator 1-alpha; shRNAs: Short hairpin RNAs

Acknowledgments
Members of the Wendt Laboratory are thanked for their critical reading of the manuscript. We kindly acknowledge the expertise of the personnel within the Purdue Center for Cancer Research Biological Evaluation Core. We also acknowledge the use of the facilities within the Bindley Bioscience Center, a core facility of the NIH-funded Indiana Clinical and Translational Sciences Institute.

Funding
This research was supported in part by the American Cancer Society (RSG-CSM130259) to MKW and the National Institutes of Health (R01CA207751) to MKW, the National Institutes of Health (R25CA128770) to DT and the Indiana Elks Charities to DT. Support was also provide by the Indiana Clinical and Translational Science Institute to MKW and DT (UL1TR001108) and the Purdue Center for Cancer Research via an NIH NCI grant (P30CA023168).

Authors' contributions
AS, HC, and TW contributed to the design of the experiments, completed experiments, and contributed to the writing of the manuscript. MKW and DT contributed to the design of the experiments, supervised experiments, and contributed to the writing of the manuscript. All authors read and approved the final manuscript.

Competing interests
The authors declare that they have no competing interests.

Author details
[1]Purdue University Center for Cancer Research, Purdue University, West Lafayette, IN 47907, USA. [2]Department of Medicinal Chemistry and Molecular Pharmacology, Purdue University, West Lafayette, IN 47907, USA. [3]Department of Nutrition Science, West Lafayette, IN 47907, USA.

References
1. Ali R, Wendt MK. The paradoxical functions of EGFR during breast cancer progression. Signal Transduct Target Ther. 2017;2:16042.

2. Chambers AF, Groom AC, MacDonald IC. Dissemination and growth of cancer cells in metastatic sites. Nat Rev Cancer. 2002;2:563–72.

3. Minn AJ, Kang Y, Serganova I, Gupta GP, Giri DD, Doubrovin M, et al. Distinct organ-specific metastatic potential of individual breast cancer cells and primary tumors. J Clin Invest. 2005;115:44–55.

4. Hoshino A, Costa-Silva B, Shen T-L, Rodrigues G, Hashimoto A, Tesic Mark M, et al. Tumour exosome integrins determine organotropic metastasis. Nature. 2015;527:329–35.

5. Hanahan D, Weinberg RA. Hallmarks of cancer: the next generation. Cell. 2011;144:646–74.

6. Heiden MGV, DeBerardinis RJ. Understanding the intersections between metabolism and cancer biology. Cell. 2017;168:657–69.

7. Simões RV, Serganova IS, Kruchevsky N, Leftin A, Shestov AA, Thaler HT, et al. Metabolic plasticity of metastatic breast cancer cells: adaptation to changes in the microenvironment. Neoplasia. 2015;17:671–84.

8. Andrzejewski S, Klimcakova E, Johnson RM, Tabariès S, Annis MG, McGuirk S, et al. PGC-1α promotes breast cancer metastasis and confers bioenergetic flexibility against metabolic drugs. Cell Metab. 2017;26:778–787.e5.

9. Phannasil P, Thuwajit C, Warnnissorn M, Wallace JC, MacDonald MJ, Jitrapakdee S. Pyruvate carboxylase is up-regulated in breast cancer and essential to support growth and invasion of MDA-MB-231 cells. PLoS One. 2015;10:e0129848.

10. Sellers K, Fox MP, Bousamra M, Slone SP, Higashi RM, Miller DM, et al. Pyruvate carboxylase is critical for non–small-cell lung cancer proliferation. J Clin Invest. 2015;125:687–98.

11. Christen S, Lorendeau D, Schmieder R, Broekaert D, Metzger K, Veys K, et al. Breast cancer-derived lung metastases show increased pyruvate carboxylase-dependent Anaplerosis. Cell Rep. 2016;17:837–48.

12. Rizwan A, Serganova I, Khanin R, Karabeber H, Ni X, Thakur S, et al. Relationships between LDH-A, lactate, and metastases in 4T1 breast tumors. Clin Cancer Res. 2013;19:5158–69.

13. Dupuy F, Tabariès S, Andrzejewski S, Dong Z, Blagih J, Annis MG, et al. PDK1-dependent metabolic reprogramming dictates metastatic potential in breast cancer. Cell Metab. 2015;22:577–89.

14. Gebäck T, Schulz MMP, Koumoutsakos P, Detmar M. TScratch: a novel and simple software tool for automated analysis of monolayer wound healing assays. BioTechniques. 2009;46:265–74.

15. Madden SF, Clarke C, Gaule P, Aherne ST, O'Donovan N, Clynes M, et al. BreastMark: an integrated approach to mining publicly available transcriptomic datasets relating to breast cancer outcome. Breast Cancer Res BCR. 2013;15:R52.

16. Pereira B, Chin S-F, Rueda OM, Vollan H-KM, Provenzano E, Bardwell HA, et al. The somatic mutation profiles of 2,433 breast cancers refines their genomic and transcriptomic landscapes. Nat Commun. 2016;7:11479.

17. Strickland LB, Dawson PJ, Santner SJ, Miller FR. Progression of premalignant MCF10AT generates heterogeneous malignant variants with characteristic histologic types and immunohistochemical markers. Breast Cancer Res Treat. 2000;64:235–40.

18. Morris VL, Tuck AB, Wilson SM, Percy D, Chambers AF. Tumor progression and metastasis in murine D2 hyperplastic alveolar nodule mammary tumor cell lines. Clin Exp Metastasis. 1993;11:103–12.

19. Aslakson CJ, Miller FR. Selective events in the metastatic process defined by analysis of the sequential dissemination of subpopulations of a mouse mammary tumor. Cancer Res. 1992;52:1399–405.

20. Lee SY, Jeon HM, Ju MK, Kim CH, Yoon G, Han SI, et al. Wnt/snail signaling regulates cytochrome c oxidase and glucose metabolism. Cancer Res. 2012; 72:3607–17.

21. Jitrapakdee S, Maurice MS, Rayment I, Cleland WW, Wallace JC, Attwood PV. Structure, mechanism and regulation of pyruvate carboxylase. Biochem J. 2008;413:369–87.

22. Kumashiro N, Beddow SA, Vatner DF, Majumdar SK, Cantley JL, Guebre-Egziabher F, et al. Targeting pyruvate carboxylase reduces gluconeogenesis and adiposity and improves insulin resistance. Diabetes. 2013;62:2183–94.

23. Wendt MK, Taylor MA, Schiemann BJ, Schiemann WP. Down-regulation of epithelial cadherin is required to initiate metastatic outgrowth of breast cancer. Mol Biol Cell. 2011;22:2423–35.

24. Shibue T, Weinberg RA. Integrin beta1-focal adhesion kinase signaling directs the proliferation of metastatic cancer cells disseminated in the lungs. Proc Natl Acad Sci U S A. 2009;106:10290–5.

25. Wendt MK, Schiemann BJ, Parvani JG, Lee Y-H, Kang Y, Schiemann WP. TGF-β stimulates Pyk2 expression as part of an epithelial-mesenchymal transition program required for metastatic outgrowth of breast cancer. Oncogene. 2013;32:2005–15.

26. Frees AE, Rajaram N, McCachren SS, Fontanella AN, Dewhirst MW, Ramanujam N. Delivery-corrected imaging of fluorescently-labeled glucose reveals distinct metabolic phenotypes in murine breast cancer. PLoS One. 2014;9:e115529.

27. Kim J, Tchernyshyov I, Semenza GL, Dang CV. HIF-1-mediated expression of pyruvate dehydrogenase kinase: a metabolic switch required for cellular adaptation to hypoxia. Cell Metab. 2006;3:177–85.

28. Wilmanski T, Zhou X, Zheng W, Shinde A, Donkin SS, Wendt M, et al. Inhibition of pyruvate carboxylase by 1α,25-dihydroxyvitamin D promotes oxidative stress in early breast cancer progression. Cancer Lett. 2017;411:171–81.

29. Davidson SM, Papagiannakopoulos T, Olenchock BA, Heyman JE, Keibler MA, Luengo A, et al. Environment impacts the metabolic dependencies of Ras-driven non-small cell lung cancer. Cell Metab. 2016;23:517–28.

30. Kim J, Gao P, Liu Y-C, Semenza GL, Dang CV. Hypoxia-inducible factor 1 and dysregulated c-Myc cooperatively induce vascular endothelial growth factor and metabolic switches hexokinase 2 and pyruvate dehydrogenase kinase 1. Mol Cell Biol. 2007;27:7381–93.

31. Lou Y, McDonald PC, Oloumi A, Chia S, Ostlund C, Ahmadi A, et al. Targeting tumor hypoxia: suppression of breast tumor growth and metastasis by novel carbonic anhydrase IX inhibitors. Cancer Res. 2011;71:3364–76.

32. Sosa MS, Bragado P, Aguirre-Ghiso JA. Mechanisms of disseminated cancer cell dormancy: an awakening field. Nat Rev Cancer. 2014;14:611–22.

33. Pontén F, Jirström K, Uhlen M. The human protein atlas–a tool for pathology. J Pathol. 2008;216:387–93.

15

Paternal malnutrition programs breast cancer risk and tumor metabolism in offspring

Raquel Santana da Cruz[1†], Elissa J. Carney[1†], Johan Clarke[1], Hong Cao[1], M. Idalia Cruz[1], Carlos Benitez[1], Lu Jin[1], Yi Fu[2], Zuolin Cheng[2], Yue Wang[2] and Sonia de Assis[1*] (ID)

Abstract

Background: While many studies have shown that maternal factors in pregnancy affect the cancer risk for offspring, few studies have investigated the impact of paternal exposures on their progeny's risk of this disease. Population studies generally show a U-shaped association between birthweight and breast cancer risk, with both high and low birthweight increasing the risk compared with average birthweight. Here, we investigated whether paternal malnutrition would modulate the birthweight and later breast cancer risk of daughters.

Methods: Male mice were fed AIN93G-based diets containing either 17.7% (control) or 8.9% (low-protein (LP)) energy from protein from 3 to 10 weeks of age. Males on either group were mated to females raised on a control diet. Female offspring from control and LP fathers were treated with 7,12-dimethylbenz[a]anthracene (DMBA) to initiate mammary carcinogenesis. Mature sperm from fathers and mammary tissue and tumors from female offspring were used for epigenetic and other molecular analyses.

Results: We found that paternal malnutrition reduces the birthweight of daughters and leads to epigenetic and metabolic reprogramming of their mammary tissue and tumors. Daughters of LP fathers have higher rates of mammary cancer, with tumors arising earlier and growing faster than in controls. The energy sensor, the AMP-activated protein kinase (AMPK) pathway, is suppressed in both mammary glands and tumors of LP daughters, with consequent activation of mammalian target of rapamycin (mTOR) signaling. Furthermore, LP mammary tumors show altered amino-acid metabolism with increased glutamine utilization. These changes are linked to alterations in noncoding RNAs regulating those pathways in mammary glands and tumors. Importantly, we detect alterations in some of the same microRNAs/target genes found in our animal model in breast tumors of women from populations where low birthweight is prevalent.

Conclusions: Our study suggests that ancestral paternal malnutrition plays a role in programming offspring cancer risk and phenotype by likely providing a metabolic advantage to cancer cells.

Keywords: Ancestral nutrition, Paternal programming, Breast cancer, AMPK pathway

* Correspondence: deassiss@georgetown.edu
†Raquel Santana da Cruz and Elissa J. Carney contributed equally to this work.
[1]Department of Oncology, Lombardi Comprehensive Cancer Center, Georgetown University, 3970 Reservoir Road, NW, The Research Building, Room E410, Washington, DC 20057, USA
Full list of author information is available at the end of the article

Background

Parental environmental exposures have been shown to affect phenotype in the next generation [1]. Given the close relationship between mother and the fetus, most of the evidence for this phenomenon comes from maternal exposures in pregnancy. However, many recent studies both in animals and humans have shown that paternal environmental exposures ranging from stress to nutrition can influence the risk of disease in the offspring. Paternal ancestral exposures have been shown to affect organ development in offspring including brain, liver, pancreas, bone, and mammary tissue [2–6]. Many of these studies also suggest that memory of past paternal exposures is transmitted to the progeny through the germline via epigenetic mechanisms. More recently, it was reported that the noncoding RNA sperm load, particularly microRNAs (miRNAs) and tRNA-derived fragments (tRFs), plays an essential role in transmitting environmental memory from fathers to offspring [7–9].

Epidemiologic and animal studies have consistently linked birthweight to cancer risk, particularly breast cancer [10–13]. Population studies generally show a U-shaped association between birthweight and breast cancer risk, with both high and low birthweight increasing risk compared with average birthweight [11, 13]. In these studies, the child's birthweight is often attributed to maternal weight gain and nutrition in pregnancy. However, paternal factors also play a role in the offspring's birthweight [14]. In line with this, we recently reported that paternal high-fat diet intake or overweight leads to increased birthweight, alterations in mammary gland development, and higher rates of breast cancer risk in daughters in two rodent models [5, 6]. While no studies in humans have directly investigated the link between paternal nutrition and breast cancer in daughters, an association between other paternal factors and cancer risk in the progeny has been reported [15–17].

Moderate paternal malnutrition such as protein restriction has been shown to impact the development of the offspring's organs and metabolism [3, 4, 7], yet its influence on mammary development is unknown. Studies in humans suggest that this may be the case as women who were conceived during a famine have increased breast cancer risk [18]. Here, we investigated whether paternal suboptimal nutrition (low--protein (LP) diet) can modulate the birthweight, mammary development, and breast cancer risk of daughters using a mouse model. We found that LP daughters have lower birthweight, alterations in mammary gland morphology, and higher rates of mammary cancer. Furthermore, we found that mammary glands and tumors of LP daughters are metabolically rewired, with alterations in the AMP-activated protein kinase (AMPK) and amino-acid metabolism pathways. These changes were associated with differential expression of miR-451a, miR-200c, and miR-92a. Importantly, some of the

same miRNAs and target gene alterations were detected in breast tumors of women from populations with high rates of a low birthweight.

Methods

Breeding and dietary exposures

The c57bl/6 strain of mice was used in all experiments. Male mice were fed AIN93G-based diets (Additional file 1: Table S1) manufactured by Envigo Teklad Diets (Madison, Wisconsin, USA) containing either 17.7% (control, $n = 11$) or 8.9% energy from protein (LP, $n = 11$) starting after weaning (3 weeks of age). Male bodyweight was recorded weekly. At 10 weeks of age, LP-fed and control-fed male mice were mated to female mice reared on the control diet to generate the female offspring (Additional file 1: Figure S1). Males were kept in female cages for 3 days. Female mice were kept on the control diet during the breeding period, for the extent of pregnancy (21 days), and after giving birth. The birthweight of pups and number of pups per litter was determined. To avoid a litter effect, pups were cross-fostered 2 days after dams gave birth. Pups from 2 to 3 dams were pooled and housed in a litter of 8–10 pups per nursing dam. All pups were weaned on postnatal day 21 and fed the control diet throughout the experiment. Pup bodyweight was recorded weekly. The female offspring of control or LP fathers were used to study birthweight, mammary gland morphology, molecular analyses, and mammary tumorigenesis as described in the following sections. The number of contributing fathers and female offspring used in each experiment is listed in Additional file 1 (Table S2). All animal procedures were approved by the Georgetown University Animal Care and Use Committee, and the experiments were performed following the National Institutes of Health guidelines for the proper and humane use of animals in biomedical research.

Mature spermatozoa collection and purification

Control and LP fathers were euthanized once mating was completed and the caudal epididymis (for sperm collection) was dissected. The cauda and vas deferens from male mice were collected, punctured, and transferred to a tissue culture dish containing M2 media (M2 medium with HEPES, without penicillin and streptomycin, liquid, sterile-filtered, and suitable for mouse embryo; SIGMA, product #M7167) where it was incubated for 1 h at 37 °C. Sperm samples were isolated and purified from somatic cells. Briefly, the samples were washed with phosphate-buffered saline (PBS), and then incubated with somatic cell lysis buffer (SCLB; 0.1% SDS, 0.5% TX-100 in diethylpyrocarbonate water) for 1 h. SCLB was rinsed off with two washes of PBS and the purified spermatozoa sample was pelleted and used for DNA and miRNA extraction. To further rule out any somatic cell contamination, quantitative polymerase chain reaction (qPCR) was performed using RNA from purified sperm samples and primers for the somatic cell marker *Actb*, or the sperm-specific marker *Smcp* (Additional file 1: Figure S2).

Bodyweight monitoring
The bodyweight of female offspring was measured at birth ($n = 10$–12 litters/group) and weekly after weaning ($n = 29$–32/group). Birthweights were analyzed by t test, and longitudinal bodyweight analyzed using two-way analysis of variance (ANOVA; group and time), with Sidak's multicomparison test used for post-hoc analyses.

Mammary gland harvesting
Inguinal mammary glands (fourth pair) of the female offspring of control and LP fathers ($n = 8$–10/group) were collected on postnatal day (PND) 50 and used for mammary gland development analysis, DNA, RNA, and protein extraction.

Small RNA-seq analysis
Total RNA (small and large transcripts) was isolated from paternal sperm and the mammary tissue of offspring ($n = 4$/group/tissue) using Qiagen's miRNeasy extraction kit according to the manufacturer's instructions. Small noncoding RNA transcript libraries were constructed according to the Illumina TrueSeq Small RNA Pre-Kit. Indexed, paired-end sequencing libraries were prepared from quality total RNA (RIN ≥ 8). For each library, 10 million reads (raw data) were generated by Illumina Hi-Seq 4000. The raw reads were subject to adapter trimming and low-quality filtering using the Trimmomatic program. The high-quality clean reads were aligned on the mouse genome. Noncoding RNA tags were mapped to the mouse genome (GRCm38/mm10 reference genome) to analyze their expression and distribution on the genome. Small RNA tags were annotated with miRNA, tRNA, piRNA, and rRNA to miRBase, Ref-seq, GenBank, and Rfam databases using blastn with standard parameters. To analyze the differential expression of small RNA between control and LP groups, different small RNA species (miRNA, tRF, etc.) were normalized to TPM (transcripts per kilobase million). When needed, cross-sample re-normalization and/or batch-effect correction were performed [19]. The P value and q value between groups was generated using model-based and/or permutation-based significance tests. Small RNA with a q value less than 0.05 were considered significant, with an appropriate correction for multiple testing [19]. Target prediction for microRNAs of interest was conducted using TargetScan (Release 6.2). The predicted targeted mRNA list was then uploaded to ingenuity pathway analysis (IPA) for gene set enrichment analysis.

Quantitative real-time PCR validation (qRT-PCR)
Differentially methylated genes (mammary tissue only) or differentially expressed miRNA (mammary tissue/tumors)

uncovered by our bioinformatics team were validated in mammary tissues ($n = 7$–10/group) and tumors ($n = 12$/group) using qRT-PCR. Briefly, cDNA was synthesized from total RNA samples using the TaqMan™ Advanced miRNA cDNA Synthesis Kit (Applied Biosystems). PCR products were amplified from cDNA using TaqMan® Fast Advanced Master Mix and sequence-specific primers from TaqMan Assays (Applied Biosystems). Fold-change was calculated from Ct values and the expression levels of specific miRNAs were determined by normalizing these values with the fold-change values for appropriate endogenous controls (miR-361 or miR-26A for miRNAs and GAPDH for genes). Fold-differences between the groups were analyzed using a t test.

Genome-wide DNA methylation analysis
Genomic DNA was isolated from paternal sperm and the mammary tissue of offspring ($n = 2$–3/group/tissue) using Qiagen's DNeasy extraction kit according to the manufacturer's instructions. Methylated DNA was eluted by the MethylMiner Methylated DNA Enrichment Kit (Invitrogen). Briefly, 1 µg of genomic DNA was sheared by sonication and captured by MBD proteins. The methylated DNA was eluted and used to generate methyl-CpG binding domain-based capture (MBDCap) libraries as previously described [20]. MBDCap coupled with massively parallel sequencing (MBDCap-seq) libraries were sequenced using the Illumina Genome Analyzer II (GA II). Image analysis and base calling were performed with the standard Illumina pipeline. Sequencing reads was mapped by the ELAND algorithm.

Data analysis
The gene promoter regions are defined as up to 5000 base pairs upstream of the transcription starting site, as described in our previous study [20], and also included the first exon, since methylation in these two regions most strongly correlate with reduced gene expression [21–23]. We used a novel statistical approach, AISAIC [20, 24, 25], to determine the significant 'driver' methylation changes between LP and control offspring. To detect significant methylation changes (against background random events), methylation intensity fold-change is used as the differential methylation measure. The total number of bases of short reads in a promoter representing regional methylation intensity are used for calculating the fold-change, the jth promoter in the ith generation, i.e., $f_{ij} = (I_{case,ij} + \beta L)/(I_{control,ij} + \beta L)$, where $I_{case,ij}$ and $I_{control,ij}$ are the methylation intensities in case and control samples, respectively. L ($= 36$) is the short-read length in MDBCap-seq data, and β ($= 10$) is an offset parameter that suppresses the effects of weak methylation signals in the denominator [20]. Due to potential imbalanced rates of hypermethylation and hypomethylation, the null distribution of M_j can be asymmetric

in some chromosomes. Thus, we adopted a one-sided test to separately evaluate the significance ($p < \alpha0$ after multiple testing correction) of hypermethylation or hypomethylation. To address the complex 'length'-dependent background rates, we exploited M_j score on flexible intervals, i.e., promoters, CpG islands, and CpG sites, to account for the potentially correlated effect by nearby CpG sites. We exploited the intrinsic correlation among nearby CpG sites and calculated and assigned an M-score to each methylation unit. Over the samples, we first merged nearby CpG sites into methylation intervals with flexible lengths, leaving the gaps of no/minimal CpG sites; then we divided each methylation interval into methylation units by the 'break points' of minimal correlation between CpG sites. Intuitively, a methylation unit contains a subset of highly correlated nearby CpG sites. In addition to permuting the promoter, CpG island, or CpG site, we permutated methylation units to account for different background rates of methylation units with varying lengths. Accordingly, we assessed the significance of length-specific methylation units, against the null hypothesis, similar to Algorithm 1 in Yuan et al. [24]. To address the biased null distribution problem, we iteratively detected significant methylation events and re-estimated an unbiased null distribution by an events-exclusive permutation scheme. This step improves the detection sensitivity Theorem 1 in Yuan et al. because conventional permutation schemes cannot distinguish between the contributions of sporadic methylations (obeying the null distribution) and true methylations (deviating from null distribution) to estimating null distributions, resulting in a theoretically conservative estimate [24].

Mammary gland development

Inguinal mammary glands (fourth pair, $n = 8$–9/group) were stretched onto a slide, placed in a fixative solution, and stained with a carmine aluminum solution (Sigma Chemical Co.) as previously described [26]. Whole mounts were examined under the microscope and ductal elongation and number of terminal end buds (TEBs; undifferentiated structure considered to be the targets of malignant transformation), as previously described [26]. In addition, whole-mount images were analyzed using the ImageJ software (National Institute of Health, Bethesda, MD, USA). The area and integrated density of a manually drawn perimeter around the mammary epithelial tree of each whole-mount were measured. The average area as well as integrated density measurements are reported for each group. Differences were statistically tested using a t test (or corresponding nonparametric test).

Mammary tumorigenesis

Mammary tumors were induced in female mice offspring ($n = 29$–32/group) by administration of medroxyprogesterone acetate (MPA; 15 mg, subcutaneously) at 6 weeks of age, followed by three weekly doses of 1 mg 7,12-dimethylbenz[a]anthracene (DMBA; Sigma, St. Louis, MO) dissolved in peanut oil by oral gavage. This established model of breast cancer has been used by us and others [5, 27]. Mice were examined for mammary tumors by palpation once per week, starting at week 2 after the last dose of DMBA and continue for a total of 20 weeks. Tumor growth was measured using a caliper, and the width and height of each tumor were recorded. The endpoints for data analysis were: i) latency to tumor appearance; ii) the number of animals with tumors (tumor incidence); and iii) the number of tumors per animal (tumor multiplicity). During follow-up, those animals in which tumor burden approximated 10% of total bodyweight were sacrificed, as required by our institution. Histopathology of tumors was evaluated commercially by Animal Reference Pathology (Salt Lake City, Utah). Differences in tumor latency and multiplicity were analyzed by a t test (or corresponding nonparametric test). Kaplan-Meier survival curves were used to compare differences in tumor incidence, followed by the log-rank test. Tumor growth was analyzed using two-way ANOVA (group and time), with Sidak's multi-comparison test used for post-hoc analyses.

Analysis of cell proliferation

Cell proliferation was evaluated in PND50 inguinal mammary glands (fourth pair, $n = 6$/group) and mammary tumors ($n = 6$/group) by Ki-67 immunohistochemistry. Briefly, tissues were fixed in 10% buffered formalin, embedded in paraffin, and sectioned (5 μm). Sections were deparaffinized with xylene and rehydrated through a graded alcohol series. Antigen retrieval was performed by immersing the tissue sections at 98 °C for 40 min in 1× Diva Decloaker (Biocare). Tissue sections were treated with 3% hydrogen peroxide and 10% normal goat serum for 10 min, and were incubated with the primary antibody (Additional file 1: Table S3) overnight at 4 °C. After several washes, sections were treated to the appropriate horseradish peroxidase (HRP)-labeled polymer for 30 min and DAB chromagen (Dako) for 5 min. Slides were counterstained with hematoxylin (Fisher, Harris Modified Hematoxylin), blued in 1% ammonium hydroxide, dehydrated, and mounted with Acrymount. The sections were photographed using an Olympus IX-71 Inverted Epifluorescence microscope at 20× magnification. The proliferation index was determined by calculating the percentage of Ki67-positive cells among 1000 cells per slides. Images were evaluated with ImageJ software (National Institute of Health, Bethesda, MD, USA). Results were analyzed by t test (or corresponding nonparametric test).

Analysis of cell apoptosis

Cell apoptosis analysis was conducted in PND50 inguinal mammary glands (fourth pair, $n = 7$–9/group) and mammary tumors ($n = 10$/group) by morphological detection. Tissues were fixed in neutral-buffered 10% formalin and stained with hematoxylin and eosin (H&E). Cells presenting loss of adhesion between adjacent cells, cytoplasmic condensation, and formation of apoptotic bodies were considered apoptotic. The sections were photographed using a Nikon E600 Epifluorescence microscope at 100× magnification. The apoptotic index was determined by the percentage of apoptotic bodies among 1000 cells per slide. Images were evaluated with ImageJ software (NIH, USA). Results were analyzed by t test (or corresponding nonparametric test).

Analysis of protein levels in LP and control offspring mammary tissues and mammary tumors

Protein levels were assessed by Western blot in mammary tissues ($n = 4$–7/group) and tumors obtained from LP or control female offspring ($n = 5$/group). Total protein was extracted from mammary tissues using RIPA buffer with Halt™ Protease Inhibitor Cocktail (Thermo Fisher). Protein extracts (10 μg) were resolved on a 4–12% denaturing polyacrylamide gel (SDS-PAGE). Proteins were transferred using the iBlot® 7-Minute Blotting System (Invitrogen, USA) and blocked with 5% nonfat dry milk for 1 h at room temperature. Membranes were incubated with the specific primary antibodies (for antibody specifications and dilutions, see Additional file 1: Table S3) at 4 °C overnight. After several washes, the membranes were incubated with HRP-conjugated secondary antibody at room temperature for 1 h. Membranes were developed using the Chemiluminescent HRP antibody detection reagent (Denville Scientific Inc., USA), and exposed to blot imaging systems (Amersham™ Imager 600, GE Healthcare Life Sciences). Optical density of the bands was quantified using Quantity-one software (BIO-RAD, USA). To control for equal protein loading, expression of the proteins of interest was normalized to the β-actin or β-tubulin signal.

Amino-acid analysis in LP and control offspring mammary tissues and mammary tumors

Tumor amino acid levels were measured using liquid chromatography/mass spectrometry (LC/MS; $n = 6$/group). Briefly, tissues were kept on ice for thawing before the extraction procedure. At total of 200 μL methanol was added prior to homogenization and 10 μl of the internal standard was added to these vials; 10 μL of calibrant standards and QC solution was then added to the respective vials. The derivatizing reagent was prepared by mixing 950 μL of water, ethanol, and pyridine along with 150 μL of phenyl isothiocyanate; 50 μL of this mixture was then added to the vials and left at room temperature for 20 min. The excess liquid was removed from the vials by drying under nitrogen for 60 min and 300 μL of 5 mM ammonium acetate in

methanol was added to the vials and kept on the shaker for 15 min. The vials were centrifuged at 13,000 rpm for 10 min at 4 °C and the supernatant transferred to mass spectrometry vials. Then 5 μL of the samples were injected onto a Waters Acquity UPLC- Xevo TQ-S system (Waters Corporation, Milford, USA). Levels of glutamine were validated in tumors ($n = 5$/group) and measured in normal mammary tissue ($n = 5$–7/group) and plasma ($n = 5$–6/group) using a colorimetric assay kit (BioVision, CA). Levels of glutamate were measured in tumors, mammary tissue, and plasma using a colorimetric assay kit (BioVision, USA). For both assays, samples were diluted in assay buffer and placed into a 96-well plate and the protocol provided by the manufacturer was then followed. Absorbance was measured at 450 nm. The concentrations of glutamine and glutamate were calculated according to their respective standard curves. LC/MS results were statistically analyzed using two-way ANOVA (group and amino-acid type), with Sidak's multicomparison test used for post-hoc analyses. Colorimetric assay results were analyzed using two-way ANOVA (group and tissue type), with Tukey's test used for post-hoc analyses.

TCGA analysis

The Cancer Genome Atlas (TCGA) database (http://cancergenome.nih.gov/) is classified by data type and data level to allow structured access to this resource with appropriate patient privacy protection. In this study, level 3 normalized gene level miRNA and mRNA next-generation sequencing data and corresponding demographic and clinical information for 1098 breast cancer patients were obtained from TCGA. Statistical analysis was conducted using DESeq2 package in R. Two kinds of comparison were made: one based on race/ethnicity, the other based on estrogen receptor (ER), progesterone receptor (PR), and human epidermal growth factor receptor (HER)2 status.

Results
Low protein consumption has no effect on paternal bodyweight but alters sperm epigenetic profile

Male mice (c57bl/6) consumed either a control or low-protein (LP) diet from 3 to 10 weeks of age (experimental design; Additional file 1: Figure S1). No difference in bodyweight gain was observed in males consuming a LP diet compared with controls ($P = 0.99$; Additional file 1: Figure S3a).

We and others have shown that the male germline can be epigenetically reprogrammed due to lifestyle and environmental exposures [2, 3, 5, 6, 9, 28]. Thus, we performed RNA-seq and MBD-seq analyses to assess small RNA and DNA methylation patterns, respectively, in mature sperm of control and LP males. Compared with controls, sperm from LP males showed several differentially methylated genes (promoter and exon1 regions).

Of these, 14 were hypomethylated and 10 were hypermethylated (Additional file 1: Figure S3b).

The two groups had similar abundance and distribution of the major small RNA species. In agreement with previous reports [7, 29], tRFs were the most abundant sperm small RNA subtype, followed by miRNAs and piRNAs (Additional file 1: Figure S3c, d and Table S4). A total of 16 miRNAs were differentially expressed, with eight down- and eight up-regulated, in sperm of LP mice compared with controls (Additional file 1: Figure S3e). In addition, a significant increase was observed in the expression of tRF5-Ile-TAT, tRF5-Arg-ACG, and tRF5-SeC-TCA, while tRF5-Pro-AGG and tRF5-Ser-CGA were significantly decreased in LP sperm compared with controls (Additional file 1: Figure S3f).

LP female offspring have decreased birthweight and increased breast cancer risk

Next, we examined the offspring of control or LP male mice mated with female mice reared on the control diet.

No differences in gender distribution were observed between litters from control and LP fathers (Additional file 1: Figure S4). Paternal LP consumption was associated with decreased birthweight of female ($P = 0.035$; Fig. 1a) but not male offspring ($P = 0.45$, data not shown). The decrease in the bodyweight of female offspring persisted through the prepubertal period when LP offspring began to gain more weight than controls animals, with LP females being slightly but significantly heavier over a 24-week monitoring period ($P < 0.0001$; Fig. 1b) compared with controls.

Low birthweight has been associated with higher risk for breast cancer in humans [11, 13] and animal models [30]. Thus, we studied the mammary cancer risk in control and LP daughters using a well-established [5, 27] carcinogen-induced mouse model of breast cancer. Tumor latency was significantly shorter in LP daughters compared with controls ($P = 0.029$; Fig. 1c). The incidence of palpable mammary tumors in the LP female mice was higher than in controls but did not reach statistical significance ($P = 0.1$;

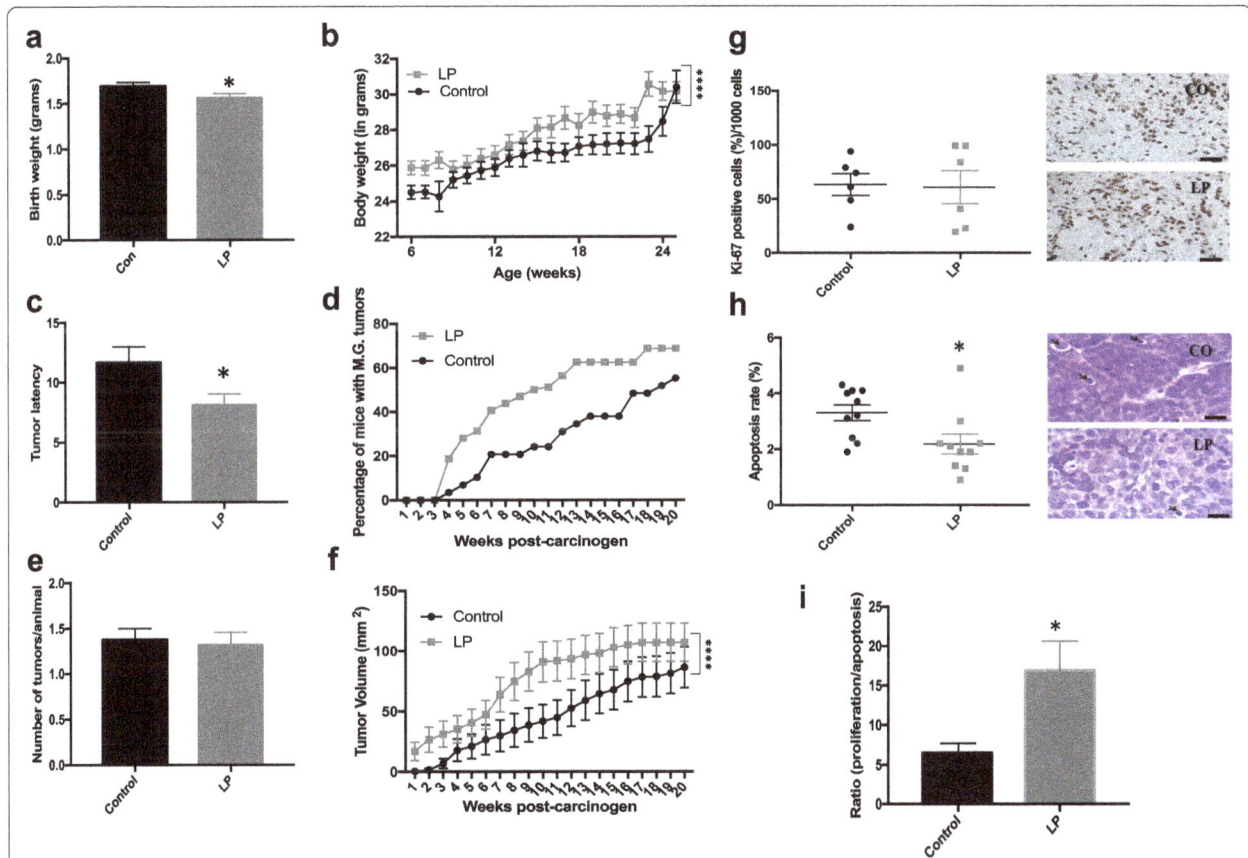

Fig. 1 Paternal low-protein (LP) diet modulates birthweight and breast cancer risk in female offspring. Body weight (mean ± SEM) of LP female offspring **a** at birth and **b** longitudinally. **c** Mammary tumor latency (mean ± SEM), **d** mammary tumor incidence, **e** mammary tumor multiplicity (mean ± SEM), and **f** mammary tumor growth (mean ± SEM) in control (Con) and LP female offspring ($n = 29–32$/group). **g** Proliferation staining (Ki-67) quantification (percentage/1000 cells) with representative control and LP mammary tumor sections (20× magnification, mean ± SEM, $n = 6$/group), **h** morphological quantification (percentage/1000 cells) of apoptotic cells with representative control and LP mammary tumor sections (100× magnification, mean ± SEM, $n = 10$/group), and **i** proliferation/apoptosis ratio in control and LP mammary tumors. Significant differences versus the control group were determined as follows: t test (birthweight, tumor multiplicity and latency, cell proliferation, and apoptosis), log-rank test (tumor incidence), and two-way ANOVA (longitudinal bodyweight and tumor growth). *$P < 0.05$, ****$P < 0.0001$. Scale bars = 20 μm (**g,h**)

Fig. 1d). Tumor multiplicity was not different between the groups ($P = 0.77$; Fig. 1e). However, tumor growth was significantly increased in LP daughters at several time points ($P < 0.0001$; Fig. 1f). All mammary tumors included in our analyses were classified as mammary carcinomas by a pathologist.

Because we observed decreased mammary tumor latency and increased tumor growth in the LP offspring, we assessed cell proliferation and apoptosis rates in their tumors. We did not find differences in rates of cell proliferation ($P = 0.89$; Fig. 1g) between the groups, but detected a significant decrease in apoptosis ($P = 0.023$; Fig. 1h) in mammary tumors of LP offspring compared with controls. Consequently, the proliferation/apoptosis ratio was increased in LP tumors compared with controls ($P = 0.018$; Fig. 1i).

Mammary gland development and epigenome of LP daughters are altered

Given that the LP offspring had increased breast cancer risk, we then analyzed the effects of paternal suboptimal nutrition on their mammary development. We used postnatal day (PND)50 inguinal mammary glands to assess number of TEBs, ductal elongation, and epithelial area/

density. Neither the number of TEBs ($P = 0.96$) nor the bodyweight-adjusted mammary ductal elongation ($P = 0.97$) was different between the groups. However, both total mammary epithelial area and epithelial density ($P = 0.02$ and $P = 0.001$, respectively; Fig. 2a, b) were significantly higher in LP offspring compared with controls.

Because we observed an increase in epithelial area as well as density in the mammary tissue of LP offspring, we tested whether this phenotype was due to a change in the balance between cell proliferation and apoptosis. Our analyses revealed that normal mammary tissue from LP offspring had lower rates of both proliferation (ki67 staining, $P = 0.02$; Fig. 2c) and apoptosis (morphologic assessment, $P = 0.05$; Fig. 2d) compared with controls. Although it was lower in LP mammary tissue, there were no statistically significant differences in the ratio of mammary proliferation/apoptosis between the groups ($P = 0.13$; Fig. 2e).

It has been shown that ancestral paternal exposures are associated with epigenetic alterations in offspring [5, 9, 31]. Our genome-wide methylation analyses revealed few changes in mammary DNA methylation patterns in the promoter/exon 1 regions (Fig. 3a). Furthermore, we were unable to detect any meaningful changes in expression levels of the differentially methylated genes or in DNA

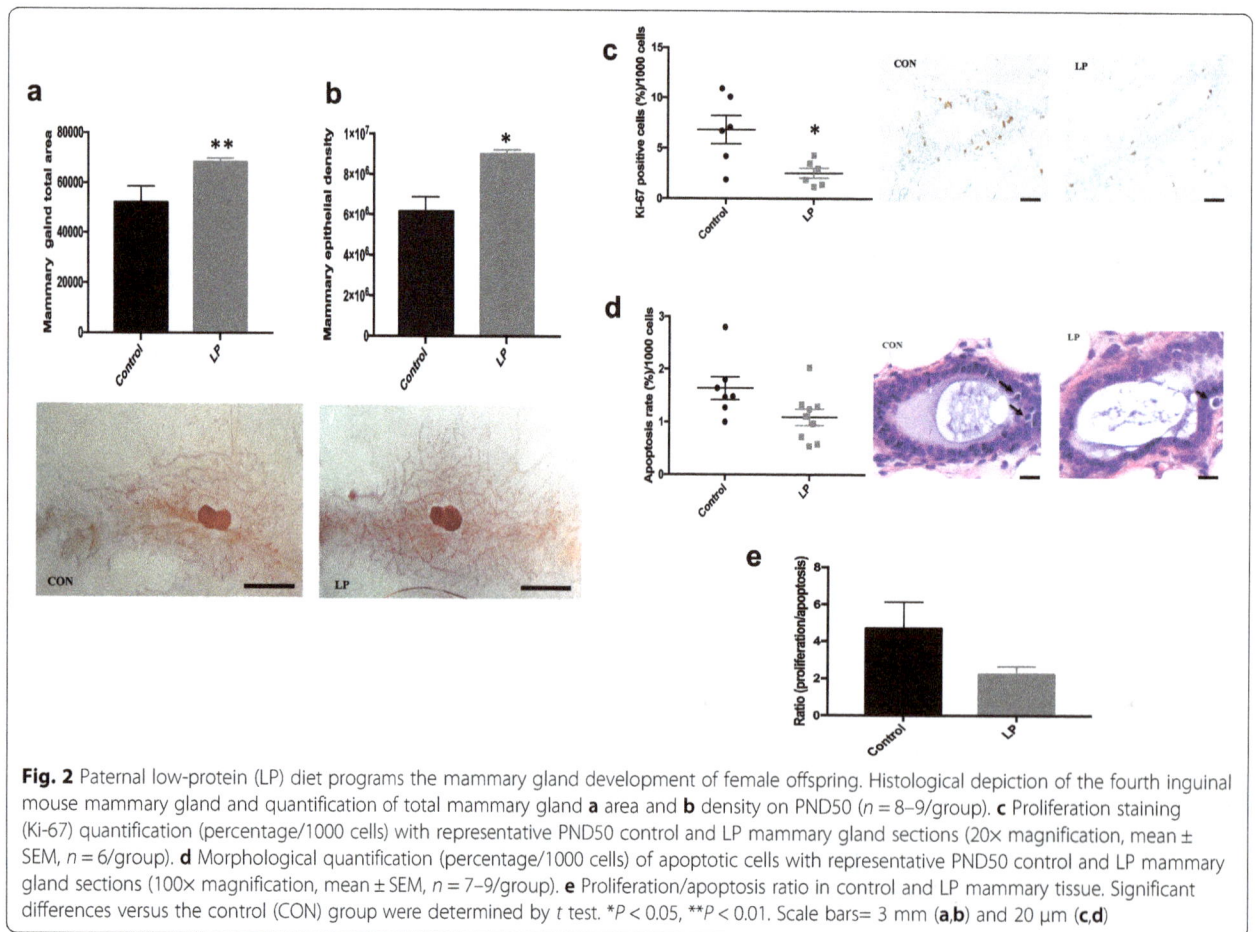

Fig. 2 Paternal low-protein (LP) diet programs the mammary gland development of female offspring. Histological depiction of the fourth inguinal mouse mammary gland and quantification of total mammary gland **a** area and **b** density on PND50 ($n = 8$–9/group). **c** Proliferation staining (Ki-67) quantification (percentage/1000 cells) with representative PND50 control and LP mammary gland sections (20× magnification, mean ± SEM, $n = 6$/group). **d** Morphological quantification (percentage/1000 cells) of apoptotic cells with representative PND50 control and LP mammary gland sections (100× magnification, mean ± SEM, $n = 7$–9/group). **e** Proliferation/apoptosis ratio in control and LP mammary tissue. Significant differences versus the control (CON) group were determined by t test. *$P < 0.05$, **$P < 0.01$. Scale bars= 3 mm (**a,b**) and 20 μm (**c,d**)

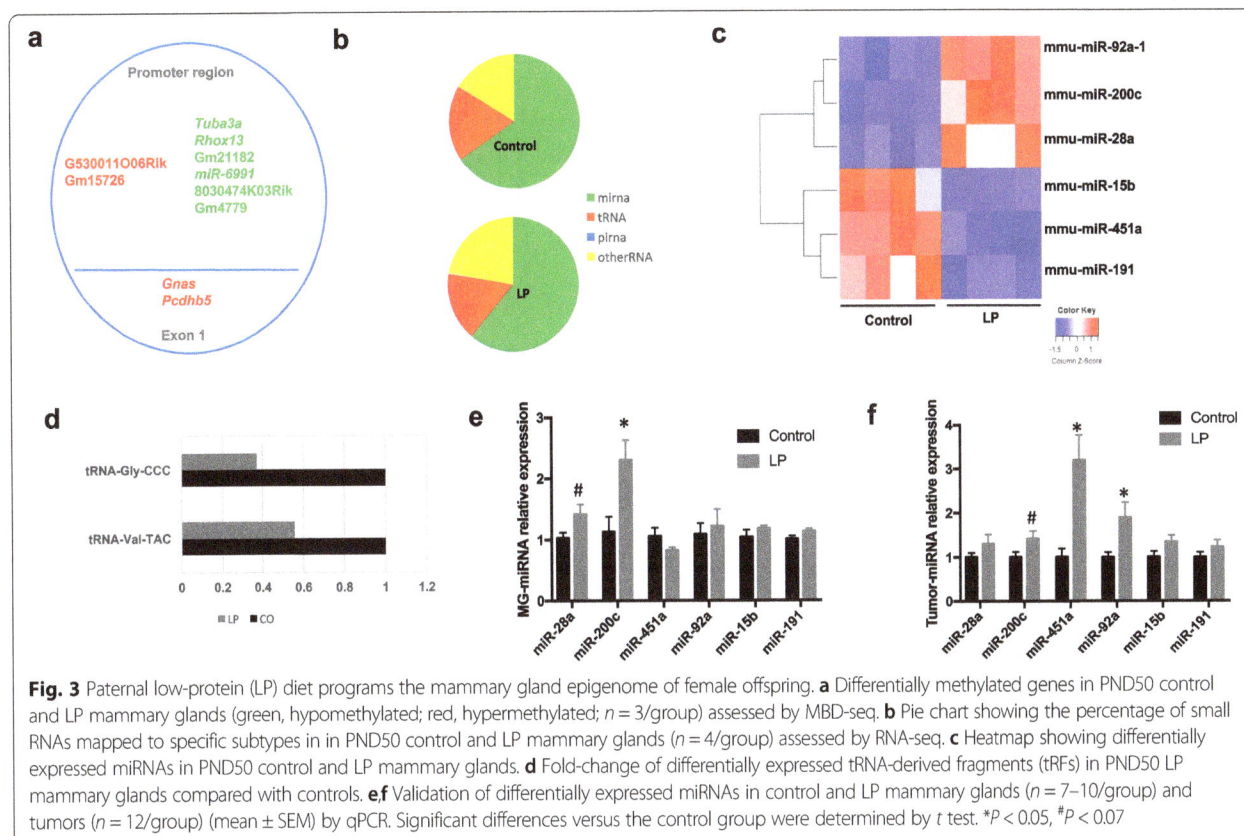

Fig. 3 Paternal low-protein (LP) diet programs the mammary gland epigenome of female offspring. **a** Differentially methylated genes in PND50 control and LP mammary glands (green, hypomethylated; red, hypermethylated; *n* = 3/group) assessed by MBD-seq. **b** Pie chart showing the percentage of small RNAs mapped to specific subtypes in in PND50 control and LP mammary glands (*n* = 4/group) assessed by RNA-seq. **c** Heatmap showing differentially expressed miRNAs in PND50 control and LP mammary glands. **d** Fold-change of differentially expressed tRNA-derived fragments (tRFs) in PND50 LP mammary glands compared with controls. **e,f** Validation of differentially expressed miRNAs in control and LP mammary glands (*n* = 7–10/group) and tumors (*n* = 12/group) (mean ± SEM) by qPCR. Significant differences versus the control group were determined by *t* test. *P* < 0.05, #*P* < 0.07

methyltransferase genes using qPCR (Additional file 1: Table S5). However, using RNA-seq analyses, we found differences in the noncoding small RNA content between control and LP mammary glands. This analysis showed that the majority of small noncoding RNAs in mammary tissue were miRNAs, followed by tRFs, and other small RNA subtypes (Fig. 3b). A total of six miRNAs (upregulated: miR-28a, miR-92a, miR-200c; downregulated: miR-451a, miR-191, miR-15b) and two tRFs (downregulated: tRF5-Gly-CCC, tRF5-Val-TAC) were differentially expressed in mammary tissues of LP offspring compared with controls (Fig. 3c, d and Additional file 1: Table S4).

Given that miRNAs were the most abundant small RNA biotype in mammary tissue and, given their reported role in breast cancer [32], we focused on these molecules and downstream pathways for the remaining experiments. Validation of miRNAs by qPCR showed patterns of expression similar to those detected by RNA-seq in LP mammary tissues, with two exceptions: miR-191 and miR-15b. However, borderline or significant differences were only found for miR-28a (*P* = 0.06) and miR-200c (*P* = 0.01) (Fig. 3e).

In LP mammary tumors, miR-451a levels had a threefold increase compared with controls (*P* = 0.002). This increase was in contrast with normal LP mammary tissue where its levels were reduced. Both mir-92a1 (*P* = 0.02) and mir-200c (*P* = 0.07) also had higher expression in LP

mammary tumors than in controls (Fig. 3f). miRNA expression can be regulated by DNA methylation [33]; however, integration of the genome-wide DNA methylation and RNA-seq data in control and LP normal mammary tissues did not reveal any statistically significant changes in DNA methylation patterns in promoter regions of differentially expressed miRNAs.

Mammary tissues and tumors of LP daughters show altered amino-acid metabolism

Low birthweight and protein restriction have been shown to affect amino acid availability and metabolism [34–36]. Accordingly, a gene set enrichment analysis using the predicted target genes of the differentially expressed miRNAs showed that the top associated bio-function is amino-acid metabolism. A complete list of functions uncovered in our analyses is shown in Additional file 1 (Table S6).

Using a LC/MS analysis, we found that total free amino acid levels were significantly lower in LP tumors compared with controls (*P* < 0.0001). This reduction was mainly due to two amino acids, glutamine and alanine, which were significantly lower in LP tumors compared with controls (*P* < 0.05; Fig. 4a). Glutamine is one of the most abundant amino acids in the circulation and in cancer cells is known to be metabolized as a source of energy [37, 38]. Using a colorimetric assay, we further

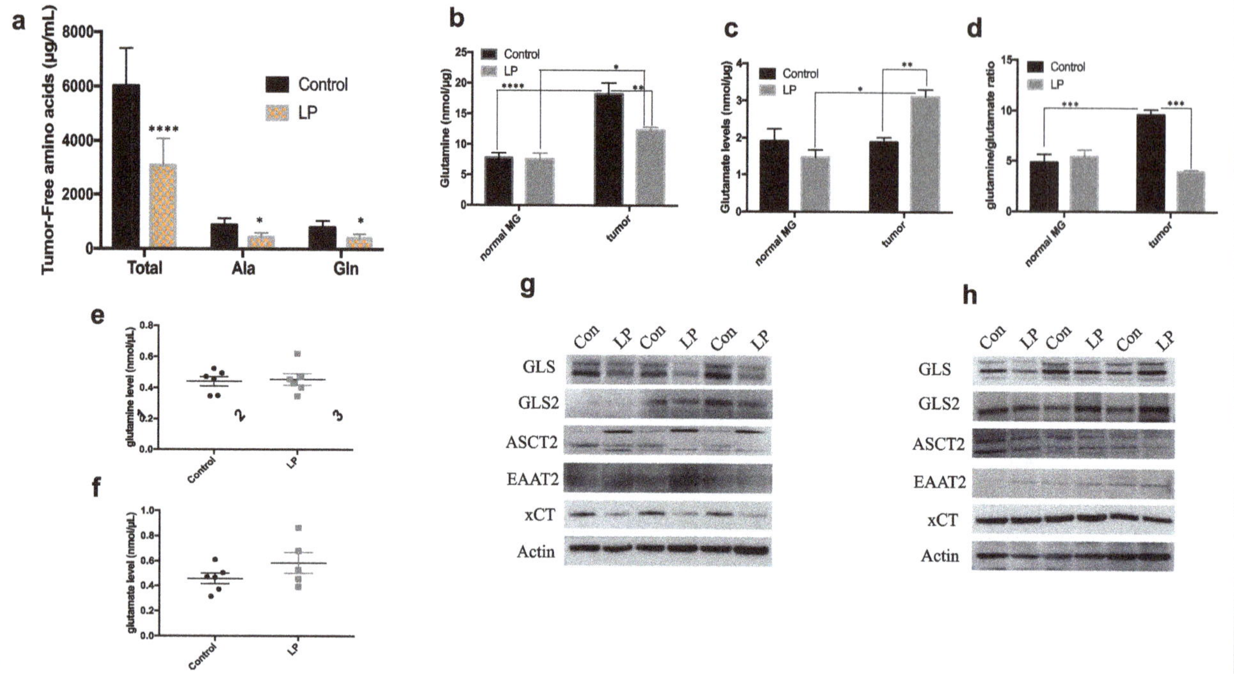

Fig. 4 Amino acid metabolism is altered in low-protein (LP) diet mammary tissues and tumors. **a** Levels of free amino acids (total, alanine (Ala), and glutamine (Gln)) in control and LP tumors assessed by LC/MS (mean ± SEM; $n = 6$/group). **b–f** Levels of glutamine and glutamate in control and LP mammary glands and tumors (**b-d**), and in circulation (**e-f**) assessed by a colorimetric assay (mean ± SEM; $n = 5$–7/group). **g, h** Representative Western blots for GLS, GLS2, ASCT2, EEAT2, and xCT on PND50 control (Con) and LP mammary tissues (**g**) ($n = 4$–7/group) and tumors (**h**) ($n = 5$/group). Protein levels were normalized by β-actin. Significant differences versus the control group were determined as follows: two-way ANOVA (total amino acid levels, glutamine/glutamate in normal mammary tissue and tumors) and t test (glutamine/glutamate circulation). $*P < 0.05$, $**P < 0.01$$***P < 0.001$, $****P < 0.0001$

confirmed levels of glutamine and its metabolite, glutamate, using cell lysates from tumors. We found that glutamine levels were significantly lower and glutamate levels significantly higher, respectively, in LP tumors ($P = 0.01$ and $P < 0.001$) compared with controls. An assessment of glutamine and glutamate in LP mammary tissue lysates and plasma showed that levels of these amino acids were unchanged compared with controls. Interestingly, intratumor levels of glutamine were higher regardless of group while intratumor levels of glutamate were only in higher in the LP group compared with normal mammary glands (Fig. 4b–f).

Glutamine is metabolized to glutamate by glutaminases (GLS and GLS-2) and are carried in and out of the cell through several transporters [37, 39]. We therefore assessed the expression of these proteins using Western blot. Surprisingly, we found that levels of GLS were decreased while GLS-2 levels were unchanged in both LP mammary tissue and tumors in comparison with controls. We also found that levels of the glutamate transporter EEAT2 were unchanged in LP mammary gland and LP tumors. However, the glycosylated form of the glutamine transporter, ASCT2, was higher in LP mammary tissue, but not in LP tumors compared with controls. Levels of the glutamate-cystine antiporter xCT (Slc7a11) were decreased in LP mammary tissue. Compared with normal mammary tissue, LP tumors had increased expression of xCT, but not compared with control tumors (Fig. 4g, h).

Mammary tissues and tumors of LP daughters have rewired nutrient-sensing mechanism

MicroRNAs 451a, 92a1, and 200c also regulate genes involved in other nutrient and energy sensing pathways. Both miR-451a and miR-200c are predicted or experimentally shown [40] to target *Cab39* mRNA, a component of the LKB1 complex which phosphorylates and activates AMPK. Furthermore, miR-92a is predicted to directly target the AMPK catalytic alpha subunit mRNA *Prkaa2*. Accordingly, we found that CAB39 expression was downregulated in LP tumors. We also found that both the expression and phosphorylation of AMPK was decreased in those tumors. In line with this, the levels of mammalian target of rapamycin (mTOR) activity and its downstream target S6 kinase were increased in LP mammary tumors. Interestingly, similar patterns of expression were detected LP mammary tissue, with reduction of CAB39 and AMPK levels compared with controls. While no increase in activity of mTOR or S6 kinase were observed in LP normal mammary tissues, an increase in 4E-BP1 phosphorylation was noted (Fig. 5).

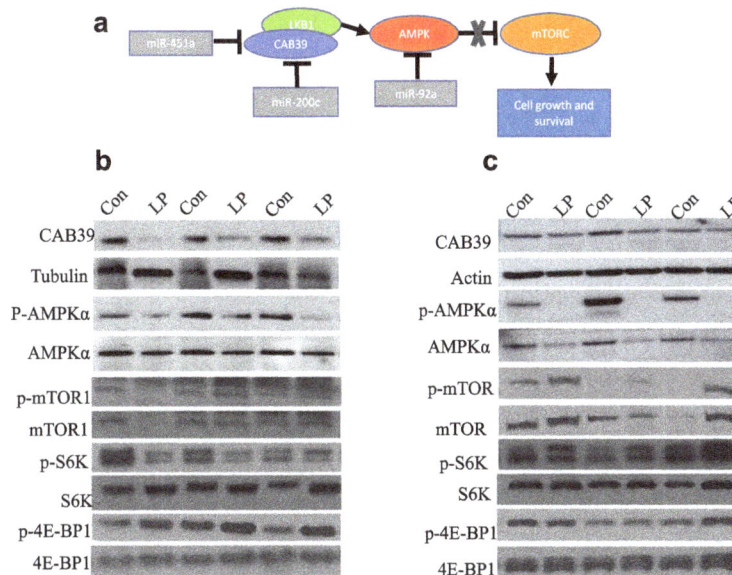

Fig. 5 The AMPK signaling pathway is suppressed in low-protein (LP) diet mammary tissues and tumors. **a** Schematic representation of the interaction between miR-200c, miR-451a, and miR-92a1 with members of the AMP-activated protein kinase (AMPK) pathway. **b,c** Representative Western blots for CAB39, phospho-AMPK, AMPK, phospho-mTOR1, and mTOR1 on PND50 control (Con) and LP mammary tissues (**b**) ($n = 4$–7/ group) and tumors (**c**) ($n = 5$/group). CAB39 protein levels were normalized by β-actin or β-tubulin. Phosphorylated proteins were normalized using the respective total protein levels

The expression of miRNAs and target genes altered in LP tumors differ by race/ethnicity and ER/PR/HER2 status in human breast tumors

Low birthweight is prevalent in minority populations, with the highest rates observed in African-Americans [41], a group that is also afflicted with more aggressive breast cancers [42]. With that in mind, we asked whether the miRNAs (451a, 92a1, and 200c) differentially expressed in LP tumors varied by race/ethnicity and tumor subtype in humans. Using the TCGA database, we found that breast cancers in African-Americans have significantly higher expression of both miR-92a1 ($P = 1.464 \times 10^{-10}$) and miR-200c ($P = 5.986 \times 10^{-8}$), but not miR-451a, compared with whites. Furthermore, the expression of both *Cab39* ($P = 2.734 \times 10^{-14}$) and *Prkaa2* (AMPK catalytic alpha subunit; $P = 1.442 \times 10^{-7}$) is lower in breast tumors of African-Americans compared with whites. We also found that miR-92a1 expression is upregulated ($P = 1.328 \times 10^{-6}$) while the expression of its target gene, *Prkaa2*, is downregulated ($P = 0.0053$) in triple-negative breast cancers compared with triple-positive breast tumors (Fig. 6).

Discussion

Using a mouse model, we found that paternal malnutrition (low-protein intake) led to reduced birthweight, alterations in mammary development, and increased mammary cancer risk in their female offspring. This phenotype was associated with differential expression of

miRNAs (miR-200c, miR-92a, and miR-451a) known to regulate the AMPK energy-sensing pathway. Furthermore, we showed that the increase in mammary cancer risk in LP female offspring is associated with amino acid metabolism alterations, particularly with an increase in the energy-generating substrate glutamate.

Reports in the literature show that maternal protein restriction in gestation and lactation are associated with decreased birthweight, catch-up growth, and increased breast cancer risk in offspring [30]. We found similar results stemming from preconception paternal protein restriction. These, as well as our previously published findings, suggest that paternal exposures may be as important as maternal ones regarding determination of birthweight and cancer risk in offspring. As noted by others [43], there is a remarkable overlap between maternal and paternal exposure effects on offspring phenotypes, and our findings support this notion.

Epidemiologic studies have consistently shown that both high and low birthweight increases a woman's breast cancer risk [11–13]. It is often assumed in those studies that birthweight is determined by maternal factors in pregnancy. Our data suggest that birthweight associated with paternal diet can also modulate breast cancer risk in offspring. Population studies have not directly investigated the link between paternal malnutrition and breast cancer, but indirect evidence exists. An analysis using the Dutch Famine Cohort has shown that women who were conceived during a famine, but not

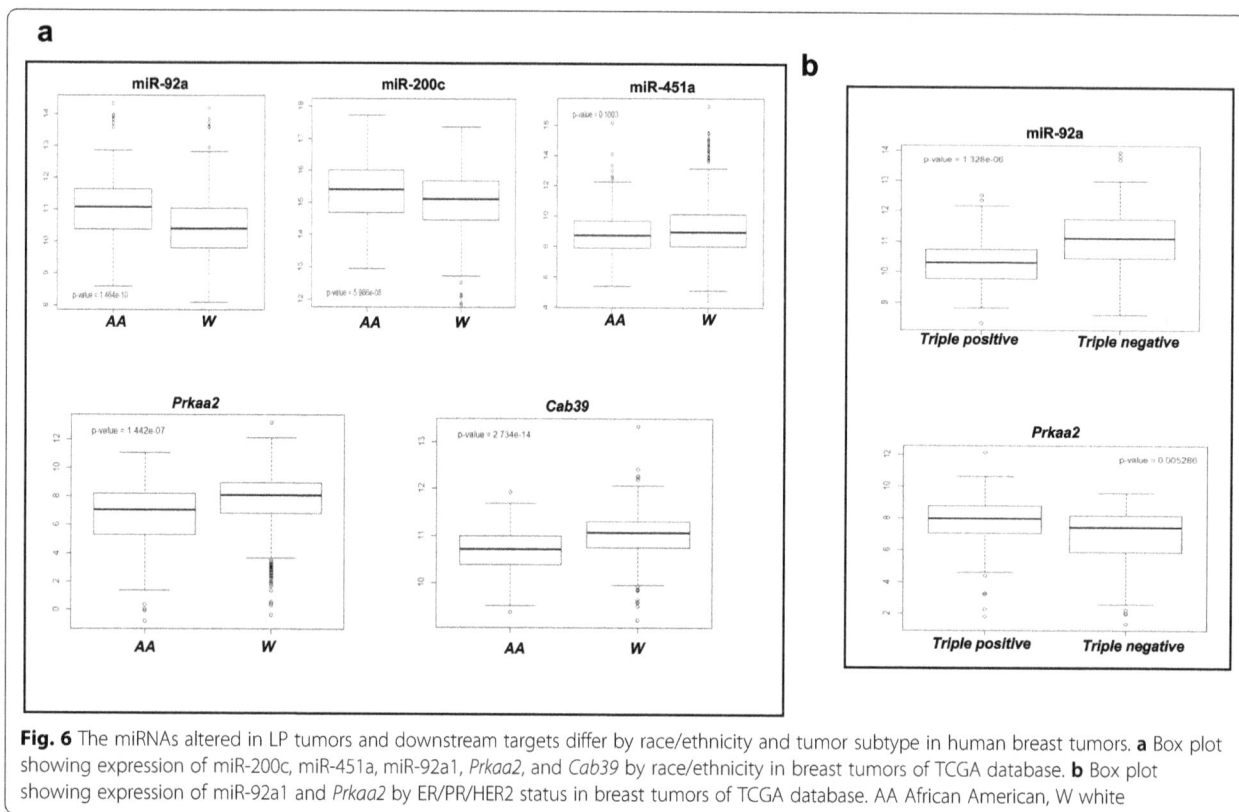

Fig. 6 The miRNAs altered in LP tumors and downstream targets differ by race/ethnicity and tumor subtype in human breast tumors. **a** Box plot showing expression of miR-200c, miR-451a, miR-92a1, *Prkaa2*, and *Cab39* by race/ethnicity in breast tumors of TCGA database. **b** Box plot showing expression of miR-92a1 and *Prkaa2* by ER/PR/HER2 status in breast tumors of TCGA database. AA African American, W white

those exposed in later gestation, have increased breast cancer risk [18]. Furthermore, the association between other paternal environmental exposures and cancer risk in the offspring has been examined. For instance, paternal ethnicity and paternal age have been linked to the risk of breast cancer and hematological malignancies in their children [15, 16, 44]. In animal models, paternal overweight increases breast cancer risk in offspring [5]. Paternal dietary intake also modulates cancer risk, with both micronutrient deficiency and high saturated fat consumption increasing breast cancer risk in offspring [6, 45]. In addition to cancer risk, studies suggest that paternal exposures affect other diseases in the offspring, and sometimes grand-offspring, in both animals and humans [2, 9, 31, 46, 47].

Although we detected epigenetic changes (noncoding RNAs, DNA methylation) in LP male sperm, we did not directly investigate the mechanisms by which ancestral undernutrition information is transmitted to the offspring and modulates their cancer risk. However, recent published studies may offer some clues. Watkins and colleagues [4] report that paternal protein restriction is associated with reduced placental weight and alterations in placental nutrient transporters. Other studies suggest that sperm small noncoding RNAs can be delivered to the oocyte during fertilization and directly regulate gene expression in the developing embryo [7, 8]. Using zygote

microinjections, Rodgers and colleagues [2] showed that miRNAs altered by paternal stress recapitulate the off-spring stress phenotype in a mouse model. More recently, it was shown that tRFs, which are abundant in sperm, can also carry ancestral exposure memory from fathers to off-spring. Others found that acquired DNA methylations patterns can be transmitted from fathers to offspring [33].

The extent by which protein restriction-induced changes in the male germline influence mammary gland development in their female progeny is also currently unknown. Our data, however, suggest that ancestral paternal protein intake is associated with changes in adult offspring mammary tissue, making this organ more prone to cancer development. The underlying rewiring of metabolism and energy-sensing mechanisms in LP mammary tissue may be partly responsible for the increase in breast cancer risk. Whether other systemic alterations in LP daughters, in addition to local mammary tissue changes, are important in determining that phenotype needs to be further explored. Previous studies report [3, 31], however, that ancestral diet can lead to metabolic abnormalities in the offspring suggesting that systemic changes may also be important. Of particular interest are reports showing that plasma amino acid levels are altered in adults who had low birthweight compared with those with normal birthweight, particularly when challenged with a high-calorie diet [36].

MicroRNAs regulate mammary tissue development [48] and tumorigenesis [32] and can act as either tumor suppressors or as oncomiRs depending on their target genes [49]. While functional studies are needed, published reports [40, 50] support the notion that miRNAs differentially expressed in mammary tumors of LP daughters target the tumor suppressive and energy-sensing AMPK pathway resulting in sustained mTOR activity and cell growth. Other alterations in nutrient metabolism were observed in LP daughters. We found that their tumors have reduced levels of total free amino acids, particularly alanine and glutamine. However, while reduced in LP tumors, the levels of glutamine are still higher compared with normal mammary tissue. This suggests that more glutamine, and possibly other amino acids, are in a bound state in LP tumor cells due to increased protein translation and cell growth. LP tumors also produce large amounts of glutamate which infers that more glutamine is being metabolized to glutamate in those tumors. Surprisingly, the levels of glutaminases were reduced (GLS) or unchanged (GLS-2) in LP mammary tumors compared with controls. This, however, is in line with inhibition of GLS expression by excess glutamate as well as protein restriction [37, 51]. Oncogenic alterations can render cancer cells addicted to glutamine, with rapidly dividing cells avidly consuming this amino acid [37]. Glutamate generated from glutamine can enter the tricarboxylic acid (TCA) cycle to produce energy and to act as a source of carbon and nitrogen to support nucleotides, fatty acids, and amino acid biosynthesis [37, 38]. Increased glutamine uptake and metabolism can further activate the mTOR pathway [52]. Together, these metabolic alterations may contribute to the higher growth rates seen in LP tumors, likely allowing cancer cells to withstand nutrient fluctuations under harsh conditions.

Our study also suggests that breast cancer phenotypes could be determined by an individual's ancestral exposures. Our TCGA analysis and published findings [53] support this notion; breast tumors of women in ethnic groups with high rates of low birthweight show miRNAs and AMPK pathway alterations similar to those found in our animal model. Furthermore, it has been reported that more aggressive breast cancer subtypes such as triple-negative cancers are dependent on glutamine/glutamate metabolism and tend to have a low glutamine/glutamate ratio compared with ER-positive cancers [54]. Paternal protein restriction has been shown to perturb AMPK signaling in embryos, potentially as an adaptive mechanism to preserve viability [4]. Our study suggests that programming of the AMPK pathway and amino acid metabolism by ancestral LP diet persists through adulthood and, while it can be adaptive, it can also provide a growth advantage to transformed cells.

Conclusions

In summary, we report that preconception paternal protein restriction can influence the birthweight, mammary gland development, and breast cancer risk and metabolism of daughters. Our findings could have important implications if confirmed in humans. First, our data support the notion that the heritable aspect of cancer risk and phenotype go beyond genetic factors. It could also result from ancestral exposures and possibly be inherited through modifiers of gene expression such as noncoding RNAs that could modulate organ development. Whether the miRNAs identified in our study are functionally responsible for increasing breast cancer risk in LP daughters still remains to be determined. However, our data strongly suggest that they may play a role in regulating tumor metabolism. Our findings could also help explain differences in breast cancer phenotypes and outcomes given that aggressive breast cancers with poor prognosis have rewired glutamine metabolism, a trait displayed by LP tumors. Finally, our results indicate that the effects of malnutrition on cancer risk go past the directly exposed individual. In humans, malnutrition and low birthweight are more prevalent in minority populations [41, 55]. Breast cancers in those populations are often more aggressive and have poorer prognosis [42]. Ancestral dietary patterns and lifestyle likely play a role in determining the breast cancer risk and outcomes in minority and low-income women, and needs to be further investigated in epidemiologic studies.

Additional file

Additional file 1: Figure S1. Experimental design. a Male mice were fed the experimental diets (control or low protein (LP)) from 3 to 10 weeks of age. b Control and LP-fed males (F0) were mated to control-fed females to generate the offspring (F1) as shown. **Figure S2.** Representative results of *Actb* (a somatic cell marker) and *Smcp* (a sperm-specific marker) gene expression patterns by qRT-PCR in purified sperm samples after treatment with somatic cell lysis buffer. **Figure S3.** a Longitudinal bodyweight of males consuming a control or low-protein (LP) diet. b Diagram showing differentially methylated genes in control and LP paternal sperm assessed by MBD-seq. c Scatter plot showing small RNA abundance (counts per million) from control (x axis) and LP sperm (y axis) for different small RNA subtypes assessed by RNA-seq. d Pie chart showing the percentage of small RNAs mapped to specific subtypes in control and LP sperm. e Heatmap showing differentially expressed miRNAs in control and LP sperm. f Fold-change of differentially expressed tRFs in control and LP sperm. **Figure S4.** Gender-specific distribution in litters from LP and control fathers. **Table S1.** Composition of experimental diets. **Table S2.** Number of contributing fathers and female offspring per experiment. **Table S3.** List of antibodies used. **Table S4.** List of differentially expressed noncoding RNAs in LP fathers' sperm and LP daughters' mammary tissue. **Table S5.** Gene expression levels verified by qRT-PCR. **Table S6.** Biofunctions regulated by the microRNAs differentially expressed in LP daughters. (DOCX 1018 kb)

Acknowledgments
We thank the Lombardi Cancer Center Shared Resources (SR) for their assistance: Animal Model SR, Histopathology and Tissue SR, Microscopy and Imaging SR, Genomics and Epigenomics SR, and Metabolomics SR. We also thank Dr. Anni Warri for insightful comments and suggestions to the

manuscript. The results shown here are in part based upon data generated by the TCGA Research Network (http://cancergenome.nih.gov/).

Funding
This study was supported in part by the Prevent Cancer Foundation (Research grant #299045 to SdA), The American Cancer Society (Research Scholar Grant to SdA), the National Institutes of Health (1P30-CA51008; Lombardi Comprehensive Cancer Center Support Grant to L. Weiner). EJC was supported in part by the National Center for Advancing Translational Sciences of the National Institutes of Health under Award TL1TR001431.

Authors' contributions
SdA conceived the study, oversaw the research, and wrote the manuscript; RS and EJC supervised the animal work and tissue collection; RS performed molecular analysis and helped to write the manuscript; JC and HC processed tissues and helped perform molecular analysis; MIC and CB assisted with animal studies; LJ performed RNA-seq data and TCGA analysis; YF and ZC performed MBD-seq data analysis; YW oversaw data analysis. All authors read and approved the final manuscript.

Competing interests
The authors declare that they no competing interests.

Author details
[1]Department of Oncology, Lombardi Comprehensive Cancer Center, Georgetown University, 3970 Reservoir Road, NW, The Research Building, Room E410, Washington, DC 20057, USA. [2]The Bradley Department of Electrical and Computer Engineering, Virginia Polytechnic Institute and State University Research Center, Arlington, VA, USA.

References
1. Jirtle RL, Skinner MK. Environmental epigenomics and disease susceptibility. Nature Review Genetics. 2007;8(4):253–62.
2. Rodgers AB, Morgan CP, Leu NA, Bale TL. Transgenerational epigenetic programming via sperm microRNA recapitulates effects of paternal stress. Proc Natl Acad Sci U S A. 2015;112(44):13699–704.
3. Caronne BRFL, Habib N, Shea JM, Hart CE, Li R, Bock C, Li C, Gu H, Zamore PD, Meissner A, Weng Z, Hofmann HA, Friedman N, Rando OJ. Paternally induced transgenerational environment reprogramming of metabolic gene expression in mammals. Cell. 2010;143(7):1084–96.
4. Watkins AJSS, Stokes B, Isaacs M, Addison O, Martin RA. Paternal low protein diet programs preimplantation embryo gene expression, fetal growth and skeletal development in mice. Biochimica et Biophysica Acta. 2017;1863(6):1371–81.
5. Fontelles CC, Carney E, Clarke J, Nguyen NM, Yin C, Jin L, Cruz MI, Ong TP, Hilakivi-Clarke L, de Assis S. Paternal overweight is associated with increased breast cancer risk in daughters in a mouse model. Sci Rep. 2016;6:28602.
6. Fontelles CC, Guido LN, Rosim MP, Andrade Fde O, Jin L, Inchauspe J, Pires VC, de Castro IA, Hilakivi-Clarke L, de Assis S, et al. Paternal programming of breast cancer risk in daughters in a rat model: opposing effects of animal- and plant-based high-fat diets. Breast Cancer Res. 2016;18(1):71.
7. Sharma UCC, Shea JM, Boskovic A, Derr AG, Bing XY, Belleannee C, Kucukural A, Serra RW, Sun F, Song L, Caronne BR, Ricci EP, Li XZ, Fauquier L, Moore MJ, Sullivan R, Mello CC, Garber M, Rando OJ. Biogenesis and function of tRNA fragments during sperm maturation and fertilization in mammals. Science. 2016;351(6271):391–6.
8. Chen QYW, Duan W. Epigenetic inheritance of acquired traits through sperm RNAs and sperm RNA modifications. Nat Rev Genet. 2016;17(12):733–43.
9. Gapp KJA, Sarkies P, Bohacek J, Pelzcar P, Prados J, Farinelli L, Miska E, Mansuy IM. Implication of sperm RNAs in transgenerational inheritance of the effects of early trauma in mice. Nat Neurosci. 2014;17(5):667–9.
10. de Assis S, Khan G, Hilakivi-Clarke L. High birth weight increases mammary tumorigenesis in rats. Int J Cancer. 2006;119(7):1537–46.
11. Mellemkjaer LOM, Sørensen HT, Thulstrup AM, Olsen J, Olsen JH. Birth weight and risk of early-onset breast cancer (Denmark). Cancer Causes Control. 2003;14(1):61–4.
12. Michels KBTD, Robins JM, Rosner BA, Manson JE, Hunter D, Colditz GA, Hankinson SE, Speizer FE, Willett WC. Birthweight as a risk factor for breast cancer. Lancet. 1996;348(9041):1542–6.
13. Sanderson M, Williams MA, Malone KE, Stanford JL, Emanuel I, White E, Daling JR. Perinatal factors and risk of breast cancer. Epidemiology. 1996;7(1):34–7.
14. Griffiths LJDC, Cole TJ. Differential paternal weight and height contributions to offspring birthweight and weight gain in infancy. Int J Epidemiol. 2007;36(1):104–7.
15. Choi JY, Lee KM, Park SK, Noh DY, Ahn SH, Yoo KY, Kang D. Association of paternal age at birth and the risk of breast cancer in offspring: a case control study. BMC Cancer. 2005;5:143.
16. Weiss-Salz I, Harlap S, Friedlander Y, Kaduri L, Levy-Lahad E, Yanetz R, Deutsch L, Hochner H, Paltiel O. Ethnic ancestry and increased paternal age are risk factors for breast cancer before the age of 40 years. Eur J Cancer Prev. 2007;16(6):549–54.
17. Ji BT, Shu XO, Linet MS, Zheng W, Wacholder S, Gao YT, Ying DM, Jin F. Paternal cigarette smoking and the risk of childhood cancer among offspring of nonsmoking mothers. J Natl Cancer Inst. 1997;89(3):238–44.
18. Painter RCDRS, Bossuyt PMM, Osmond C, Barker DJP, Bleker OP, Roseboom TJ. A possible link between prenatal exposure to famine and breast cancer: a preliminary study. Am J Hum Biol. 2006;18:853–6.
19. Clarke R, Ressom HW, Wang A, Xuan J, Liu MC, Gehan EA, Wang Y. The properties of high-dimensional data spaces: implications for exploring gene and protein expression data. Nat Rev Cancer. 2008;8(1):37–49.
20. de Assis SWA, Cruz MI, Laja O, Tian Y, Zhang B, Wang Y, Huang T, Hilakivi-Clarke L. High-fat or ethinyl-oestradiol intake during pregnancy increases mammary cancer risk in several generations of offspring. Nat Commun. 2012;3
21. Brenet FMM, Funk P, Feierstein E, Viale AJ, Socci ND, Scandura JM. DNA methylation of the first exon is tightly linked to transcriptional silencing. PLoS One. 2011;6(1)
22. Jones PA. Functions of DNA methylation: islands, start sites, gene bodies and beyond. Nature Review Genetics. 2012;13(7):484–92.
23. Rhee JKKK, Chae H, Evans J, Yan P, Zhang BT, Gray J, Spellman P, Huang TH, Nephew KP, Kim S. Integrated analysis of genome-wide DNA methylation and gene expression profiles in molecular subtypes of breast cancer. Nucleic Acids Res. 2013;41(18):8464–74.
24. Yuan XYG, Shih IM, Clarke R, Zhang J, Hoffman EP, Wang RR, Zhang Z, Wang Y. Genome-wide identification of significant aberrations in cancer genome. BMC Genomics. 2012;13(342)
25. Zhang BHX, Yuan X, IeM S, Zhang Z, Clarke R, Wang RR, Fu Y, Madhavan S, Wang Y, Yu G. AISAIC: a software suite for accurate identification of significant aberrations in cancers. Bioinformatics. 2014;30(3):431–3.
26. de Assis S, Warri A, Cruz MI, Hilakivi-Clarke L. Changes in mammary gland morphology and breast cancer risk in rats. J Vis Exp. 2010;44:2260.
27. Apostoli AJ, Skelhorne-Gross GE, Rubino RE, Peterson NT, Di Lena MA, Schneider MM, SenGupta SK, Nicol CJ. Loss of PPARγ expression in mammary secretory epithelial cells creates a pro-breast tumorigenic environment. Int J Cancer. 2014;134(5):1055–66.
28. Donkin IVS, Ingerslev LR, Qian K, Mechta M, Nordkap L, Mortensen B, Appel EV, Jørgensen N, Kristiansen VB, Hansen T, Workman CT, Zierath JR, Barrès R. Obesity and bariatric surgery drive epigenetic variation of spermatozoa in humans. Cell Metab. 2016;23(2):369–78.
29. Chen QYM, Cao Z, Li X, Zhang Y, Shi J, Feng GH, Peng H, Zhang X, Zhang Y, Qian J, Duan E, Zhai Q, Zhou Q. Sperm tsRNAs contribute to intergenerational inheritance of an acquired metabolic disorder. Science. 2016;351(6271):397–400.
30. Fernandez-Twinn DSES, Martin-Gronert MS, Terry-Adkins J, Wayman AP, Warner MJ, Luan JA, Gusterson BA, Ozanne SE. Poor early growth and excessive adult calorie intake independently and additively affect mitogenic signaling and increase mammary tumor susceptibility. Carcinogenesis. 2010;31(10):1873–81.
31. Ng SF, Lin RC, Laybutt DR, Barres R, Owens JA, Morris MJ. Chronic high-fat diet in fathers programs β-cell dysfunction in female rat offspring. Nature. 2010;467(7318):963–6.
32. Yu Z, Pestell RG. Small non-coding RNAs govern mammary gland tumorigenesis. J Mammary Gland Biol Neoplasia. 2012;17(1):59–64.

33. Wu L, Lu Y, Jiao Y, Liu B, Li S, Li Y, Xing F, Chen D, Liu X, Zhao J, et al. Paternal psychological stress reprograms hepatic gluconeogenesis in offspring. Cell Metab. 2016;23(4):735–43.

34. Cetin IMA, Bozzetti P, Sereni LP, Corbetta C, Pardi G, Battaglia FC. Umbilical amino acid concentrations in appropriate and small for gestational age infants: a biochemical difference present in utero. Am J Obstet Gynecol. 1988;158(1):120–6.

35. Master JSTG, Harvey AJ, Sheedy JR, Hannan NJ, Gardner DK, Wlodek ME. Fathers that are born small program alterations in the next-generation preimplantation rat embryos. J Nutr. 2015;145(5):876–83.

36. Ribel-Madsen A, Hellgren LI, Brons C, Ribel-Madsen R, Newgard CB, Vaag AA. Plasma amino acid levels are elevated in young, healthy low birth weight men exposed to short-term high-fat overfeeding. Physiol Rep. 2016;4(23)

37. Altman BJ, Stine ZE, Dang CV. From Krebs to clinic: glutamine metabolism to cancer therapy. Nat Rev Cancer. 2016;16(10):619–34.

38. Pavlova NN, Thompson CB. The emerging hallmarks of cancer metabolism. Cell Metab. 2016;23(1):27–47.

39. Taylor PM. Role of amino acid transporters in amino acid sensing. Am J Clin Nutr. 2014;99(1):223S–30S.

40. Godlewski JNM, Bronisz A, Nuovo G, Palatini J, De Lay M, Van Brocklyn J, Ostrowski MC, Chiocca EA, Lawler SE. MicroRNA-451 regulates LKB1/AMPK signaling and allows adaptation to metabolic stress in glioma cells. Mol Cell. 2010;37(1):620–32.

41. Lumpkins CY, Saint Onge JM. Reducing low birth weight among African Americans in the midwest: a look at how faith-based organizations are poised to inform and influence health communication on the Developmental Origins of Health and Disease (DOHaD). Healthcare (Basel). 2017;5(1).

42. Kohler BA, Sherman RL, Howlader N, Jemal A, Ryerson AB, Henry KA, Boscoe FP, Cronin KA, Lake A, Noone AM, et al. Annual report to the nation on the status of cancer, 1975–2011, featuring incidence of breast cancer subtypes by race/ethnicity, poverty, and state. J Natl Cancer Inst. 2015;107(6):djv048.

43. Rando OJ, Simmons RA. I'm eating for two: parental dietary effects on offspring metabolism. Cell. 2015;161(1):93–105.

44. Teras LR, Gaudet MM, Blase JL, Gapstur SM. Parental age at birth and risk of hematological malignancies in older adults. Am J Epidemiol. 2015;182(1):41–8.

45. Guido LN, Fontelles CC, Rosim MP, Pires VC, Cozzolino SM, Castro IA, Bolanos-Jimenez F, Barbisan LF, Ong TP. Paternal selenium deficiency but not supplementation during preconception alters mammary gland development and 7,12-dimethylbenz[a]anthracene-induced mammary carcinogenesis in female rat offspring. Int J Cancer. 2016;139(8):1873–82.

46. Kaati GBL, Pembrey M, Sjöström M. Transgenerational response to nutrition, early life circumstances and longevity. Eur J Hum Genet. 2007;15(7):784–90.

47. Pembery MEBL, Kaati G, Edvinsson S, Northstone K, Sjöström M, Golding J, ALSPAC Study Team. Sex-specific, male-line transgenerational responses in humans. Eur J Hum Genet. 2006;14(2):159–66.

48. Piao HL, Ma L. Non-coding RNAs as regulators of mammary development and breast cancer. J Mammary Gland Biol Neoplasia. 2012;17(1):33–42.

49. Mulrane L, McGee SF, Gallagher WM, O'Connor DP. miRNA dysregulation in breast cancer. Cancer Res. 2013;73(22):6554–62.

50. Izreig S, Samborska B, Johnson RM, Sergushichev A, Ma EH, Lussier C, Loginicheva E, Donayo AO, Poffenberger MC, Sagan SM, et al. The miR-17 approximately 92 microRNA cluster is a global regulator of tumor metabolism. Cell Rep. 2016;16(7):1915–28.

51. Curthoys NP, Watford M. Regulation of glutaminase activity and glutamine metabolism. Annu Rev Nutr. 1995;15:133–59.

52. Efeyan ACW, Sabatini DM. Nutrient-sensing mechanisms and pathways. Nature. 2015;517(7534):302–10.

53. Sugita B, Gill M, Mahajan A, Duttargi A, Kirolikar S, Almeida R, Regis K, Oluwasanmi OL, Marchi F, Marian C, et al. Differentially expressed miRNAs in triple negative breast cancer between African-American and non-Hispanic white women. Oncotarget. 2016;7(48):79274–91.

54. Cao MD, Lamichhane S, Lundgren S, Bofin A, Fjosne H, Giskeodegard GF, Bathen TF. Metabolic characterization of triple negative breast cancer. BMC Cancer. 2014;14:941.

55. Wang Y, Beydoun MA. The obesity epidemic in the United States—gender, age, socioeconomic, racial/ethnic, and geographic characteristics: a systematic review and meta-regression analysis. Epidemiol Rev. 2007;29:6–28.

16

Effect of exercise and/or reduced calorie dietary interventions on breast cancer-related endogenous sex hormones in healthy postmenopausal women

Martijn de Roon[1], Anne M. May[1], Anne McTiernan[2,3], Rob J. P. M. Scholten[1,4], Petra H. M. Peeters[1,5], Christine M. Friedenreich[6,7,8] and Evelyn M. Monninkhof[1]*

Abstract

Background: Physical inactivity and being overweight are modifiable lifestyle risk factors that consistently have been associated with a higher risk of postmenopausal breast cancer in observational studies. One biologic hypothesis underlying this relationship may be via endogenous sex hormone levels. It is unclear if changes in dietary intake, physical activity, or both, are most effective in changing these hormone levels.

Objective: This systematic review and meta-analysis examines the effect of reduced caloric dietary intake and/or increased exercise levels on breast cancer-related endogenous sex hormones.

Methods: We conducted a systematic literature search in MEDLINE, Embase, and Cochrane's Central Register of Controlled Trials (CENTRAL) up to March 2017. Main outcome measures were breast cancer-related endogenous sex hormones.
Randomized controlled trials (RCTs) reporting effects of reduced caloric intake and/or exercise interventions on endogenous sex hormones in healthy, physically inactive postmenopausal women were included. Studies including women using hormone therapy were excluded. The methodological quality of each study was assessed by the Cochrane's risk of bias tool.

Results: From the 2599 articles retrieved, seven articles from six RCTs were included in this meta-analysis. These trials investigated 1588 healthy postmenopausal women with a mean age ranging from 58 to 61 years. A combined intervention of reduced caloric intake and exercise, with durations ranging from 16 to 52 weeks, compared with a control group (without an intervention to achieve weight loss) resulted in the largest beneficial effects on estrone treatment effect ratio (TER) = 0.90 (95% confidence interval (CI) = 0.83–0.97), total estradiol TER = 0.82 (0.75–0.90), free estradiol TER = 0.73 (0.66–0.81), free testosterone TER = 0.86 (0.79–0.93), and sex hormone biding globulin (SHBG) TER = 1.23 (1.15–1.31). A reduced caloric intake without an exercise intervention resulted in significant effects compared with control on total estradiol TER = 0.86 (0.77–0.95), free estradiol TER = 0.77 (0.69–0.84), free testosterone TER = 0.91 (0.84–0.98), and SHBG TER = 1.20 (1.06–1.36). Exercise without dietary change, versus control, resulted in borderline significant effects on androstenedione TER = 0.97 (0.94–1.00), total estradiol TER = 0. 97 (0.94–1.00), and free testosterone TER = 0. 97 (0.95–1.00).

(Continued on next page)

* Correspondence: E.Monninkhof@umcutrecht.nl
[1]Department of Epidemiology, Julius Center for Health Sciences and Primary Care, University Medical Center Utrecht, PO Box 85500, 3508 GA Utrecht, the Netherlands
Full list of author information is available at the end of the article

(Continued from previous page)

Conclusions and relevance: This meta-analysis of six RCTs demonstrated that there are beneficial effects of exercise, reduced caloric dietary intake or, preferably, a combination of exercise and diet on breast cancer-related endogenous sex hormones in physically inactive postmenopausal women.

Keywords: Breast cancer, Postmenopausal women, Exercise, Caloric restriction, Prevention, Sex hormones, Weight loss

Background

Breast cancer is the most common invasive cancer among women worldwide with 1.67 million new cases diagnosed in 2012 [1]. Although numerous breast cancer risk factors are known, most are not easily amenable to intervention. Low levels of physical activity and being overweight are modifiable lifestyle risk factors for breast cancer that have been consistently associated with a higher risk of postmenopausal breast cancer in observational epidemiologic studies [2–5]. One of the pathways, with one of the largest bodies of evidence, is via endogenous sex hormones [6].

High levels of sex serum hormones, including estrogens and androgens, and low levels of sex hormone binding globulin (SHBG) are associated with higher postmenopausal breast cancer risk [4, 7]. SHBG binds to estradiol and testosterone and thereby reduces their harmful free fractions [8, 9]. In postmenopausal women, the main source of estrogens and androgens is via conversion of precursors in peripheral fat tissue [10, 11]. Postmenopausal women who are overweight and/or physically inactive have been shown to have higher levels of circulating endogenous sex hormones [12, 13].

Physical activity might affect sex hormonal levels by reducing the amounts of adipose tissue [14–16]. Normal-weight women show lower levels of estrogens and higher levels of SHBG causing decreased levels of free estradiol compared with overweight/obese women [14–16]. Two large multi-armed randomized controlled trials (RCTs) (n = 439 and n = 243, respectively) have also shown that weight loss and fat loss can be achieved by reduced caloric intake, also affecting sex hormonal levels [17, 18]. However, it is unclear what the most effective method is to reduce postmenopausal endogenous sex hormones.

The aim of this systematic review was to summarize the evidence and to compare the effectiveness of reduced caloric intake and/or exercise on endogenous sex steroid hormones in postmenopausal women.

Methods

In February 2018 we searched MEDLINE, Embase, and the Cochrane Central Register of Controlled Trials (CENTRAL) for eligible studies. The following MeSH terms, keywords, and synonyms of those terms were used: physical activity, exercise, weight loss, diet, postmenopausal, sex hormones. A more detailed description

of the search strategies is presented in Additional file 1. We additionally checked the references of the included studies.

This meta-analysis was registered in Prospero, the international register of systematic reviews, with registration number CRD42015026094.

Selection of studies

Study selection was performed by two authors (MdR, EMM) independently. Studies were first screened on title. After screening on title, a second screening on the remaining potentially eligible abstracts was performed. Of potentially eligible studies, definite selection was based on a full-text copy of the study. Disagreements between the two authors were resolved by discussion. If no consensus could be achieved, a third author (AMM) was consulted.

We included RCTs comparing a reduced calorie dietary intervention, an exercise intervention, or both, with each other or with a control group in healthy postmenopausal women with endogenous sex hormones as outcome measurements. In this meta-analysis, trial arms were considered controls if they did not receive any form of intervention or received only a stretching/relaxation program. Furthermore, studies were excluded when the study population consisted of women using hormone therapy, contained less than 20 women, or the intervention period was less than 12 weeks (since physiologically it is unlikely to expect a meaningful reduction in adipose tissue, which is one mechanism by which physical activity affects sex hormone levels, in such a short time frame [19]).

Data extraction

One author (MdR) extracted data using a predefined data extraction form. Data extracted included: 1) author(s), year, study nationality; 2) details of the study design, size, study duration; 3) characteristics of the study population (age, bodyweight, body mass index (BMI), etc.); 4) details of the interventions; and 5) study results. Extractions of study results were checked by a second author (EMM). For data extraction and quality assessment, both the paper and, if available, the study protocol were used. If data were missing or further information was required, we contacted the study authors to request further information.

Quality assessment

A risk of bias assessment was performed with Cochrane's risk of bias tool by two authors (MdR and EMM) independently [20]. This tool addresses the following domains: 1) randomization; 2) concealment of allocation; 3) blinding of participants and personnel; 4) blinding of outcome assessment; 5) incomplete outcome data; 6) selective outcome reporting; and 7) other biases. Each item was scored as low, unclear, or high risk of bias. For other biases, three topics were scored: were blood samples of the same women analyzed in the same batch, were the participants instructed to avoid exercise 24 h before blood sampling, and was adherence to the exercise and/or reduced calorie diet program monitored. If one or more of these three topics was not met studies were scored as high risk of bias for this item. When information regarding these potential sources of bias was missing in the publication or the study protocol, the study authors were contacted.

Data synthesis and analysis

We analyzed the data for six comparisons: 1) exercise intervention versus control; 2) combined exercise and reduced calorie diet versus no intervention; 3) reduced calorie diet versus no intervention; 4) combined exercise and reduced calorie diet versus reduced calorie diet alone; 5) combined exercise and reduced calorie diet versus exercise alone; and 6) exercise intervention versus reduced calorie diet. When at least two studies were available for a comparison and no substantial heterogeneity was present, meta-analysis was performed according to the generic inverse variance method by the use of Cochrane's Review Manager (RevMan®) version 5.3.5 [21]. Studies reported either geometric means of sex hormone levels at the end of the study or a treatment effect ratio (TER) (i.e., the ratio of the geometric means of the study arms). For meta-analysis, we used the log-transformed value of these measures. For log(TER), we derived the standard error (SE) from the 95% confidence interval (CI) of TER. When geometric means were reported per study arm, we calculated the difference of the log-transformed geometric means (which is equal to the log(TER)) and derived the SE of the log(TER) from the 95% CIs of the geometric means of the respective study arms. For calculation of these values, we used the built-in calculator of RevMan. If the required values were not reported, we contacted the study authors. All tables and figures in this meta-analysis are original for this article.

For each meta-analysis, a random effects model was used. Heterogeneity between studies was assessed by visual inspection of the forest plots (i.e., whether confidence intervals overlap), the Chi-square test for homogeneity, and the I^2 statistic. Values of 25%, 50%, and 75% indicate low, moderate, and high heterogeneity, respectively.

Results

The search resulted in 4027 articles (Fig. 1). After removing duplicates, 2881 references remained. After screening titles and abstracts, 47 references remained for full text screening. Of these, 40 references were excluded. Reasons for exclusion were: did not address our outcomes of interest ($n = 26$), sample size per study arm was < 20 ($n = 5$), no full text available ($n = 6$), no control group (control group was offered an intervention other than stretching/relaxation; $n = 2$), study was not an original (randomized) trial ($n = 1$). Finally, we included seven articles from six randomized controlled trials [3, 17, 18, 22–25].

The main characteristics of the six included studies are shown in Tables 1 and 2. These studies were published between 2004 and 2015, and investigated a total of 1588 postmenopausal women with a mean age ranging from 57.8 to 61.2 years. Five of the six studies included a control group that did not receive any intervention. The control group of the Physical Activity for Total Health (PATH) trial received a stretching program (that was not assumed to affect weight loss or measures of fitness) [22, 23]. Two studies compared two or three interventions with control.

A summary of the risk of bias of the included studies is presented in Additional file 2. We scored five studies as high quality [3, 17, 18, 23, 24] and one as low quality [25]. All studies scored high risk of bias on blinding of personnel since blinding of personnel was not applicable during the exercise interventions.

Interventions

The six studies applied a range of intervention programs varying in duration from 16 weeks to 12 months (Tables 1 and 2). Five studies reported supervised sessions in their exercise program [3, 17, 18, 22–24]. The frequency of the exercise sessions varied from 2 to 5 days per week. The exercise sessions consisted of a warm up of 5–10 min and aerobic exercises guided by the maximum heart rate (MHR) or heart rate reserve (HRR) while intensity increased during the intervention program. The duration of aerobic exercises varied from 15 to 45 min per session. Most exercise interventions started with approximately the same intensity, 50–60% of MHR or HRR. Only the PATH trial intervention started at 40% MHR [22, 23]. Intensity at the end of the aerobic intervention period ranged between 70 and 90% of MHR or HRR in all studies. The Sex Hormone and Physical Exercise (SHAPE) 1 and 2 studies and the study by Orsatti et al. also included strength training in the exercise program [3, 18, 25].

Both SHAPE-2 and the Nutrition and Exercise for Woman (NEW) trial reduced calorie intake interventions and had specific weight loss goals. SHAPE-2 aimed for 5–6 kg of weight loss in both intervention groups (exercise

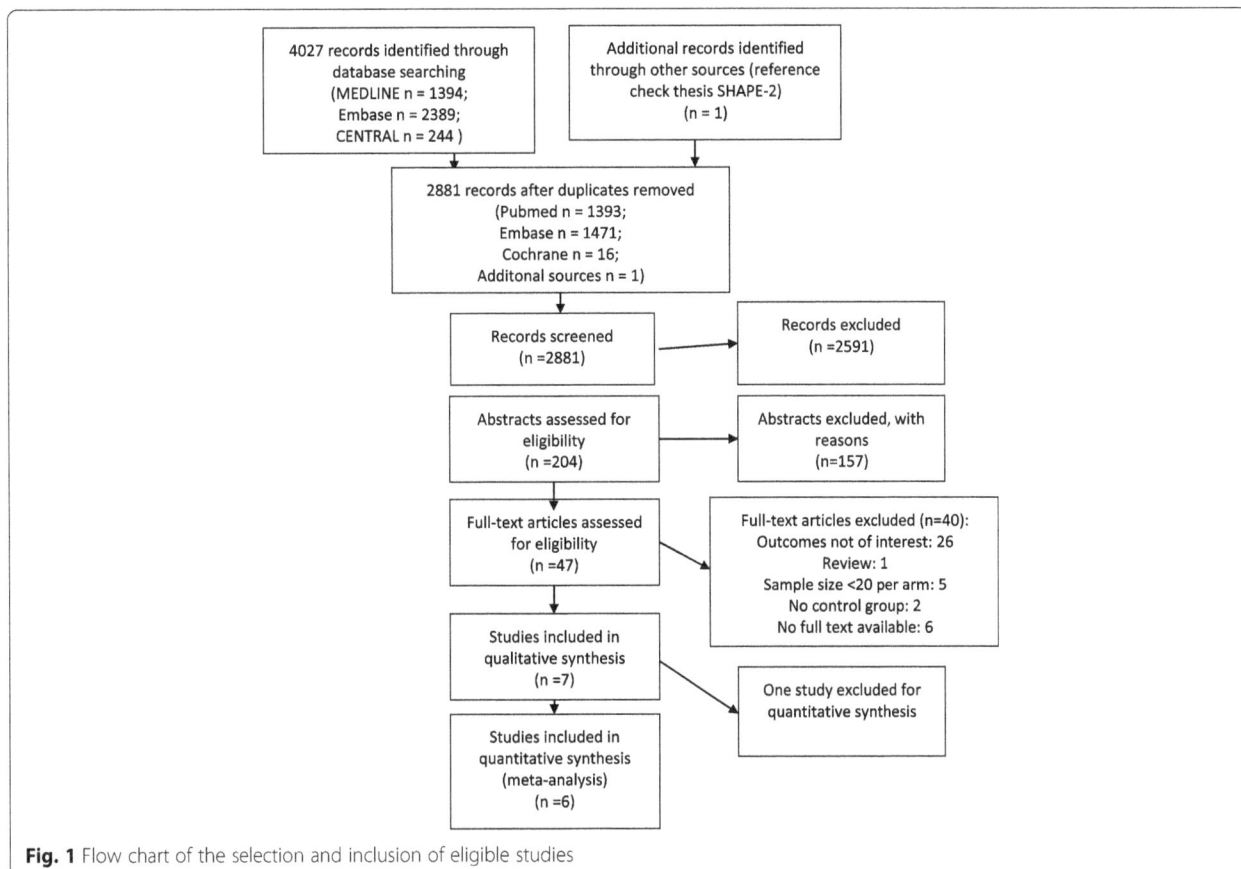

Fig. 1 Flow chart of the selection and inclusion of eligible studies

group and exercise + diet group) while the NEW trial's reduced calorie intake arms aimed for a 10% reduction in body weight at 6 months with maintenance thereafter to 12 months. In the SHAPE-2 trial, the diet group was prescribed a caloric restriction of 3500 kcal/week (or 500 kcal/day). In the NEW trial, the dietary intervention comprised a modification of the dietary component of the Diabetes Prevention Program [26, 27] and Look Ahead lifestyle intervention programs [27, 28], with the following goals: total daily energy intake of 1200–2000 kcal based on baseline weight, less than 30% daily intake from fat, and a 10% reduction in body weight.

Body weight

All studies measured the effect of the intervention on weight or BMI. As shown in Table 3, the SHAPE-2 and NEW trials found the greatest amount of weight loss within the diet (SHAPE-2 −4.9%, NEW −9.1%) and exercise + diet group (SHAPE-2 −5.5%, NEW −9.8%) [17, 18]. The exercise groups (not intended to lose weight) in the SHAPE-1 study (−1.4%), the PATH trial (−1.6%), and the Alberta Physical Activity and Breast Cancer (ALPHA) trial (−2.3%) achieved modest decreases in weight and BMI [3, 17, 24]. The study by Orsatti et al. showed a small increase in body weight in the exercise group (+0.6%) [25].

Sex hormone levels

Five studies reported geometric means for the relevant sex hormone levels (i.e., total estradiol, free estradiol, estrone, SHBG, total testosterone, free testosterone, and androstenedione) [3, 17, 18, 22–24]. One study reported data only on total estradiol and total testosterone (means not based on log transformed data) and no other sex hormones [25]. The reported measure of association varied by trial. Both the SHAPE trials [3, 18] and the ALPHA trial [24] reported absolute change, percentage change, TER, and the 95% CI of the TER. Both the PATH and NEW trials reported absolute change, percentage change, and the p values for between-group differences [17, 22, 23]. The study of Orsatti et al. could technically not be included in the meta-analysis because arithmetic means were reported and geometric means could not be re-estimated [25].

Table 4, Fig. 2, and Additional file 3 show the treatment effects and CIs of all our analyses. Below, we describe our results. We report only statistically significant TERs and 95% CIs.

Exercise versus control

Four studies compared an exercise intervention with no intervention (Table 3) [3, 17, 22–24]. Pooled TERs were

Table 1 Characteristics of the six included studies

Study	Study arms	Mean age (SD) (years)	Sample size, n; drop out, n (%)	Sex hormone outcomes	Methods for sex hormone evaluation	Intervention period
SHAPE-2 [18], 2015, The Netherlands	Ex + D	59.5 (4.9)	98; 9 (9%)	Total estradiol, estrone, free estradiol, total testosterone, free testosterone, SHBG, androstenedione	Determined by liquid chromatography-mass spectrometry (LC-MC). SHBG by double-antibody radioimmunoassay (RIA) kits[b]	16 weeks[a]
	D	60.5 (4.6)	97; 6 (6%)			
	C	60.0 (4.9)	48; 3 (6%)			
NEW trial [17], 2012, United States	Ex + D	58.0 (4.4)	117; 9 (8%)	Total estradiol, estrone, free estradiol, total testosterone, free testosterone, SHBG, androstenedione	Quantified by RIA after organic solvent extraction and Celite column partition chromatography. SHBG via chemiluminescent immunometric assay using Immulite Analyzer[b]	6 months, 12 months
	Ex	58.1 (5.0)	117; 11 (9%)			
	D	58.1 (5.9)	118; 13 (11%)			
	C	57.4 (4.4)	87; 7 (8%)			
ALPHA trial [24], 2010, Canada	Ex	61.2 (5.4)	160; 6 (4%)	Total estradiol, estrone, free estradiol, total testosterone, free testosterone, SHBG, androstenedione	Quantified by RIA after organic solvent extraction and Celite column partition chromatography. SHBG via immunometric assay using Immulite Analyzer[b]	6 months, 12 months
	C	60.6 (5.7)	160; 6 (4%)			
SHAPE-1, 2009 [3], The Netherlands	Ex	58.9 (4.6)	96; 1 (1%)	Total estradiol, estrone, free estradiol, total testosterone, free testosterone, SHBG, androstenedione	Double-antibody RIA kits were used for determining sex hormones, also for SHBG[b]	4 months, 12 months
	C	58.4 (4.2)	93; 5 (5%)			
Orsatti et al. [25], 2008, Brazil	Ex	57.8 (8.0)	27; 6 (22%)	Total testosterone, total estradiol	Measured by the Immulite System, automated immunoassay.	16 weeks
	C	59.3 (6.2)	23; 1 (4%)			
PATH trial [22, 23], 2004, United States	Ex	60.7 (6.7)	87; 3 (3%)	Total estradiol, estrone, free estradiol, total testosterone, free testosterone, SHBG, androstenedione	Quantified by RIA after organic solvent extraction and Celite column partition chromatography. SHBG via immunometric assay using Immulite Analyzer[b]	12 months
	C	60.6 (6.8)	86; 0			

ALPHA Alberta Physical Activity and Breast Cancer, *C* control, *D* reduced calorie diet, *Ex* exercise, *NEW* Nutrition and Exercise for Woman, *PATH* Physical Activity for Total Health, *SHAPE* Sex Hormone and Physical Exercise, *SHBG* sex hormone binding globulin
[a]Although this study took 16 weeks, results were pooled with the other studies
[b]Free estradiol/free testosterone were calculated using the measured values for estradiol, testosterone, and SHBG, and assumed constant for albumin

borderline statistically significant for androstenedione (0.97, 95% CI 0.94–1.00; $P = 0.05$), for total estradiol (0.97, 95% CI 0.94–1.00; $P = 0.06$), and free testosterone (0.97, 95% CI 0.95–1.00; $p = 0.09$) in favor of the exercise group (Table 4 and Fig. 2). Pooled TERs for estrone, free estradiol, total testosterone, and SHBG were in favor of the exercise group, although not statistically significant.

Combined exercise and reduced calorie diet versus control

Two studies compared combined reduced calorie diet and exercise interventions versus controls [17, 18]. The control groups in both studies were requested not to change their diet (NEW trial) [17] or follow a standardized diet (SHAPE-2) and maintain their exercise habits [18]. Both control groups were offered alternative weight loss programs after study completion. Pooled TERs showed a statistically significant effect for total estradiol (0.82, 95% CI 0.75–0.90), for free estradiol (0.73, 95% CI 0.66–0.81), for estrone (0.90, 95% CI 0.83–0.97), for free testosterone (0.86, 95% CI 0.79–0.93), and for SHBG (1.23, 95% CI 1.15–1.31) in favor of the combined exercise and reduced calorie intervention. Pooled effects for total testosterone showed a favorable effect for the exercise and reduced calorie group, although this was not

statistically significant. No statistically significant effects were found for androstenedione.

Reduced calorie diet versus control

Meta-analysis of two studies resulted in a statistically significant decrease in favor of the reduced calorie group for total estradiol (0.86, 95% CI 0.77–0.95), for free estradiol (0.77, 95% CI 0.69–0.84), for free testosterone (0.91, 95% CI 0.84–0.98), and an increase for SHBG (1.20, 95% CI 1.06–1.36), and a favorable but not statistically significant decrease in estrone [17, 18]. No statistically significant effects were found for total testosterone and androstenedione.

Combined exercise and reduced calorie diet versus diet

Meta-analysis of two studies showed a statistically significant decrease in free testosterone (0.94, 95% CI 0.88–1.00) for a combination of exercise and reduced calorie diet compared with reduced calorie diet only. A favorable decrease, although not statistically significant, was shown for estrone (0.94, 95% CI 0.88–1.01), total testosterone (0.95, 95% CI 0.89–1.01), and androstenedione (0.94, 95% CI 0.87–1.02) [17, 18]. No statistically significant effects were found on SHBG, total, or free estradiol.

Table 2 Intervention characteristics of included studies

Study	Intervention	Start intervention	Duration of program	Frequency and duration of sessions	Intensity	Adherence	Control group
SHAPE-2 [18], 2015	Ex + D D	4-6 week run-in period. Standardized diet to maintain stable weight and to achieve a comparable diet composition among all participants	4-6 run period + 16 week intervention	4 h/week, two 1-h group sessions of combined strength and endurance, two 1-h sessions of Nordic walking. Two individual consultations of 30 min with dietician. Five 1-h group sessions spread over the study period	20-25 min of endurance training (60-90% of HRR), 25 min strength training, 5-10 min WU/CD, caloric restriction was 1750 kcal/ week. Moderate to vigorous Nordic walking (60-65% of HRR). Diet group was prescribed a caloric restriction of 3500 kcal/week (or 500 kcal/day)	Group sessions were supervised. Participants kept an exercise log that the physiotherapist regularly checked. Telephone calls every other week	The control group was asked to maintain a stable weight by continuing the standardized diet and their habitual physical activity patterns. After study completion the control group was offered a weight loss intervention
NEW trial [17], 2012	Ex D Ex + D		A 10% reduction in body weight at 6 months with maintenance thereafter to 12 months	5 days/225 min per week for 12 months. Weekly group meetings with a dietician for the first 6 months, thereafter dieticians contacted participants twice a month, including one face to face contact and one additional phone call or e-mail. Women in the diet + exercise group received both interventions	Exercise started with a 15 min session at 60-70% of MHR and progressed to 70-85% of MHR for 45 min by the 7th week where it was maintained for the rest of the study. The dietary intervention comprised a modification of the dietary component of the dietary prevention program and Look Ahead lifestyle intervention programs, with the following goals: total daily energy intake of 1200-2000 kcal/day based on baseline weight, less than 30% daily intake from fat, and a 10% reduction in bodyweight. Women in the diet + exercise group received both interventions	Participants attended at least three supervised sessions per week. In home sessions they recorded mode and duration of the exercise. Women were asked to record all food eaten daily for at least 6 months. Journaling, weekly weighing, and sessions attendance were tracked to promote adherence	The control group was asked not to change their diet or exercise habits. After study completion the control group was offered a weight loss intervention
ALPHA trial [24], 2010	Ex	Started with three sessions per week of 15 to 20 min	During the first 3 months the frequency, duration and intensity increased and maintained for 9 more months	5 days per week of at least 45 min of aerobic exercise	During the first 3 months frequency, duration and intensity were increased from three sessions a week of 15 to 20 min in duration at an intensity of 50 to 60% of HRR to five sessions per week of at least 45 min at 70-80% of HRR	Three sessions per week were facility based. Adherence was monitored through weekly participant- and trainer- administered exercise logs	Controls were asked to maintain their inactive lifestyle. All participants were instructed not to change their usual diet
SHAPE-1 [3], 2009	Ex		12 months	Twice per week a 1-h exercise intervention, once per week home-based exercise	10 min WU, 25 min moderate to vigorous aerobic exercise at 60-85% of MHR, 25 min strength training, 5 min CD. Home-based exercise session contained 30 min	Sport instructors register the attendance of the subjects. Study coordinator	Controls were requested to retain their habitual exercise pattern

Table 2 Intervention characteristics of included studies (Continued)

Study	Intervention	Start intervention	Duration of program	Frequency and duration of sessions	Intensity	Adherence	Control group
					of brisk walking or cycling with an intensity of moderate to vigorous intensity (60–80% of MHR)	performed visits per exercise group to control adherence of the protocol	
Orsatti et al. [25], 2008	Ex	Before training, subjects in the exercise group attended a 4-week adaptation period to become familiarized with the protocol	16 weeks	3 weekly session on nonconsecutive days, under supervision.	Initially lighter loads were used and subjects performed 1 set of 15 repetitions at 40–50% of 1-RM, progression was gradual till 3 sets of 8–12 repetitions at 60–80% of 1-RM were performed. Protocol consisted of dynamic exercises for both lower and upper limbs for a total of 50–60 min. Loads were periodically adjusted at the end of each month	Attendance was recorded by the trainers	Controls were advised to keep their habitual diets and asked not to change their exercise habits
PATH trial [22, 23], 2004	Ex		12 months	At least 45 min of moderate-intensity exercise, 5 days/week for 12 months	The training program started at 40% of observed MHR for 16 min/session and gradually increased to 60–75% of MHR for 45 min/session by week 8	Participants were required to attend the three offered supervised sessions/week during months 1–3 and to exercise on 2 days/week at home. For months 4–12, they were required to attend at least one of the three offered sessions/week at a study facility and to exercise 4 days per week at home or at the facility	Control participants attended 1 weekly 45-min stretching session for 12 months and were asked not to change other exercise habits. Both groups were asked to maintain their usual diet

1-RM one-repetition maximum, ALPHA Alberta Physical Activity and Breast Cancer, CD cooling down, D reduced calorie diet, Ex exercise, HRR heart rate reserve, MHR maximal heart rate, NEW Nutrition and Exercise for Woman, PATH Physical Activity for Total Health, SHAPE Sex Hormone and Physical Exercise, WU warming-up

Table 3 Effect of the interventions on body weight and on serum sex hormones levels

Name, duration	Baseline value[a]	Postintervention[a]	Within-group difference (%)	Between-group difference[b]	Between-group difference[b]
Weight (kg) or BMI[c]					
SHAPE-2 [18], 2015, 16 weeks					
Exercise + diet (Ex+WL)	80.4	74.9	−5.5	−5.58 (−6.32 to −4.84)	Ex+WL vs WL
Reduced calorie diet (WL)	80.3	75.4	−4.9	− 4.95 (−5.69 to −4.21)	−0.63 (−1.23 to −0.04)
Control	80.4	80.4	0.1	Referent	
NEW trial [17], 2012, 12 months					
Exercise + diet	82.5	72.7	−9.8	$P < 0.001$	Ex+WL vs WL, $P = 0.1$
Exercise	83.7	80.9	−2.8	$P = 0.02$	Ex+WL vs Ex, $P < 0.001$
Reduced calorie diet	84.0	74.9	−9.1	$P < 0.001$	Ex vs WL, $P < 0.001$
Control	84.2	83.7	−0.5	Referent	
ALPHA trial [24], 2010, 12 months					
Exercise			−2.3	−1.80 (−2.60 to −1.00)	
Control			−0.5	Referent	
SHAPE-1 [3], 2009, 12 months					
Exercise	73.6	72.2	−1.4	N/A	
Control	74.8	74.0	−0.8		
Orsatti et al. [25], 2008, BMI, 16 weeks					
Exercise	28.8[c]	29.6[c]	0.6[c]	$P = 0.57$	
Control	27.6[c]	27.1[c]	−0.5[c]	Referent	
PATH trial [22, 23], 2004, 12 months					
Exercise	81.6	80.3	−1.6	$P = 0.1$	
Control	81.7	81.8	0.1	Referent	
Total estradiol (pg/ml)					
SHAPE-2 [18], 2015					
Exercise + diet	3.69	3.22	−12.7	0.83 (0.73–0.95)	Ex+WL vs WL
Reduced calorie diet	4.20	3.62	−13.8	0.86 (0.75–0.98)	0.97 (0.87–1.08)
Control	3.89	4.01	3.11	Referent	
NEW trial [17], 2012					
Exercise + diet	11.5	9.2	−20.3	$P < 0.001$	Ex+WL vs WL, $P = 0.07$
Exercise	11.5	11.0	−4.9	$P = 0.1$	Ex+WL vs Ex, $P < 0.001$
Reduced calorie diet	11.6	9.7	−16.2	$P < 0.001$	Ex vs WL, $P = 0.002$
Control	10.9	11.4	4.9	Referent	
ALPHA trial [24], 2010					
Exercise	10.1	8.7		0.93 (0.88–0.98)	
Control	10.2	9.9		Referent	
SHAPE-1 [3], 2009					
Exercise	8.8	8.1	−7.3	0.99 (0.95–1.02)	
Control	9.8	8.8	−10.2	Referent	
Orsatti et al. [25], 2008					
Exercise	21.5	23.2		$P = 0.56$	
Control	25.1	27.4		Referent	
PATH trial [22, 23], 2004					

Table 3 Effect of the interventions on body weight and on serum sex hormones levels *(Continued)*

Name, duration	Baseline value[a]	Postintervention[a]	Within-group difference (%)	Between-group difference[b]	Between-group difference[b]
Exercise	18.3	17.5	−4.4	P = 0.32	
Control	17.9	17.8	−0.6	Referent	
Estrone (pg/ml)					
SHAPE-2 [18], 2015					
Exercise + diet	19.9	18.5	−6.67	0.92 (0.82:1.02)	Ex+WL vs WL
Reduced calorie diet	20.4	20.1	−1.26	0.98 (0.88:1.08)	0.94 (0.86:1.02)
Control	20.1	20.4	3.11	Referent	
NEW trial [17], 2012					
Exercise + diet	33.9	30.2	−11.1	P < 0.001	Ex+WL vs WL, P = 0.17
Exercise	34.8	32.9	−5.5	P < 0.01	Ex+WL vs Ex, P = 0.1
Reduced calorie diet	35.2	31.8	−9.6	P < 0.001	Ex vs WL, P = 0.3
Control	32.0	34.6	8.1	Referent	
ALPHA trial [24], 2010	31.4	29.4			
Exercise	31.3	30.6		0.99 (0.94–1.03)	
Control				Referent	
SHAPE-1 [3], 2009					
Exercise	30.6	27.6	−9.7	0.97 (0.92–1.04)	
Control	28.0	27.3	−3.4	Referent	
PATH trial [22, 23], 2004					
Exercise	44.2	42.5	−1.8	P = 0.13	
Control	43.9	45.4	3.9	Referent	
Free estradiol (pg/ml)					
SHAPE-2 [18], 2015					
Exercise + diet	0.09	0.07	−19.1	0.77 (0.67–0.88)	Ex+WL vs WL
Reduced calorie diet	0.10	0.08	−17.7	0.80 (0.70–0.92)	0.96 (0.85–1.02)
Control	0.09	0.10	3.23	Referent	
NEW trial [17], 2012					
Exercise + diet	0.32	0.23	−26	P < 0.001	Ex+WL vs WL, P = 0.06
Exercise	0.30	0.29	−4.7	P = 0.08	Ex+WL vs Ex, P < 0.001
Reduced calorie diet	0.31	0.24	−21.4	P < 0.001	Ex vs WL, P < 0 .001
Control	0.30	0.33	6.3	Referent	
ALPHA trial [24], 2010					
Exercise	0.24	0.21		0.91 (0.87–0.96)	
Control	0.25	0.24		Referent	
SHAPE-1 [3], 2009					
Exercise	0.22	0.21	−7.3	1.00 (0.96–1.04)	
Control	0.25	0.23	−10.2	Referent	
PATH trial [22, 23], 2004					
Exercise	0.49	0.46	−6.2	P = 0.2	
Control	0.47	0.47	0.0	Referent	
Testosterone (pg/ml)					
SHAPE-2 [18], 2015					

Table 3 Effect of the interventions on body weight and on serum sex hormones levels *(Continued)*

Name, duration	Baseline value[a]	Postintervention[a]	Within-group difference (%)	Between-group difference[b]	Between-group difference[b]
Exercise + diet	186	172	−7.63	0.96 (0.87–1.05)	Ex+WL vs WL
Reduced calorie diet	197	189	−3.76	1.01 (0.92–1.10)	0.95 (0.88–1.02))
Control	194	186	4.07	Referent	
NEW trial [17], 2012					
Exercise + diet	239	225	−5.9	$P = 0.02$	Ex+WL vs WL, $P = 0.07$
Exercise	248	236	−4.9	$P = 0.24$	Ex+WL vs Ex, $P = 0.24$
Reduced calorie diet	239	236	−0.9	$P = 0.4$	Ex vs WL, $P = 0.67$
Control	228	232	1.8	Referent	
ALPHA trial [24], 2010					
Exercise	239	234		0.99 (0.95–1.03)	
Control	231	237		Referent	
SHAPE-1 [3], 2009					
Exercise	528	507	−4.0	0.98 (0.94–1.01)	
Control	535	526	−1.6	Referent	
PATH trial [22, 23], 2004					
Exercise	211	208		$P = 0.94$	
Control	223	218		Referent	
Androstenedione (pg/ml)					
SHAPE-2 [18], 2015					
Exercise + diet	573	488	−14.7	0.87 (0.76–1.00)	Ex+WL vs WL
Reduced calorie diet	562	537	−4.5	0.97 (0.85–1.12)	0.90 (0.80–1.01)
Control	575	560	−2.6	Referent	
NEW trial [17], 2012					
Exercise + diet	526	508	−3.5	$P = 0.22$	Ex+WL vs WL, $P = 0.26$
Exercise	502	496	−1.2	$P = 0.75$	Ex+WL vs Ex, $P = 0.25$
Reduced calorie diet	511	518	1.4	$P = 0.83$	Ex vs WL, $P = 0.93$
Control	487	494	1.5	Referent	
ALPHA trial [24], 2010					
Exercise	578	572		0.98 (0.93–1.03)	
Control	553	577		Referent	
SHAPE-1 [3], 2009					
Exercise	1146	1115	−2.7	0.97 (0.93–1.01)	
Control	1172	1199	2.3	Referent	
PATH trial [22, 23], 2004					
Exercise	533	480		$P = 0.89$	
Control	585	525		Referent	
Free testosterone (pg/ml)					
SHAPE-2 [18], 2015					
Exercise + diet	2.44	2.01	−17.7	0.84 (0.76–0.93)	Ex+WL vs WL
Reduced calorie diet	2.53	2.25	−11.2	0.91 (0.83–1.01)	0.92 (0.85–0.99)
Control	2.71	2.61	−3.9	Referent	
NEW trial [17], 2012					

Table 3 Effect of the interventions on body weight and on serum sex hormones levels *(Continued)*

Name, duration	Baseline value[a]	Postintervention[a]	Within-group difference (%)	Between-group difference[b]	Between-group difference[b]
Exercise + diet	5.3	4.5	−15.6	$P < 0.001$	Ex+WL vs WL, $P = 0.02$
Exercise	5.1	4.9	−4.5	$P = 0.2$	Ex+WL vs Ex, $P < 0.001$
Reduced calorie diet	5.1	4.6	−10.0	$P < 0.001$	Ex vs WL, $P = 0.02$
Control	4.9	5.1	2.6	Referent	
ALPHA trial [24], 2010					
Exercise	3.5	3.3		0.96 (0.92–1.01)	
Control	3.5	3.5		Referent	
SHAPE-1 [3], 2009					
Exercise	8.7	8.5	−2.9	0.99 (0.95–1.03)	
Control	8.7	8.5	−1.8	Referent	
PATH trial [22, 23], 2004					
Exercise	4.6	4.3		$P = 0.42$	
Control	4.7	4.6		Referent	
SHBG (nmol/l)					
SHAPE-2 [18], 2015					
Exercise + diet	49.3	58.6	19.0	1.21 (1.12–1.30)	Ex+WL vs WL
Reduced calorie diet	50.7	57.1	12.6	1.14 (1.07–1.23)	1.05 (1.00–1.12)
Control	44.2	44.0	−0.30	Referent	
NEW trial [17], 2012					
Exercise + diet	34.1	42.9	25.8	$P < 0.001$	Ex+WL vs WL, $P = 0.41$
Exercise	39.1	38.8	0.7	$P = 0.41$	Ex+WL, vs Ex $P < 0.001$
Reduced calorie diet	35.8	43.8	22.4	$P < 0.001$	Ex vs WL, $P < 0.001$
Control	34.7	33.7	−2.7	Referent	
ALPHA trial [24], 2010					
Exercise	40.3	41.9		1.04 (1.02–1.07)	
Control	38.1	38.4		Referent	
SHAPE-1 [3], 2009					
Exercise	33.9	33.6	−0.7	0.98 (0.92–1.04)	
Control	34.7	33.6	−3.3	Referent	
PATH trial [22, 23], 2004					
Exercise	35.2	38.3	8.8	$P = 0.10$	
Control	35.8	36.7	2.5	Referent	

ALPHA Alberta Physical Activity and Breast Cancer, *NEW* Nutrition and Exercise for Woman, *PATH* Physical Activity for Total Health, *SHAPE* Sex Hormone and Physical Exercise, *SHBG* sex hormone binding globulin
[a]Geometric means reported
[b]Values are given as either treatment effect ratios (95% confidence intervals) or as P values
[c]Body mass index (BMI) was reported when bodyweight was not available

Combined exercise and reduced calorie diet versus exercise
One study compared exercise combined with a reduced calorie diet to exercise alone [17]. Since only one study performed this comparison, original study data are shown instead of estimating the TER. When compared with the exercise-only intervention, the exercise combined with a reduced calorie intervention showed significant beneficial changes for estrone (−1.9 pg/ml, $P = 0.01$), total estradiol (−1.7 pg/ml, $P < 0.001$), free estradiol (−0.07 pg/ml, $P < 0.01$),

SHBG (+9.1 nmol/l, $P = < 0.01$), and free testosterone (−0.59 pg/ml, $P < 0.01$) [17]. For total testosterone and androstenedione no statistically significant results were found [17].

Exercise versus reduced calorie diet
This comparison was also only investigated in one study [17]. The reduced calorie intervention showed beneficial statistically significant results when compared with the exercise intervention for total estradiol (−1.3 pg/ml, $P =$

Table 4 Pooled mean differences of the four comparisons on the different sex hormone outcomes and sex hormone binding globulin (SHBG)

Pooled effects[a]	Treatment effect ratios (95% confidence interval)
Estrone	
Exercise vs control	0.97 (0.94–1.01)
Exercise + diet vs control	0.90 (0.83–0.97)
Diet vs control	0.95 (0.88–1.03)
Exercise + diet vs diet	0.94 (0.88–1.01)
Total estradiol	
Exercise vs control	0.97 (0.94–1.00)
Exercise + diet vs control	0.82 (0.75–0.90)
Diet vs control	0.86 (0.77–0.95)
Exercise + diet vs diet	0.96 (0.89–1.04)
Free estradiol	
Exercise vs control	0.95 (0.87–1.01)
Exercise + diet vs control	0.73 (0.66–0.81)
Diet vs control	0.77 (0.69–0.84)
Exercise + diet vs diet	0.96 (0.87–1.06)
Total testosterone	
Exercise vs control	0.98 (0.95–1.01)
Exercise + diet vs control	0.96 (0.89–1.04)
Diet vs control	1.01 (0.94–1.09)
Exercise + diet vs diet	0.95 (0.89–1.01)
Free testosterone	
Exercise vs control	0.97 (0.95–1.00)
Exercise + diet vs control	0.86 (0.79–0.93)
Diet vs control	0.91 (0.84–0.98)
Exercise + diet vs diet	0.94 (0.88–1.00)
Androstenedione	
Exercise vs control	0.97 (0.94–1.00)
Exercise + diet vs control	0.95 (0.80–1.12)
Diet vs control	1.01 (0.93–1.11)
Exercise + diet vs diet	0.94 (0.87–1.02)
SHBG	
Exercise vs control	1.03 (0.99–1.08)
Exercise + diet vs control	1.23 (1.15–1.31)
Diet vs control	1.20 (1.06–1.36)
Exercise + diet vs diet	1.03 (0.97–1.09)

[a] For readability reduced calorie diet is labeled as "diet"

0.002), free estradiol (−0.06 pg/ml, $P < 0.001$), free testosterone (−0.28 pg/ml, $P = 0.02$), and SHBG (+8.3 nmol/l, $P < 0.001$) [17]. No statistically significant effects were found for estrone, total testosterone, or androstenedione [17].

Discussion

This systematic review and meta-analysis found beneficial effects on endogenous estrogen levels and free testosterone

from interventions that were designed to change either dietary caloric intake, exercise levels, or both, in postmenopausal healthy women, which is relevant for breast cancer risk reduction in this population. No beneficial effects were found for any of these interventions on total testosterone levels (only in free testosterone). Our meta-analysis suggests that weight loss is important for achieving effects on hormone levels, and caloric restriction (with or without an

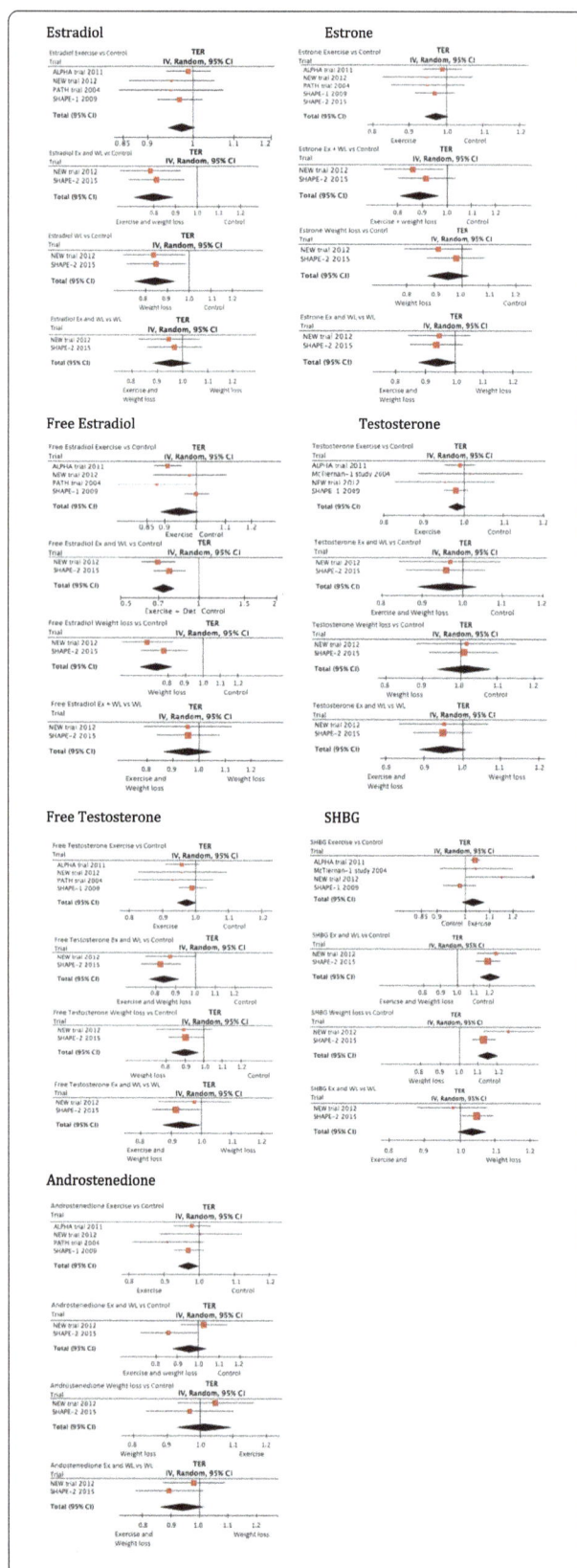

Fig. 2 Forest plots per sex hormone. Plots per comparison: 1) exercise compared with control; 2) exercise (Ex) and diet (WL) versus control; 3) diet (WL) versus control; 4) exercise (Ex) and diet (WL) versus diet (WL). ALPHA Alberta Physical Activity and Breast Cancer, CI confidence interval, NEW Nutrition and Exercise for Woman, PATH Physical Activity for Total Health, SHAPE Sex Hormone and Physical Exercise, TER treatment effect ratio

exercise component) affects weight loss to a larger extent than exercise only in physically inactive postmenopausal women. We found that caloric restriction combined with exercise seems to be most beneficial for lowering sex hormone levels. Comparing the combination of exercise and caloric restriction with caloric restriction only, all results favored the combination even when weight loss between the groups was comparable. An additional important advantage of combining caloric restriction with exercise is that the exercise component maintains or increases muscle mass and cardiovascular fitness.

The studies in this meta-analysis mostly showed beneficial effects of exercise and/or caloric restriction on endogenous sex hormones, although the magnitude of effects varied. There are several underlying factors that can explain this variation. First, varying types, doses, and duration of interventions might be responsible for differences between studies. Second, inclusion criteria across studies were largely comparable, but differences in baseline BMI and other differences in study populations might have contributed to varying results on endogenous sex hormones. The SHAPE-1, the ALPHA trial, and the study of Orsatti et al. included normal-weight women [3, 24, 25], while the other studies excluded these women. Women with normal weight might have less room for improvement in sex hormone levels since this change depends on the amount of fat mass. Similarly, although all studies included "inactive" women, the definition of "inactive" varied between studies. Third, the studies varied by the mean weight loss in the intervention group(s), with larger weight loss in the studies that explicitly aimed for weight loss. On average, stronger effects were found in the NEW trial and in the SHAPE-2 study [17, 18]. Contrary to the ALPHA, PATH, and SHAPE-1 trials, the interventions in the NEW and SHAPE-2 trials targeted weight loss, with goals of −10% of body weight and 5 to 6 kg, respectively [3, 17, 18, 22–24]. This difference might explain the larger effects since all studies found that women who lost larger amounts of weight showed larger effects on sex hormone levels [16, 28, 29]. Results of the trials studying the effect of exercise without aiming for weight loss show that exercise only is not sufficient to affect the hormone levels substantially [3, 17, 18, 22–24]. After stratifying for fat loss, the SHAPE-1 and PATH trials both reported larger effects on hormone levels in women who lost > 2% of body fat [3, 22, 23]. Hence, it is important to achieve weight loss to affect sex hormone levels [16, 28, 29]. Pooled effects for diet (compared with control groups) showed statistically significant results for several hormones, which was not observed for interventions with mainly exercise.

Although our meta-analysis showed beneficial effects of exercise and/or caloric restriction on most endogenous sex hormones, null associations were found for total testosterone. This result was an unexpected finding because of the earlier observed associations between increased adiposity and increased androgen levels and because of effects for free testosterone that were statistically significant [30–32]. A potential reason for this null association might be the large variation in testosterone values and the extremely low levels, which complicate detecting effects.

It is still a challenge to estimate the magnitude of the clinical impact of the observed effects on sex hormones, since there are no absolute cut-off values defined that correspond with a certain change in future breast cancer risk. Until now, it is assumed that the distributions and rankings of sex hormone levels, rather than the absolute values, correspond with breast cancer risk. Observational studies that linked sex hormone levels to breast cancer risk mainly show that women whose hormone levels are in the highest quintiles of the distribution have an up to twofold increased risk when compared with women with levels in the lowest quintiles [12, 33]. However, the absolute values corresponding to these quintiles vary largely between studies. For example, the Endogenous Hormones and Breast Cancer Collaborative Group evaluated nine prospective studies that measured sex hormones in postmenopausal breast cancer cases and samples of healthy postmenopausal controls [12]. Median hormone levels varied substantially; for example, estradiol levels differed up to fivefold between the studies, ranging from 22 pmol/l to 101 pmol/l in control women. Besides population heterogeneity (in ages, BMI, and other determinants of hormone levels such as reproductive factors and nutritional habits), the large variation in absolute values is probably mainly caused by differences in laboratory assays [34, 35]. These issues might, in addition to the different intervention programs, explain the differences in magnitude of effects across the studies included in this meta-analysis.

The focus of this meta-analysis is on breast cancer-related endogenous sex hormones, but there might be additional beneficial effects of adding exercise to a dietary intervention. It has been shown that exercise interventions have beneficial effects on cardiopulmonary fitness, may prevent diabetes, increase muscular strength, and lower the risk of osteoporosis. For example, the SHAPE-2 study showed a small loss of muscle mass in the reduced calorie group, which should be avoided [18]. Therefore, including an exercise component in the intervention is highly recommended rather than a reduction in caloric intake alone.

The strength of this meta-analysis is that the separate trials were each of high quality with large sample sizes. This meta-analysis also has some limitations. First, results might not be generalizable to all postmenopausal women, since only physically inactive women with a BMI > 22 kg/m^2 were included in this meta-analysis. We were not able to stratify our results in this meta-analysis for physical activity levels because the interventions differed in duration, intensity, and type of exercises.

There are several topics for further research. First, studies considering the long-term maintenance of the effect on endogenous sex hormones are lacking. For the sustainability of intervention effects, behavioral changes in food intake and daily physical activity are necessary. A follow-up study from the SHAPE-2 trial found that the participants were able to maintain weight loss and increase physical activity levels in both study groups 1 year after trial completion, but sex hormone levels were not measured again at the 1-year follow-up time point [36]. A second topic of interest is whether or not the effects are found in different population subgroups, such as women of different race/ethnic origin, or women at risk for breast cancer because of familial predisposition (e.g., breast cancer (BRCA)1 and BRCA2 genes). Third, future research should consider different biologic mechanisms that have not yet been investigated, such as immune function.

Conclusions
In conclusion, the combined data from six randomized controlled trials demonstrate that there are beneficial effects when weight loss was achieved by a reduced calorie diet intervention with or without exercise on breast cancer-related endogenous sex hormones in overweight, physically inactive postmenopausal women. Our results suggest that the most beneficial effects on endogenous sex hormones were found with a combined exercise and reduced caloric dietary intervention. Exercise interventions without a reduced caloric intake showed small effects on endogenous sex hormone levels. To reduce breast cancer-related endogenous sex hormones, we recommend combining a reduced calorie diet with exercise to increase weight loss and maintain or increase muscle mass and cardiovascular fitness.

Abbreviations
ALPHA: Alberta Physical Activity and Breast Cancer; BMI: Body mass index; CI: Confidence interval; HRR: Heart rate reserve; MHR: Maximum heart rate; NEW: Nutrition and Exercise for Woman; PATH: Physical Activity for Total Health; RCT: Randomized controlled trial; SE: Standard error; SHAPE: Sex Hormone and Physical Exercise; SHBG: Sex hormone binding globulin; TER: Treatment effect ratio

Authors' contributions

MdR participated in the study design, setting up and adjusting eligibility criteria, carried out searches in all databases, study selection and quality assessment, carried out data-analysis, and participated in interpretation of the results and drafting the manuscript. AMM participated in the study design, setting up and adjusting eligibility criteria, consulting when disagreements occurred in study selection, participated in interpretation of the results, and helped to draft the manuscript. AM participated in setting up and adjusting eligibility criteria, interpretation of the results, and completing the manuscript. RJPMS carried out data analysis and reviewed the study protocol and methods. PHMP participated in the interpretation of the results and drafting the manuscript. CMF participated in the study design, study selection and quality assessment, and participated in interpretation of the results and drafting the manuscript. EMM participated in the study design, setting up and adjusting eligibility criteria, study selection and quality assessment, participated in data-analysis, and participated in interpretation of the results and drafting the manuscript. All authors read and approved the final manuscript.

Competing interests

The authors declare that they have no competing interests.

Author details

[1]Department of Epidemiology, Julius Center for Health Sciences and Primary Care, University Medical Center Utrecht, PO Box 85500, 3508 GA Utrecht, the Netherlands. [2]Epidemiology Program, Division of Public Health Sciences, Fred Hutchinson Cancer Research Centre, Seattle, Washington, USA. [3]Department of Epidemiology, School of Public Health, and Department of Medicine, School of Medicine, University of Washington, Seattle, Washington, USA. [4]Cochrane Netherlands, University Medical Center Utrecht, Utrecht, the Netherlands. [5]MRC-PHE Centre for Environment and Health, Department of Epidemiology and Biostatistics, School of Public Health, Imperial College, London, UK. [6]Department of Cancer Epidemiology and Prevention Research, CancerControl Alberta, Alberta Health Services, Alberta, Canada. [7]Department of Oncology, Cumming School of Medicine, University of Calgary, Calgary, Canada. [8]Department of Community Health Sciences, Cumming School of Medicine, University of Calgary, Calgary, Canada.

References

1. Ferlay J, Steliarova-Foucher E, Lortet-Tieulent J, Rosso S, Coebergh JW, Comber H, et al. Cancer incidence and mortality patterns in Europe: estimates for 40 countries in 2012. Eur J Cancer. 2013;49(6):1374–403.
2. Lynch BM, Neilson HK, Friedenreich CM. Physical activity and breast cancer prevention. Recent Results Cancer Res. 2011;186:13–42. https://doi.org/10.1007/978-3-642-04231-7_2.
3. Monninkhof EM, Velthuis MJ, Peeters PH, Twisk JW, Schuit AJ. Effect of exercise on postmenopausal sex hormone levels and role of body fat: a randomized controlled trial. J Clin Oncol. 2009;27(27):4492–9. https://doi.org/10.1200/JCO.2008.19.7459.
4. Monninkhof EM, Elias SG, Vlems FA, van der Tweel I, Schuit AJ, Voskuil DW, et al. Physical activity and breast cancer: a systematic review. Epidemiology. 2007;18(1):137–57.
5. World Cancer Research Fund, American Institute for Cancer Research(AICR). Continuous update project report. Food, nutrition, physical activity, and the prevention of breast cancer. 2010. Washington DC: AICR; 2010. https://www.wcrf.org/sites/default/files/Breast-Cancer-2010-Report.pdf. Accessed 9 July 2018.
6. Neilson HK, Conroy SM, Friedenreich CM. The influence of energetic factors on biomarkers of postmenopausal breast cancer risk. Curr Nutr Rep. 2014;3(1):22–34.
7. Cust AE, Armstrong BK, Friedenreich CM, Slimani N, Bauman A. Physical activity and endometrial cancer risk: a review of the current evidence, biologic mechanisms and the quality of physical activity assessment methods. Cancer Causes Control. 2007;18(3):243–58.
8. Schwartz MW, Woods SC, Porte D Jr, Seeley RJ, Baskin DG. Central nervous system control of food intake. Nature. 2000;404(6778):661 71.
9. Neilson HK, Conroy SM, Friedenreich CM. The influence of energetic factors on biomarkers of postmenopausal breast cancer risk. Curr Nutr Rep. 2013;3: 22–34. https://doi.org/10.1007/s13668-013-0069-8.
10. Judd HL, Shamonki IM, Frumar AM, Lagasse LD. Origin of serum estradiol in postmenopausal women. Obstet Gynecol. 1982;59(6):680–6.
11. Deslypere JP, Verdonck L, Vermeulen A. Fat tissue: a steroid reservoir and site of steroid metabolism. J Clin Endocrinol Metab. 1985;61(3):564–70.
12. Key T, Appleby P, Barnes I, Reeves G, Endogenous Hormones and Breast Cancer Collaborative Group. Endogenous sex hormones and breast cancer in postmenopausal women: reanalysis of nine prospective studies. J Natl Cancer Inst. 2002;94(8):606–16.
13. Friedenreich CM, Cust AE. Physical activity and breast cancer risk: impact of timing, type and dose of activity and population subgroup effects. Br J Sports Med. 2008;42(8):636–47.
14. van Gils CH, Peeters PH, Schoenmakers MC, Nijmeijer RM, Onland-Moret NC, van der Schouw YT, et al. Physical activity and endogenous sex hormone levels in postmenopausal women: a cross-sectional study in the Prospect-EPIC cohort. Cancer Epidemiol Biomark Prev. 2009;18(2):377–83. https://doi.org/10.1158/1055-9965.EPI-08-0823.
15. Bjornerem A, Straume B, Midtby M, Fonnebo V, Sundsfjord J, Svartberg J, et al. Endogenous sex hormones in relation to age, sex, lifestyle factors, and chronic diseases in a general population: the Tromso study. J Clin Endocrinol Metab. 2004;89(12):6039–47.
16. Verkasalo PK, Thomas HV, Appleby PN, Davey GK, Key TJ. Circulating levels of sex hormones and their relation to risk factors for breast cancer: a cross-sectional study in 1092 pre- and postmenopausal women (United Kingdom). Cancer Causes Control. 2001;12(1):47–59.
17. Campbell KL, Foster-Schubert KE, Alfano CM, Wang CC, Wang CY, Duggan CR, et al. Reduced-calorie dietary weight loss, exercise, and sex hormones in postmenopausal women: randomized controlled trial. J Clin Oncol. 2012; 30(19):2314–26. https://doi.org/10.1200/JCO.2011.37.9792.
18. van Gemert WA, Schuit AJ, van der Palen J, May AM, Iestra JA, Wittink H, et al. Effect of weight loss, with or without exercise, on body composition and sex hormones in postmenopausal women: the SHAPE-2 trial. Breast Cancer Res. 2015;17:120. 015–0633-9
19. McTiernan A. Mechanisms linking physical activity with cancer. Nat Rev Cancer. 2008;8(3):205–11.
20. Higgins JPT, Altman DG, Sterne JAC. Chapter 8: assessing risk of bias in included studies. In: Higgins JPT, Altman DG, Sterne JAC, editors. Cochrane Handbook for Systematic Reviews of Interventions. Version 5.1.0 (updated March 2011): The Cochrane Collaboration; 2011. Available from www.handbook.cochrane.org.
21. Review Manager (RevMan) [Computer program]. Version [5.3.5]. Copenhagen: The Nordic Cochrane Centre, The Cochrane Collaboration; 2014.
22. McTiernan A, Tworoger SS, Rajan KB, Yasui Y, Sorenson B, Ulrich CM, et al. Effect of exercise on serum androgens in postmenopausal women: a 12-month randomized clinical trial. Cancer Epidemiol Biomark Prev. 2004;13(7):1099–105.
23. McTiernan A, Tworoger SS, Ulrich CM, Yasui Y, Irwin ML, Rajan KB, et al. Effect of exercise on serum estrogens in postmenopausal women: a 12-month randomized clinical trial. Cancer Res. 2004;64(8):2923–8.
24. Friedenreich CM, Woolcott CG, McTiernan A, Ballard-Barbash R, Brant RF, Stanczyk FZ, et al. Alberta physical activity and breast cancer prevention trial: sex hormone changes in a year-long exercise intervention among postmenopausal women. J Clin Oncol. 2010;28(9):1458–66. https://doi.org/10.1200/JCO.2009.24.9557.
25. Orsatti FL, Nahas EA, Maesta N, Nahas-Neto J, Burini RC. Plasma hormones, muscle mass and strength in resistance-trained postmenopausal women. Maturitas. 2008;59(4):394–404. https://doi.org/10.1016/j.maturitas.2008.04.002.
26. Knowler WC, Barrett-Connor E, Fowler SE, Hamman RF, Lachin JM, Walker EA, et al. Reduction in the incidence of type 2 diabetes with lifestyle intervention or metformin. N Engl J Med. 2002;346(6):393–403.
27. Ryan DH, Espeland MA, Foster GD, Haffner SM, Hubbard VS, Johnson KC, et al. Look AHEAD (action for health in diabetes): design and methods for a clinical trial of weight loss for the prevention of cardiovascular disease in type 2 diabetes. Control Clin Trials. 2003;24(5):610–28.
28. Chan MF, Dowsett M, Folkerd E, Bingham S, Wareham N, Luben R, et al. Usual physical activity and endogenous sex hormones in postmenopausal women: the European prospective investigation into cancer—Norfolk population study. Cancer Epidemiol Biomark Prev. 2007;16(5):900–5.
29. McTiernan A, Wu L, Chen C, Chlebowski R, Mossavar-Rahmani Y, Modugno F, et al. Relation of BMI and physical activity to sex hormones in postmenopausal women. Obesity (Silver Spring). 2006;14(9):1662 77.

17

Metastatic breast cancer cells overexpress and secrete miR-218 to regulate type I collagen deposition by osteoblasts

Xuxiang Liu[2], Minghui Cao[1], Melanie Palomares[3], Xiwei Wu[4], Arthur Li[5], Wei Yan[1], Miranda Y. Fong[6], Wing-Chung Chan[7] and Shizhen Emily Wang[1*] (iD)

Abstract

Background: Bone is one of the most frequent metastatic sites of advanced breast cancer. Current therapeutic agents aim to inhibit osteoclast-mediated bone resorption but only have palliative effects. During normal bone remodeling, the balance between bone resorption and osteoblast-mediated bone formation is essential for bone homeostasis. One major function of osteoblast during bone formation is to secrete type I procollagen, which will then be processed before being crosslinked and deposited into the bone matrix.

Methods: Small RNA sequencing and quantitative real-time PCR were used to detect miRNA levels in patient blood samples and in the cell lysates as well as extracellular vesicles of parental and bone-tropic MDA-MB-231 breast cancer cells. The effects of cancer cell-derived extracellular vesicles isolated by ultracentrifugation and carrying varying levels of miR-218 were examined in osteoblasts by quantitative real-time PCR, Western blot analysis, and P1NP bone formation marker analysis. Cancer cells overexpressing miR-218 were examined by transcriptome profiling through RNA sequencing to identify intrinsic genes and pathways influenced by miR-218.

Results: We show that circulating miR-218 is associated with breast cancer bone metastasis. Cancer-secreted miR-218 directly downregulates type I collagen in osteoblasts, whereas intracellular miR-218 in breast cancer cells regulates the expression of inhibin β subunits. Increased cancer secretion of inhibin βA results in elevated Timp3 expression in osteoblasts and the subsequent repression of procollagen processing during osteoblast differentiation.

Conclusions: Here we identify a twofold function of cancer-derived miR-218, whose levels in the blood are associated with breast cancer metastasis to the bone, in the regulation of type I collagen deposition by osteoblasts. The adaptation of the bone niche mediated by miR-218 might further tilt the balance towards osteolysis, thereby facilitating other mechanisms to promote bone metastasis.

Keywords: Breast cancer, Bone metastasis, miRNA, Cytokines, Osteoblasts, Type I collagen

Background

The "Seed and Soil" hypothesis first brought up by Stephen Paget highlights the importance of matching between cancer and its metastatic niche, and implies the requirement of niche adaptation during cancer metastasis [1]. The bone tropism of breast cancer cells is in part mediated by chemokines and their receptors, exemplified by C-X-C chemokine receptor type 4 (CXCR4) expressed as one of the signature genes on bone-seeking cancer cells and its ligand stromal-derived-factor-1 expressed by cells within the bone environment including osteoblasts [2, 3]. The adaption of bone metastatic niche involves exchange of factors between breast cancer cells and cells naturally residing in the bone niche. Previous studies have shown that the osteolytic bone lesion, which is induced by metastatic breast cancer cells through secretion of bone catabolic factors including parathyroid hormone-related protein (PTHrP), interleukin (IL)-11, IL-8, and IL-6, in turn exacerbates this tropism by promoting cancer cell growth in the bone

* Correspondence: emilywang@ucsd.edu
[1]Department of Pathology, University of California San Diego, 9500 Gilman Drive, La Jolla, CA 92093-0612, USA
Full list of author information is available at the end of the article

via growth factors released from the degraded bone matrix [4, 5].

In addition to cytokines, extracellular vesicles (EVs) that contain biomaterials such as microRNA (miRNA), mRNA, and proteins, including exosomes, are important vehicles for intercellular communication in short or long range [6]. Our lab has previously shown that breast cancer-secreted EVs target endothelial cells and fibroblasts to induce vascular permeability and metabolic reprogramming, respectively [7–9]. Stromal cells in the metastatic niche can also secrete EVs to regulate cancer cells [10]. Bone marrow mesenchymal stem cells secrete miR-23b-containing exosomes, which induce breast cancer dormancy by targeting a cell cycle regulator myristoylated alanine rich protein kinase C substrate (MARCKS) [11]. Interestingly, a recent study found that exosomes also exhibited organotropism, which was regulated by the integrin profile of these exosomes [12].

Human adult bones constantly undergo turnover and remodeling to replace old bones and to repair damaged ones [13]. Osteoclast-mediated bone resorption can be regulated by osteoblasts, which secrete osteoclast differentiation-inducing factor receptor activator of nuclear factor kappa-B ligand (RANKL) and its decoy receptor osteoprotegerin (OPG) [14]. Conversely, recent studies revealed that osteoclasts could also secrete coupling factors to regulate proliferation, migration and differentiation of osteoblasts during new bone formation [15]. Osteoblasts secrete type I procollagen into the matrix during differentiation and bone formation [16]. A disintegrin-like and metalloprotease with thrombospondin type 1 motif, 2 (ADAMTS2) procollagenase then cleaves and releases the N′-terminus of type I procollagen [17], which is often referred to as P1NP and widely used as a marker for bone formation [18]. Crosslinked type I collagens then constitute 90% of the organic matrix of the bone [16].

The transforming growth factor beta (TGF-β) superfamily has been shown to regulate bone physiology [19]. TGF-β can either enhance or repress osteoclast differentiation dependent on dose and the presence of other cell types [20, 21]. TGF-β1 has also been reported to induce bone formation through regulating bone mesenchymal stem cell migration [22]. Different bone morphogenetic proteins (BMPs) are implicated in the positive or negative regulation of bone formation [23]. Activin A and activin B, which also belong to the TGF-β superfamily, are homodimers of inhibin βA and inhibin βB, respectively [24]. They bind to type II receptors on plasma membrane and subsequently activate type I receptors. Mothers against DPP homolog (SMAD)2 and SMAD3 are then phosphorylated and bind with SMAD4, which translocates to the nucleus and regulates target gene transcription. Inhibins, which are heterodimers of inhibin α and β subunits,

usually antagonize the effect of activins. Blockade of activin signaling by a soluble activin receptor type IIA fusion protein can promote osteoblast-mediated bone formation and inhibit breast cancer bone metastasis in a murine model [25], indicating an important role of activins in bone homeostasis and bone metastasis.

Here we set out to understand the function of miR-218, which is detected at a higher level in the sera from stage IV breast cancer patients with bone metastasis and in the EVs of bone-tropic breast cancer cells, in mediating the profound interplay between breast cancer and bone cells. Our data suggest a model through which cancer-derived miR-218 inhibits osteoblast function of collagen deposition though direct targeting of collagen type I alpha 1 chain (COL1A1) and regulation of inhibin βA expression.

Methods
Clinical specimens
Human serum specimens were obtained from voluntarily consenting breast cancer patients between February 2006 and December 2011 at the City of Hope National Medical Center (Duarte, CA, USA) under institutional review board-approved protocols. All 47 patients involved in this study had stage IV disease with or without bone metastases at the time metastatic disease was diagnosed. Among them, 33 patients had bone metastases, in most cases with concurrent metastases to other organs, whereas the other 14 patients had distant metastases to other organs without the involvement of bone. The two groups exhibited balanced age, tumor subtype, and sample collection time. Serum specimens examined in this study were collected at the time metastasis was initially diagnosed or the earliest draw available. Clinical characteristics are summarized in Additional file 1: Table S1. Trizol LS reagent (Thermo Fisher Scientific; Waltham, MA, USA) was used to extract total RNA from ~ 0.5 ml of serum; RNA pellet was dissolved in 10 μl of RNase-free water and subjected to Solexa sequencing and RT-qPCR as previously described [26].

Cells
Human breast cancer cell line MDA-MB-231, MCF-7, human non-cancerous mammary epithelial cell line MCF10A, and mouse preosteoblast cell line MC3T3-E1 were obtained from American Type Culture Collection (Manassas, VA, USA) and cultured in the recommended media. The bone-tropic subline of MDA-MB-231 was a kind gift from Dr. T. Yoneda. All cells used herein were tested to be free of mycoplasma contamination and authenticated by using the short tandem repeat profiling method. MDA-MB-231 cells were stably transduced with control and miR-218 lentiviral constructs purchased from GeneCopoeia (Rockville, MD, USA). miRIDIAN miR-218

mimic and the corresponding negative control were purchased from GE Dharmacon (Lafayette, CO, USA). LNA oligonucleotides against miR-218 and control were purchased from Exiqon (Woburn, MA, USA). Cell transfection, reporter assays, production of viruses, infection and selection of transduced cells, as well as flow cytometry for cell characterization, were carried out as previously described [7–9, 27]. Osteoblast differentiation was induced by 50 µg/ml L-ascorbic acid, 10 mM β-glycerolphosphate, and 0.1 µM dexamethasone for 16–21 days with medium change every 3–4 days. Conditioned medium was collected by passing through 0.45 µm filters. Conditioned medium concentration was performed using Vivaspin 20 columns from Sartorius (Bohemia, NY, USA).

Primary bone marrow cell isolation and induction of osteoclast differentiation

One million bone marrow cells isolated from C57BL/ 6 mice were bulk cultured in a six-well plate and 40 ng/ml M-CSF was added to induce adherence for 3 days. Osteoclast differentiation was induced by adding 40 ng/ml M-CSF and 100 ng/ml RANKL (R&D Systems; Minneapolis, MN, USA) and culturing the cells for 3–7 days. Tartrate-resistant acid phosphatase (TRAP) staining was performed using an Acid Phosphatase, Leukocyte (TRAP) Kit (Sigma-Aldrich; St. Louis, MO, USA).

Constructs

PCR primers 5′- GATCAACTCGAGGTACACGGTGG GCTGAGTA and 5′- GATCAAGCGGCCGCCCGTG GCACTCAATCTTTTA were used to clone the wild-type 3′ untranslated region (UTR) of human INHBB. The PCR-amplified fragments were digested with XhoI and NotI and then inserted into the same sites of psiCHECK-2 reporter vector (Promega; Madison, WI, USA) downstream of the Renilla luciferase gene. PCR primers 5′- AATTGCGCCTTCCGAGCACACATAA**CTCAGAT**AA GACAGAGACGCAGAGA and 5′- CTCTCTCTCTCT GCGTCTCTGTCTT**ATCTGAG**TTATGTGTGCTCGGA AGG (mutated nucleotides underlined) were used to clone the miR-218-site-mutant of INHBB 3′UTR. Similarly, human Yin and Yang 1 (YY1) 3′UTR was cloned into psiCheck-2 vector using primers 5′-GATCAACTCGAGTT CTCGACCACGGGAAGCA, 5′-GATCAAGCGGCCGCT GAAATTAAGCTACTGGCACTCAA, and mutagenesis primers 5′-AAGAATATGGCAGAACAAGATCTGT**CTC AGAT**GTCTTATTTTCTTTTGTT and 5′-TCTGGACA ACAAAAGAAAATAAGA**CATCTGAG**ACAGATCTTGT TCTGCCA. The YY1 overexpression plasmid was constructed by cloning the full-length YY1 cDNA amplified by primers 5′-GATCAGAATTCATGGCCTCGGGCGAC A and 5′- AATAGGATCCTCACTGGTTGTTTTTGGCC

T from MDA-231 cells, and inserting the cDNA into the EcoRI/BamHI sites of pSG5 vector. All constructs were verified by sequencing.

EV purification and characterization

EVs secreted by MDA-MB-231 and derived cell lines were prepared as previously reported [7–9]. Conditioned medium was first collected after incubating cells in growth medium containing 10% EV-depleted FBS (prepared by overnight ultracentrifugation of medium-diluted FBS at 100,000 × g at 4 °C) for 48 h, and pre-cleared by centrifugation at 500 × g for 15 min and then at 10,000 × g for 20 min. EVs were isolated by ultracentrifugation at 110,000 × g for 70 min, and washed in PBS using the same ultracentrifugation conditions. When indicated, DiI (1,1′-Dioctadecyl-3,3,3′,3′-tetramethylindocarbocyanine perchlorate; Sigma-Aldrich) was added into the PBS at 1 µM and incubated for 20 min before the washing spin, followed by an additional wash to remove the excess dye. The pelleted EVs were resuspended in ~ 100 µl of PBS for cell treatment. For cell treatment, 2 µg of EVs (equivalent to those collected from ~ 5 × 10^6 producer cells) based on protein measurement using Pierce™ BCA protein assay kit (Thermo Fisher Scientific) were added to 2 × 10^5 recipient cells. For EV characterization, EVs were subjected to nanoparticle tracking analysis using a NanoSight NS300 (Malvern; Westborough, MA,USA), or further fractionated by gradient separation following a modified protocol [28]. EVs isolated by ultracentrifugation were loaded onto a 5-step OptiPrep (Sigma-Aldrich) gradient consisted of 40, 30, 20, 10, and 5% iodixanol in 20 mM Hepes (pH 7.2), 150 mM NaCl, 1 mM Na_3VO_4, and 50 mM NaF. After centrifugation in a SW 40 Ti rotor (Beckman Coulter; Indianapolis, IN, USA) at 110,000 × g at 4 °C for 16 h, 12 1-mL fractions were collected and washed in PBS by another spin at 110,000 × g for 70 min before Western analysis and RNA extraction for RT-qPCR.

RNA extraction and quantitative reverse transcription PCR

These procedures were performed as described previously [7–9]. Primers used in RT-qPCR are indicated in Additional file 2: Table S2. The miR-218, miR-140-3p (as internal control for miR-218 in EVs and sera), and U6 primers (as internal control for intracellular miR-218) were purchased from Qiagen (Valencia, CA, USA). An annealing temperature of 57.5 °C was used for all primers.

Western blot analysis

Protein extracts were separated by SDS-PAGE. Protein detection was performed using the following antibodies: Collagen alpha-1(I) chain carboxy-telopeptide (LF68) (Kerafast; Boston, MA, USA, ENH018), Inhibin βA (Novus, NBP1–30928), Inhibin βB (Thermo Fisher Scientific, PA5–28814), Inhibin α (Santa Cruz Biotechnology; Dallas, TX, USA, SC-22048), YY1 (Abcam; Cambridge, MA, USA, ab109228), Phospho-Smad2 (Ser465/467) (Cell Signaling Technology; Danvers, MA, USA, 3108S), SMAD2 (Cell Signaling Technology, 3122S), Phospho-Smad3 (Ser423/425) (Cell Signaling Technology, 9520S), SMAD3 (Cell Signaling Technology, 9523S), tissue inhibitor of metalloproteinases 3 (TIMP3) (Abcam, ab155749), β-actin (Sigma-Aldrich, A1978), as well as anti-rabbit, anti-mouse, and anti-goat HRP-conjugated secondary antibodies (Santa Cruz Biotechnology).

ELISA
Bone formation marker P1NP was detected by a rat/mouse P1NP enzyme immunoassay kit (Immunodiagnostic Systems; Boldons, UK). Bone resorption marker C-terminal telopeptide (CTX-1) was detected by a RatLaps EIA kit (Immunodiagnostic Systems).

Animals
All animal experiments were approved by the institutional animal care and use committee at the Beckman Research Institute of the City of Hope. Female NOD/SCID/IL2Rγ-null (NSG) mice of 6-month-old were used in this study. EVs from ~ 10^7 cancer cells were used to treat mice through tail vein injection with 27G needles twice a week for 4 weeks. Serum was collected 1 week after the last EV injection via retro-orbital bleeding.

smRNA-seq and RNA-seq
Illumina sequencing was performed by the City of Hope Integrative Genomics Core using RNA samples from patient sera, EVs from parental and bone-tropic MDA-231, and MDA-231 transduced with miR-218-overexpressing or control vector. For smRNA-seq, each serum sample was independently subjected to library preparation and deep sequencing. All small RNAs of 15–52 nts were selected and sequenced using the Hiseq 2500 system, following the manufacturer's protocol (Illumina; San Diego, CA, USA). Raw counts were normalized by trimmed mean of M value (TMM) method and differentially expressed miRNAs between patients with and without bone metastasis or between different cell lines were identified using Bioconductor package "edgeR". The miRNAs will be regarded as differentially expressed when their P values were less than 0.05, minimum expression value more than 50 and log2 fold change more than 1. For RNA-seq, poly(A) RNA was enriched and reverse-transcribed into cDNA, followed by end repair, A-tailing, and linker ligation. The ligated material was amplified by PCR and then analyzed on a HiSeq2500 (Illumina) for parallel sequencing. Sequences were aligned to human genome assembly hg19. Quantification of RefSeq mRNAs was performed using customized R scripts. Counts were normalized by TMM method and differential expression analysis was performed using Bioconductor package "edgeR".

Statistics
All quantitative data are presented as mean ± standard deviation (s.d.) unless stated otherwise. Two-sample two-tailed Student t tests were used for comparison of means of quantitative data between two groups. For multiple independent groups, one-way ANOVA with post hoc Tukey tests were used. Values of $P < 0.05$ were considered significant. Sample size was generally chosen based on preliminary data indicating the variance within each group and the differences between groups. All samples/animals that have received the proper procedures with confidence were included for the analyses. For experiments in which no quantification is shown, images representative of at least three independent experiments are shown.

Results
miR-218 is associated with breast cancer bone metastasis
To search for miRNAs that might be functionally relevant to breast cancer bone metastasis, we obtained sera from 47 stage IV breast cancer patients with ($n = 33$) or without ($n = 14$) bone metastases and performed small RNA sequencing. In addition, to identify miRNAs characteristically secreted by bone-metastasizing breast cancer cells, we profiled the miRNAs in the EVs secreted by the metastatic breast cancer cell line MDA-MB-231 (MDA-231) as well as its bone-seeking variant designated as MDA-231-bone [29]. hsa-miR-218-5p (miR-218) was significantly higher in the sera from patients with bone metastases compared to those without (Additional file 3: Table S3), and was > 5-fold higher in the EVs from MDA-231-bone cells compared to those from parental MDA-231 (Additional file 4: Table S4). These results were confirmed by qRT-PCR using a selected internal reference miR-140-3p, which was consistent among all serum samples tested and between EVs from the two cell lines based on the smRNA-seq data (Fig. 1a and b). In contrast, levels of circulating miR-218 were not significantly different when the same cohort of patients was stratified by the presence or absence of brain metastases (Fig. 1a, right panel). In addition, miR-218 was also expressed at a higher intracellular level in the bone-tropic MDA-231 cells compared to parental MDA-231 and the non-cancerous mammary epithelial cells MCF10A (Fig. 1b). Thus, we focused on miR-218 in the subsequent studies for its potential role in breast cancer bone metastasis.

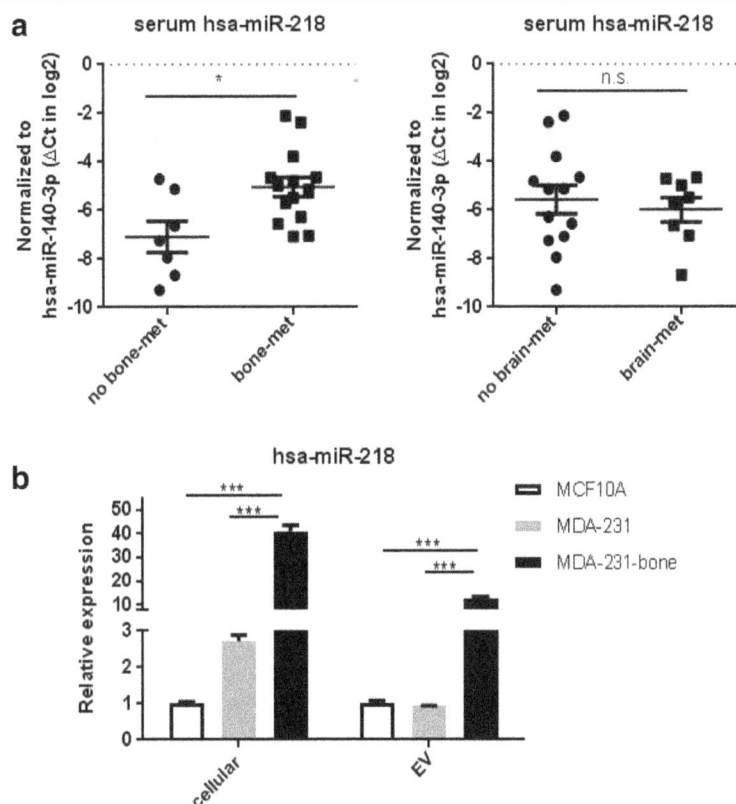

Fig. 1 miR-218 is associated with breast cancer bone metastasis. **a** Relative RNA level of miR-218 normalized to miR-140-3p in sera from stage IV breast cancer patients with or without bone metastases (bone-met) (*left panel*), or patients with or without brain metastases (brain-met) (*right panel*). *$P < 0.05$. n.s. not significant. **b** Relative RNA level of intracellular and EV miR-218 normalized to U6 and miR-140-3p, respectively, in indicated cell lines. ***$P < 0.001$

Cancer-secreted miR-218 directly targets *Col1a1* in preosteoblasts and decreases type I collagen secretion by differentiated osteoblasts

To determine the specific effects of miR-218 we established a stable cell line of MDA-231 that overexpresses miR-218 (MDA-231-miR-218) or control vector (MDA-231-miR-ctrl) (Fig. 2a). Compared to the control cells, the miR-218-overexpressing cells also secreted a higher level of miR-218 into the EVs. Upon density gradient fractionation of the EVs, miR-218 was found to be enriched in the fractions containing exosomes and with a density between ~ 1.10 and ~ 1.145 g/mL (Additional file 5: Figure S1). When fluorescently labeled EVs from MDA-231-miR-ctrl, MDA-231-miR-218, and MDA-231-bone were added to preosteoblast cells MC3T3, a high EV uptake efficiency was observed with all types of EVs (Fig. 2b). We also detected transfer of miR-218 into recipient MC3T3 cells upon EV treatment in the presence of an RNA polymerase II inhibitor DRB to block endogenous miR-218 transcription (Fig. 2c). *COL1A1* has been reported as a direct target of miR-218 in gastric cancer cells and human stellate cells [30, 31]. We found that *Col1a1*, but not collagen type I alpha 2 chain (*Col1a2*), was significantly downregulated by EVs from

the two high-miR-218-secreting cell lines at the mRNA level (Fig. 2d), and that this effect on type I collagen expression was more dramatic at the protein level (Fig. 2e). Consistent with the lower levels of all forms of type I collagen, the bone formation marker P1NP was also decreased in the conditioned medium (CM) from differentiated MC3T3 treated with high-miR-218 EVs (Fig. 2f). To test the effect of secreted miR-218 in vivo, we injected EVs from MDA-231-miR-ctrl or MDA-231-miR-218 into NSG mice through the tail vein twice a week for 4 weeks. The bone formation marker P1NP was significantly decreased in the serum from mice treated with MDA-231-miR-218 EVs, whereas the bone resorption marker CTX-1 was not affected (Fig. 2g and h). Taken together, cancer-secreted miR-218 encapsulated in the EVs downregulated type I collagen expression and deposition by osteoblasts. In comparison, breast cancer-secreted EVs were found incapable of regulating osteoclast differentiation (Additional file 6: Figure S2).

miR-218 regulates the expression of inhibin β subunits in breast cancer cells

To identify other genes regulated by miR-218, we performed RNA-seq to compare the gene expression profile

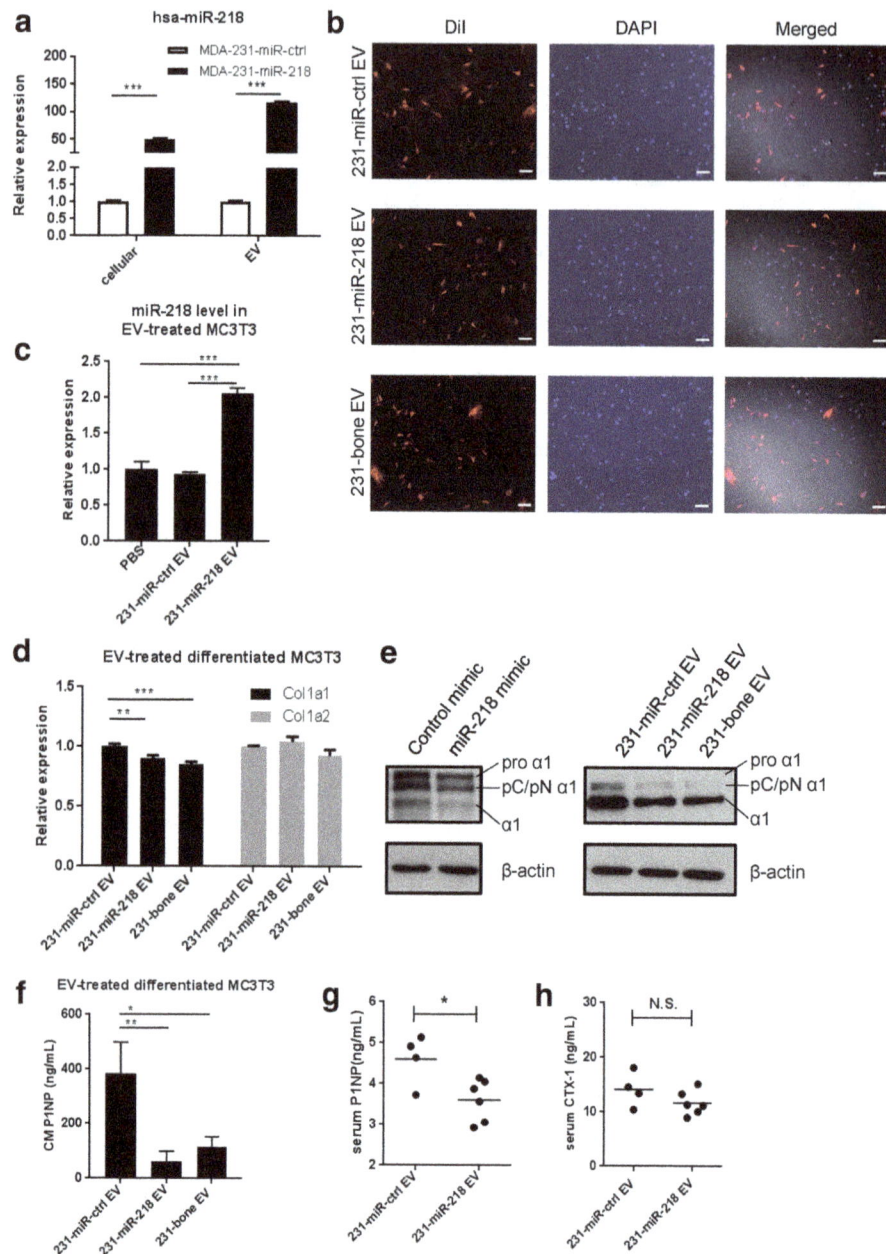

Fig. 2 EV miR-218 directly targets Col1a1 and downregulates type I collagen in differentiated MC3T3. **a** Relative RNA level of intracellular and EV miR-218 normalized to U6 and miR-140-3p, respectively, in indicated cell lines. ***$P < 0.001$. **b** DiI-labeled EV was used to treat MC3T3 cells seeded in a chamber slide for 48 h. Cells were fixed and imaged with fluorescent microscope Zeiss Observer II. Scale bar indicates 100 μm. **c** Relative RNA level of miR-218 normalized to U6 in MC3T3 cells treated with indicated EV or PBS for 24 h in the presence of 10 μM DRB (5,6-dichloro-1-β -D-ribofuranosylbenzimidazole). **d** Relative RNA level of Col1a1, Col1a2 normalized to Actb in differentiated MC3T3 cells treated with indicated EVs. Osteoblast differentiation medium with EV was replenished every 3 to 4 days for 16 days. ***$P < 0.001$. **e** Western blot analyses of type I collagen in the CM from EV-treated differentiated MC3T3 at day 18. CM of miR-218 mimic-transfected differentiated MC3T3 was also examined. The top band (pro α1), second band (pC/pN α1) and third band (α1) indicates type I procollagen, type I procollagen with either N′ terminus or C′ terminus cleaved, and mature type I collagen with both N′ and C′ termini cleaved, respectively. Cellular β-actin was used as control. **f** P1NP in CM collected from EV-treated differentiated MC3T3 at day 3 was measured by ELISA. *$P < 0.05$. **g** and **h** Bone formation marker P1NP (**g**) and bone resorption marker CTX-1 (**h**) in the sera from EV-treated mice were measured by ELISA. *$P < 0.05$; n.s. not significant

in MDA-231-miR-ctrl and MDA-231-miR-218 cells. Among the genes showing significantly different expression between the two cell lines, we found that inhibin beta A subunit (INHBA) was upregulated and inhibin beta B subunit (INHBB) downregulated by miR-218 overexpression (Additional file 7: Table S5). This was also observed at both mRNA and protein levels in parental MDA-231 cells upon transient transfection of a miR-218 mimic (Fig. 3a and b). Similar results were observed in another breast cancer cell line MCF-7, where miR-218 also upregulated INHBA but downregulated INHBB expression (Additional file 8: Figure S3a). In contrast, transfection of an antagomiR against miR-218 into MDA-231 bone cells led to a lower mRNA level of INHBA and a higher level of INHBB (Fig. 3c). Since INHBB is predicted to be a direct target of miR-218 by TargetScan (Fig. 3d), we performed dual luciferase reporter assay using psiCheck2 vector to confirm that the 3'UTR of INHBB containing the wild-type, but not mutated, miR-218 binding site responded to miR-218

(Fig. 3e). In search of the mechanism through which INHBA was upregulated by miR-218, we focused on *YY1*, a transcriptional repressor that is also a putative miR-218 target (Fig. 3d) and has been associated with Inhba expression in ovaries [32]. *YY1* mRNA was downregulated by miR-218 in MDA-231 cells (Fig. 3f). Ectopic expression of YY1 abolished the effect of miR-218 on inducing inhibin βA (Fig. 3g). Furthermore, dual luciferase assay revealed that *YY1* was directly targeted by miR-218 through the predicted binding site in the 3'UTR (Fig. 3h). Thus, miR-218 regulates the expression of two TGFβ superfamily cytokines in breast cancer cells by directly targeting *YY1* and *INHBB*.

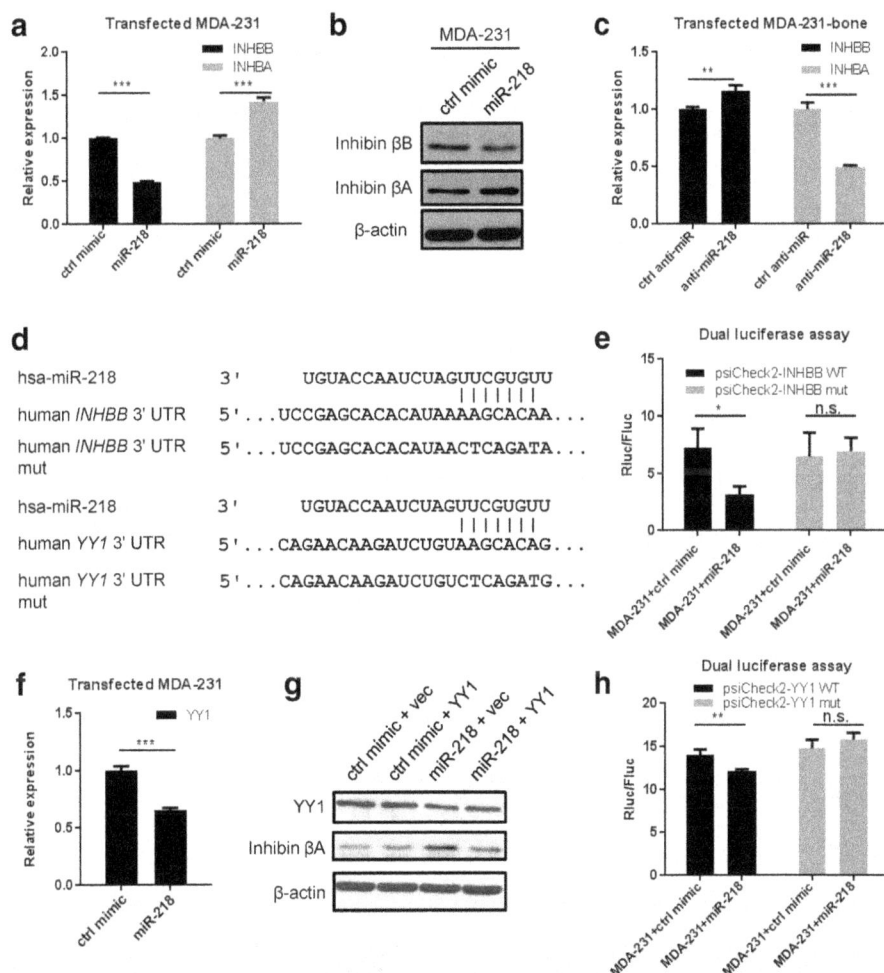

Fig. 3 miR-218 directly targets INHBB and YY1, and increases INHBA expression. **a** Relative RNA level of INHBB and INHBA normalized to 18S in MDA-231 transfected with miR-218 or control miRNA mimic at 24 h and 72 h, respectively. ***$P < 0.001$. **b** Western blot analyses of inhibin βB and inhibin βA in mimic-transfected MDA-231 cells at 48 h. **c** Relative RNA level of INHBB and INHBA normalized to 18S in MDA-231-bone transfected with anti-miR-218 or control antagomiR at 24 h and 48 h, respectively.. **$P < 0.01$; ***$P < 0.001$. **d** Sequence alignment of miR-218 and its predicted targets INHBB and YY1. **e** psiCheck2 reporter plasmids and miR-218 mimic or its corresponding control were transfected into indicated cell lines. Renilla and firefly luciferase activity was measured at 48 h. *$P < 0.05$; n.s. not significant. **f** Relative RNA level of YY1 normalized to 18S in mimic-transfected MDA-231 cells at 24 h. ***$P < 0.001$. **g** Western blot analyses of YY1 and inhibin βA in MDA-231 cells co-transfected with miR-218 mimic and YY1-overexpressing plasmid, or the corresponding controls at 72 h. **h** psiCheck2 reporter plasmids and miR-218 mimic or its corresponding control vector were transfected into MDA-231 cells. Renilla and firefly luciferase activity was measured at 48 h. **$P < 0.01$; n.s. not significant

Cancer-secreted inhibin βA regulates SMAD2/3 signaling differently in cancer and preosteoblast cells

We continued to test how miR-218-mediated differential expression of inhibin β subunits in breast cancer cells potentially influences the surrounding cancer cells and preosteoblasts to respectively establish autocrine and paracrine signaling. We treated serum-starved MDA-231 or MC3T3 with EV-depleted CM collected from miR-218-transfected MDA-231 cells or anti-miR-218-transfected MDA-231-bone cells. To our surprise, CM from miR-218-overexpressing breast cancer cells induced SMAD2/3 phosphorylation in MDA-231 cells (Fig. 4a), whereas the same CM treatment to MC3T3 cells suppressed the level of phospho-SMAD2/3 (Fig. 4b). Similarly, CM from miR-218-overexpressing MCF-7 cells also induced SMAD2 phosphorylation in untransfected MCF-7 cells (Additional file 8: Figure S3b). Conversely,

anti-miR inhibition of miR-218 in CM-producing MDA-231-bone cells led to reduction of SMAD2/3 phosphorylation in cancer cells (Fig. 4a) and de-repression of SMAD2/3 signaling in preosteoblasts (Fig. 4b) at the 2-h time point.

To explain the differential response of SMAD signaling in cancer or bone stromal cells to CM from breast cancer cells with varying levels of miR-218, we concentrated the CM from MDA-231 cells and found that the inhibin βA subunit was secreted at a higher level by miR-218-transfected MDA-231 cells compared to control group while inhibin βB was undetectable in the concentrated CM (Fig. 4c). Moreover, we also detected increased secretion of activin A in the CM from MDA-231 cells transfected with miR-218 (Fig. 4d). Interestingly, concentrated CM from MC3T3 preosteoblast cells contained inhibin α subunits (Fig. 4e), which was not expressed by

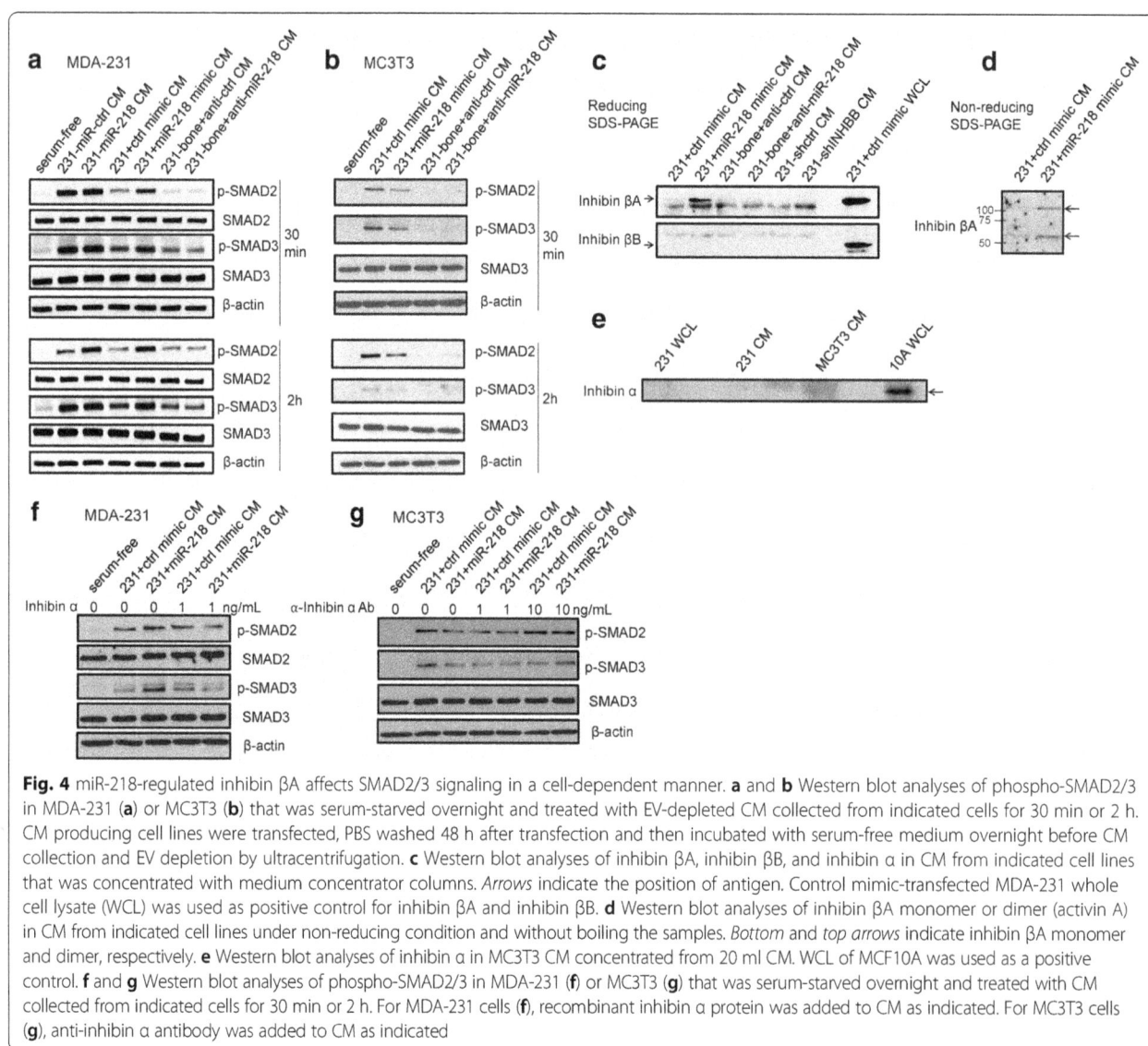

Fig. 4 miR-218-regulated inhibin βA affects SMAD2/3 signaling in a cell-dependent manner. **a** and **b** Western blot analyses of phospho-SMAD2/3 in MDA-231 (**a**) or MC3T3 (**b**) that was serum-starved overnight and treated with EV-depleted CM collected from indicated cells for 30 min or 2 h. CM producing cell lines were transfected, PBS washed 48 h after transfection and then incubated with serum-free medium overnight before CM collection and EV depletion by ultracentrifugation. **c** Western blot analyses of inhibin βA, inhibin βB, and inhibin α in CM from indicated cell lines that was concentrated with medium concentrator columns. *Arrows* indicate the position of antigen. Control mimic-transfected MDA-231 whole cell lysate (WCL) was used as positive control for inhibin βA and inhibin βB. **d** Western blot analyses of inhibin βA monomer or dimer (activin A) in CM from indicated cell lines under non-reducing condition and without boiling the samples. *Bottom* and *top arrows* indicate inhibin βA monomer and dimer, respectively. **e** Western blot analyses of inhibin α in MC3T3 CM concentrated from 20 ml CM. WCL of MCF10A was used as a positive control. **f** and **g** Western blot analyses of phospho-SMAD2/3 in MDA-231 (**f**) or MC3T3 (**g**) that was serum-starved overnight and treated with CM collected from indicated cells for 30 min or 2 h. For MDA-231 cells (**f**), recombinant inhibin α protein was added to CM as indicated. For MC3T3 cells (**g**), anti-inhibin α antibody was added to CM as indicated

MDA-231 or MCF-7 breast cancer cells (Additional file 7: Table S5, Fig. 4e, Additional file 8: Figure S3c). We thereby hypothesized that the presence of inhibin α in the environment led to a functional switch of cancer-secreted inhibin βA from activin-mediated SMAD2/3 activation to inhibin-mediated suppression. Indeed, addition of recombinant inhibin α into the CM from miR-218-overexpressing cells reversed the activation of SMAD2/3 phosphorylation in recipient cancer cells (Fig. 4f), whereas adding neutralizing antibody against inhibin α into the CM to treat MC3T3 cells led to de-repression of SMAD2/3 signaling (Fig. 4g). Therefore, secreted inhibin βA, which is upregulated by miR-218 in breast cancer cells, autocrinally activates SMAD signaling in MDA-231 cancer cells but paracrinally represses this pathway in bone stromal cells, due to the different expression status of inhibin α in the environment.

Paracrinal inhibin βA controls type I collagen processing of differentiating osteoblasts by regulating Timp3 expression

We next examined the downstream effect of cancer-secreted inhibin βA on preosteoblasts. Tissue inhibitor of metalloproteinases 3 (TIMP3) has been shown to inhibit the activity of ADAMTS2, which is the processing enzyme of type I procollagen during osteoblast differentiation [33]. We found that Timp3 was upregulated in differentiating MC3T3 cells following the treatment with EV-depleted CM from miR-218-overexpressing MDA-231 cells, and was downregulated when miR-218 was inhibited in CM-producing cells (Fig. 5a and b). As a result, the processing of type I procollagen was suppressed during osteoblast differentiation when miR-218 level was high in breast cancer cells, and vice versa (Fig. 5a). To confirm that this effect was caused by higher level of inhibin βA in the CM from miR-218-overexpressing MDA-231 cells, which contributed to the upregulation of Timp3 expression, we added neutralizing antibody against inhibin βA into the CM and detected restoration of Timp3 level in differentiating MC3T3 (Fig. 5c and d). Taken together, we show that paracrinal inhibin βA secretion by breast cancer cells, which is regulated by miR-218, alters the processing of procollagen during osteoblast differentiation through regulating Timp3 expression.

Discussion

Bone matrix is composed of inorganic and organic materials deposited and mineralized mainly by osteoblasts. Of the organic components of the bone matrix, 90% are type I collagen [16]. During osteoblast differentiation, type I procollagen is expressed and secreted into the bone matrix where ADAMTS2 and BMP1 cleave the N′- and C′-terminus of procollagen, respectively, to generate mature collagens before they are crosslinked and stabilized [17]. Due to the abundance of type I collagen and the importance of its processing in bone formation, P1NP is one of the most commonly used marker for bone formation [18]. Our study identified miR-218 as a miRNA associated with breast cancer bone metastasis, which can inhibit the deposition of type I collagen through two mechanisms (Fig. 5e): (1) miR-218 secretion into the EVs and transfer to osteoblasts during differentiation, where miR-218 directly downregulates COL1A1 expression; (2) direct targeting of YY1 in cancer cells to induce inhibin βA expression and secretion, which then represses procollagen processing by inducing TIMP3, an inhibitor of the N-procollagenase ADAMTS2.

The first mechanism could be initiated at an early tumor stage before bone metastasis occurs, as miR-218-containing EVs secreted by breast cancer cells in situ could travel through the blood stream to the bone environment where miR-218 could exert its effect on osteoblasts after being taken up. The second mechanism would require close proximity of cancer cells and osteoblasts because a previous study has shown that most circulating activins are bound by their endogenous antagonist follistatin [34]. However, several studies found that serum activin A level was elevated in patients with breast cancer bone metastasis [35, 36], indicating a possible long-range effect of activin A on bone cells including osteoblasts. These two mechanisms, acting both distantly and locally, might have synergistic effects on the inhibition of collagen deposition and bone formation, thereby undermining the quality of newly formed bone. Considering the large amount of collagen within the bone environment, the blockade of collagen deposition by miR-218 might require time to take effect on bone formation and breast cancer bone metastasis. Therefore, miR-218 may be insufficient to induce bone metastasis by itself but may facilitate other cancer-autonomous mechanisms to promote breast cancer bone metastasis.

Our study shows that secreted inhibin βA regulates SMAD2/3 signaling in cancer cells and osteoblasts in opposite directions, which is dependent on the absence or presence of inhibin α subunit. We show that inhibin βA, when encountering inhibin α to form inhibin A, inhibits phosphorylation of SMAD2/3 in osteoblasts, and thereby blocks an important function of these cells by inducing the expression and secretion of TIMP3. As for the consequences of SMAD2/3 activation in cancer cells, a study has reported intense immunohistochemical staining of phosphorylated SMAD2 in metastatic breast tumors in the bone and that knockdown of SMAD4, the downstream effector of activated SMAD2/3, was able to decrease bone metastasis of breast cancer in mice [37]. On the other hand, activin A has been shown to inhibit breast cancer proliferation [38]. Therefore, it is possible

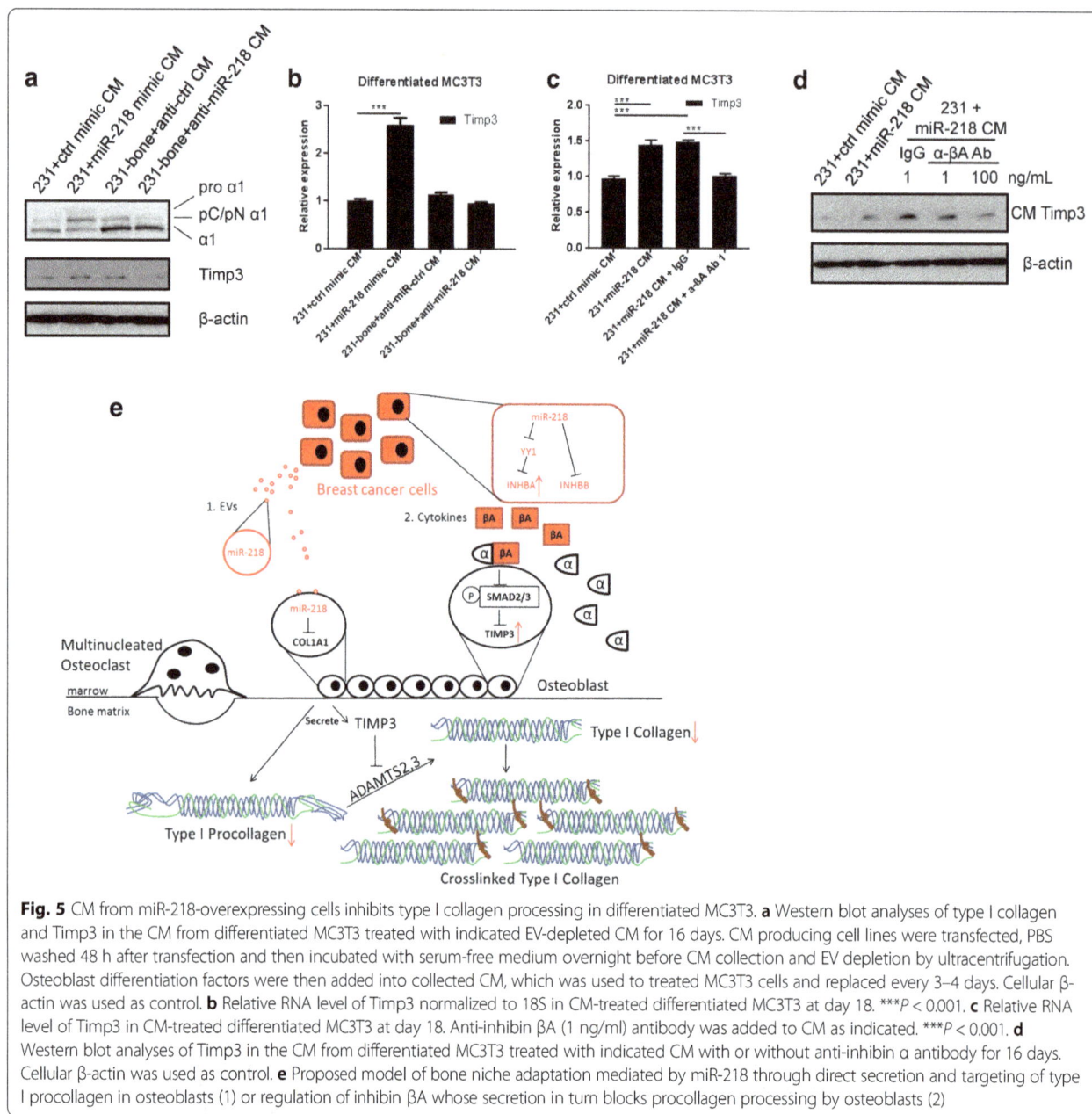

Fig. 5 CM from miR-218-overexpressing cells inhibits type I collagen processing in differentiated MC3T3. **a** Western blot analyses of type I collagen and Timp3 in the CM from differentiated MC3T3 treated with indicated EV-depleted CM for 16 days. CM producing cell lines were transfected, PBS washed 48 h after transfection and then incubated with serum-free medium overnight before CM collection and EV depletion by ultracentrifugation. Osteoblast differentiation factors were then added into collected CM, which was used to treated MC3T3 cells and replaced every 3–4 days. Cellular β-actin was used as control. **b** Relative RNA level of Timp3 normalized to 18S in CM-treated differentiated MC3T3 at day 18. ***$P < 0.001$. **c** Relative RNA level of Timp3 in CM-treated differentiated MC3T3 at day 18. Anti-inhibin βA (1 ng/ml) antibody was added to CM as indicated. ***$P < 0.001$. **d** Western blot analyses of Timp3 in the CM from differentiated MC3T3 treated with indicated CM with or without anti-inhibin α antibody for 16 days. Cellular β-actin was used as control. **e** Proposed model of bone niche adaptation mediated by miR-218 through direct secretion and targeting of type I procollagen in osteoblasts (1) or regulation of inhibin βA whose secretion in turn blocks procollagen processing by osteoblasts (2)

that the formation of inhibin A in the bone microenvironment, as a result of osteoblast-derived inhibin α, could alleviate or even reverse the growth inhibitory effect of activin A in the outer layer of tumor mass growing in the bone. Together, increased secretion of inhibin βA might promote breast cancer bone metastasis by regulating SMAD signaling differently in cancer and bone stromal cells.

A recent study on miR-218 also implicated this miRNA in breast cancer metastasis [39]. It also found that miR-218 level was higher in breast cancer metastasized to the bone. In consistent with this, we show that miR-218 is not only overexpressed in bone-tropic breast cancer cells,

but also more abundant in EVs from these cells as well as in the sera from breast cancer patients with bone metastases. Mechanistically, this previous study found that miR-218 directly targeted Wnt inhibitors to promote PTHrP expression, which in turn stimulated osteoclastogenesis and osteolytic bone lesion. Another study on miR-218 suggested that this miRNA had a role in the induction of osteomimicry phenotype of breast cancer cells [40]. Therefore, it is possible that miR-218 contributes to a pro-metastatic bone environment through regulating the function of both osteoclasts and osteoblasts, thereby tilting the balance towards osteoclast-mediated bone resorption and providing a permissive environment for cancer growth in the bone. Based on the association between miR-218 and breast cancer bone metastasis, it would be of interest to test the possibility of using miR-218 as a diagnostic and/or prognostic marker for the disease.

Conclusions

In summary, our study showed that miR-218, which exhibited higher levels in the blood of breast cancer patients with bone metastases, and which was overexpressed and highly secreted by bone-tropic MDA-MB-231 breast cancer cells, could contribute to the adaption of bone niche. Cancer cell-secreted miR-218 directly downregulated type I collagen expression by osteoblasts, whereas intracellular miR-218 in breast cancer cells elevated inhibin βA expression, whose secretion in turn inhibited the processing of type I collagen during collagen deposition and osteoblast differentiation. Together, compromised collagen deposition might further enhance the vicious cycle of osteolysis and thereby facilitate other cancer-autonomous mechanisms to promote breast cancer colonization in the bone environment.

Additional files

Additional file 1: Table S1. Clinical characteristics of the patients. (XLSX 23 kb)

Additional file 2: Table S2. Sequences of the PCR primers. (XLSX 9 kb)

Additional file 3: Table S3. miRNAs detected in patient sera. (XLSX 122 kb)

Additional file 4: Table S4. Cellular and EV miRNAs detected in MDA-231-bone and parental MDA-231 cells. (XLSX 128 kb)

Additional file 5: Figure S1. EV characterization. **a** EVs pelleted at 110,000 × g were analyzed by nanoparticle tracking analysis. **b** Density measurement and Western blot of EV fractions collected from indicated cell lines to detect EV markers. **c** Density measurement and RT-qPCR of EV fractions collected from indicated cell lines to detect miR-218 levels. (PDF 1060 kb)

Additional file 6: Figure S2. Breast cancer-secreted EVs did not regulate osteoclast differentiation. Mouse bone marrow cells were cultured in 40 ng/ml M-CSF for 3 days before EV treatment and further induction of osteoclast differentiation with 40 ng/ml M-CSF and 100 ng/ml RANKL for up to 7 days. **a** Representative TRAP staining images of EV-treated osteoclasts after 7 days of differentiation. **b** Quantitative analysis of TRAP staining in (**a**). Mature osteoclasts were identified as multinucleated TRAP$^+$ cells. **c** Relative RNA level of osteoclast differentiation marker genes *Trap* and *Ctsk* normalized to *Rpl19* in primary pre-osteoclast cells treated with indicated EVs and induced for osteoclast differentiation for 5 days. (PDF 318 kb)

Additional file 7: Table S5. Gene expression in MDA-231-miR-218 and MDA-231-miR-ctrl cells. (XLSX 1093 kb)

Additional file 8: Figure S3. miR-218 regulated inhibin β expression and enhanced SMAD signaling in MCF-7 cells. **a** Western blot analyses of inhibin βB and inhibin βA in miRNA mimic-transfected MCF-7 cells at 48 h after transfection. **b** Western blot analyses of phospho-SMAD2/3 in MCF-7 cells that were serum-starved overnight and then treated with CM collected from indicated cells for 30 min. The CM-producing cells were transfected, PBS washed at 48 h after transfection, and then incubated with serum-free medium overnight before CM collection. **c** Western blot analysis of inhibin α in MCF-7 cells. WCL of MCF10A was used as a positive control. (PDF 145 kb)

Abbreviations

ADAMTS2: A disintegrin-like and metalloprotease with thrombospondin type 1 motif, 2; BMPs: Bone morphogenetic proteins; CM: Conditioned medium; COL1A1: Collagen type I alpha 1 chain; COL1A2: Collagen type I alpha 2 chain; CTX-1: C-terminal telopeptide; CXCR4: C-X-C chemokine receptor type 4; DiI: 1,1'-Dioctadecyl-3,3,3',3'-tetramethylindocarbocyanine perchlorate; DRB: 5,6-dichloro-1-β -D-ribofuranosylbenzimidazole; EV: Extracellular vesicle; IL: Interleukin; INHBA: Inhibin beta A subunit; INHBB: Inhibin beta B subunit; MARCKS: Myristoylated alanine rich protein kinase C substrate; M-CSF: Macrophage colony-stimulating factor; MDA-231: MDA-MB-231; miRNA: microRNA; NSG: NOD-scid IL2Rgamma(null); OPG: Osteoprotegerin; P1NP: Procollagen type 1 amino terminal propeptide; PTHrP: Parathyroid hormone-related protein; RANKL: Receptor activator of nuclear factor kappa-B ligand; SMAD: Mothers against DPP homolog; TGF-β: Transforming growth factor beta; TIMP3: Tissue inhibitor of metalloproteinases 3; TRAP: Tartrate-resistant acid phosphatase; UTR: Untranslated region; YY1: Yin and Yang 1

Acknowledgements
We thank Drs. Marcin Kortylewski, Ching-cheng Chen, and Vu Ngo for valuable suggestions.

Funding
This work was supported by the National Institutes of Health (NIH)/National Cancer Institute (NCI) grants to SEW. (R01CA206911 and R01CA218140). Research reported in this publication included work performed in Core facilities supported by the NIH/NCI under grant number P30CA23100 (UCSD Cancer Center) and P30CA33572 (City of Hope Cancer Center).

Authors' contributions
SEW, XL and MP conceived ideas, and WCC contributed to project planning. XL and SEW designed and performed most of the experiments. MC and MYF assisted with cell line construction and mouse experiments. MYF and WY assisted with Western blot analysis. XW and AL assisted with RNA-seq and data analyses. XL and SEW wrote the manuscript. All authors read and approved the final manuscript.

Competing interests
The authors declare that they have no competing interests.

Author details
[1]Department of Pathology, University of California San Diego, 9500 Gilman Drive, La Jolla, CA 92093-0612, USA. [2]City of Hope Irell & Manella Graduate School of Biological Sciences, Duarte, CA 91010, USA. [3]Cancer Prevention Movement, Arcadia, CA 91006, USA. [4]Department of Molecular and Cellular Biology, Beckman Research Institute of the City of Hope, Duarte, CA 91010, USA. [5]Division of Biostatistics, Beckman Research Institute of the City of Hope, Duarte, CA 91010, USA. [6]Department of Cancer Biology, Beckman Research Institute of the City of Hope, Duarte, CA 91010, USA. [7]Department of Pathology, City of Hope National Medical Center, Duarte, CA 91010, USA.

References
1. Paget S. The distribution of secondary growths in cancer of the breast. 1889. Cancer Metastasis Rev. 1989;8(2):98–101.
2. Kang Y, Siegel PM, Shu W, Drobnjak M, Kakonen SM, Cordón-Cardo C, Guise TA, Massagué J. A multigenic program mediating breast cancer metastasis to bone. Cancer Cell. 2003;3(6):537–49.
3. Brenner S, Whiting-Theobald N, Kawai T, Linton GF, Rudikoff AG, Choi U, Ryser MF, Murphy PM, Sechler JM, Malech HL. CXCR4-transgene expression significantly improves marrow engraftment of cultured hematopoietic stem cells. Stem Cells. 2004;22(7):1128–33.
4. Lu X, Kang Y. Organotropism of breast cancer metastasis. J Mammary Gland Biol Neoplasia. 2007;12(2–3):153–62.
5. Weilbaecher KN, Guise TA, McCauley LK. Cancer to bone: a fatal attraction. Nat Rev Cancer. 2011;11(6):411–25.

6. Valadi H, Ekström K, Bossios A, Sjöstrand M, Lee JJ, Lötvall JO. Exosome-mediated transfer of mRNAs and microRNAs is a novel mechanism of genetic exchange between cells. Nat Cell Biol. 2007;9(6):654–9.

7. Fong MY, Zhou W, Liu L, Alontaga AY, Chandra M, Ashby J, Chow A, O'Connor STF, Li S, Chin AR. Breast-cancer-secreted miR-122 reprograms glucose metabolism in premetastatic niche to promote metastasis. Nat Cell Biol. 2015;17(2):183–94.

8. Zhou W, Fong MY, Min Y, Somlo G, Liu L, Palomares MR, Yu Y, Chow A, O'Connor STF, Chin AR. Cancer-secreted miR-105 destroys vascular endothelial barriers to promote metastasis. Cancer Cell. 2014;25(4):501–15.

9. Yan W, Wu X, Zhou W, Fong MY, Cao M, Liu J, Liu X, Chen C-H, Fadare O, Pizzo DP. Cancer-cell-secreted exosomal miR-105 promotes tumour growth through the MYC-dependent metabolic reprogramming of stromal cells. Nat Cell Biol. 2018;20(5):597.

10. Kahlert C, Kalluri R. Exosomes in tumor microenvironment influence cancer progression and metastasis. J Mol Med (Berl). 2013;91(4):431–7.

11. Ono M, Kosaka N, Tominaga N, Yoshioka Y, Takeshita F, Takahashi R-u, Yoshida M, Tsuda H, Tamura K, Ochiya T. Exosomes from bone marrow mesenchymal stem cells contain a microRNA that promotes dormancy in metastatic breast cancer cells. Sci Signal. 2014;7(332):63.

12. Hoshino A, Costa-Silva B, Shen T-L, Rodrigues G, Hashimoto A, Mark MT, Molina H, Kohsaka S, Di Giannatale A, Ceder S. Tumour exosome integrins determine organotropic metastasis. Nature. 2015;527(7578):329–35.

13. Sims NA, Gooi JH. Bone remodeling: Multiple cellular interactions required for coupling of bone formation and resorption. Semin Cell Dev Biol. 2008; 19(5):444-51. (https://doi.org/10.1016/j.semcdb.2008.07.016; https://www.ncbi.nlm.nih.gov/pubmed/18718546).

14. Teitelbaum SL. Bone resorption by osteoclasts. Science. 2000;289(5484):1504–8.

15. Sims NA, Martin TJ. Coupling the activities of bone formation and resorption: a multitude of signals within the basic multicellular unit. Bonekey Rep. 2014;3:481.

16. Hlaing TT, Compston JE. Biochemical markers of bone turnover - uses and limitations. Ann Clin Biochem. 2014;51(Pt 2):189–202.

17. Bekhouche M, Colige A. The procollagen N-proteinases ADAMTS2, 3 and 14 in pathophysiology. Matrix Biol. 2015;44:46–53.

18. Ferreira A, Alho I, Casimiro S, Costa L. Bone remodeling markers and bone metastases: From cancer research to clinical implications. Bonekey Rep. 2015;4:668.

19. Janssens K, ten Dijke P, Janssens S, Van Hul W. Transforming growth factor-beta1 to the bone. Endocr Rev. 2005;26(6):743–74.

20. Galvin RJS, Gatlin CL, Horn JW, Fuson TR. TGF-β enhances osteoclast differentiation in hematopoietic cell cultures stimulated with RANKL and M-CSF. Biochem Biophys Res Commun. 1999;265(1):233–9.

21. Shinar DM, Rodan GA. Biphasic effects of transforming growth factor-β on the production of osteoclast-like cells in mouse bone marrow cultures: the role of prostaglandins in the generation of these cells. Endocrinology. 1990; 126(6):3153–8.

22. Tang Y, Wu X, Lei W, Pang L, Wan C, Shi Z, Zhao L, Nagy TR, Peng X, Hu J. TGF-β1–induced migration of bone mesenchymal stem cells couples bone resorption with formation. Nat Med. 2009;15(7):757–65.

23. Wang RN, Green J, Wang Z, Deng Y, Qiao M, Peabody M, Zhang Q, Ye J, Yan Z, Denduluri S. Bone Morphogenetic Protein (BMP) signaling in development and human diseases. Gene Dis. 2014;1(1):87–105.

24. Stenvers KL, Findlay JK. Inhibins: from reproductive hormones to tumor suppressors. Trends Endocrinol Metab. 2010;21(3):174–80.

25. Chantry AD, Heath D, Mulivor AW, Pearsall S, Baud'huin M, Coulton L, Evans H, Abdul N, Werner ED, Bouxsein ML. Inhibiting activin-A signaling stimulates bone formation and prevents cancer-induced bone destruction in vivo. J Bone Miner Res. 2010;25(12):2633–46.

26. Wu X, Somlo G, Yu Y, Palomares MR, Li AX, Zhou W, Chow A, Yen Y, Rossi JJ, Gao H, et al. De novo sequencing of circulating miRNAs identifies novel markers predicting clinical outcome of locally advanced breast cancer. J Transl Med. 2012;10:42.

27. Tsuyada A, Chow A, Wu J, Somlo G, Chu P, Loera S, Luu T, Li X, Wu X, Ye W. CCL2 mediates crosstalk between cancer cells and stromal fibroblasts that regulates breast cancer stem cells. Cancer Res. 2012;3567:2011.

28. Kowal J, Arras G, Colombo M, Jouve M, Morath JP, Primdal-Bengtson B, Dingli F, Loew D, Tkach M, Thery C. Proteomic comparison defines novel markers to characterize heterogeneous populations of extracellular vesicle subtypes. Proc Natl Acad Sci U S A. 2016;113(8):E968–77.

29. Yoneda T, Williams PJ, Hiraga T, Niewolna M, Nishimura R. A bone-seeking clone exhibits different biological properties from the MDA-MB-231 parental human breast cancer cells and a brain-seeking clone in vivo and in vitro. J Bone Miner Res. 2001;16(8):1486–95.

30. Zhang Y, Peng Z, Chen L. Co-regulation of miR-143, miR-218 and miR-338-3pin inhibits gastric cancer migration and invasion by targeting collagen type I. Int J Clin Exp Pathol. 2016;9(6):6127–35.

31. Ogawa T, Iizuka M, Sekiya Y, Yoshizato K, Ikeda K, Kawada N. Suppression of type I collagen production by microRNA-29b in cultured human stellate cells. Biochem Biophys Res Commun. 2010;391(1):316–21.

32. Griffith GJ, Trask MC, Hiller J, Walentuk M, Pawlak JB, Tremblay KD, Mager J. Yin-yang1 is required in the mammalian oocyte for follicle expansion. Biol Reprod. 2011;84(4):654–63.

33. Wang W-M, Ge G, Lim N, Nagase H, Greenspan DS. TIMP-3 inhibits the procollagen N-proteinase ADAMTS-2. Biochem J. 2006;398(3):515–9.

34. Welt C, Sidis Y, Keutmann H, Schneyer A. Activins, inhibins, and follistatins: from endocrinology to signaling. A paradigm for the new millennium. Exp Biol Med. 2002;227(9):724–52.

35. Leto G, Incorvaia L, Badalamenti G, Tumminello FM, Gebbia N, Flandina C, Crescimanno M, Rini G. Activin A circulating levels in patients with bone metastasis from breast or prostate cancer. Clin Exp Metastasis. 2006;23(2):117–22.

36. Reis FM, Cobellis L, Tameirao LC, Anania G, Luisi S, Silva IS, Gioffre W, Di Blasio AM, Petraglia F. Serum and tissue expression of activin a in postmenopausal women with breast cancer. J Clin Endocrinol Metab. 2002;87(5):2277–82.

37. Kang Y, He W, Tulley S, Gupta GP, Serganova I, Chen C-R, Manova-Todorova K, Blasberg R, Gerald WL, Massagué J. Breast cancer bone metastasis mediated by the Smad tumor suppressor pathway. Proc Natl Acad Sci U S A. 2005;102(39): 13909–14.

38. Burdette JE, Jeruss JS, Kurley SJ, Lee EJ, Woodruff TK. Activin A mediates growth inhibition and cell cycle arrest through Smads in human breast cancer cells. Cancer Res. 2005;65(17):7968–75.

39. Taipaleenmäki H, Farina NH, van Wijnen AJ, Stein JL, Hesse E, Stein GS, Lian JB. Antagonizing miR-218-5p attenuates Wnt signaling and reduces metastatic bone disease of triple negative breast cancer cells. Oncotarget. 2016;7(48):79032.

40. Hassan MQ, Maeda Y, Taipaleenmaki H, Zhang W, Jafferji M, Gordon JA, Li Z, Croce CM, Van Wijnen AJ, Stein JL. miR-218 directs a Wnt signaling circuit to promote differentiation of osteoblasts and osteomimicry of metastatic cancer cells. J Biol Chem. 2012;287(50):42084–92.

Permissions

List of Contributors

Hao-Ching Hsiao, Xuejun Fan, Robert E. Jordan, Ningyan Zhang and Zhiqiang An
Texas Therapeutics Institute, Brown Foundation Institute of Molecular Medicine, the University of Texas Health Science Center at Houston, 1825 Pressler St., Suite 532, Houston, TX 77030, USA

Tian Du, Matthew J. Sikora, Kevin M. Levine, Nilgun Tasdemir, Stacy G. Wendell, Bennett Van Houten and Steffi Oesterreich
Women's Cancer Research Center, UPMC Hillman Cancer Institute, Magee Womens Research Institute, 204 Craft Avenue, Pittsburgh, PA 15213, USA

Tian Du
School of Medicine, Tsinghua University, Beijing 100084, China

Matthew J. Sikora
Department of Pathology, University of Colorado Anschutz Medical Campus, Aurora, CO 80045, USA

Kevin M. Levine
Department of Pathology, University of Pittsburgh, Pittsburgh, PA 15213, USA

Nilgun Tasdemir, Stacy G. Wendell, Bennett Van Houten and Steffi Oesterreich
Department of Pharmacology and Chemical Biology, University of Pittsburgh, Pittsburgh, PA 15213, USA

Rebecca B. Riggins
Department of Oncology, Georgetown-Lombardi Comprehensive Cancer Center, Georgetown University Medical Center, Washington, DC 20057, USA

Cecilia W. Huo, Grace Chew, Michael A. Henderson and Erik W. Thompson
Department of Surgery, St. Vincent's Hospital, University of Melbourne,Melbourne, Australia

Prue Hill
Department of Pathology, St Vincent's Hospital, Melbourne, Australia

Paul J. Neeson
Pathology Department, University of Melbourne, Melbourne, Australia

Paul J. Neeson, Heloise Halse, Michael A. Henderson and Kara L. Britt
Peter MacCallum Cancer Centre, Melbourne, Australia

Elizabeth D. Williams and Erik W. Thompson
Institute of Health and Biomedical Innovation and School of Biomedical Sciences, Queensland University of Technology, Brisbane, Australia
Translational Research Institute, Brisbane, Australia

Paul J. Neeson and Kara L. Britt
The Sir Peter MacCallum Department of Oncology, University of Melbourne, Melbourne, Australia

Takuya Osada, Zachary C. Hartman, Junping Wei, Gangjun Lei, Amy C. Hobeika, William and H. Kim Lyerly
Division of Surgical Sciences, Department of Surgery, Duke University Medical Center, MSRB Research Drive, Box 2714, Durham, NC 27710, USA

William R. Gwin
Division of Medical Oncology, Department of Medicine, University of Washington, Seattle, WA, USA

Marcio A. Diniz
Biostatistics and Bioinformatics Research Center, Samuel Oschin Comprehensive Cancer Institute, Cedars-Sinai Medical Center, Los Angeles, CA, USA

Neil Spector and Michael A. Morse
Division of Medical Oncology, Department of Medicine, Duke University Medical Center, Durham, NC, USA

Timothy M. Clay
Cell and Gene Therapy Discovery Research, PTS, GlaxoSmithKline, Collegeville, PA, USA

Wei Chen
Division of Gastroenterology, Department of Medicine, Duke University Medical Center, Durham, NC, USA

Timothy M. Clay
Division of General Surgery, Department of Surgery, Duke University Medical Center, Durham, NC, USA

Asra N. Shaik, Julie J. Ruterbusch and Michele L. Cote
Department of Oncology, Wayne State University School of Medicine, 4100 John R Street, MM04EP, Detroit, MI 48201, USA

Eman Abdulfatah, Resha Shrestha, M. H. D. Fayez Daaboul, Visakha Pardeshi and Rouba Ali-Fehmi
Department of Pathology, Wayne State University School of Medicine, Detroit, MI, USA

Daniel W. Visscher
Department of Laboratory Medicine and Pathology, Mayo Clinic, Rochester, MN, USA

Sudeshna Bandyopadhyay, Rouba Ali-Fehmi and Michele L. Cote
Barbara Ann Karmanos Cancer Institute, Detroit, MI, USA

Dustin W. Shipp and Ioan Notingher
School of Physics and Astronomy, University of Nottingham, Nottingham NG7 2RD, UK

Emad A. Rakha and Ian O. Ellis
Division of Oncology, School of Medicine, University of Nottingham, Nottingham NG5 1PB, UK

Alexey A. Koloydenko
Mathematics Department, Royal Holloway, University of London, Egham TW20 0EX, UK

R. Douglas Macmillan
Nottingham Breast Institute, Nottingham University Hospitals NHS Trust, Nottingham NG5 1PB, UK

Liu Yang, Wei Yang, Meiqi Wang, Xinle Wang, Baoen Shan and Zhengchuan Song
Breast Center, Fourth Hospital of Hebei Medical University, Shijiazhuang 050035, China

Yanhua Tian
Peking-Tsinghua Center for Life Sciences, Academy for Advanced Interdisciplinary Studies, Peking University, Beijing 100871, China

Wei Sun Leong and Jing Kong
Department of Electrical Engineering and Computer Science, Massachusetts Institute of Technology, Cambridge, MA 02139, USA

Heng Song
Laboratory of Experimental Pathology, Hebei Medical University, Shijiazhuang, China

Mao Yang, Xuesen Li, Bo Luo, Wenli Yang, Yan Lin, Dabing Li, Zhonglin Gan and Tao He
Institute for Cancer Medicine and School of Basic Medical Sciences, Southwest Medical University, Luzhou Sichuan, 646000, China

Xiaobin Yu and Jianming Xu
Department of Molecular and Cellular Biology, Baylor College of Medicine, Houston, TX 77030, USA

Safiah Olabi, Ahmet Ucar, Keith Brennan and Charles H. Streuli
Faculty of Biology, Medicine and Health, University of Manchester, Manchester M13 9PT, UK

Maj-Britt Jensen
Danish Breast Cancer Cooperative Group, Rigshospitalet, Copenhagen University Hospital, DBCG Secretariat, Bldg. 2501 Rigshospitalet, Blegdamsvej 9, DK-2100 Copenhagen, Denmark

Anne-Vibeke Lænkholm, Jens Ole Eriksen and Pernille Wehn
Department of Surgical Pathology, Zealand University Hospital, Slagelse, Denmark

Torsten O. Nielsen
Department of Pathology and Laboratory Medicine, University of British Columbia, Vancouver, BC, Canada

Tressa Hood, Namratha Ram, Wesley Buckingham and Sean Ferree
NanoString Technologies, Inc, Seattle, WA, USA

Bent Ejlertsen
Danish Breast Cancer Cooperative Group, Department of Oncology, Rigshospitalet, Copenhagen University Hospital, Copenhagen, Denmark

Chuying Wang and Enxiao Li
Department of Medical Oncology, The First Affiliated hospital of Xi'an Jiaotong University, Xi'an, Shaanxi 710061, People's Republic of China

Chuying Wang, Feng Bai, Li-han Zhang, Alexandria Scott and Xin-Hai Pei
Molecular Oncology Program, Division of Surgical Oncology, Dewitt Daughtry Family Department of Surgery, University of Miami, Miami, FL 33136, USA.

Xin-Hai Pei
Sylvester Comprehensive Cancer Center, Miller School of Medicine, University of Miami, Miami, FL 33136, USA

Sruthi Ravindranathan, Samantha L. Kurtz, Sean G. Smith, Bhanu prasanth Koppolu, Narasimhan Rajaram and David A. Zaharoff
Department of Biomedical Engineering, University of Arkansas, Fayetteville, AR, USA

Khue G. Nguyen and David A. Zaharoff
Cell and Molecular Biology Program, University of Arkansas, Fayetteville, AR, USA
Department of Microbiology and Immunology, University of North Carolina, Chapel Hill, NC, USA

Haven N. Frazier and David A. Zaharoff
Honors College, University of Arkansas, Fayetteville, AR, USA

Sean G. Smith, Bhanu prasanth Koppolu and David A. Zaharoff
Joint Department of Biomedical Engineering, University of North Carolina, Chapel Hill, NC and North Carolina State University, Raleigh, NC, USA

Suzan Vreemann, Jan C. M. van Zelst, Nico Karssemeijer, Albert Gubern-Mérida and Ritse M. Mann
Department of Radiology and Nuclear Medicine, Radboud University Medical Center, Geert Grooteplein 10, 6525 GA Nijmegen, the Netherlands

Margrethe Schlooz-Vries
Department of Surgery, Radboud University Medical Center, Nijmegen, the Netherlands

Peter Bult
Department of Pathology, Radboud University Medical Center, Nijmegen, the Netherlands

Nicoline Hoogerbrugge
Department of Human Genetics, Radboud University Medical Center, Nijmegen, the Netherlands

Aparna Shinde, Tomasz Wilmanski, Hao Chen, Dorothy Teegarden and Michael K. Wendt
Purdue University Center for Cancer Research, Purdue University, West Lafayette, IN 47907, USA

Aparna Shinde, Hao Chen and Michael K. Wendt
Department of Medicinal Chemistry and Molecular Pharmacology, Purdue University, West Lafayette, IN 47907, USA

Tomasz Wilmanski and Dorothy Teegarden
Department of Nutrition Science, West Lafayette, IN 47907, USA

Raquel Santana da Cruz, Elissa J. Carney, Johan Clarke, Hong Cao, M. Idalia Cruz, Carlos Benitez, Lu Jin and Sonia de Assis
Department of Oncology, Lombardi Comprehensive Cancer Center, Georgetown University, 3970 Reservoir Road, NW, The Research Building, Room E410, Washington, DC 20057, USA

Yi Fu, Zuolin Cheng and Yue Wang
The Bradley Department of Electrical and Computer Engineering, Virginia Polytechnic Institute and State University Research Center, Arlington, VA, USA

Martijn de Roon, Anne M. May, Rob J. P. M. Scholten, Petra H. M. Peeters and Evelyn M. Monninkhof
Department of Epidemiology, Julius Center for Health Sciences and Primary Care, University Medical Center Utrecht, 3508 GA Utrecht, the Netherlands

Anne McTiernan
Epidemiology Program, Division of Public Health Sciences, Fred Hutchinson Cancer Research Centre, Seattle, Washington, USA
Department of Epidemiology, School of Public Health, and Department of Medicine, School of Medicine, University of Washington, Seattle, Washington, USA

Rob J. P. M. Scholten
Cochrane Netherlands, University Medical Center Utrecht, Utrecht, the Netherlands

Petra H. M. Peeters
MRC-PHE Centre for Environment and Health, Department of Epidemiology and Biostatistics, School of Public Health, Imperial College,London, UK

Christine M. Friedenreich
Department of Cancer Epidemiology and Prevention Research, CancerControl Alberta, Alberta Health Services, Alberta, Canada
Department of Oncology, Cumming School of Medicine, University of Calgary, Calgary, Canada
Department of Community Health Sciences, Cumming School of Medicine, University of Calgary, Calgary, Canada

Minghui Cao, Wei Yan and Shizhen Emily Wang
Department of Pathology, University of California San Diego, 9500 Gilman Drive, La Jolla, CA 92093-0612, USA

Xuxiang Liu
City of Hope Irell & Manella Graduate School of Biological Sciences, Duarte, CA 91010, USA

Melanie Palomares
Cancer Prevention Movement, Arcadia, CA 91006, USA

Xiwei Wu
Department of Molecular and Cellular Biology, Beckman Research Institute of the City of Hope, Duarte, CA 91010, USA

Arthur Li
Division of Biostatistics, Beckman Research Institute of the City of Hope, Duarte, CA 91010, USA

Miranda Y. Fong
Department of Cancer Biology, Beckman Research Institute of the City of Hope, Duarte, CA 91010, USA

Wing-Chung Chan
Department of Pathology, City of Hope National Medical Center, Duarte, CA 91010, USA

Index

www.ingramcontent.com/pod-product-compliance
Lightning Source LLC
Chambersburg PA
CBHW080523200326
41458CB00012B/4317